D1348429

WITHDRAWN

Updates in Surgery

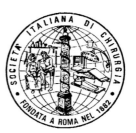

Walter Siquini

Surgical Treatment of Pancreatic Diseases

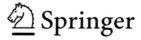 Springer

Walter Siquini
Department of Surgery
Ospedali Riuniti University Hospital
Polytechnic University of Marche
Ancona, Italy

Translated and adapted from the original title
Il trattamento chirurgico delle patologie pancreatiche
© Alpes Italia Srl 2008

The publication and the distribution of this volume have been supported by the Italian Society of Surgery

Library of Congress Control Number: 2008936506

ISBN 978-88-470-0855-7 Springer Milan Berlin Heidelberg New York
e-ISBN 978-88-470-0856-4

Springer is a part of Springer Science+Business Media
springer.com
© Springer-Verlag Italia 2009

This work is subject to copyright. All rights are reserved, whether the whole or part of the material is concerned, specifically the rights of translation, reprinting, re-use of illustrations, recitation, broadcasting, reproduction on microfilms or in other ways, and storage in data banks. Duplication of this publication or parts thereof is only permitted under the provisions of the Italian Copyright Law in its current version, and permission for use must always be obtained from Springer. Violations are liable for prosecution under the Italian Copyright Law.

The use of general descriptive names, registered names, trademarks, etc., in this publication does not imply, even in the absence of a specific statement, that such names are exempt from the relevant protective laws and regulations and therefore free for general use.
Product liability: The publisher cannot guarantee the accuracy of any information about dosage and application contained in this book. In every individual case the user must check such information by consulting the relevant literature.

Cover design: Simona Colombo, Milan, Italy
Typesetting: Graphostudio, Milan, Italy
Printing and binding: Arti Grafiche Nidasio, Assago, Italy

Printed in Italy
Springer-Verlag Italia S.r.l. – Via Decembrio 28 – I-20137 Milan

"...ηγήσασθαι μέν τόν διδσζαντα τήν τέχνην ταύτην γενέτησιν εμοισι"

"...*to consider dear to me as my parents him who taught me this art*"
(The Hippocratic Oath, 400 B.C.)

To my Father, who recently departed this life,
and to Professor Eduardo Landi, my teacher

Foreword

Although many advances have been made in the diagnosis and management of pancreatic disease, this field remains one of the most challenging for surgeons. In this book, young Italian surgeons, with contributions from experienced authorities, have attempted to review in a systematic way the history, surgical anatomy, physiology, pathology, and treatment of pancreatic disease.

Taken as a whole, this book is designed to provide clinicians with an up-to-date, informative, and accurate summary of the present problems and positions. The contents have been skillfully harmonized to create a balanced account of the areas of importance in pancreatic disease, providing practitioners with a good basis of knowledge and specialists with more detailed information.

It has been a great pleasure for the Italian Society of Surgery to provide an environment which was conducive to the development of this book.

Rome, October 2008

Roberto Tersigni
President, Italian Society of Surgery

Preface

The surgical treatment of pancreatic diseases is a topic of increasing interest, both because of its epidemiological significance and because of the complexity and fascination which the pancreas – the last organ to enter the domain of abdominal surgery – holds for abdominal surgeons.

The treatment of pancreatitis and pancreatic tumors, the incidence of which is slowly but relentlessly increasing, remains a challenge for the surgeon. This book aims to delineate the state of the art in the surgical treatment of both inflammatory and neoplastic pancreatic diseases, discussing which surgical strategy to opt for and detailing operating techniques. Ample space has also been devoted to imaging techniques, in particular operational endoscopy and ultrasonography. These techniques have now proved indispensable both in the diagnostic work-up and subsequently during interventional radiology and endoscopic procedures, which now play a crucial role when it comes to the management of pancreatitis and the palliative care of patients with pancreatic tumors.

Last, but certainly not least in terms of their importance, we describe both adjuvant and neoadjuvant therapies used for either treatment or palliative care, looking also at the use and potential of new and promising biologics with molecular targets. Only a multidisciplinary approach involving all these professionals (radiologist, surgeon, endoscopist, interventional radiologist, oncologist, radiotherapist) can produce the comprehensive and integrated overview which today constitutes a winning strategy for the optimization of results.

What we hope we have achieved is a flexible, up-to-date, exhaustive publication, rich in illustrations and consistent with evidence-based medicine.

My sincere thanks go to Professor Davide D'Amico, Professor Gianluigi Melotti, and Dr. Fausto Catena for their support for the Italian edition, and to all the co-authors, experts in pancreatic surgery at the most prestigious Italian institutions, who have offered their valuable contributions and honored us by participating in the making of this volume.

My very deep thanks are also due to the Board of the Italian Society of Surgery and particularly to its President, Professor Roberto Tersigni, for the tremendous opportunity and honor accorded to me and to the Eduardo Landi Young Surgeons' Association in having our written works taken up into the prestigious "Updates in Surgery" series.

Special thanks to Dr. Gianpaolo Balzano for his availability and help in the planning of the various chapters of the manuscript, and for his help in enriching it with beautiful illustrations.

Finally, with deep gratitude and devotion, I wish to celebrate and honor the memory of Professor Eduardo Landi, my unforgettable master and teacher. This book is dedicated to my Father and to him.

Ancona, October 2008   *Walter Siquini*

Contents

Contributors

Erica Adrario
Department of Neuroscience, Anesthesia and Resuscitation Unit, Ospedali Riuniti
University Hospital, Polytechnic University of Marche, Ancona, Italy

Luca Ansaloni
Department of Surgery, Sant'Orsola-Malpighi University Hospital, University of
Bologna, Bologna, Italy

Ettore Antico
Vascular and Interventional Radiology Unit, Department of Radiology, Torrette
Hospital, Ancona, Italy

Nicola Antonacci
Department of Surgery, 1st Surgical Clinic, Sant'Orsola-Malpighi Hospital,
University of Bologna, Bologna, Italy

Paolo Giorgio Arcidiacono
Endoscopic Ultrasonography Unit, Gastroenterology Department, San Raffaele
Scientific Institute, Milan, Italy

Gianpaolo Balzano
Pancreas Unit, Department of Surgery, San Raffaele Scientific Institute, Milan,
Italy

Claudio Bassi
Endocrine and Pancreatic Unit, Department of Gastroenterology and Surgery,
G.B. Rossi Hospital, University of Verona, Italy

Nicolò Bassi
4th Division of Surgery, Regional Reference Center of Hepato-Biliary-Pancreatic
Surgery, Regional Hospital Ca' Foncello, Treviso, Italy

Fiorenza Belli
Department of Surgery, Hepato-Biliary-Pancreatic Unit, Galliera Hospital, Genoa,
Italy

Emanuele Bendia
Department of Gastroenterology, Ospedali Riuniti University Hospital,
Polytechnic University of Marche, Ancona, Italy

Antonio Benedetti
Department of Gastroenterology, Ospedali Riuniti University Hospital,
Polytechnic University of Marche, Ancona, Italy

Aldo Alberto Beneduce
Pancreas Unit, Department of Surgery, Scientific Institute San Raffaele, Milan,
Italy

Rossella Bettini
Endocrine and Pancreatic Unit, Department of Gastroenterology and Surgery,
G.B. Rossi Hospital, University of Verona, Italy

Alberto Biondi
Department of General Surgery, Medical School A. Gemelli, University of the
Sacred Heart, Rome, Italy

Cinzia Boemo
Endoscopic Ultrasonography Unit, Gastroenterology Department, San Raffaele
Scientific Institute, Milan, Italy

Ugo Boggi
Division of General and Transplant Surgery in Uremic and Diabetic Patients, Pisa
University Hospital, Pisa, Italy

Letizia Boninsegna
Endocrine and Pancreatic Unit, Department of Gastroenterology and Surgery,
G.B. Rossi Hospital, University of Verona, Italy

Marco Braga
Pancreas Unit, Department of Surgery, San Raffaele Scientific Institute, Milan,
Italy

Giovanni Butturini
Endocrine and Pancreatic Unit, Department of Gastroenterology and Surgery,
G.B. Rossi Hospital, University of Verona, Italy

Linda Cacciamani
Department of Radiology, General and Pediatric Radiology, Ospedali Riuniti
University Hospital, Polytechnic University of Marche, Ancona, Italy

Stefano Cappato
Department of Surgery, Hepato-Biliary-Pancreatic Unit, Galliera Hospital, Genoa,
Italy

Michela Cappelletti
Division of Surgery, U. Sestilli Hospital, Polytechnic University of Marche,
Ancona, Italy

Ezio Caratozzolo
4th Division of Surgery, Regional Reference Center of Hepato-Biliary-Pancreatic
Surgery, Regional Hospital Ca' Foncello, Treviso, Italy

Silvia Carrara
Endoscopic Ultrasonography Unit, Gastroenterology Department, San Raffaele
Scientific Institute, Milan, Italy

Riccardo Casadei
Department of Surgery, 1st Surgical Clinic, Sant'Orsola-Malpighi Hospital,
University of Bologna, Bologna, Italy

Stefano Cascinu
Department of Oncology, Ospedali Riuniti University Hospital, Polytechnic
University of Marche, Ancona, Italy

Fausto Catena
Department of Surgery, S. Orsola-Malpighi University Hospital, University of
Bologna, Bologna, Italy

Nicola Cautero
Hepato-Biliary-Pancreatic and Transplantation Unit, Department of Medical and
Surgical Sciences, Polytechnic University of Marche, Ancona, Italy

Sara Cecchini
Department of Radiology, General and Pediatric Radiology, Ospedali Riuniti
University Hospital, Polytechnic University of Marche, Ancona, Italy

Luigi Ciccoritti
Department of General Surgery, A. Gemelli Hospital, Catholic University of the
Sacred Heart, Rome, Italy

Lorenzo Copparoni
Department of Neuroscience, Anesthesia and Resuscitation Unit, Ospedali Riuniti
University Hospital, Polytechnic University of Marche, Ancona, Italy

Roberto Coppola
General Surgery, Biomedical Campus University, Rome, Italy

Gabriele Corradini
Division of General Surgery, A. Murri Hospital, Fermo (AP), Italy

Leonardo Costarelli
Vascular and Interventional Radiology Unit, Department of Radiology, Torrette
Hospital, Ancona, Italy

Antonio Crucitti
Department of General Surgery, A. Gemelli Hospital, Catholic University of the
Sacred Heart, Rome, Italy

Pierfilippo Crucitti
General Surgery, Biomedical Campus University, Rome, Italy

Federico Crusco
Department of Radiology, Polytechnic University of Marche, Ancona, Italy

Domenico D'Ugo
Department of General Surgery, Medical School A. Gemelli, University of the
Sacred Heart, Rome, Italy

Despoina Daskalaki
Endocrine and Pancreatic Unit, Department of Gastroenterology and Surgery,
G.B. Rossi Hospital, University of Verona, Italy

Antonio De Bonis
Department of General Surgery, Abdominal Surgery Unit, Casa Sollievo della
Sofferenza, IRCCS, San Giovanni Rotondo, Italy

Diego Dedola
Department of Surgery, Hepato-Biliary-Pancreatic Unit, Galliera Hospital, Genoa,
Italy

Marco Del Chiaro
Division of General and Transplant Surgery in Uremic and Diabetic Patients, Pisa
University Hospital, Pisa, Italy

Stefano De Luca
Hepato-Biliary-Pancreatic and Transplantation Unit, Department of Medical and
Surgical Sciences, Polytechnic University of Marche, Ancona, Italy

Angelo de Sanctis
Division of Minimally Invasive Surgery, Ospedali Riuniti University Hospital,
Polytechnic University of Marche, Ancona, Italy

Valerio Di Carlo
Pancreas Unit, Department of Surgery, San Raffaele Scientific Institute, Milan,
Italy

Fabrizio di Francesco
Hepato-Biliary-Pancreatic and Transplantation Unit, Department of Medical and
Surgical Sciences, Polytechnic University of Marche, Ancona, Italy

F. Francesco di Mola
Department of General Surgery, Abdominal Surgery Unit, Casa Sollievo della
Sofferenza, IRCCS, San Giovanni Rotondo, Italy

Saverio Di Palo
Department of Surgery, San Raffaele Scientific Institute, Milan, Italy

Antonio Di Sario
Department of Gastroenterology, Ospedali Riuniti University Hospital,
Polytechnic University of Marche, Ancona, Italy

Salomone Di Saverio
Department of Surgery, Sant'Orsola-Malpighi University Hospital, University of
Bologna, Bologna, Italy

Pierluigi di Sebastiano
Department of General Surgery, Abdominal Surgery Unit, Casa Sollievo della
Sofferenza, IRCCS, San Giovanni Rotondo, Italy

Giancarlo Fabrizzi
Department of Radiology, General and Pediatric Radiology, Ospedali Riuniti
University Hospital, Polytechnic University of Marche, Ancona, Italy

Massimo Falconi
Endocrine and Pancreatic Unit, Department of Gastroenterology and Surgery,
G.B. Rossi Hospital, University of Verona, Italy

Giuseppe Feliciangeli
Department of Gastroenterology, Ospedali Riuniti University Hospital,
Polytechnic University of Marche, Ancona, Italy

Aroldo Fianchini
Department of Surgery, C. e G. Mazzoni County Hospital, Ascoli Piceno, Italy

Marco Filauro
Department of Surgery, Hepato-Biliary-Pancreatic Unit, Galliera Hospital, Genoa,
Italy

Domitilla Foghetti
Division of General Surgery, Santa Croce Hospital, Fano (PU), Italy

Andrea Garberini
General Surgery, Biomedical Campus University, Rome, Italy

Francesca Gavazzi
Pancreas Unit, Department of Surgery, San Raffaele Scientific Institute, Milan,
Italy

Gian Massimo Gazzaniga
Department of Surgery, Hepato-Biliary-Pancreatic Unit, Galliera Hospital, Genoa,
Italy

Guido Cesare Gesuelli
Department of General Surgery, Macerata Hospital, Macerata, Italy

Roberto Ghiselli
Division of Surgery, U. Sestilli Hospital, Polytechnic University of Marche,
Ancona, Italy

Andrea Giovagnoni
Department of Radiology, Polytechnic University of Marche, Ancona, Italy

Pier Cristoforo Giulianotti
Department of General and Minimally Invasive Surgery, Misericordia Hospital,
Grosseto, Italy

Maurizio Grillo
Division of General Surgery, San Giovanni di Dio e Ruggi d'Aragona Hospital,
Salerno, Italy

Gianluca Guercioni
Division of General Surgery, C. e G. Mazzoni County Hospital, Ascoli Piceno,
Italy

Mario Guerrieri
Division of Minimally Invasive Surgery, Ospedali Riuniti University Hospital, Polytechnic University of Marche, Ancona, Italy

Shigeki Kusamura
Department of Surgery, San Raffaele Scientific Institute, Milan, Italy

Luciano Landa
Division of General Surgery, Santa Croce Hospital, Fano (PU), Italy

Arianna Lorenzoni
Department of Radiology, General and Pediatric Radiology, Ospedali Riuniti University Hospital, Polytechnic University of Marche, Ancona, Italy

Giampiero Macarri
Department of Gastroenterology, Ospedali Riuniti University Hospital, Polytechnic University of Marche, Ancona, Italy

Domenico Marchi
Division of General Surgery, Nuovo Ospedale Civile Sant'Agostino Estense, Baggiovara (MO), Italy

Daniele Marrelli
Department of Human Pathology and Oncology, Unit of Surgical Oncology, University of Sienna, Sienna, Italy

Marco Marzioni
Department of Gastroenterology, Ospedali Riuniti University Hospital, Polytechnic University of Marche, Ancona, Italy

Giuseppe Mascetta
Department of General Surgery, Abdominal Surgery Unit, Casa Sollievo della Sofferenza, IRCCS, San Giovanni Rotondo, Italy

Marco Massani
4th Division of Surgery, Regional Reference Center of Hepato-Biliary-Pancreatic Surgery, Regional Hospital Ca' Foncello, Treviso, Italy

Gianluigi Melotti
Division of General Surgery, Nuovo Ospedale Civile Sant'Agostino Estense, Baggiovara (MO), Italy

Luciano Minestroni
Division of General Surgery, A. Murri Hospital, Fermo (AP), Italy

Francesco Minni
Department of Surgery, 1st Surgical Clinic, Sant'Orsola-Malpighi Hospital,
University of Bologna, Bologna, Italy

Federico Mocchegiani
Division of Surgery, U. Sestilli Hospital, Polytechnic University of Marche,
Ancona, Italy

Franco Mosca
Department of Oncology, Transplantation and New Technologies Medicine, 1st
Division of General Surgery, Pisa University Hospital, Pisa, Italy

Barbara Mullineris
Division of General Surgery, Nuovo Ospedale Civile Sant'Agostino Estense,
Baggiovara (MO), Italy

Carmine Napolitano
Division of General Surgery, San Giovanni di Dio e Ruggi d'Aragona Hospital,
Salerno, Italy

Elena Orsenigo
Department of Surgery, San Raffaele Scientific Institute, Milan, Italy

Enrico Ortolano
Pancreas Unit, Department of Surgery, San Raffaele Scientific Institute, Milan,
Italy

Enrico Paci
Vascular and Interventional Radiology Unit, Department of Radiology, Torrette
Hospital, Ancona, Italy

Alessandra Pagliacci
Department of Oncology, Ospedali Riuniti University Hospital, Polytechnic
University of Marche, Ancona, Italy

Ivo Patrizi
Department of General Surgery, Macerata Hospital, Macerata, Italy

Paolo Pederzoli
Endocrine and Pancreatic Unit, Department of Gastroenterology and Surgery,
G.B. Rossi Hospital, University of Verona, Italy

Corrado Pedrazzani
Department of Human Pathology and Oncology, Unit of Surgical Oncology,
University of Sienna, Sienna, Italy

Paolo Pelaia
Department of Neuroscience, Anesthesia and Resuscitation Unit, Ospedali Riuniti
University Hospital, Polytechnic University of Marche, Ancona, Italy

Graziano Pernazza
Department of General and Minimally Invasive Surgery, Misericordia Hospital,
Grosseto, Italy

Roberto Persiani
Department of General Surgery, Medical School A. Gemelli, University of the
Sacred Heart, Rome, Italy

Maria Chiara Petrone
Endoscopic Ultrasonography Unit, Gastroenterology Department, San Raffaele
Scientific Institute, Milan, Italy

Micaela Piccoli
Division of General Surgery, Nuovo Ospedale Civile Sant'Agostino Estense,
Baggiovara (MO), Italy

Chiara Pierantoni
Department of Oncology, Ospedali Riuniti University Hospital, Polytechnic
University of Marche, Ancona, Italy

Antonio Daniele Pinna
Department of Surgery, Sant'Orsola-Malpighi University Hospital, University of
Bologna, Bologna, Italy

Enrico Pinto
Department of Human Pathology and Oncology, Unit of Surgical Oncology,
University of Sienna, Sienna, Italy

Claudio Ricci
Department of Surgery, 1st Surgical Clinic, Sant'Orsola-Malpighi Hospital,
University of Bologna, Bologna, Italy

Raffaella Ridolfo
Department of Surgery, C. e G. Mazzoni County Hospital, Ascoli Piceno, Italy

Massimiliano Rimini
Division of Minimally Invasive Surgery, Ospedali Riuniti University Hospital,
Polytechnic University of Marche, Ancona, Italy

Andrea Risaliti
Hepato-Biliary-Pancreatic and Transplantation Unit, Department of Medical and
Surgical Sciences, Polytechnic University of Marche, Ancona, Italy

Simona Irma Rocchetti
Pancreas Unit, Department of Surgery, Scientific Institute San Raffaele, Milan,
Italy

Marco Romiti
Division of General Surgery, A. Murri Hospital, Fermo (AP), Italy

Franco Roviello
Department of Human Pathology and Oncology, Unit of Surgical Oncology,
University of Sienna, Sienna, Italy

Vittorio Saba
Division of Surgery, U. Sestilli Hospital, Polytechnic University of Marche,
Ancona, Italy

Roberto Santoro
Division of General Surgery and Transplantation, San Camillo-Forlanini Hospital,
Rome, Italy

Massimo Sartelli
Department of General Surgery, Macerata Hospital, Macerata, Italy

Mario Scartozzi
Department of Oncology, Ospedali Riuniti University Hospital, Polytechnic
University of Marche, Ancona, Italy

Rodolfo Scibé
Department of General Surgery, Macerata Hospital, Macerata, Italy

Emidio Senati
Division of General Surgery, C. e G. Mazzoni County Hospital, Ascoli Piceno,
Italy

Walter Siquini
Department of Surgery, Ospedali Riuniti University Hospital, Polytechnic
University of Marche, Ancona, Italy

Carlo Staudacher
Department of Surgery, San Raffale Scientific Institute, Milan, Italy

Silvia Taffetani
Department of Gastroenterology, Ospedali Riuniti University Hospital,
Polytechnic University of Marche, Ancona, Italy

Sergio Valeri
General Surgery, Biomedical Campus University, Rome, Italy

Luca Valvano
Division of General Surgery, San Giovanni di Dio e Ruggi d'Aragona Hospital, Salerno, Italy

Paola Verdenelli
Department of Neuroscience, Anesthesia and Resuscitation Unit, Ospedali Riuniti University Hospital, Polytechnic University of Marche, Ancona, Italy

Alessandro Zerbi
Pancreas Unit, Department of Surgery, San Raffaele Scientific Institute, Milan, Italy

Marco Zoccali
Department of General Surgery, Medical School A. Gemelli, University of the Sacred Heart, Rome, Italy

Chapter 1

The History of Pancreatic Surgery

Gian Massimo Gazzaniga, Stefano Cappato

Introduction

"We can measure the attainments of the past but we can never measure the inevitable advances of the future." Thus Allen Whipple in his book *The Evolution of Surgery in the United States*. That the progress achieved to date is a quantifiable entity, whereas our future potential is simply unknowable, is all too true. Not only this, but it is quite curious to note that we surgeons – markedly more so than any other category of medical practitioner – have throughout history always labored under the impression of having attained all that is possible to attain, thereby ruling out prospects of future improvements.

History has clearly proved us wrong and taught us a salutary lesson. Progress, true progress, is born of curiosity, and is spurred on by a healthy dose of ambition. Therefore, when we look back, it is no surprise to see that significant contributions have come from the younger generation. Young people, curious, tireless, and resistant to dogma and preconceptions, have often provided answers to the most intractable questions.

Regnier de Graaf was 22 years old when in 1663 in Leiden he demonstrated unequivocally that the pancreas is an exocrine gland. Johann Brunner was a student when in 1673 in Paris he started to conduct the first experimental pancreatectomies in animals. Abraham Vater was 27 when he described the duodenal papilla, and Ruggero Oddi was 23 when in Perugia in 1887 he described what became called after him the "sphincter of Oddi."

It has been, therefore, a real pleasure to recall some historical milestones in surgery, since even though it is true that contemporary history has probably produced more than 95% of the publications and surgical operations of the pancreas, it is no less true that the foundations were laid some 130 years ago.

The Building Blocks of History

For a long time, the pancreas remained off limits to surgeons because of its anatomical position. Furthermore, up until a few decades ago, the diagnosis of

W. Siquini (Ed.), *Surgical Treatment of Pancreatic Diseases*.
©Springer-Verlag Italia 2009

pancreatic diseases was entrusted to intuition, and more often than not, to the post mortem. The history of pancreatic surgery is therefore relatively young and is comprised largely of two periods.

The first historical period comes in the second half of the nineteenth century, a period in which "major surgery" became a reality. In reality only minor surgical operations were carried out on the pancreas, but they formed the basis (the so-called building blocks) upon which subsequent major operations could be developed, thanks to the introduction of anesthesia, microscopy, infection control, and radiology.

The second period, which can be pinned down to around the beginning of the twentieth century, is the period of results, thanks to the key contributions of Whipple and other surgical pioneers.

The First Biliary Reconstructive Operations

"April 18th, 10 A.M.: There was great tenderness and pain in the region of the tumour, aggravated by pressure [...]. Dr. Hayden gave ether, and Dr. Bremond and Dr. Pratt assisted me. The operation was performed under proper antiseptic precautions [...] an incision [...] the peritoneal membrane was soon reached, but was not opened till all bleeding from divided vessels was controlled [...]. A Dieulafoy's trocar of the largest size was thrust into the tumour, and twenty-four ounces of a dark-brown fluid was withdrawn, which I supposed to be bile. As soon as the cyst was emptied [...] it was seized with forceps and drawn out [...] the finger was passed into the peritoneal cavity [...] it was ascertained [...] to be the gall-bladder [...] the gall-bladder was then incised [...] sixty gall-stones were removed [...] a fistulous outlet [was created, suturing the open gall bladder to the abdominal walls]."

This account, by James Marion Sims, was published in the *British Medical Journal*, and describes the first cholecystostomy carried out for obstructive jaundice in pancreatic carcinoma. The patient died 8 days later following a hemorrhage and a medicolegal autopsy was conducted. No elements of blame were found.

In 1880 William Halsted performed a cholecystostomy on his mother – at home – who had cholecystic empyema. She recovered from the operation, and died 2 years later from obstructive jaundice. Seven years later, a Swiss surgeon by the name of Kappeler performed a cholecystojejunostomy on a tumor of the head of the pancreas, and the patient survived for 18 months. Other surgeons, especially of the French school, preferred to anastomose the gallbladders to the stomach; this technique was performed for the first time in 1886 by Felix Terrier, a surgeon from Paris.

At the end of the nineteenth century the palliative treatment of jaundice in patients with cancer of the head of the pancreas was developed. A succession of technical innovations followed: in 1897 Cesar Roux, a pupil of Emil Theodor

Kocher, described the creation of a segment of small intestine, isolated from the intestinal transit – a technique which came to be universally known as the Roux-en-Y technique. This procedure was initially developed for gastric reconstruction after gastric resection, and it was only from the beginning of the 1900s that it became used for biliodigestive anastomosis.

Another technical innovation was introduced by Kocher, who won the Nobel prize in 1909 for his pioneering activity in the field of thyroid surgery. Kocher described the mobilization of the duodenum and of the head of the pancreas in order to facilitate surgery in this region.

The First Resections Start from the Tail

At this point, the surgeons were technically prepared to tackle the pancreas. The tail of the pancreas was the right place to start: technically simpler, no associated visceral resections, and no phenomena related to obstructive jaundice. Bleeding in jaundiced patients was at the time a fatal complication, as the then knowledge regarding the dynamics and pathophysiology of coagulation events was fragmentary and incomplete.

On 16 July 1882, Friedrich Trendelenburg, professor of surgery in Bonn, performed the first distal splenopancreatectomy. The patient died several weeks after being discharged and Trendelenburg did not publish anything. Only 4 years later, one of his assistants (Witzel) published the case in full. Nevertheless, from that point on, reviewing the literature over more than 20 years (1882–1905) shows that only 21 surgeons performed a total of 24 pancreatic resections, and no single surgeon performed more than three such operations.

After Trendelenburg, it was the turn of Giuseppe Ruggi, the chief of the Maggiore Hospital, Bologna, on 4 September 1889. One year later it was the turn of Briggs of the Beaumont Hospital of St. Louis. Billroth himself is credited with having performed two pancreatic resections during gastric cancer surgery. All the resections described, however, were limited to the body–tail region or were simply enucleations of the mass.

Resections of the Head of the Pancreas

It was only logical that sooner or later developments in resection techniques would lead to the resective treatment of cancers of the head of the pancreas. On 9 February 1898 Alessandro Codivilla, a surgeon from Imola, Italy, and pioneer of orthopedic surgery (he was to become director of the Rizzoli Orthopedic Institute of Bologna) performed the first ever pancreaticoduodenectomy. Codivilla had already published extensively on resective surgery, extending it to gastric cancer. In these writings, resections associated with the stomach, colon, and pancreas were also described. Nevertheless, he never published this first experience, which in fact was described in *The Medical Writings of Alessandro Codivilla* (*Scritti medici di Alessandro Codivilla*) published by Putti and Nigrisoli in 1912. Surgery comprised resection of the pylorus, part of the duodenum, and the head of the pancreas, with closure of the duodenal stump and ligation of the main biliary duct. In accordance with the practice of the time, a cholecystojejunostomy and a gastroenterostomy were performed. We have no description of the treatment applied to the pancreatic stump in this specific case. Presumably it was closed by means of a suture and left in situ. The patient died on the 24th day.

Eleven years were to pass before the second pancreaticoduodenectomy was performed, this one by Walter Kausch, 5 days after Codivilla performed his operation, William Halsted at the Johns Hopkins Hospital in Baltimore carried out the first ampullectomy with reconstruction of the continuity of the common bile duct and of the duct of Wirsung (main pancreatic duct) directly in the duodenum. After the patient had remained in hospital from 3 months, Halsted decided to reoperate since the common bile duct–duodenal anastomosis was not draining. He therefore performed a "cystico-duodenoanastomosis" which carried out its task right up until the patient's death due to recurrence (at 6 months from the initial surgery). Codivilla and Halsted made no further contributions to pancreatic surgery, but they had nonetheless opened up a new field of endeavor. Ampullectomies were, however, performed with increasing frequency, yet survival was always the exception rather than the rule.

Finally, in the summer of 1909, Walter Kausch, a pupil of Mikulicz, and chief surgeon at the municipal hospital of Berlin-Schöneberg, performed a pancreaticoduodenectomy in two stages on a 49-year-old patient with ampullary cancer. The first stage comprised a cholecystojejunostomy anastomosis and a jejunojejunostomy, employing the so-called Murphy's button for both anastomoses. Nine weeks later he operated again on the patient and performed the pancreaticoduodenectomy, closing the distal biliary pathway duct and carrying out a gastrojejunostomy. The pancreas was invaginated into the distal duodenum and preserved. The patient survived for several months before dying of cholangitis. Further resective attempts by Kausch met with failure, and, inundated by criticism, he published no further work on resective surgery of the pancreas.

In spite of this "relative" success, few surgeons, and certainly few patients, had the courage to repeat the experience in the short term. In 1914 Hirschel, a surgeon from Heidelberg, performed a pancreaticoduodenectomy for cancer of the ampulla, reconstructing the biliary duct by interposing a rubber tube. Surprisingly, the patient survived for 1 year.

In 1918, the Italian Ottorino Tenani, in Bellagio, in the northern Italian province of Como, during the First World War, performed a pancreaticoduodenectomy in two stages for ampullary cancer, and appears to have been the first to employ transfusions in pancreatic surgery and to use extracts of animal pancreas as orally administered replacements.

The era of revolutionary discoveries was under way: in 1922 Frederick Banting and Charles Best discovered insulin and in 1929 Henrik Dam discovered Vitamin K ("K" from the Danish *Koagulation*). From 1939, thanks to the determination of its molecular structure by Edward Doisy, Vitamin K entered into clinical use.

The Pancreaticoduodenectomy of Allen Whipple

On 16 March 1934 Allen O. Whipple, Director of the Surgical Service at the Presbyterian Hospital in New York, performed the first pancreaticoduodenectomy of his career. The patient was a 60-year-old woman with cholestatic jaundice and ampullary neoplasia. In the first operation, a choledochoduodenostomy and cholecystostomy were performed. After several weeks the patient underwent resective surgery with excision of a duodenal window and of the pancreas head. The remnant pancreas was anastomosed to the duodenal window with catgut. The patient died after 30 h as a result of massive dehiscence of the pancreatico-duodenal anastomosis.

Whipple's second patient, a man aged 53, underwent a three-stage procedure in July 1934 (the remnant pancreas was left without anastomosis) and the patient survived for 8 months. He died of cholangitis.

The third – and most effective – resection was performed in July 1935 on a 49-year-old man. The first-stage procedure consisted of gastroenterostomy and cholecystogastrostomy, with inversion and closure of the distal bile duct (Fig. 1.1). In the second stage, the patient underwent resection of the duodenopancreatic bloc and the remnant pancreatic stump was closed with a whip-stitched silk suture (Fig. 1.2). The patient was reoperated on 1 month later because of an abscess and a pancreatic fistula. He survived the disease for 25 months.

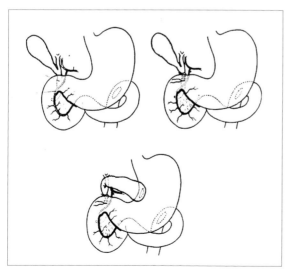

Fig. 1.1 First stage Whipple's procedure

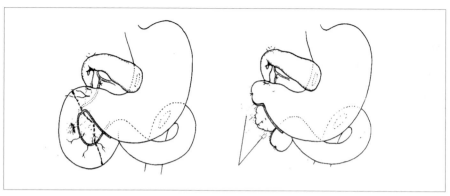

Fig. 1.2 Second stage Whipple's procedure

In 1935 Whipple published these three clinical cases in the *Annals of Surgery* and drew up the first guidelines for the treatment of neoplasia of the head of the pancreas. This work underlined that surgery was relatively safe if performed in two stages and without anastomosing the pancreas.

Five years later, in 1940, Whipple conducted the first pancreaticoduodenectomy in a single stage only, in a patient with glucagonoma of the head of the pancreas. The patient had been diagnosed with a neoplasm of the gastric antrum and was not jaundiced. In the light of this unexpected intraoperative finding Whipple decided to perform a pancreaticoduodenectomy and the patient survived for 9 years.

Whipple published his experiences in 1945: he had performed 19 one-stage resections with a 31% mortality rate and 8 two-stage resections with a 38% mortality rate. He concluded that the one-stage procedure was safer for the patient and urged in favor of pancreaticojejunostomy, which was only to be performed with silk sutures.

Pancreaticoduodenectomy: The Procedure of a Thousand Variations

The wider use of pancreatic resection and the manner in which the three anastomoses were performed underwent numerous variations in the years to come with a view to increased surgical radicality and safety. Let us begin with biliodigestive anastomosis.

Initially, Whipple was an advocate of cholecystogastrostomy, but he rapidly became a convert to cholecystojejunostomy. Cholecystojejunostomy was abandoned from 1950 onward because of the excessive frequency of anastomotic stenoses, and was replaced with hepaticojejunostomy, which had in fact been suggested some time previously by Desjardins on the basis of his work with animal models.

The treatment of the remnant pancreatic stump was, however, the issue which caused the greatest problems. Ligation and sinking of the pancreatic stump was soon abandoned in favor of anastomosis with the jejunum. In 1948 Richard Cattell of the Lahey Clinic transferred a technique into the clinical arena, which had been developed by Patrie in 1917 using the animal model: the Wirsung-jejunostomy. Furthermore, Cattell used a transanastomotic drain in order to protect the anastomosis and avoid stenosis. Other surgeons subsequently employed this very type of anastomosis, often using removable drainages, exteriorized via the jejunum (Imanaga in 1960 and Madden in 1964).

Postoperative fistula formation continued to remain, however, the cause of significant morbidity and mortality. In 1993 Johnson conducted a meta-analysis on a total of 1,828 pancreaticoduodenectomies, showing a fistula incidence of 13.6% and a mortality rate in the fistula group of 12.5%. Therefore, anastomosis with invagination of the pancreatic stump came to be proposed over time (Brinkley in 1951 and Nagakawa in 1992) and in 1978 the German school of Erlangen (Gebhardt and Stolte) revived the idea of occlusion of the pancreatic duct, this time by means of an adhesive amino acid solution (Ethibloc). The results did not confirm expectations and the incidence of fistula did not decrease. Other groups (Machado of Brazil) then proposed that a defunctionalized loop be used for pancreatic anastomosis alone, with a view to isolating the pancreas in case of fistula formation.

The final problem to be solved concerned gastrojejunal anastomosis. In the first "pioneering" operations, the stomach was closed at the level of the pylorus and intestinal continuity was achieved by means of a gastrojejunostomy created on the posterior wall. Warren of the Lahey Clinic proposed gastroresection to reduce the incidence of ulcers and this became standard procedure. Nonetheless, over time evidence revealed that that the problem of anastomotic ulcer seemed to have been overestimated, and the pendulum swung back again to preserving the pylorus: in 1978 Traverso and Longmire put forward the "principle" of preservation of the stomach, initially in cases of chronic pancreatitis and subsequently in oncology patients. The results proved Traverso and Longmire to be correct: the incidence of anastomotic ulcer was low, and, conversely, digestive function was markedly improved, even though this type of procedure occasionally provoked problems of gastric emptying.

The succession of the different anastomoses has also been the subject of debate; today a "theoretical" advantage is recognized in reconstruction upstream from the pancreatic and biliary anastomoses, in order to minimize the acidity in the jejunal loop, which contains the biliopancreatic anastomoses. Furthermore, in the event of fistula there is no spread of the alimentary bolus into the abdomen. The delicate nature of the problem has, however, led to a series of variants (approximately 100) being employed, without arrival at a conclusive answer.

Results of the Second Half of the Twentieth Century: Improvement of Postoperative Mortality

In 1969, 271 pancreaticoduodenectomies were carried out in the United States, with a mortality rate of 32%, equivalent to the results obtained by Whipple 30 years earlier. Finally, John Howard of the University of Ohio published the results of a consecutive series of 72 patients with no postoperative mortality, and Crile in 1979 stated that in order to be acceptable, postoperative mortality should be contained within 10%.

At the end of the twentieth century, the centers of excellence reported mortality rates of less than 5% in long positive series without any mortality whatsoever (Trede 118 cases, 1990; Cameron 145 cases, 1993).

The Unresolved Problems

In 1970 George Crile of the Cleveland Clinic published an article entitled "The advantages of bypass operations over radical pancreatoduodenectomy in the treatment of pancreatic carcinoma," in which he maintained that survival after bypass surgery was better than that after so-called radical surgery, and obviously had a lower mortality burden. From that point on, several surgical schools adopted Crile's ideas, treating only patients affected with ampullary neoplasia and performing bypass procedures on those with cancers of the head of the pancreas.

In 1978 Gudjonsson continued this disillusioning task, publishing the results of a meta-analysis on 15,000 patients with cancer of the pancreas. Of these only 65 became "long-term survivors", and surprisingly 8 did not undergo surgery. In addition 7 underwent simple bypass, and so the cure rate for resected patients fell to 0.3%.

Improvements in diagnostic imaging and surgical experience have however led to a change in the results. A 1994 report from the French Association of Surgery documented a survival rate of 15% in a group of 550 patients who underwent resection over the period 1982–1988, and an American report covering the same period indicated a survival rate of 12% (US Veterans Affairs Hospital, 1994).

In the 1980s, the Japanese school of surgery moved towards an "aggressive" surgical treatment which came to be known as "extended" pancreatoduodenectomy. The skeletonization of the celiac trunk, the superior mesenteric artery, preaortic lymphatic tissue and fat tissue, and a wide peripancreatic area, including Gerota's fascia, should have guaranteed greater radicality. The preliminary results, presented in June 1989 in Toledo, Ohio, seemed to prove them correct: Manabe, Osaki, and Hiraoka reported an actuarial survival of between 25 and 35% at 5 years. However, in 1981 the Japanese Pancreatic Cancer Registry was created. From 1981 to 1985, 17, 130 patients were registered from 350 national referral centers. This registry has represented a formidable analytical tool in the analysis of pancreatic cancer and has clearly indicated that the 5-year survival rate in patients who undergo resection does not exceed 18%, even if one modifies the "degree of extension" of the surgery.

The Lessons of History

Although the history of pancreatic surgery is relatively short, 130 years having elapsed since the first pancreatic surgical operation was performed on a human, and 350 years since the functions of the pancreas were discovered, progress has been slow. Two hundred years have passed from the discovery of the duct of Wirsung to the exploration of glandular function by Claude Bernard. Forty years passed between Codivilla's first unsuccessful pancreaticoduodenectomy and Whipple's first procedure. Periods of stagnation alternated with periods of rapid growth, thanks to the introduction of the microscope, anesthesiological techniques, more sophisticated imaging, and the introduction of intensive therapy. But history, unlike the Nobel Committee, is not obliged to honor only those who have made steps forward, since each and every step is supported by foundations built by "unknown" precursors, the "shoulders" of science. Furthermore, it behooves history to recognize the value of the industriousness and ingenuity which has provided essential support to the development of surgery. Motivation (at an economic level), the key resources, and the quality of multidisciplinary teams have provided an essential complement to creative, talented individuals in order to ensure that their discoveries have become widely known.

The history of recent decades has, taken all together, demonstrated an important fact, namely the centralization of major surgical procedures, particularly those in development. Codivilla and Kausch possessed great initiative, but they met with failure due to lack of adequate resources. Whipple, on the other hand, met with success thanks to the unconditional support of the Columbia Presbyterian Medical Center. Centralization, therefore, enables more efficient and effective treatment, with consequent savings, not only financially, but also, and above all, in terms of human lives.

As Leriche wrote, surgeons should be proud of what they have achieved over the course of these centuries. We must, however, also be aware that we have a long road ahead. Diabetes, pancreatitis, and pancreatic cancer are increasingly present in the population in the twenty-first century. Severe acute pancreatitis is always accompanied by high mortality, chronic pancreatitis is always incapacitating, and pancreatic cancer is always diagnosed too late.

Fortunately, today, unlike Galen, we are aware of our ignorance. And this is already progress.

Suggested Reading

Child CG III (1948) Radical one stage pancreatoduodenectomy. Surgery 23:492–500

Desjardins A (1907) Technique de la pancreatectomie. Rev Chir 35:945–973

Gordon-Taylor G (1934) The radical surgery of cancer of the pancreas. Ann Surg 100:206–214

Gudjonnson B, Livingstone E, Spiro H (1978) Cancer of the pancreas; diagnostic accuracy and survival statistics. Cancer 42:2494–2506

Howard J (1997) Pancreatojejunostomy: leakage is a preventable complication of the Whipple resection. J Am Coll Surg 184:454–457

Howard JM, Freiss R (2002) History of the pancreas. Mysteries of a hidden organ. Springer, Berlin Heidelberg New York

Kausch W (1912) Das carcinom der Papilla Vateri und seine radikale Entfernung. Beitr Klin Chir 78:439–450

Trede M, Schwall G, Saeger HD (1990) Survival after duodenopancreatectomy: 118 consecutive resections without an operative mortality. Ann Surg 211:447–458

Whipple AO (1945) Pancreatoduodenectomy for islet cell carcinoma. Ann Surg 121:847–852

Whipple AO, Parsons WB, Mullins CR (1935) Treatment of carcinoma of the ampulla of Vater. Ann Surg 102:763–779

Chapter 2

Surgical Anatomy of the Pancreas

Massimo Sartelli, Rodolfo Scibé, Guido Cesare Gesuelli, Ivo Patrizi

The pancreas is a lobular gland, grayish-pink in color and 12–15 cm in length. It extends crosswise along the posterior abdominal wall, behind the stomach, between the duodenum and the spleen.

Embryology

The pancreas grows in the part of the intestine situated directly under the stomach, cranial to the connection between the duodenum and the yolk-sac. In this region the intestinal epithelium becomes thicker, forming the so-called hepatopancreatic ring. From this thicker part, dorsal epithelial buds form, giving origin to the dorsal pancreas, and ventral epithelial buds, from which the ventral pancreas derives (Fig. 2.1).

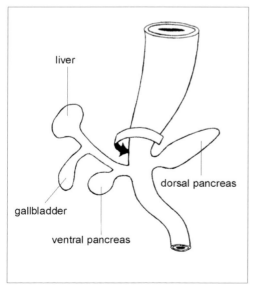

Fig. 2.1 Embryology of the pancreas. Formation of the dorsal and ventral pancreatic buds

W. Siquini (Ed.), *Surgical Treatment of Pancreatic Diseases.*
©Springer-Verlag Italia 2009

When the duodenum grows and rotates clockwise, the ventral bud is dragged dorsally, integrating with the dorsal bud (Fig. 2.2). The superior portion of the head, the body, and the tail of the pancreas originate from the larger, dorsal bud, whereas the lesser pancreas forms from the ventral bud. When the pancreatic buds merge, the ducts fuse. The main pancreatic duct (duct of Wirsung) originates from the duct of the ventral bud and from the distal portion of the duct of the dorsal bud. The proximal portion of the dorsal bud duct remains in the form of the pancreatic accessory duct (Fig. 2.3).

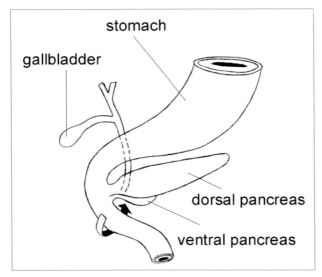

Fig. 2.2 As the duodenum grows and rotates, the ventral bud is dragged dorsally, becoming integrated with the dorsal bud

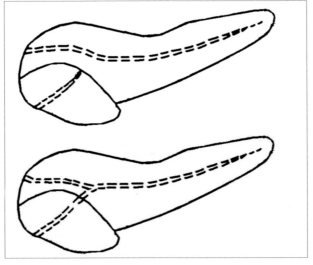

Fig. 2.3 Formation of pancreatic ducts

Connection with Other Organs

The head of the pancreas is included in the bend of the duodenum (Fig. 2.4). The lesser pancreas detaches from the inferior left portion of the pancreatic head. It moves up and to the left, behind the superior mesenteric vessels. The lesser pancreas (Winslow's pancreas, uncinate process of pancreas) can be more or less developed. In half of the cases it covers the mesenteric vein and it may sometimes extend beyond the superior mesenteric artery.

The anterior surface of the head is connected with the transverse mesocolon and the transverse colon. The pancreatic head is posteriorly connected with the inferior vein cava, the last segment of the kidney veins, and the right pillar of the diaphragm. The lesser pancreas passes ahead of the aorta. The choledochus (common bile duct) runs in a groove of the superior and lateral portion of the posterior surface of the head.

The isthmus connects the head with the body. Since there are numerous vascular anastomoses at this level, it is difficult to extract. Anteriorly it is linked with the pylorus. The gastroduodenal and pancreatic duodenal superior and anterior arteries run in front of the gland on the right of the passage between the head and the isthmus. The posterior surface is connected with the superior mesenteric vein and the beginning of lymph nodes near the celiac trunk, the superior mesenteric artery and the superior mesenteric vein as well as on the right and left of the aorta.

The body of the pancreas is placed over the transverse mesocolon, behind the stomach and in front of the aorta. It is connected to the first segment of the superior mesenteric artery, to the left pillar of the diaphragm, the left adrenal gland, the left kidney and its vessels. It is also linked with the splenic vein.

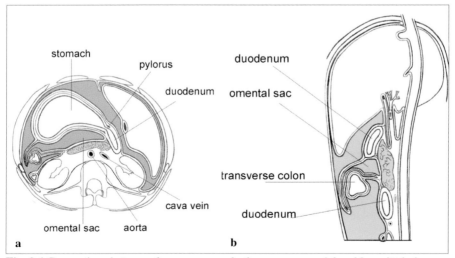

Fig. 2.4 Connections between the pancreas and other organs: **a** axial and **b** sagittal views

The pancreatic tail is surgically far more reachable. Posteriorly it is also connected with the posterior wall of the stomach. It is held between the two layers of the lienorenal ligament together with the splenic vessels.

Surgical Access

The pancreas is a relatively firm organ and it is possible to determine the surgical routes of access by studying its connections:
–   When the transverse mesocolon is lifted, it is possible to palpate through its roots the body and the tail of the pancreas, the lesser pancreas, and the superior mesenteric vein.
–   With the Kocher maneuver it is possible to mobilize completely the duodenopancreatic bloc. This type of maneuver begins with mobilization of the hepatic flexure of the colon downward and medially, followed by sectioning of the peritoneal lamina which fixes the hepatic fold to the duodenum and to the anterior side of the pancreas. Sectioning the peritoneum laterally from the second portion of the duodenum, the duodenum itself and the pancreatic head are separated from the posterior structure. In this way the bulk of the pancreatic head and the duodenum are lifted, thus exposing the right kidney, the right renal vein, the inferior vena cava, and the beginning of the left renal vein.
–   Through the lesser omentum you can reach the pancreatic body from the top and from the front aspect. Separating the vascular part from the lesser omentum, going back down the lesser gastric curvature you can obtain a reasonable view of the pancreatic body.
–   A more complete view of the pancreatic body can be obtained by opening the gastrocolic ligament. Extending this movement towards the right in the pyloric area by tying up and sectioning the beginning of the righthand vessels, it is possible to obtain a good view of the front aspect of the isthmus.
–   Mobilization of the spleen and the left pancreas is possible on an avascular plane of cleavage which allows exploration of the body and tail.

Pancreatic and Common Bile Ducts

The main pancreatic duct goes through the pancreas from left to right. It begins to unite the small globular ducts of the tail. Passing along the body it receives the globular ducts which form the gland, and they arrange themselves in a herringbone pattern. It then reaches the neck of the pancreas, turning downwards beside the choledochus or common bile duct, and at this point it confluences with it.
    The type of confluence and the connections of flow can vary:
–   *Type I:* The two ducts flow into a shared ampulla which protrudes into the duodenum in the form of a papilla (70% of cases) (Fig. 2.5a).

- *Type II:* The two ducts confluence near the papilla (21% of cases) (Fig. 2.5b).
- *Type III:* The two ducts flow down separately to the outlet (8.5% of cases) (Fig. 2.5c).
- *Type IV:* The two ducts confluence together at a certain distance from the duodenum without forming an ampulla (Fig. 2.5d).

The other duct which receives the lobular ducts of the superior portion of the head is called the pancreatic accessory duct. This is in front of the main pancreatic duct, with which it is connected by a communicating duct, and it opens into the duodenum around 2 cm above and a little in front of the main duodenal papilla on a small duodenal papilla. The accessory duct is sometimes partially present either as a self-governing outlet into the duodenum or as a rudimentary accessory duct of the main duct (Fig. 2.6).

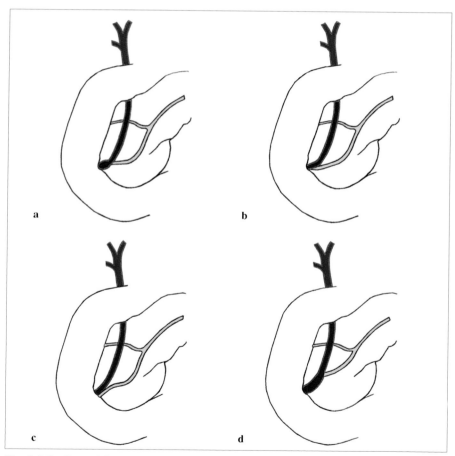

Fig. 2.5 Outflow of the common bile duct and of the main ducts. **a** The two ducts flow into a shared ampulla. **b** The two ducts confluence near the papilla. **c** The two ducts flow down separately to the outlet. **d** The two ducts confluence together at a certain distance from the duodenum without forming an ampulla

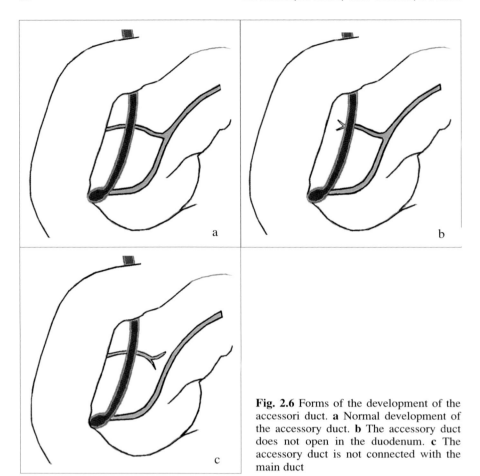

Fig. 2.6 Forms of the development of the accessori duct. **a** Normal development of the accessory duct. **b** The accessory duct does not open in the duodenum. **c** The accessory duct is not connected with the main duct

Arterial Vascularization

The arterial vascularization is established by a thick anastomotic net coming from the celiac trunk and from the mesenteric superior artery (Fig. 2.7).

The gastroduodenal artery is the descending branch of the common hepatic artery. It courses in front of the portal vein. Its starting point can vary: it can originate from the accessory left hepatic artery, from the right branch of the main hepatic artery, or from the superior mesenteric artery.

The first big branch that comes off from the gastroduodenal artery is nearly always the superior posterior pancreaticoduodenal artery, also defined as the posterior duodenal artery. It generally begins at the top of the duodenum. It crosses the common bile duct at the superior level of the head of the pancreas, leaves it on the left, and continues in a caudal direction to meet it again during its course going down and forming a posterior arch with a posterior branch of the

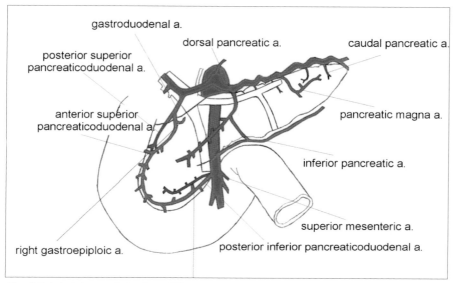

gastroduodenal a.

dorsal pancreatic a.

caudal pancreatic a.

posterior superior
pancreaticoduodenal a.

anterior superior
pancreaticoduodenal a.

pancreatic magna a.

inferior pancreatic a.

superior mesenteric a.

right gastroepiploic a.

posterior inferior pancreaticoduodenal a.

Fig. 2.7 Arterial vascularization of the pancreas

inferior pancreaticoduodenal artery. Sometimes a supraduodenal artery can leave the gastroduodenal artery before the posterior superior pancreaticoduodenal artery.

The superior anterior pancreaticoduodenal artery together with the gastroepiploic artery represents the final second branch of the gastroduodenal artery. It lies in the center of the head of the pancreas, often running along the bend of the duodenum in a concavity partially or totally situated in the glandular parenchyma. It forms an anterior arch with the anterior branch of the inferior pancreaticoduodenal artery.

The inferior pancreaticoduodenal artery begins behind the uncinate process of the pancreas as the first right branch of the mesenteric superior artery and divides after a short distance into an anterior and a posterior branch. The anterior branch runs behind the uncinate process and comes out onto the anterior surface of the pancreas in the zone where it fuses with the superior anterior pancreaticoduodenal artery. The posterior branch of the inferior pancreaticoduodenal artery runs along the back of the head of the pancreas at a greater distance from the duodenum than that of the anterior branch and fuses with the posterior pancreaticoduodenal artery.

The dorsal pancreatic artery originates from the celiac trunk as the first branch of the splenic artery near its origin, or directly from the celiac trunk or from the common hepatic artery. The inferior pancreatic artery runs dorsally and in the body of the pancreas and along its inferior margin. In the majority of cases it starts at the left main branch of the dorsal pancreatic artery or at the superior mesenteric artery.

The great pancreatic artery takes off from the splenic artery and joins into the glandular parenchyma at the level of the passage from the middle part to the left third of the tail of the pancreas.

The artery of the tail of the pancreas is represented by four arterial trunks which surround the pancreatic tail. They originate from the left gastroepiploic artery or from the so-called main inferior trunk of the splenic artery.

Venous Drainage

It is normally said, in view of the embryonic development, that the blood from the glandular parenchyma which begins in the ventral bud flows into the superior mesenteric vein, while that coming from the dorsal bud flows in part into the mesenteric vein and in part into the splenic vein or directly into the portal vein.

The superior anterior pancreaticoduodenal vein begins halfway down the descending portion of the duodenum and is situated on the head of the pancreas near the duodenum (Fig. 2.8). It goes towards the right gastroepiploic vein, into which it flows. The superior posterior pancreaticoduodenal vein begins in the posterior surface of the pancreatic head. It generally courses behind the common bile duct and flows into the portal vein.

The inferior anterior pancreaticoduodenal vein begins between the pancreas and the duodenum. It courses for a short distance in the pancreatic parenchyma and flows into the superior mesenteric vein. The inferior posterior pancreatico-

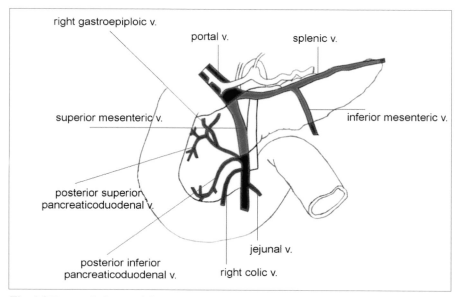

Fig. 2.8 Venous drainage of the pancreas

duodenal vein begins at the same height as the inferior anterior one and courses behind the head. Generally it flows into the superior mesenteric vein.

The splenic vein courses behind the pancreas near the superior margin. The small pancreatic veins fuse among themselves and flow into the splenic vein at various distances.

The inferior pancreatic vein courses along the inferior margin of the pancreas and receives different small veins. It flows into the inferior or the superior mesenteric vein.

Lymphatic Drainage

The lymphatic ducts which drain the pancreas course towards the lymph nodes situated near the gland, following the artery. Generally one can distinguish a first position made up of peripancreatic lymph nodes (Fig. 2.9a) and a second position made up of a collection of lymph nodes near the celiac trunk the mesenteric artery and the superior mesenteric vein let alone on the right and left of the aorta (Fig. 2.9b).

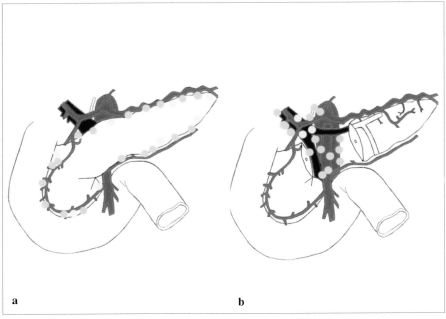

a   b

Fig. 2.9 Lymphatic drainage of the pancreas. **a** The main duct and the accessory duct are separated. **b** The main pancreatic duct and the accessory duct anastomose after the fusion of the dorsal and the ventral buds

Suggested Reading

Balboni GC (1975) Anatomia umana, vol 1. Edi-ermes, Milan

Chiarugi G (1944) Istituzioni di anatomia dell'uomo, vol 3. Società Editoriale Libraria, Milan

Kremer K Lierse W, Platzer W et al (1993) Colecisti, vie biliari, pancreas. Grande Atlante di tecnica chirurgica. UTET, Turin

Moore KM (1980) Lo sviluppo dell'uomo. Zanichelli, Bologna

Testut L, Jacob O (1922) Trattato di anatomia topografica, vol 2. UTET, Turin

Chapter 3

Pancreatic Trauma

Fausto Catena, Salomone Di Saverio, Luca Ansaloni, Antonio Daniele Pinna

Epidemiology, Etiology, and Pathogenesis

Traumatic injuries of the pancreas are rare. Epidemiological studies in a Scandinavian population have reported an incidence of 0.4 cases per 100,000 head of population per year, accounting for 7% of laparotomies performed for abdominal trauma [1]. An earlier study reported the same incidence of pancreatic injuries (7.4%) among trauma laparotomies performed in the Los Angeles urban area [2].

The mechanisms leading to pancreatic injury can be divided into the blunt and the penetrating. While an injury caused by a penetrating stab wound is limited to the trajectory of the blade path, the passage of a high velocity bullet, because of the pressure it exerts on the surrounding tissue, can cause a worse and wider injury, the more so since it may burst and shatter, spreading itself around the area. All penetrating trauma requires careful evaluation of the integrity of the main pancreatic duct, for ductal injuries occur in 15% of cases of pancreatic trauma and are almost always associated with penetrating injuries [3].

Blunt pancreatic injuries are associated with high-energy impact because of the deep retroperitoneal and relatively protected location of the gland. In adults most blunt injuries occur in motor vehicle accidents, and usually (60% of such cases) the underlying mechanism is high-energy impact between the steering wheel and the epigastrium or hypochondrium, resulting in crushing of the retroperitoneal structures against the vertebral column. The anatomy of the injuries can vary widely from just a contusion of the pancreas up to complete transection of the glandular body and duct. In children the most common traumatic mechanism is a handlebar injury [4].

Diagnosis

In the diagnostic work-up of the polytrauma patient with probable pancreatic injury, it is essential to prioritize early control of hemorrhage and prevention of any bacterial contamination from associated vascular or hollow-visceral lesions.

W. Siquini (Ed.), *Surgical Treatment of Pancreatic Diseases.*
©Springer-Verlag Italia 2009

Severe associated vascular and/or intra-abdominal injuries dramatically increase early morbidity and mortality. The next step should be to look carefully for any pancreatic lesion, paying particular attention to the possible presence of major ductal injury, since this is the strongest single prognostic factor. Patients in whom exploratory trauma laparotomy is clearly mandatory because of associated lesions of other intra-abdominal organs (those who are hemodynamically unstable, and/or have signs of peritonism, and/or with intra-abdominal free fluid shown by ultrasound) do not require further investigation to assess the integrity of the pancreas, but for all other patients without evident indications for immediate laparotomy, the diagnosis of an isolated pancreatic injury can be insidious and challenging. Patients with an isolated pancreatic injury – even with ductal transection – can be initially asymptomatic or present only minor signs.

The finding of a high serum concentration of amylase is not a reliable indicator of pancreatic injury, having low sensitivity and specificity. A recent review showed that the serum amylase concentration after pancreatic trauma has a positive predictive value ranging from 8 to 100% and a negative predictive value ranging from 0 to 99% [5]. However, the enzyme levels later than 3 h after injury and repeated measurements can improve the diagnostic accuracy [6]. The retroperitoneal posterior location of the pancreas makes it remarkably difficult to explore by ultrasound, particularly in obese patients; in addition, after abdominal trauma the presence of reflex post-traumatic ileus can mask the underlying organs.

Abdominal CT seems to be the most reliable diagnostic tool for identifying pancreatic injuries. Sensitivities and specificities as high as 80% have been reported, although the accuracy is largely interpreter-dependent and is affected by the quality of the images and the time elapsed since the injury [7, 8]. The CT signs of pancreatic injury may not be clear and evident, even immediately after injury or in the initial phase; some authors have reported a false negative rate of CT diagnosis of up to 40%, even when pancreatic damage is significant [9]. A repeat CT scan in the presence of continuing symptoms can improve the sensitivity. CT findings indicating a pancreatic injury are direct visualization of a parenchymal fracture, intrapancreatic hematoma, fluid in the lesser sac, fluid between the splenic vein and the body of the gland, thickening of the left anterior renal fascia, and, finally, retroperitoneal hematoma or fluid.

Endoscopic retrograde cholangiopancreatography (ERCP) can play an important and useful role in the diagnosis and treatment of pancreatic trauma, in two different phases. In the acute phase, in patients who are hemodynamically stable and in whom pancreatic involvement is suspected, especially in the presence of unexplained abdominal pain, hyperamylasemia, and abnormal or suspicious CT findings, ERCP can demonstrate a disruption of the pancreatic duct [10]. When a disrupted duct is found, laparotomy is mandatory. On the other hand, an early ERCP showing an intact ductal tree without extravasation may, if there are no associated lesions of other organs, allow observation and nonoperative management [11–13]. In a later phase, ERCP can be useful in the diagnosis and, sometimes, treatment of late complications presenting months to years after an initially missed pancreatic injury.

Finally, MRI, although usually used in the elective setting, seems to be a safe and effective, noninvasive alternative to ERCP in the careful assessment of the main pancreatic duct after pancreatic traumatic injury [14].

Intraoperative pancreatography to visualize the main duct is helpful particularly when ductal injury is suspected, or when the assessment of its integrity during the intraoperative inspection is difficult and uncertain. Technically, intraoperative pancreatography can be performed by transduodenal catheterization of the ampulla, distal cannulation of the duct in the tail of the pancreas, or even by a needle cholecystocholangiogram [5].

Treatment

The current worldwide accepted classification of pancreatic trauma is that of the American Association for the Surgery of Trauma (AAST) Committee on Organ Injury Scaling. Focusing on whether the injury is proximal or distal, parenchymal and/or ductal, it suggests useful if nonspecific guidelines for treatment. In particular, parenchymal contusions or lacerations without ductal injury and with minimal or small tissue loss (grade I or II) can be safely managed with adequate external drainage alone. Distal transections of the gland with ductal injury (grade III) require a distal pancreatectomy. Proximal injuries involving the head of the pancreas, especially if involving the ampulla or duodenum (grade IV or V), may require a pancreaticoduodenectomy or other complex reconstructive procedure: however, in patients with this kind of injury and in those in critical general condition, such complex procedures are preferably delayed until definitive surgery can be carried out, and a less aggressive therapeutic strategy of damage control is preferred. As a matter of fact, patients with severe pancreatic or combined pancreaticoduodenal injury (grade IV and V) are usually not stable enough to undergo complex definitive procedures at the time of trauma laparotomy. A damage-control approach focusing on the control of hemorrhage and bacterial contamination, packing, and external drainage is highly preferable in these situations. Placement of a draining tube directly into the duct can be helpful, both for drainage and to allow easier isolation of the duct at a later operation [15].

Minor pancreatic contusions, hematomas, and capsular lacerations (grade I) represent 60% of all post-traumatic pancreatic injuries. Major parenchymal lacerations and contusions without ductal disruption or substantial tissue loss (grade II) account for an additional 20%. Appropriate treatment of these lesions is based on hemostasis and effective external drainage [16]; any attempt to repair capsular lacerations should be avoided because their closure may result in formation of a pancreatic pseudocyst, whereas even if a pancreatic fistula develops, it is usually self-limiting if adequately drained and controlled [5]. Soft closed-suction drains (e.g., Jackson Pratt) should be preferred owing to the lower incidence of intra-abdominal abscesses and collections. It is not advisable to attempt to achieve hemostasis of the bleeding vessels by suturing the injured parenchyma, because this is not effective for reliable hemostasis and only leads to necrosis of the pancreatic tissue. Bleeding vessels should be ligated individually and an omental patch can be added.

The distinction between the proximal and distal parts of the pancreas is usually defined by the passage of the superior mesenteric vessels behind the pancreas, dividing the head and the body of the gland. In a patient with distal parenchymal transection or major parenchymal injury with ductal disruption, or even a major parenchymal lesion of the distal pancreas regardless of the degree of ductal involvement (grade II and III), the best surgical option is distal pancreatectomy. The degree of ductal involvement and the status of the remaining, proximal part of the main pancreatic duct can be assessed by intraoperative pancreatography. The vessels should be carefully ligated, the glandular stump can be sutured and the duct ligated separately or closed using a stapling device [17]. The reported occurrence of postoperative fistula from the transection stump is as high as 14% [16].

Traumatic injuries to the head of the pancreas pose a challenging therapeutic dilemma. The priority is the definition of the anatomy and status of the pancreatic duct. Surgical exploration and intraoperative pancreatography are mandatory if feasible. If ductal involvement cannot be assessed by direct inspection and pancreatography cannot be performed, a wide external drainage with several closed-suction drains followed by postoperative ERCP (with duct stenting if a major proximal ductal injury is confirmed) or magnetic resonance cholangiopancreatography (MRCP) is advisable. Pancreatic head and neck injuries that spare the major pancreatic duct can be safely and effectively managed by adequate external drainage alone, which is even more recommended in unstable patients (with postoperative ERCP). Some authors suggest external closed-suction drainage alone for any proximal pancreatic injury, rather than wide resection. They obtained a 13.5% fistula and abscess formation rate [18]; however, it has to be noted that the patients in this study did not undergo pancreatography and could not be assessed as to whether true major pancreatic ductal injury was present.

Severe combined pancreaticoduodenal injuries are rare (less than 10% of pancreatic traumatic injuries) and are usually caused by penetrating trauma and associated with multiple severe intra-abdominal injuries, frequently of the inferior vena cava [19]. Therapeutic and operative management must be based on the integrity of the common bile duct and ampulla on cholangiography and the severity of duodenal injury [5]. In a review of 129 patients with combined pancreaticoduodenal injury, 24% of them were treated with simple repair and drainage and 50% underwent repair and pyloric exclusion, while only 10% required a pancreaticoduodenectomy (Whipple's procedure) [19]. Because of the broad spectrum of injuries in these cases, and the strategies required to treat them, any patient with pancreaticoduodenal trauma needs to undergo a cholangiogram, pancreatogram, and careful evaluation of the status of the ampulla as well. In massive injuries with destruction of the proximal duodenum and pancreatic head involving the ampulla and/or distal common bile duct and proximal duct of Wirsung, any reconstructive attempt is precluded (also because the head of the pancreas and the duodenum have a common arterial supply) and a pancreaticoduodenectomy is unavoidable. A wide-ranging review of 184 cases of Whipple's procedure performed for trauma between 1961 and 1994 showed high morbidity and mortality rates (14% intraoperative and 36% overall mortality) [20].

Some authors have suggested nonoperative management for grade I–II injuries, combined with early ERCP to identify the presence of ductal injury requiring surgery [21]. In selected cases of ductal injury in adults, proximal stenting of the pancreatic duct has been employed successfully [22]. Further investigations are needed before any recommendations or guidelines can be made about nonoperative management of pancreatic traumatic injuries in adults. The use of somatostatin and its analogues (octreotide) is common in patients with acute pancreatitis in order to reduce the exocrine secretions; however, several studies failed to show a benefit or reported just a slight reduction of the complication rate [23]. The use of these drugs is frequent in cases of traumatic injury of the pancreas but is not supported by evidence-based studies.

Adequate nutritional support is a priority in the management of severe pancreatic trauma and should be considered and planned intraoperatively. A feeding jejunostomy 15–30 cm distal to the duodenojejunal flexure, allowing early enteral feeding, should be performed routinely. Elemental diets are preferred because they are less stimulating to the pancreas and are cheaper [24]. Total parenteral nutrition is a more expensive alternative if enteral access is unavailable.

Pancreatic traumatic injuries are associated with a postoperative complication rate from 20 up to 42%; the more severe the injury, the higher the morbidity. With multiple associated injuries of other intra-abdominal organs the complication rate rises up to 62% [25]. Furthermore, the development of sepsis and multiple organ failure accounts for 30% of the deaths after pancreatic trauma. Although the majority of the complications of pancreatic trauma are self-limiting or at least treatable, careful intraoperative inspection of the pancreas and assessment of the status of the duct of Wirsung can reduce morbidity by up to one-half. Complications can occur early and late. The onset of transient abdominal pain associated with elevation of the serum amylase concentration may indicate the development of postoperative pancreatitis, which occurs in 7–18% of patients [26–28]. Most patients with this form of post-traumatic pancreatitis are well treated with bowel rest, nasogastric tube decompression, and parenteral nutritional support. The severity may vary from just a transient biochemical and self-limiting peak of amylase up to fulminant, usually deadly hemorrhagic pancreatitis. The latter is fortunately rare, occurring in less than 2% of operated patients with pancreatic trauma, but the mortality can approach 80% in these cases [29].

Postoperative pancreatic fistula development is the most common complication following pancreatic trauma, with an incidence of 7–20% [26] but rising to 26–37% in cases where there is ductal involvement or combined pancreatico-duodenal injury [18, 30, 31]. Most of these fistulas are minor (output less than 200 ml/day) and are self-limiting within 2 weeks given effective and adequate external drainage. A recent multicenter review of post-traumatic distal pancrea-tectomy reported a 14% rate of postoperative fistula, with spontaneous closure in 6–54 days [27]. High-output fistulas (more than 700 ml/day) are rare and require either surgical intervention or a prolonged period of external drainage combined with nutritional support (preferably enteral feeding via jejunostomy) as well as medical treatment of the underlying cause (such as sepsis) and octreotide to reduce the glandular secretions. However, the efficacy of octreotide is uncertain and octreotide treatment does not obviate the necessity of eradicat-ing any infection and excluding obstruction or stenosis of the pancreatic duct [32]. If a high-output fistula persists for more than 10 days and/or fails to decrease in volume of output, ERCP (or MRCP/CT) can be done to establish the underlying cause sustaining the fistula. A documented ductal lesion requires sur-gical reoperation; otherwise transpapillary duct stenting is an option [33].

The incidence of post-traumatic abscess formation, usually peripancreatic, ranges from 10 to 25%, depending on the number and type of associated lesions, especially if they involve the liver and the intestine. Early operative or percuta-neous evacuation is mandatory since the mortality in patients with such abscess-es is as high as 25% [34, 35]. The abscesses are most often subfascial or peri-pancreatic: a true pancreatic abscess is unusual, resulting from inadequate debridement of necrotic tissue. For this reason, abscesses of this kind are not treatable with percutaneous drainage and require prompt surgical debridement and drainage; percutaneous decompression allows an abscess to be distinguished from a pseudocyst.

Early diagnosis and correct treatment of pancreatic trauma should guarantee a pseudocyst formation rate not higher than 2–3%. Despite this, a report on 42 patients with blunt pancreatic trauma treated nonoperatively showed pseudocyst formation in more than half of them [36]. The main prognostic factor for pseudo-cysts, both predicting outcome and suggesting further treatment, is the status of the pancreatic duct as assessed using either ERCP or MRCP. If the duct is intact, percutaneous drainage of the pseudocyst should be effective. If on the other hand the pseudocyst is caused by major pancreatic duct disruption, previously unrec-ognized, simple percutaneous drainage will only convert the pseudocyst to a chronic fistula and the definitive treatment should include either partial gland resection or an internal Roux-en-Y drainage, or cystogastrostomy (open or endo-scopic), or endoscopic transpapillary ductal stenting [37]. Surgery is usually pre-ferred for the larger sizes of cyst, because of the risk of stent migration [10].

The morbidity and mortality after gunshot wound, especially with high-ener-gy impact, are clearly higher than those following a stab-wound penetrating injury. The amount of energy involved is therefore a discriminant factor in deter-mining the severity of injuries, ranging from a small contusion or superficial lac-eration of the gland up to massive destruction of the pancreas with complete ductal transection.

The mortality associated with pancreatic trauma is mostly in patients who die within the first 48 h, primarily because of exsanguinating injuries to the major vessels, liver, or spleen [38]. For example, in penetrating wounds of the pancreas, the aorta, portal vein, or vena cava are involved in the injury in more than 75% of cases. In blunt trauma, associated injuries of a parenchymal or hollow viscus are also common. In a multicenter review of more than 1,000 patients with pancreatic injuries, the incidence and type of the associated lesions were respectively 47% involving the liver, 42% the stomach, 41% major vessels, 28% spleen and 23% kidneys, 19% the duodenum, 17% the colon, and 15% the small bowel [5, 30]. The presence and severity of associated injuries is strongly and significantly related to the mortality, which is 2.5% when there is no associated injury or only one lesion involving the adjacent organs, but rises to 13.6% when there are two or three associated lesions, and goes up again to 29.6% with four or more lesions [31]. Late deaths (later than 48 h after trauma) are usually related to the development of sepsis and multiple organ failure secondary to the associated duodenal or pancreatic injury [32, 39]. The most common complications are anastomotic breakdown, fistula, pseudocyst, intra-abdominal abscess, and pneumonia.

The time elapsed from injury to definitive treatment is a further prognostic factor. A mortality rate of 50% has been reported in six patients with pancreatic trauma in whom surgical treatment was delayed until 17 up to 60 days after injury [40]. Other authors have reported mortality rates ranging from 50 to 90% without surgical treatment, and the onset for surviving patients of long-term problems such as pancreatitis, abdominal pain, and pseudocyst formation [25, 41, 42].

Finally, the last but not the least prognostic factor is the status of the pancreatic duct. A ductal lesion – more so if initially missed and treated late – can strongly and significantly increase morbidity and mortality [21]. The last few decades have shown the importance of a careful assessment for the presence of a ductal lesion; a distal pancreatectomy including the injured duct reduced mortality from 19 to 3%, compared with nonoperative management [43]. A further study showed a significant decrease in the complication rate from 55 to 15% using intraoperative pancreatography for accurate investigation of the ductal status in cases of suspected proximal injury [43].

References

1. Nilsson E, Norrby S, Skullman S et al (1986) Pancreatic trauma in a defined population. Acta Chir Scand 152: 647–651
2. White PH, Benfield JR (1972) Amylase in the management of pancreatic trauma. Arch Surg 105:158–163
3. Graham JM, Mattox KL, Jordan GL Jr et al (1978) Traumatic injuries of the pancreas. Am J Surg 136:144–148
4. Arkovitz MS, Johnson N, Garcia VF (1997) Pancreatic trauma in children: mechanisms of injury. J Trauma 42:49–53
5. Moore E, Feliciano D, Mattox K (2004) Trauma, 5th edn. McGraw-Hill, New York
6. Takishima T, Sugimoto K, Hirata M et al (1997) Serum amylase level on admission in the diagnosis of blunt injury to the pancreas: its significance and limitations. Ann Surg 226:70–76

7.   Jeffrey RB Jr, Federle MP, Crass RA et al (1983) CT of pancreatic trauma. Radiology 147:491–494
8.   Peitzman AB, Makaroun MS, Slasky BS et al (1986) Prospective study of CT in initial man-agement of blunt abdominal trauma. J Trauma 26:585–592
9.   Wilson RH, Moorehead RJ (1991) Current management of trauma to the pancreas. Br J Surg 78:1196–1202
10. Buccimazza I, Thomson SR, Anderson F et al (2006) Isolated main pancreatic duct injuries spectrum and management. Am J Surg 191:448–452
11. Heitsch RC, Knutson CO, Fulton RC, Jones CE (1976) Delineation of critical factors in the treatment of pancreatic trauma. Surgery 80:523–539
12. Whittwell AE, Gomez GA, Byers P et al (1989) Blunt pancreatic trauma: prospective eval-uation of early endoscopic retrograde pancreatography. South Med J 82:586–591
13. Wisner DH, Wold RL, Fray CF (1990) Diagnosis and treatment of pancreatic injuries. An analysis of management principles. Arch Surg 125:1109–1113
14. Soto TA, Alvarez O, Mùnera F et al (2001) Traumatic disruption of the pancreatic duct: diag-nosis with MR pancreatography. AJR Am J Roentgenol 176:175–178
15. Boffard K (ed) (2003) Manual of definitive surgical trauma care. Arnold, London
16. Nowak MM, Baringer DC, Ponsky JL (1986) Pancreatic injuries: effectiveness of debride-ment and drainage for nontransecting injuries. Am Surg 52:599–602
17. Andersen DK, Bolman RM et al (1980) Management of penetrating pancreatic injuries: subtotal pancreatectomy using the auto-suture stapler. J Trauma 20:347–349
18. Patton JH jr, Lyden SP, Croce MA et al (1997) Pancreatic trauma: a simplified management guideline. J Trauma 43:234–239
19. Feliciano DV, Martin TD, Cruse PA et al (1987) Management of combined pancreatoduode-nal injuries. Ann Surg 205:673–680
20. Delcore R, Stauffer JS, Thomas JH et al (1994) The role of pancreatogastrostomy following pancreatoduodenectomy for trauma. J Trauma 37:395–400
21. Bradley EL, Young PR Jr, Chang MC et al (1998) Diagnosis and initial management of blunt pancreatic trauma: guidelines from a multi-institutional review. Ann Surg 227:861–869
22. Kim HS, Lee DK, Kim IW et al (2001) The role of endoscopic retrograde pancreatography in the treatment of traumatic pancreatic duct injury. Gastroint Endosc 54:49–55
23. McKay C, Baxter J, Imrie C (1997) A randomised controlled trial of octreotide in the man-agement of patients with acute pancreatitis. Int J Pancreatol 21:13–19
24. Kellum JM, Holland GF, McNeill P (1988) Traumatic pancreatic cutaneous fistula: compar-ison of enteral and parenteral feeding. J Trauma 28:700–714
25. Leppaniemi A, Haapiainer R, Kiviluoto T, Lempinen M (1988) Pancreatic trauma: acute and late manifestations. Br J Surg 75:165–167
26. Akhrass R, Yaffe MB, Brandt CP et al (1997) Pancreatic trauma: a 10-year multi-institution-al experience. Am Surg 63:598–604
27. Cogbill TH, Moore EE, Moris JA Jr et al (1991) Distal pancreatectomy for trauma: a multi-center experience. J Trauma 31:1600–1606
28. Moore JB, Moore EE (1984) Changing trends in the management of combined pancreato-duodenal injuries. World J Surg 8:791–797
29. Graham JM, Mattox KL, Jordan GL Jr (1978) Traumatic injuries of the pancreas. Am J Surg 136:744–748
30. Graham JM, Mattox KL, Vaughan GD 3rd, Jordan GL Jr (1979) Combined pancreatoduo-denal injuries. J Trauma 19:340
31. Balasegaram M (1979) Surgical management of pancreatic trauma. Curr Prob Surg 16(12):1–59
32. Prinz RA, Pickleman J, Hoffman JP (1988) Treatment of pancreatic cutaneous fistula with a somatostatin analog. Am J Surg 155:36–42
33. Kozarek RA, Traverso LW (1996) Pancreatic fistulas: etiology, consequences and treatment. Gastroenterologist 4:238–244
34. Feliciano DV, Martin TD, Cruse PA et al (1987) Management of combined pancreatoduode-

nal injuries. Ann Surg 205:673–680

35. Wynn M, Hill DM, Miller DR et al (1985) Management of pancreatic and duodenal trauma Am J Surg 150:327–332

36. Kudsk KA, Temizer D, Ellison EC et al (1986) Post-traumatic pancreatic sequestrum: recognition and treatment. J Trauma 26:320–324

37. Kozarek RA, Ball TJ, Patterson DJ et al (1991) Endoscopic transpapillary therapy for disrupted pancreatic duct and peripancreatic fluid collections. Gastroenterology 100:1362–1370

38. Blaisdell FW, Trunkey DD (eds) (1982) Trauma to the pancreas and duodenum. In: Abdominal trauma. Thieme-Stratton, New York, pp 87–122

39. Jones RC (1985) Management of pancreatic trauma. Am J Surg 150:698–704

40. Bach RD, Frey CF (1971) Diagnosis and treatment of pancreatic trauma. Am J Surg 121:20–29

41. Glancy KE (1989) Review of pancreatic trauma. West J Med 151:45–51

42. Carr ND, Cairns SJ, Lees WR (1989) Late complications of pancreatic trauma. Br J Surg 76:1244–1246

43. Smego DR, Richardson JD, Flint LM (1985) Determinants of outcome in pancreatic trauma. J Trauma 25:771–776

Chapter 4

Epidemiology, Classification, Etiopathogenesis, and Diagnosis of Acute Pancreatitis

Gianluca Guercioni, Walter Siquini, Emidio Senati

Introduction

In 1925, Moynihan described the dramatic nature of acute pancreatitis as the "most terrible of all calamities that occurs in connection with the abdominal viscera. The suddenness of its onset, the illimitable agony which accompanies it, and the mortality attendant upon it renders it the most formidable of catastrophes" [1]. From mild and self-limiting disease to multiorgan failure and sepsis, acute pancreatitis is a disorder that has numerous causes, an obscure pathogenesis, few effective remedies, and an often unpredictable outcome. The anatomopathological alterations of the pancreatic parenchyma vary from interstitial edema and very limited necrosis of the parenchymal fat to extensive areas of pancreatic necrosis and bleeding.

Epidemiology

Several authors have noted that the incidence of acute pancreatitis has significantly increased in the last 40 years [2–5]. In the United States the incidence of acute pancreatitis ranges from 5 to 25 cases per 100,000 population, and between 166,000 and 224,000 patients are admitted each year with a diagnosis of acute pancreatitis [6, 7]. Estimates of the incidence in Europe range from about 10 to 15 cases per 100,000 population; more women than men are affected (2:1), perhaps due to the prevalence of cholelithiasis in women [2, 3]. In Italy the incidence of acute pancreatitis has been reported at between 5 and 10 cases per 100,000 population, with a greater frequency in the north than in the central and southern regions [2]. The age of peak incidence is between 45 and 55 years in men and between 55 and 65 years in women [2–7].

Although acute pancreatitis has a benign disease course, the global mortality rate is around 5% [8], being less than 1% in the mild form [6, 9] and 20–25% in the severe ones [10].

Definition, Classification, and Terminology

Acute pancreatitis is an acute inflammatory process of the pancreas with variable involvement of other regional tissues or remote organ systems [11]. The most significant factor in classifying acute pancreatitis is the presence of pancreatic necrosis, which is the major risk factor.

The most useful and widely accepted classification system for describing the clinical course of acute pancreatitis was developed during the consensus conference of Atlanta in 1992. Table 4.1 shows the clinically based classification system for acute pancreatitis derived from this symposium [11].

From the pathological viewpoint, the following can be distinguished (pathologic classification of acute pancreatitis) [12]:

- Edematous acute pancreatitis
- Edematous pancreatitis with focal areas of steatonecrosis, bleeding, or necrosis
- Necrotic–hemorrhagic pancreatitis
- Suppurative pancreatitis

Table 4.1 Clinically-based classification system for acute pancreatitis (Atlanta Conference 1992)

Term	Definition
Mild acute pancreatitis	Acute inflammation of the pancreas with minimal distant organ dysfunction and uneventful recovery
Severe acute pancreatitis	Acute pancreatitis associated with organ failure and/or local complications, such as necrosis, abscess, or pseudocyst
Acute fluid collections	Fluid collections that occur early in the course of acute pancreatitis located within or near the pancreas, without a wall of granulation or fibrous tissue
Pancreatic necrosis	Diffuse or focal areas of nonviable pancreatic parenchyma typically associated with peripancreatic fat necrosis
Pseudocyst	Collection of pancreatic juice enclosed by a wall of granulation or fibrous tissue which arises as a consequence of acute pancreatitis, pancreatic trauma, or chronic pancreatitis
Pancreatic abscess	Circumscribed intra-abdominal collection of pus, usually in proximity to the pancreas, containing little or no pancreatic necrosis which arises as a consequence of acute pancreatitis or pancreatic trauma

Etiology

Many factors have been implicated as cause of acute pancreatitis (Table 4.2), although gallstone disease and alcoholism together are responsible for 70–80% of all cases.

Table 4.2 Causes of acute pancreatitis

Gallstones
Alcoholism
Metabolic causes
    Hypertriglyceridemia
    Hypercalcemia
Genetic mutations
    Hereditary pancreatitis
    Cystic fibrosis
    Autoimmune pancreatitis
Pancreas divisum
Drugs
    Azathioprine
    6-Mercaptopurine
    Pentamidine
    Didanosine
    Sulfonamides
    Valproic acid
    Furosemide
    Aminosalicylates
    Metronidazole
    Acetaminophen
Toxins
    Organophosphate insecticides
Scorpion's venom
    Trauma
    ERCP
Infections
    Viruses:
–   Cytomegalovirus
–   Mumps
–   Rubella
–   Coxsackievirus B
–   Hepatitis A, B, and non-A, non-B
    Bacteria:
–   *Klebsiella* spp.
–   *E. coli*
–   *Mycobacterium tuberculosis* (AIDS)
–   *Mycobacterium avium complex* (AIDS)
    Fungi:
–   *Cryptosporidium* spp.
–   *Cryptococcus* spp.
–   *Candida* spp.
    Worms:
–   *Ascaris lumbricoides*
–   *Clonorchis sinensis*
Ischemia
Tumors
Idiopathic

Cholelithiasis

Gallstones are the principal cause of acute pancreatitis in Europe (up to 70%) [12]. The exact mechanism remains unclear. In 1856 Claude Bernard reported, in an experimental model, that injection of bile into the duct of Wirsung (main pancreatic duct) produced acute pancreatitis. In 1901 Eugene Lindsay Opie at the Johns Hopkins Hospital in Baltimore documented a gallstone impacted in the ampulla of Vater during the postmortem examination of a patient operated on by Halsted, who died of gallstone pancreatitis. He proposed that a gallstone obstructing the prepapillary common channel shared by the common bile duct and the pancreatic duct would lead to bile reflux into the pancreatic tree (Fig. 4.1). The diffusion of bile into the Wirsung douct would cause acute pancreatitis ("common channel theory") [13].

The etiologic role of gallstones has been well established: acute pancreatitis affects between 3 and 8% of all patients with symptomatic gallstones and up to 30% of those with microlithiasis (stones smaller than 3 mm in diameter). Moreover, several studies have documented the retrieval of gallstones in the stools of approximately 90% of patients with acute gallstones pancreatitis [14].

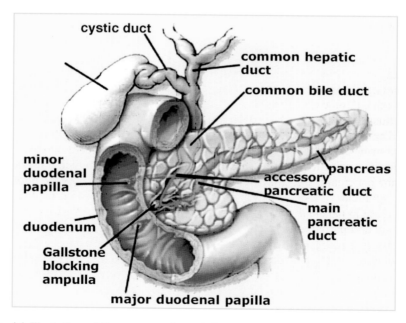

Fig. 4.1 Illustration of the common channel theory outlined by Opie in 1901 (the *green arrow* shows the reflux of bile into the pancreatic duct after a gallstone has lodged in the ampulla of Vater)

Nevertheless, the etiological model theorized by Opie has been critically reviewed, because a common channel shared between the common bile duct and the pancreatic duct is present in 10% of population (from autopsy series) [14].

It is common belief that the passage of a gallstone through the ampulla of Vater is an important factor that enhances pancreatitis because it is associated with reactive spasm of the sphincter of Oddi and with ampullary edema. The ampullary obstruction causes a reduction in exocrine pancreatic secretion with hypertension in the pancreatic ductal tree and a decrease of duodenal pH that causes hyperproduction of secretin and CCK; these enteral hormones are responsible for an increase in pancreatic secretion that leads to worsening of the pancreatic intracanalicular hypertension (obstruction–hypersecretion theory) [15]. These two phenomena may lead to inadequacy of "wall function" of the mucosa in the duct of Wirsung, with diffusion of activated proteolytic enzymes produced by acinar cells within the pancreas, thus triggering the autodigestive mechanism of acute pancreatitis.

Alcoholism

Alcohol abuse is the most common cause of acute pancreatitis in USA and the second in Western Europe (up to 50–60% of cases in the USA and 30% in Europe) [16]. Chronic alcohol abuse is the most frequent factor that causes acute pancreatitis in a patient with preexisting chronic pancreatitis. Only in a minority of patients is a large alcoholic binge the initiating event for acute pancreatitis and no evidence found of preexisting chronic damage to the gland.

Symmers was the first to establish, in 1917, that alcohol was an important pathogenetic factor in the development of acute pancreatitis [17], but the exact mechanism by which alcohol consumption produce pancreatitis is still unknown. Ethanol and its metabolites (acetaldehyde, acetate, and nonesterified fatty acids) show a direct toxic effect against the acinar pancreatic cells and seem to promote the diffusion of activated proteolytic enzymes into the gland, increasing the permeability of the epithelium in the pancreatic ductal tree. Moreover, ethanol is a well-known stimulant of gastric acid secretion, and the resultant duodenal acidification is a stimulus for the release of secretin and CCK, which increases the exocrine pancreatic secretion; at the same time, ethanol increases the basal tone of the sphincter of Oddi, resulting in activated enzyme diffusion, facilitated by an increase in pancreatic ductal permeability, in the presence of exocrine hypersecretion and partial ampullary obstruction (obstruction–hypersecretion theory) [18]. Another mechanism to explain the etiologic role of alcohol suggests that alcohol may initiate enzyme diffusion and cause pancreatic injury as a result of protein plugging of pancreatic plug [18]. An adjunctive mechanism to explain alcohol-induced pancreatitis involves injury generated by oxygen-derived free radicals produced by intrapancreatic degradation of ethanol; superoxide and hydroxyl radicals may lead to alterations of membrane permeability and of the microcirculatory bed with worsening of pancreatic injury deriving from proteolytic enzymes [18].

Finally, alcohol may induce hypertriglyceridemia; free fatty acids produced from the lipolysis of triglycerides may induce pancreatic injury by causing acinar cell or capillary endothelial cell injury [18].

Metabolic Causes

Serum triglyceride levels higher than 1000 mg/dl are usually required to cause acute pancreatitis [19]. Severe hypertriglyceridemia is most commonly observed in type V hyperlipoproteinemia (less commonly in type I and IV), nephritis, hypothyroidism, pregnancy, and drug administration (e.g., diuretics, β-blockers, retinoids, estrogens). The mechanism of pancreatic injury caused by hyperlipidemia is uncertain, but it may involve the free fatty acids released from triglycerides by lipase in the pancreatic microcirculation, with subsequent microvascular ischemic injury and increase of membrane permeability due to alteration in membrane lipoprotein balance [20].

Hypercalcemia is a rare metabolic cause of acute pancreatitis and is usually associated with hyperparathyroidism (1–2% of cases). The mechanism of hypercalcemia-related pancreatitis may involve calcium-induced trypsinogen activation and subsequent parenchymal autodigestion. Alternatively, calcium precipitation in the pancreatic duct could cause ductal obstruction associated with calcium-stimulated pancreatic exocrine hypersecretion. (obstruction–hypersecretion theory) [14].

Hereditary Pancreatitis

Patients with acute hereditary pancreatitis present with typical features. They have a family history of chronic pancreatitis and they complain of symptoms since childhood (in more than 90% of patients the first manifestations are observed before the end of the second decade of life).

In 1996, Whitcomb and colleagues identified the third exon of the cationic trypsinogen gene (*PRSS1*) on chromosome 7q35 as the gene responsible for hereditary pancreatitis [21]. This disorder is autosomal dominant, with a penetrance of about 80%. The mutation identified consisted of an arginine-to-histidine substitution at codon 122 (R122H). This mutation causes a conformational change in the three-dimensional structure of the trypsinogen-SPINK1 complex and might impair activity of the SPINK1 (serine protease inhibitor Kazal type 1, also known as pancreatic secretory trypsin inhibitor [PSTI].), which reversibly inhibits activated trypsin as a defense mechanism against hyperactivity of activated trypsin. This gene defect could enhance trypsin activity by promoting autoactivation of trypsinogen or reduction of active trypsin degradation. Patients with this defect usually develop chronic pancreatitis, and up to 40% of those with hereditary pancreatitis may develop pancreatic cancer [21, 22]. Other mutations associated with lower penetrance disorders have been identified.

The relationship between pancreatitis and mutation in the *CFTR* (cystic fibrosis transmembrane regulator) gene remains incompletely understood. Most patients with cystic fibrosis develop pulmonary diseases and pancreatic failure but not pancreatitis. These patients are not homozygous for *CFTR* mutations [23].

Autoimmune Pancreatitis

Also known as sclerosing pancreatitis, autoimmune pancreatitis is a benign disease characterized by diffuse enlargement of the whole pancreas, irregular narrowing of the pancreatic duct, swelling of the parenchyma, lymphoplasmacytic infiltration, and fibrosis [24].

Most patients with autoimmune pancreatitis present high serum levels of ANA (antinuclear antibodies), IgE, and IgG4. These alterations permit this disorder to be distinguished from other diseases of the pancreas and biliary tract. Because obstructive jaundice and computed tomographic (CT) images suggestive of focal pancreatic masses can accompany autoimmune pancreatitis, this condition can be misdiagnosed as pancreatic cancer. The clinical presentation of autoimmune pancreatitis is the same as that of acute pancreatitis. Patients with autoimmune pancreatitis generally have a favorable response to corticosteroid treatment [24].

Pancreas Divisum

On the basis of autopsy series, pancreas divisum occurs in approximately 5–7% of the population [25, 26] and represents a rare cause of acute pancreatitis. Pancreas divisum is a congenital anatomic variant in which the dorsal (Santorini duct) and ventral (Wirsung duct) pancreatic buds fail to fuse. As a consequence, the majority of pancreatic secretions enter the duodenum through the minor papilla (Santorini) [25, 26]. In a few cases the minor papilla may be inadequate to drain the pancreatic juice and creates a blockage that may lead to acute or chronic pancreatitis [25, 26].

Drugs

A lot of drugs have been implicated in causing acute pancreatitis. In fact drug-induced acute pancreatitis is a relatively rare event, and many pathogenetic mechanisms have been reported [27].

Acute pancreatitis secondary to azathioprine, 6-mercaptopurine (which have the highest attack rate, up to 4%), metronidazole, aminosalicylates, and sulfonamides is usually idiosyncratic. The pancreatic damage is evident within about 1 month from the administration [27].

Acute pancreatitis secondary to pentamidine, valproic acid, and didanosine is caused by the accumulation of toxic metabolites. The onset of pancreatic drug injury requires weeks or several months before its appearance [23, 27].

Acetaminophen may cause acute pancreatitis after a single massive dose through a direct toxic effect [23, 27].

Finally, there are several toxins that may cause acute pancreatitis. They hyperstimulate pancreatic secretion through a cholinergic mechanism and include organophosphate insecticides and venom from certain Central and South American scorpions [23, 27].

Trauma

Blunt or penetrating trauma that injures the pancreatic duct may cause acute pancreatitis. Blunt trauma to the abdomen may cause contusion, laceration, and partial or complete transaction of the pancreatic gland. In most cases of major trauma damage occurs in the mid-body of the pancreas, where the gland is crushed against the vertebral bodies (generally L2). Acute pancreatitis develops rapidly in most patients with such injuries and has a severe clinical course. Less extensive injuries cause pancreatic edema or minor contusions that may be asymptomatic or become evident after weeks or months, when late complications appear (pseudocysts, chronic fluid collections, and chronic pancreatitis) [23, 28].

Iatrogenic Pancreatitis

From 1 to 5% of ERCP procedures with sphincterotomy are complicated by acute pancreatitis. This is as a consequence of obstruction, inflammation, and edema of the pancreatic duct orifice. Barotrauma to the acinar cells secondary to the insertion of contrast into the duct of Wirsung is also implicated [29].

Infections

Many infections (viral, bacterial, and parasitic) may cause acute pancreatitis. Viral agents include cytomegalovirus, mumps, rubella, coxsackievirus B, and hepatitis A, B, and non-A, non-B [30].

AIDS patients commonly show increased serum amylase levels in the absence of acute pancreatitis and less commonly develop acute pancreatitis secondary to opportunistic infections (Cytomegalovirus spp., Cryptosporidium spp., Cryptococcus spp., Toxoplasma gondii, Mycobacterium tuberculosis, and Mycobacterium avium complex) or as a side effect of a medication (didanosine, pentamidine, and trimethoprim-sulfamethoxazole) [31].

The migration of worms (Ascaris lumbricoides and Clonorchis sinensis) from duodenum through the ampulla may be a rare cause of acute pancreatitis [32].

Ischemia

Ischemic injury to the pancreas may occur during many surgical procedures, because the pancreatic vasculature has very limited ability to vasodilate. Postoperative pancreatitis is often quite severe. It mostly occurs after cardiac surgery or cardiopulmonary bypass. Pancreatic ischemia may be secondary also to severe systemic hypotension, embolism, or visceral vasculitis [14].

Neoplasms

Primitive and metastatic pancreatic neoplasms can cause acute pancreatitis through an obstructive mechanism. Underlying pancreatic ampullary malignancy should be searched for after a pancreatitis episode in the absence of gallstones or alcohol abuse, in patients older than 45–50 years. About 1–2% of cases of acute pancreatitis are secondary to malignancy [23].

Idiopathic Pancreatitis

About 25% of cases of acute pancreatitis remain without a specific etiology. Many studies have shown idiopathic pancreatitis to be the third most common form after gallstone and alcoholic pancreatitis. Some of patients in these cases may deny alcohol dependence, but many of them are affected by a forme fruste of gallstone disease [30]. Two large studies have documented the presence of microscopic gallstones (microlithiasis) in 60–70% of patients with apparently idiopathic acute pancreatitis. The importance of microlithiasis is underscored because cholecystectomy, ERCP with sphincterotomy, and agents used to dissolve gallstones (ursodeoxycholic acid) reduce the frequency of recurrent attacks of acute pancreatitis in patients enrolled in these studies [33, 34].

Pathogenesis and Physiopathology

The pathogenesis of acute pancreatitis remains poorly understood. A large number of factors can apparently initiate this process: obstruction–overdistention of the pancreatic duct, hypertriglyceridemia, hypercalcemia, increased permeability of the pancreatic duct, gland hyperstimulation, and exposure to ethanol and other toxins. How these factors initiate a disturbance of cellular metabolism, with presumed premature intrapancreatic activation of digestive enzymes, is not clear. Once triggered, the acinar cell follows an unpredictable cascade of events that can lead to anywhere on a spectrum from mild, localized, interstitial inflammation to severe necrosis with spread into the peripancreatic spaces and the release of toxic factors into the systemic circulation or peritoneal space, leading to multiorgan failure.

The intra-acinar conversion of the inactive proenzyme trypsinogen to its active form trypsin with the release of trypsinogen activation peptide (TAP) appears to be the critical early step in the development of pancreatitis. Trypsin can activate most of the other digestive proenzymes enhancing the autodigestive process of acute pancreatitis (Fig 4.2) [35, 36]. Some of the digestive enzymes (e.g., amylase, lipase, DNAase, RNAase) are synthesized and secreted by acinar cells in the form of active enzymes. Others, including most of the potentially harmful digestive enzymes (e.g., trypsin, chymotrypsin, phospholipase, elastase, carboxypeptidase) are synthesized as inactive proenzymes or zymogens [37].

The acinar cells are protected from the injury caused by activated digestive enzymes by several features [37]:

1. Most of the potentially harmful digestive enzymes are normally present within acinar cells as inactive zymogens.
2. Throughout their intracellular trafficking within the cell, digestive enzymes and their zymogens are sequestered and enclosed within organelles of membrane with an alkalinic pH that inhibits their activation.
3. Potent inhibitors of trypsin are synthesized and co-transported through the cell along with trypsinogen:

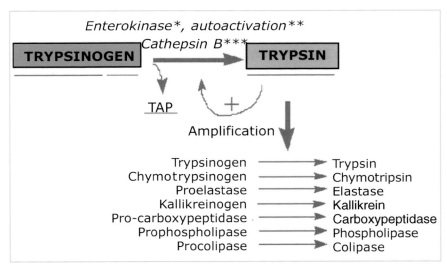

Fig. 4.2 Trypsinogen activation and cascade of activation of the digestive proenzymes into the pancreatic acinar cells. Trypsinogen activation peptide (TAP, a 7- to 10-amino-acid peptide) corresponds to the *N*-terminal region of the peptide released by the activation of trypsinogen into active trypsin. * Normally enterokinase is located on the brush border of the small intestine. ** Trypsinogen autoactivation is a unique feature of human trypsinogen. *** Abnormal pathway: cathepsin B is located within acinar cells and co-localized with digestive proenzymes in zymogen granules

(a) SPINK1 (serine protease inhibitor Kazal type 1, also known as pancreatic secretory trypsin inhibitor [PSTI]) blocks up to 20% of trypsin in the pancreas if trypsinogen becomes prematurely activated.

(b) α_1-Antitrypsin.

(c) α_2-Macroglobulin.

4. Trypsin and trypsin-like enzymes – e.g., mesotrypsin – through a feedback mechanism hydrolyze the chain connecting the two globular domains of the trypsin at R122H, resulting in permanent inactivation of trypsin and preventing subsequent activation of other proenzymes.

Acinar cells also synthesize many other types of proteins, including the hydrolytic enzymes that are designed to digest unnecessary material within intracellular lysosomes.

Both types of enzymes (secretory digestive ones and lysosomal hydrolase ones) are assembled on ribosomes attached to the rough endoplasmic reticulum (ER): the enzymes destined for secretion are carried within small transport vesicles to the Golgi stacks. Here they are post-translationally modified and then packed within condensing vacuoles known as zymogen granules that mature and migrate towards the luminal surface of the cell [38]. Their secretion, upregulated by neurohormonal secretagogue stimulus, is realized by a mechanism of fusion/fission of the granule with the luminal plasmalemma and the formation of pores of fusion, which allow the granule contents to be discharged into the extracellular (i.e., ductal) space [39]. Under physiological conditions, the activation of these zymogens does not occur until they reach the duodenum, where the brush border enzyme (enterokinase, enteropeptidase) catalytically activates trypsinogen and trypsin, then catalyzes the activation of the other zymogens. Activation involves cleavage of the zymogen and release of an "activating peptide" which, prior to its release, had maintained the zymogen in its inactive state. The quantification of free activating peptide levels may provide information regarding the extent of zymogen activation prior to that measurement [40].

The lysosomal hydrolases are a group of more than 50 dissimilar acid hydrolases, the function of which function is to degrade unneeded cellular material as well as material taken up by cells via either endocytosis or phagocytosis. As noted for other proteins, many of the lysosomal hydrolases are also synthesized as inactive proenzymes (prohydrolases) within the cisternae of the rough ER. Like other newly synthesized proteins, the lysosomal hydrolases are transported to the Golgi system, where they are recognized by specific ligands (free receptors) and follow other types of processing. Lysosomal hydrolases are activated during their transportation to the prelysosomal compartment. Once arrived at the prelysosomal compartment, where dissociation of the hydrolase-receptor complex occurs as a result of an acid pH environment, the lysosomal hydrolases are enclosed in cytoplasmic vacuoles. At this point, depending on the enzymatic components of the vacuoles they are transformed in lysosomes, endosomes, phagosomes, and autophagosomes that work as an interconnected network of organelles containing a wide variety of acid hydrolases capable of degrading nucleic acids, proteins, carbohydrates, and lipids [41–43].

The exact mechanism that leads to the early intracytoplasmic activation of digestive enzymes is not clearly elucidated. However, according to the so-called "co-localization theory" (Fig. 4.3), the digestive enzymes seem to be activated by lysosomal hydrolases due to an altered stockage that leads both types of enzymes (hydrolase and zymogen) to coexist in the same vacuoles [37, 44–46].

Cathepsin B (and, most likely, other lysosomal hydrolases) is the main hydrolase that activates trypsinogen into trypsin [47, 48]. Studies in experimental animal models suggested that perturbation of normal intracellular trafficking of digestive zymogens and lysosomal hydrolases is not simply a reaction to injury or a protective response but in fact a very early and critical event during the evolution of pancreatitis, and that, as a result of this perturbation, digestive enzyme zymogens become co-localized with lysosomal hydrolases within acinar cell cytoplasmic vacuoles [49]. Trypsin can catalyze a cascade of trypsinogen activation as well as activate all other proenzymes into the secretory vacuoles, leading to destruction of the vacuoles and liberation within the acinar cell of the proteolytic enzymes activated. Acinar cell injury induced by active trypsin allows the release of trypsin into the pancreatic parenchyma, where it activates more trypsin and other digestive enzymes leading and amplifying to the autodigestion of the gland. Larger amounts of liberated trypsin exceed the mechanisms of defense of the pancreas and of the whole system (PSTI, circulating α_2-macroglobulin, and α_1-antitrypsin) and activate other enzymes such as [50, 51]:

– Phospholipase A (phospholipase A_2 is the most important) and B, which can

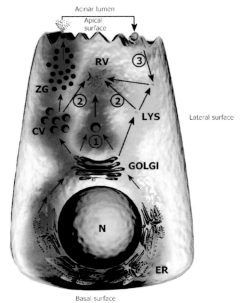

Fig. 4.3 The co-localization theory. Digestive enzyme zymogens are activated by lysosomal hydrolases when the two types of enzymes become co-localized within the same intracellular compartment. *Green:* normal intracellular path of digestive enzymes. *Yellow:* normal intracellular path of lysosomal hydrolases. *Red:* co-localization of digestive proenzymes and lysosomal hydrolases. *ER* endoplasmic reticulum; *N,* nucleus; *LYS,* lysosomes; *CV,* condensing vacuoles; *ZG,* zymogen granules, *RV,* ruptured co-localization vacuoles

induce cell necrosis by converting the lecithin of cellular membranes into more toxic lysolecithin compounds which cause the loss of membrane stability. Phospholipases are also responsible for destroying pulmonary surfactant and releasing nitric oxide from alveolar macrophages, which may contribute to the pulmonary injury.

- Elastase, which leads to digestion of the elastic components of pancreatic blood vessels, contributing to intrapancreatic bleeding.
- Carboxypeptidase A and B and chymotrypsin, which are the main responsible for the digestion of proteins within the pancreatic gland.
- Kallikrein, which leads to the release of bradykinin and kallidin, with consequent production of large amounts of prostaglandins, which may cause vascular instability and edema.
- Complement factors, which lead to the activation of the coagulative cascade with microthrombosis and deficits of the pancreatic and systemic microcirculation, promoting and aggravating the development of tissue necrosis.
- Lipase, in both the peripancreatic region and the systemic circulation, which leads to fat necrosis.
- Production of free oxygen radicals (ROS – reactive oxygen species – such as superoxide, singlet oxygen, hydroxyl radical, hydrogen peroxide, other peroxides and hypohalites), which may exacerbate the cell damage, causing lesions of cell membranes and cytoskeleton, impairing functions of intracellular proteins, damaging DNA, evoking lipid peroxidation, decreasing the level of antioxidants, and activating NF-κB. The translocation of NF-κB into the nucleus results in intra-acinar transcription of chemokines and cytokines that lead to invasion and activation of inflammatory cells, which produce more ROS and are responsible for acinar necrosis and amplification of the inflammation in the pancreas [52].

The intra-acinar activation of proteolytic enzymes and the inflammatory cascade leads to the autodigestive process in the pancreas with severe damage of acinar cells, pancreatic interstices, and vascular endothelium.

The factors that determine the severity of acute pancreatitis, e.g., whether the autodigestive process remains self-limiting and confined to the pancreas or progresses to necrotic process with development of late complications, remain poorly understood. The advance of pancreatic parenchymal damage stimulates intrapancreatic migration of lymphocytes, macrophages, and polymorphonuclear leukocytes, producing large amounts of proinflammatory cytokines and oxygen free radicals (Fig. 4.4).

The main cytokines involved in the development of pancreatic injury and systemic inflammatory response syndrome (SIRS) during acute pancreatitis are [53–55]:

- PAF (platelet activating factor)
- TNF-α (tumor necrosis factor α)
- IL-1 (interleukin 1)
- IL 6 (interleukin 6)
- IL 8 (interleukin 8)

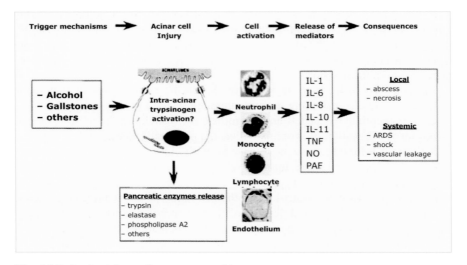

Fig. 4.4 Pathophysiology of acute pancreatitis

PAF (platelet activating factor): PAF seems to be very important in the development of severe acute pancreatitis. It is produced by a variety of cells, such as monocytes/macrophages, polymorphonuclear leukocytes, eosinophils, basophils, platelets, mast cells, vascular endothelial cells, and lymphocytes, which participate in the inflammatory reaction. PAF promotes platelet aggregation, directly modulates microvascular permeability, and increases venular permeability, causing sequestration of macromolecules and fluid in the interstices and recruitment of leukocytes through the interaction of CD11b (leukocytes) and ICAM 1 (endothelial cells). In addition, PAF causes loss of endothelial integrity, which results in edema and necrosis formation, vasospasm, and microthrombus formation (due to hypercoagulability). It can also lead to deterioration of the pancreatic microcirculation and to pancreatic necrosis. Finally, PAF seems to be directly involved in bacterial translocation due to its ability to induce gut endothelial barrier dysfunction [56].

TNF-α (tumor necrosis factor α): TNF-α is a pleiotrophic, predominantly macrophage-derived cytokine which is believed to play a major role in mediating many of the pathophysiologic responses of the organism to injury and sepsis. TNF-α promotes the production of acute-phase proteins and stimulates the production of other inflammatory mediators such as IL-1, IL-6, IL-8, and PAF. Moreover, TNF-α has chemotactic and activating effects on granulocytes, in particular stimulating the production of oxygen free radicals. Finally, in serious injury and shock, TNF-α can cause extensive autoimmune pathological reactions and promote apoptosis of pancreatic acinar cells [57].

IL-1 (interleukin 1): IL-1 is a proinflammatory cytokine produced during acute and chronic inflammation and responsible for many symptoms during sepsis. IL-1, mainly IL-1β, shows biological activities similar to those of TNF-α. In addition, IL-1β [58]:

- Has pyrogenic functions
- Promotes cell catabolism
- Promotes endothelial cells secretion of PGI₂, which increases capillary permeability
- Promotes the hepatic production of the acute-phase proteins

IL-6 (interleukin 6): IL-6, released by mononuclear macrophages in response to tissue injury, is a mediator responsible for the synthesis of the acute-phase proteins, including fibrinogen and C-reactive protein (CRP). IL-6 has extensive inflammation-promoting effects such as promoting B-cell activation, proliferation, and final differentiation into plasmocyte; increasing immunoglobulin synthesis; and promoting T-cell differentiation and proliferation. Finally, IL-6 leads to adhesion of leukocytes to the surface of endothelium. In this way the leukocytes can release toxic substances such as elastase and oxygen free radicals that injure the surface of vascular endothelial cells [59].

IL 8 (interleukin 8): IL-8 is a potent neutrophilic-granulocyte chemotactic and activating factor mainly generated by neutrophilic granulocytes. These are produced by mononuclear macrophages and endothelium cells and can activate and induce T-cell and B-cell differentiation, enhance NK (natural killer) cell activity, and promote phagocytosis [60]. In the course of severe pancreatitis, there is a massive release of a great number of inflammatory mediators, cytokines, and activated digestive enzymes into the systemic circulation. These enzymes overwhelm the normal circulating protective mechanism and cause direct damage. The resulting clinical scenarios may be SIRS, multiple organ dysfunction (MODS), and multiple organ failure (MOF).

Cardiac Failure and Shock

During severe acute pancreatitis many cardiocirculatory complications, such as cardiac failure, myocardial infarction, arrhythmias and shock may develop [51]. Hypotension represents the most common clinical sign and is mainly secondary to the fluid loss in the third space (retroperitoneal fluid collections). A diffuse increase in capillary permeability causes the systemic capillary leak syndrome (SCLS): the migration of albumin and fluids into the interstices contributes to the occurrence of hypovolemia, which worsens with the generalized vasodilatation induced by cytokines and inflammatory mediators, with the decrease in oral fluid intakes, and with the increase of oral fluid loss by vomiting. In very severe clinical courses, myocardial depressant factor (MDF) produced in response to the sepsis causes contractile myocardial dysfunction, which aggravates hypovolemia and hypotension. The signs of shock in these cases are tachycardia, hypotension, and cold, pale, and marbled sweaty skin [51].

Respiratory Dysfunction

Pulmonary complications are the most frequent and serious that can occur in acute pancreatitis [61]. They range from hypoxemia due to ventilation/perfusion (V/Q) mismatch (with acute respiratory failure without radiological abnormalities) to pulmonary infiltrates or atelectasis, pleural effusion, pulmonary edema, and acute respiratory distress syndrome (ARDS).

Phospholipase A_2 (PLA2), which is activated by trypsin in the duodenum, is known for its ability to remove fatty acids from phospholipids. One of the main components of surfactant is phospholipid dipalmitoyl phosphatidylcholine, which is a perfect substrate for PLA2. The reduction of surfactant may be a significant cause of atelectasis development because it lines the surface of the alveoli and prevents the alveoli from collapsing by maintaining the surface tension.

The presence of pleural effusion is currently considered an indication of severe pancreatitis. The majority of pleural effusions (68%) are left-sided, 22% are bilateral, and 10% are right-sided. Pleural effusions in acute pancreatitis are usually moderate, occasionally bloody, and are characterized by high levels of amylase (up to 30 times higher than the corresponding serum value), protein (>30 g/l), and lactic acid dehydrogenase (>0.6 serum value). Transdiaphragmatic lymphatic blockage and pancreatic–pleural fistulae secondary to leak and disruption of the pancreatic duct or pseudocyst contribute to cause pleural effusions.

The most dangerous complication of the pulmonary system is ARDS, which is lethal in 50% of cases. ARDS seems to be secondary to thrombosis of alveolar microcirculation due to coagulatory alterations, alveolar injury from lipase and phospholipase activity, opening of arteriovenous shunts due the action of kinins, leaking of protein-rich transudate into the alveolar space, and action of shock lung factor (SLF).

Clinical features of pulmonary symptoms range from tachypnea, mild respiratory alkalosis, and hypoxemia to severe dyspnea, cyanosis, and extreme hypoxemia refractory to a high inspired oxygen concentration.

Renal Failure

Renal failure in severe acute pancreatitis is secondary to acute tubular necrosis due to systemic hypotension and circulating toxic substances [51]. Vasoactive circulating substances, hypovolemia, and thromboembolism of the microcirculatory renal bed due to coagulatory alterations also cause a reduction in glomerular filtration. Clinical signs of renal failure during severe acute pancreatitis are oligoanuria, acidosis, and fluid-electrolyte alterations [51].

Encephalopathy

The central nervous system symptoms accompanying severe acute pancreatitis in the early stages are described as pancreatic encephalopathy [62]. The main neuropsychiatric symptoms are disorientation, restlessness, delusions, unconsciousness or slowed reaction, apathy, and depression. Pathological examination shows diffuse cerebral demyelinization.

The main pathological changes in brain tissue during severe acute pancreatitis complicated with pancreatic encephalopathy are toxic edema of neurons, hemorrhagic foci, and zones of malacia; factors such as hyponatremia, hypophosphoremia, hypoxemia, hyperazotemia, blood sugar disturbance, and infection may be triggers.

Recent studies founded multiple pathogenesis for patients with severe acute pancreatitis with pancreatic encephalopathy [62]:

- Activated PLA2 transforms enkephalin and lecithin into highly cytotoxic hemolytic enkephalin and hemolytic lecithin. It can also damage the blood–brain barrier; dissolve the phospholipid structure of the cell membrane; hydrolyze mitochondria, causing brain dysmetabolism and edema; cause severe demyelinization changes in axons; and damage acetylcholine vesicles, inhibiting acetylcholine release and leading to disturbance of nerve-muscle transmission.
- Cytokines such as TNF-α, IL-1β, and IL-6 increase the permeability of the blood–brain barrier by damaging it; promote leukocyte activation and aggregation, with direct neuronal and endothelial injury; induce inflammatory injury to the myelin sheath; and stimulate the generation of PAF, which promotes platelet aggregation, inducing cerebral capillary thrombosis and endotheliocyte injury.
- Oxygen free radicals produced by inflammatory cells in response to brain hypoxia pass the blood–brain barrier and directly injure brain tissue.
- Severe hypoxemia can cause microcirculatory disturbance and tissue ischemia, which can further aggravate brain ischemia, hypoxia, and injury.

Liver Failure

The hepatic injury caused by severe acute pancreatitis can not only aggravate the state of pancreatitis, but also develop into hepatic failure and cause patient death [63]. Its complicated pathogenic mechanism is an obstacle to clinical treatment. Among many pathogenic factors, the changes of vasoactive substances, the participation of inflammatory mediators as well as oxygen free radicals and endotoxins, and the activity of inflammatory cells may play important roles in the onset and progression of hepatocellular injury. Hepatic apoptosis could be one of the factors leading to liver failure [63].

Infective Complications

Pancreatic necrosis infection occurs in 40–70% of patients with severe acute pancreatitis and is the main life-threatening complication of the disease; subsequent sepsis and related multiple organ failure are responsible for a mortality rate of up to 50% [64]. Many clinical studies suggest that systemic infections and multiple organ failure in critically ill or injured patients often originate from intestinal floral migration, probably through the failed intestinal barrier (so-called bacterial translocation). The bowel wall undergoes ischemic injury during the hypovolemic shock of severe acute pancreatitis: in this phase vasoconstriction of the splanchnic circulation represents a compensatory reaction to maintain normal pressure in the central vascular district. When normovolemia is reached, the injury from ischemia/reperfusion syndrome is the main factor affecting the integrity of bowel wall.

Bacteria may enter the pancreas through the hematogenous route, the peritoneum, the lymphatic system, the biliary duct tree, and the duodenum via the main pancreatic duct [64].

Abdominal Compartment Syndrome

Increase in capillary permeability due endothelial damage from cytokines and oxygen free radical injury, shock, visceral and retroperitoneal edema, and bowel dilatation secondary to paralytic ileus cause intra-abdominal hypertension that may lead to abdominal compartment syndrome.

Clinical Manifestations

Abdominal pain is the main symptom of pancreatitis [14, 15, 23, 30, 51]. It is caused by acute stretching of the pancreas capsule and is experienced by about 95% of patients. Pain generally begins in the epigastrium, and in two out of three patients it has a posterior irradiation, to the dorsal-lumbar region, as a belt-like pain. Sometimes the pain can spread to the inferior abdominal areas or to the left shoulder. Generally it is severe, heavy, subcontinuous, sudden, and sometimes violent. The pain reaches a peak in the first hours and persists for days. Nausea and vomiting are also common, both produced from vagal activities due to pain and paralytic ileus. Acute pancreatitis without pain is rare. It has been observed during peritoneal dialysis, after surgery (in particular renal transplant), during legionnaires' disease, and in the course of necrotizing panniculitis. However, pain can be lacking in those cases of severe pancreatitis which onset is characterized by coma, delirium, and multiorgan failure. Fever can be present. The timing of the onset of fever is very important: during the 1st week it is generally an "inflammatory-toxic" fever, caused by proinflammatory cytokines relapse; fever that rises after the 2nd week can be the sign of pancreatic necrosis infection or extrapancreatic infections (pneumonia, cholangitis, urinary tract infections) [14, 15, 51].

The clinical examination reveals epigastric or diffuse abdominal pain; peritoneal irritation can also be found in severe pancreatitis. The abdomen is distended and tympanic and peristalsis is reduced or absent. Jaundice is infrequent at the onset but it can be present in case of gallstone pancreatitis or when the pancreatic edema compresses the distal part of the common bile duct. Vital signs can be normal, but tachycardia, hypotension, and tachypnea are present in severe pancreatitis. Early hypotension, tachycardia, dyspnea, and shock are indicators of a relevant fluid collection in the retroperitoneal third space. These cases have a severe prognosis and the patients generally need to be treated in the intensive care unit. The presence of ecchymosis in the hips (Grey Turner's sign), in the periumbilical region (Cullen's sign) and in the groin (Fox's sign) is rare: they come from retroperitoneal bleedings that reach the surface. These signs characterize very severe pancreatitis [23, 30].

Laboratory Tests

At the present time, a specific diagnostic laboratory test does not exist for acute pancreatitis [65]. Amylase and lipase are the most important biohumoral parameters.

Serum Amylase

From a long time the serum amylase concentration has been used to confirm the diagnosis of acute pancreatitis. At least 75–80% of patients with acute pancreatitis have hyperamylasemia at disease onset [66].

The serologic levels of amylase rise within a few hours from the onset, reaching a peak at between 36 and 72 h. High levels persist for 3–5 days in uncomplicated cases [67]; high levels continuing after the 1st week are associated with the development of complications such as pseudocysts, pancreatic ascites, and abscess. Amylase concentrations can normalize within 24 h from the onset because of the short half-life of the enzyme.

Serum amylase levels three times higher than the normal value indicate a diagnosis of acute pancreatitis [68]. Levels may be higher in patients with renal failure because amylase is eliminated by the kidney.

In 19–32% of cases of acute pancreatitis hyperamylasemia is not be found. This may be due to [69]:

– Massive gland destruction
– Hyperlipidemic pancreatitis (because of amylase inactivation)
– Low levels of amylase in gland in normal conditions (alcoholic pancreatitis)

(FO)Thus, absence of hyperamylasemia does not exclude a diagnosis of pancreatitis.

Hyperamylasemia may be present in different pathological conditions (Table 4.3). Although most of them cannot be confused with acute pancreatitis, some intra-abdominal diseases can mimic the clinical scenario of acute pancreatitis: intestinal ischemia, perforation, or obstruction; choledocholithiasis; acute cholecystitis; acute appendicitis; and some tubo-ovarian diseases (extrauterine pregnancy, acute salpingitis). The concentration of the pancreatic isoenzyme to amylase can improve the diagnostic accuracy of amylasemia. Pancreatic isoamylase represents 40% of all serum amylase and is only produced by the pancreas. The salivary isoamylase may be produced by the salivary glands, tubes, ovaries, endometrium, prostate, breast, lung, and liver [14].

The severity of hyperamylasemia does not correlate with the severity of pancreatitis [65]. High hyperamylasemia is more common in gallstone pancreatitis than in alcoholic pancreatitis [70].

Table 4.3 Conditions in which high serum amylase levels are found without pancreatitis

Abdominal acute disorders:
    Acute appendicitis
    Acute cholecystitis
    Common bile duct obstruction
    Intestinal ischemia
    Intestinal obstruction
    Intestinal perforation

Gynecological acute disorders:
    Acute salpingitis
    Ectopic pregnancy

Salivary gland disorders:
    Mumps
    Sialoadenitis
    Alcohol-induced salivary hyperamylasemia

Extrapancreatic tumors:
    Ovarian cysts and malignancies
    Lung cancer

Renal insufficiency

Miscellaneous:
    AIDS
    Anorexia nervosa
    Diabetic ketoacidosis
    Head trauma

Serum Lipase

Lipases are produced mainly by the pancreas and for this reason they are a more accurate diagnostic marker of pancreatitis than amylase [66]. Lipases have an half-life longer than that of amylase and remain elevated in the serum until 5–10 days, when amylase has normalized [71].

High serologic levels of lipase can be found in other pathological conditions, but a lipase concentration three times higher than the normal range is very suggestive of pancreatitis [68]. Lipases are secreted by the kidney. For this reason a lipase level five times higher than normal is considered diagnostic of pancreatitis in patients with chronic renal failure [71].

Further Investigations

Several biohumoral abnormalities can be found in acute pancreatitis. They have poor diagnostic significance but can be useful in determining the severity of pancreatitis [14, 15, 51].

Neutrophil leukocytosis is often present and is a sign of severe disease; hematocrit can be normal but increases in severe pancreatitis and when there is a large amount of fluid lost in the third space.

Fluid-electrolyte disorders relate in particular to calcium metabolism. Hypocalcemia is caused by albumin depletion (relative hypocalcemia) or, in particular, by calcium precipitation in the intra- and peripancreatic steatonecrosis due to saponification of fatty acids (real hypocalcemia). Tetany is, however, infrequent because the ionized calcium level is usually normal.

Hyperglycemia is secondary to the relative hypoinsulinemia and to the concomitant hyperglucagonemia associated with α-insular cell degranulation.

GOT and GPT alterations are more common in gallstone pancreatitis. GPT levels three time higher than the normal value correlate strongly with a gallstone etiology. The concentrations of LDH, urea, CRP, and PCT (procalcitonin) are very important for the prognosis.

Radiology

Abdominal radiography, ultrasonography, and computed tomography (CT) are usually employed when pancreatitis is suspected. CT is the most important examination because it provides very useful information for the diagnosis of pancreatitis and the severity of pancreatic damage. Magnetic resonance imaging (MRI) and MR-cholangiography offer better definition of the gland and of the biliary tree, but the high cost in terms of both time and financial resources mean that this technique is not used routinely.

Diagnosis

Diagnostic suspicion of pancreatitis is based on the clinical presentation. According to general agreement, the diagnosis of acute pancreatitis needs at least two of the following three elements [72, 73]:

1. Typical acute abdominal pain (it arises in the epigastrium and reaches a peak after a few hours after onset; it radiates into the dorsolumbar region as a "belt-like" pain; it can be more intensive in the upper abdomen, right or left)
2. Serum amylase and lipase concentrations three time higher than normal (in the absence of renal failure; lipasemia seems to be the more significant)
3. Typical abnormalities on CT

Acute pancreatitis must be distinguished from other diseases with a similar presentation such as biliary colic, acute cholecystitis, bowel occlusion, gastric or bowel perforation, bowel ischemic infarction, and, among extra-abdominal diseases, myocardial infarction (inferior type), dissection or rupture of aortic aneurysm, lower-lobe pneumonia.

Natural Course

The clinical presentation of pancreatitis ranges from a mild, self-limiting disease to severe or fatal forms. In about 80–85% of patients pancreatitis is mild and passes off spontaneously in 3–5 days (some authors call this form "1-week-disease") [74]. Neither intensive therapies nor surgery are needed for this form, and morbidity and mortality are lower than 1%. The other 15–20% of patients develop a severe form of the disease characterized by local complications (necrosis, abscesses. or pseudocysts) and organ failure that can progress to MOF [75].

Severe acute pancreatitis can be divided in two phases [8]:

First stage (SIRS). In the first week of disease, the acute inflammation causes release of the proinflammatory mediators (protease, antiprotease, cytokines, and oxygen free radicals), followed by SIRS. The systemic damage caused by acute pancreatitis (cardiovascular, respiratory, and renal failure) depends on the severity of the pancreatic process and on the volume of mediators released into the retroperitoneum, the peritoneum, and the systemic circulation. Most cases of severe pancreatitis go on to the second stage; treatment is effective in only a few cases with complete recovery.

Second stage (phase of infected necrosis). Pancreatic necrosis and complications appear between the 3rd and 5th weeks of disease. The development of necrosis (which can begin as early as the end of the 1st week) is the key to this phase. The disease severity and prognosis depend on the extent of infection in the necrotic tissue. The pancreatic exudate produced in the first phase progresses to peripancreatic fluid collections that generally develop a fibrotic wall typical of pseudocysts. The necrotic process can resolve in a few weeks or can be complicated by infection, usually between the 2nd and the 3rd week from onset. Translocation of bacteria from the colon and passing through the portal circulation seem to be primarily responsible for the infection. Fungal infection (in particular by *Candida* spp.) is infrequent. Noninfected pancreatic necrosis resolves in the 4th to 5th weeks with total recovery of the pancreas. Late infections with development of pancreatic abscess are rare.

Determination of Disease Severity

Early determination of the disease severity is fundamental to the management of acute pancreatitis, to prevent and cure complications and to determine the prognosis. The severity can be predicted with good accuracy using multiparametric score systems (Ranson, Glasgow, APACHE II), laboratory parameters (CRP, PCT), or CT features (Balthazar).

Multiparameter Scoring Systems

As mentioned, various multiparameter scoring systems have been introduced and validated to determine the severity of acute pancreatitis. They are all characterized by a high sensitivity but a low specificity.

Ranson Criteria

In 1974 John H.C. Ranson had a first intuition that the severity of a case of acute pancreatitis could be predicted by evaluating certain clinical and laboratory parameters [76]. From a trial of 100 patients with acute pancreatitis, he selected 11 clinical and laboratory parameters, 5 at admission and 6 48 h later, as a basis for classifying acute pancreatitis into mild or severe (Table 4.4). Patients with fewer than three positive criteria had very low mortality rate (<1%), while those with more than three positive criteria had progressively increasing morbidity and mortality rates. Those with a score of 3–5 had a 15% mortality rate, those with a score of 5–6 had 40–50% mortality, and in those with a score up to 6 the mortality rate was 80–100% [76, 77]. On the basis of these data Ranson concluded that with fewer than three positive criteria at 48 h from admission, a mild disease course could be expected, whereas with a score of 3 or more, a severe disease course could be expected.

The need to wait for 48 h is the main limitation of the Ranson criteria.

Glasgow (Imrie) Scoring System

In 1978 Imrie analyzed a series of patients affected by gallstone pancreatitis and determined a new score system based on nine clinical and laboratory parameters assessed in the first 48 h (Table 4.5). Again, the presence of three or more parameters is indicative of severe acute pancreatitis [78].

Table 4.4 Ranson prognostic scoring system for acute pancreatitis

Type	On admission	Within 48 h
Nongallstone acute pancreatitis	Age >55 years WBC count >16,000/μl Glucose >200 mg/dl LDH >350 U/l AST >250 U/l	Decrease in Hct >10 points Increase in BUN >5 mg/dl Serum calcium <8 mg/dl P_aO_2 <60 mmHg Base deficit >4 mmol/l Fluid deficit >6 l
Gallstone acute pancreatitis	Age >70 years WBC count >18,000/μl Glucose >220 mg/dl LDH >400 U/l AST >500 U/l	Decrease in Hct >10 points ncrease in BUN >2 mg/dl Serum calcium <8 mg/dl Base deficit >5 mmol/l Fluid deficit >4 l

AST, aspartate aminotransferase; *BUN*, blood urea nitrogen; *Hct*, hematocrit; *LDH*, lactate dehydrogenase; P_aO_2, arterial oxygen tension; *WBC*, white blood cell count

Table 4.5 Glasgow (Imrie) prognostic scoring system for acute pancreatitis

Age >55 years
WBC >15,000/μl
Glucose >180 mg/dl
BUN >45 mg/dl
LDH <600 U/l
AST and/or ALT > 200 U/l
Albumin <3.2 g/dl
Serum calcium <8 mg/dl
P_aO_2 <60 mmHg

APACHE II

APACHE (Acute Physiologic And Chronic Health Evaluation) is a complex prognostic system that evaluates many clinical and laboratory variables (Table 4.6). The APACHE II prognostic score results from the summary of three partial scores: vital parameters, age, and the presence of chronic diseases (renal, hepatic, etc.). This system can predict the severity of several diseases and it was applied to acute pancreatitis for the first time in 1989 by Larvin and McMahon. An APACHE II score higher than 7 is strongly indicative of severe acute pancreatitis [79].

Today the APACHE II is the most accurate score system: in severe pancreatitis it has a sensitivity of 60–70%, a specificity of 80–85%, a positive predictive value of 57%, and a negative predictive value of 88% [80, 81]. This system can be applied at any moment from admission and thus permits continuous re-evaluation.

Table 4.6 APACHE II scoring system. (Physiologic score + Glasgow coma score + Age score + Chronic health score)

a. Physiologic score = sum of the individual variable points for all variables

Individual variable points	+4	+3	+2	+1	0	+1	+2	+3	+4
Rectal temperature (°C)	>41	39–40.9	–	38.5–38.9	36–38.4	34–35.9	32–33.9	30–31.9	<29.9
Mean arterial pressure (mmHg)	>160	130–159	110–129	–	70–109	–	50–69	–	<49
Heart rate	>180	140–179	110–139	–	70–109	–	55–69	40–54	<39
Respiratory rate	>50	35–49	–	25–34	12–24	10–11	6–9	–	<5
AaDo$_2$ FIo$_2$>0.5 (record only Pao$_2$)	>500	350–499	200–349	–	<200	–	–	–	–
FIo$_2$<0.5	–	–	–	–	Po$_2$ >70	Po$_2$ 61–70	–	Po$_2$ 55–60	Po$_2$ <55
Arterial pH	>7.7	7.6–7.69	–	7.5–7.59	7.33–7.49	–	7.25–7.32	7.1–7.24	<7.15
Serum sodium (mmol/l)	>180	160–179	155–159	150–154	130–149	–	120–129	111–119	<110
Serum potassium (mmol/l)	>7.0	6.0–6.9	–	5.5–5.9	3.5–5.4	3.0–3.4	2.5–2.9	–	<2.5
Serum creatinine (mg/dl)	>3.5	2.0–3.4	1.5–1.9	–	0.6–1.4	<0.6	–	–	–
Hematocrit (%)[a]	>60	–	50.0–59.9	46.0–49.9	30.0–45.9	–	20.0–29.9	–	<20
White blood cell count (× 1000/μl)	>40	–	20.0–39.9	15.0–19.9	3.0–14.9	–	1.0–2.9	–	<1.0
Serum HCO$_3^-$ (mmol/l)	>52	41.0–51.9	–	32.0–40.9	22.0–31.9	18.0–21.9	14.0–17.9	–	<15

continue ↑

continue **Table 4.6**

b. *Glasgow Coma points = 15 Glasgow - Coma Scale*

Individual variable points	+4	+3	+2	+1	0	+1	+2	+3	+4

c. *Age score: Age points = points for the age of patient*

Age(years)	Points
≤44	0
45–54	2
55–64	3
65–75	5
≥75	6

d. *Chronic health score*

Hepatic	Biopsy-proven cirrhosis and portal hypertension; past episodes of upper gastrointestinal bleeding due to portal hypertension; past episodes of hepatic failure or hepatic encephalopathy
Cardiovascular	IV NYHA (New York Hearth Association) class IV
Respiratory	Class III–IV dyspnea (severe exercise restriction) due to chronic restrictive, obstructive, or vascular disease; documented chronic hypoxia, hypercapnia, secondary polycythemia, severe pulmonary hypertension (<40 mmHg) or respirator dependency
Renal	Long-term dialysis
Immunocompromise	Therapy that suppresses resistance to infections (immunosuppression, chemotherapy, radiation, high-dose steroids); advanced disease suppressing resistance to infections (leukemia, lymphoma, AIDS)

Total chronic health points: 5 points for each chronic disease in nonoperative or emergency postoperative patients; 2 points for each chronic disease in elective postoperative patients

$AaDO_2$, alveolar-arterial oxygen tension difference; FIO_2, fraction of inspired oxygen; PaO_2, arterial oxygen tension
[a] Double point score for acute renal failure

The APACHE II system has two limitations: it is complex to calculate, and it has low accuracy in identifying local complications.

Laboratory Parameters

In recent years several laboratory parameters have been proved to be accurate in predicting the severity of acute pancreatitis. These tests are cheap, easy to use, available early on, and very reliable. The main parameters used are:

- *CRP (C-reactive protein)*. CRP belongs to the group of acute-phase reactive proteins and its concentrations are high in several inflammatory conditions. This protein is produced by hepatocytes in response to inflammatory mediators. CRP is very reliable and is the most important single laboratory parameter in predicting the severity of pancreatitis [82]. The serum CRP level reaches its peak after 2–3 days from disease onset (24–48 h after IL-1 and IL-6). Most authors consider levels higher than 15 mg/dl (range 12–21 mg/dl [79, 83, 84]) at 48 h from disease onset to be highly indicative of severe pancreatitis and pancreatic necrosis [85].
- *PCT (procalcitonin)*. Procalcitonin is the propeptide of the active hormone calcitonin. In 1993 Assicot et al. described for the first time high plasma levels of PCT during bacterial/fungal infections with sepsis [86]. In the course of pancreatitis, high levels of PCT are associated with infected necrosis and a high mortality rate [87]. The threshold for the presence of infected pancreatic necrosis is 1.8–2 ng/ml; many studies have documented that PCT levels increase significantly between the 2nd and the 4th day from disease onset [88].
- *Other parameters [82, 89]*. Further laboratory parameters able to predict acute pancreatitis have been described. However, they are not currently employed because they are difficult to use, costly, and, in particular, because they do not improve upon the reliability of CRP, PCT, and the multiparametric systems. They can be divided into inflammatory markers (TNF-α IL-6, IL-8), trypsinogen activation markers (trypsin activation peptide, TAP; carboxypeptidase-B activation peptide, CAPAP-B), and pancreatic damage markers (trypsinogen-2, pancreatic elastase, and lipase).

References

1. Moynihan B (1925) Acute pancreatitis. Ann Surg 81:132–142
2. Cavallini G, Riela A, Brocco G et al (1987) Epidemiology of acute pancreatitis. In: Beger HG, Büchler M (eds) Acute pancreatitis: research and clinical management. Springer, Berlin Heidelberg New York, pp 25–31
3. Thomson SR, Hendry WS, McFarlane GA, Davidson AI (1987) Epidemiology and outcome of acute pancreatitis. Br J Surg 74:398–401
4. Bourke JB (1975) Variation in annual incidence of primary acute pancreatitis in Nottingham, 1969–74. Lancet 2:967–969

5. Wilson C, Imrie CW (1980) Changing patterns of incidence and mortality from acute pancreatitis in Scotland, 1961–1985. Br J Surg 77:731–734
6. Russo MW, Wei JT, Thiny MT et al (2004) Digestive and liver diseases statistics, 2004. Gastroenterology 126:1448–1453
7. DeFrances CJ, Hall MJ, Podgornik MN (2005) 2003 National Hospital Discharge Survey. Advance data from vital and health statistics. No. 359. Hyattsville, Md: National Center for Health Statistics
8. Werner J, Uhl W, Büchler MW (2004) Acute pancreatitis. In: Cameron JL (ed) Current surgical therapy, 8th edn. Mosby, Philadelphia
9. Triester SL, Kowdley KV (2002) Prognostic factors in acute pancreatitis. J Clin Gastroenterol 34:167–176
10. McKay CJ, Imrie CW (2004) The continuing challenge of early mortality in acute pancreatitis. Br J Surg 91:1243–1244
11. Bradley EL (1993) A clinically based classification system for acute pancreatitis: summary of the Atlanta symposium. Arch Surg 128:586–590
12. Rigamonti M, Ferraro A, Madau A, Simonini L (2001) Stadiazione e monitoraggio della pancreatite acuta. In: D'Amico DF, Favia G, Eccher C (eds) Pancreatite acuta. Aspetti diagnostico-terapeutici. Atti del convegno Pancreatite acuta, Trento. La Garangola, Padua
13. Opie EL (1901) The relation of cholelithiasis to disease of the pancreas and to fat necrosis. Am J Med Sci 121:27–43
14. Yeo CJ, Cameron JL (2001) Exocrine pancreas. In: Townsend CM, Beauchamp RD, Evers BM, Maddox KL (eds) Sabiston textbook of surgery, 16th edn. Saunders, Philadelphia, pp 1112–1143
15. Favia G, Polistina F (2000) Pancreas. In: D'amico DF (ed) Manuale di Chirurgia. McGraw Hill, Milan, pp 674–675
16. Amman RW, Muelhaut B (1994) Progression of alcoholic acute to chronic pancreatitis. Gut 35:552–556
17. Symmers WSC (1917) Acute alcoholic pancreatitis. Dublin J Med Sci 143:244–247
18. Hanck C, Whitcomb DC (2004) Alcoholic pancreatitis. Gastroenterol Clin North Am 33:751
19. Yadav D, Pitchumoni CS (2005) Issues in hyperlipidemic pancreatitis. J Clin Gastroenterol 36:54
20. Fortson MR, Freedman SN, Webster PD III (1995) Clinical assessment of hyperlipidemic pancreatitis. Am J Gastroenterol 90:2134–2139
21. Whitcomb DC, Gorry MC, Preston RA et al (1996) Hereditary pancreatitis is caused by a mutation in the cationic trypsinogen gene. Nat Genet 14:141–45
22. Varallyay E, Pal G, Patthy A et al (1998) Two mutations in rat trypsin confer resistance against autolysis. Biochem Biophys Res Commun 243:56–60
23. Whang EE (2006) Acute pancreatitis. In: Greenfield LJ, Mulholland MW, Oldham KT et al. (ed) Greenfield's surgery: scientific principles and practice, 4th edn. Lippincott Williams and Wilkins, Philadelphia
24. Lora LP, Chari ST (2005) Autoimmune pancreatitis. Curr Gastroenterol Rep 7:101
25. Klein SD, Affronti JP (2004) Pancreas divisum, an evidence-based review: part I, pathophysiology. Gastrointest Endosc 60:419
26. Klein SD, Affronti JP (2004) Pancreas divisum, an evidence-based review: part II, patient selection and treatment. Gastrointest Endosc 60:585
27. Trivedi CD, Pitchumoni CS (2005) Drug-induced pancreatitis: an update. J Clin Gastroenterol 239:709
28. Wilson RH, Moorhead RJ (1991) Current management of trauma to the pancreas. Br J Surg 78:1196–1202
29. Pezzulli R, Romboli E, Campana D, Corinaldesi R (2002) Mechanisms involved in the onset of post-ERCP pancreatitis. JOP. J Pancreas (Online) 3(6):162–168
30. Draganov P, Forsmark CE (2006) Gastroenterology V: Diseases of the pancreas. ACP Medicine online. WebMD Inc. http://www.apicella.com/pancreas.pdf [accessed 17 June 2008]

31. Reisler RB, Murphy RL, Redfield RR et al (2005) Incidence of pancreatitis in HIV-1 infected individuals enrolled in 20 adult AIDS clinical trials group studies: lessons learned. J Acquir Immune Defic Syndr 37:565

32. Khuroo MS, Zargar SA, Yattoo GN et al (1992) Ascaris-induced acute pancreatitis. Br J Surg 79:1335–1338

33. Ros E, Navarro S, Bru C et al (1991) Occult microlithiasis in "idiopathic" acute pancreatitis: prevention of relapses by cholecystectomy or ursodeoxycholic acid therapy. Gastroenterology 101:1701

34. Lee Sp, Nichols JP, Park Hz (1992) Biliary sludges as a cause of acute pancreatitis. N Engl J Med 326:589

35. Halangk W, Lerch MM (2004) Early events in acute pancreatitis. Gastroenterol Clin North Am 33:717

36. Bathia M, Wong Fl, Cao Y et al (2005) Pathophysiology of acute pancreatitis. Pancreatology 5:132

37. van Acker G JD, Perides G, Steer ML (2006) Co-localization hypothesis: a mechanism for the intrapancreatic activation of digestive enzymes during the early phases of acute pancreatitis. World J Gastroenterol 12:1985–1990

38. Palade G (1975) Intracellular aspects of the process of protein synthesis. Science 189:347–358

39. Kelly RB (1985) Pathways of protein secretion in eukaryotes. Science 230:25–32

40. Karanjia ND, Widdison AL, Jehanli A et al (1993) Assay of trypsinogen activation in the cat experimental model of acute pancreatitis. Pancreas 8:189–195

41. Kornfeld S (1986) Trafficking of lysosomal enzymes in normal and disease states. J Clin Invest 77:1–6

42. Andrews NW (2000) Regulated secretion of conventional lysosomes. Trends Cell Biol 10:316–321

43. Ishidoh K, Kominami E (2002) Processing and activation of lysosomal proteinases. Biol Chem 383:1827–1831

44. Saluja A, Hashimoto S, Saluja M et al (1987) Subcellular redistribution of lysosomal enzymes during caerulein-induced pancreatitis. Am J Physiol 253:G508–G516

45. Hofbauer B, Saluja AK, Lerch MM et al (1998) Intra-acinar cell activation of trypsinogen during caerulein-induced pancreatitis in rats. Am J Physiol 275:G352–G362

46. Otani T, Chepilko SM, Grendell JH, Gorelick FS (1998) Codistribution of TAP and the granule membrane protein GRAMP–92 in rat caerulein-induced pancreatitis. Am J Physiol 275:G999–G1009

47. Greenbaum LM, Hirshkowitz A, Shoichet I (1959) The activation of trypsinogen by cathepsin B. J Biol Chem 234:2885–2890

48. Figarella C, Miszczuk-Jamska B, Barrett AJ (1988) Possible lysosomal activation of pancreatic zymogens. Activation of both human trypsinogens by cathepsin B and spontaneous acid. Activation of human trypsinogen 1. Biol Chem Hoppe Seyler 369(Suppl): 293–298

49. Watanabe O, Baccino FM, Steer ML, Meldolesi J (1984) Supramaximal caerulein stimulation and ultrastructure of rat pancreatic acinar cell: early morphological changes during development of experimental pancreatitis. Am J Physiol 246:G457–G467

50. Gennaro A, Stefanelli N, Vassiliadis A (2001) Quadro clinico e fisiopatologia della pancreatite acuta. In: D'Amico DF, Favia G, Eccher C (eds) Pancreatite acuta. Aspetti diagnostico-terapeutici. Atti del convegno Pancreatite acuta, Trento. La Garangola, Milan

51. Pederzoli P, Giardino A, Bandoni L et al (2005) Pancreatite acuta. In: Staudacher C (ed) Chirurgia d'urgenza. Masson, Milan, pp 115-131

52. Chvanov M, Petersen OH, Tepikin A (2005) Free radicals and the pancreatic acinar cells: role in physiology and pathology. Philos Trans R Soc Lond B Biol Sci 360:2273–2284

53. Lipsett PA (2001) Serum cytokines, proteins, and receptors in acute pancreatitis: mediators, marker, or more of the same? Crit Care Med 29:1642–1644

54. Hirota M, Nozawa F, Okabe A et al (2000) Relationship between plasma cytokine concentration and multiple organ failure in patients with acute pancreatitis. Pancreas 21:141–146

55. Ogawa M (1998) Acute pancreatitis and cytokines: "second attack" by septic complication leads to organ failure. Pancreas 16:312–315
56. Liu LR, Xia SH (2006) Role of platelet-activating factor in the pathogenesis of acute pancreatitis. World J Gastroenterol 12:539–545
57. Gukovskaya AS, Gukovsky I, Zaninovic V et al (1997) Pancreatic acinar cells produce, release, and respond to tumor necrosis factor-α. Role in regulating cell death and pancreatitis. J Clin Invest 100:1853–1862
58. Denham W, Norman J (1999) The potential role of therapeutic cytokine manipulation in acute pancreatitis. Surg Clin North Am 79:767–781
59. Pezzilli R, Billi P, Miniero R et al (1995) Serum interleukin-6, interleukin-8, and beta 2-microglobulin in early assessment of severity of acute pancreatitis. Comparison with serum C-reactive protein. Dig Dis Sci 40:2341–2348
60. Gross V, Andreesen R, Leser HG et al (1992) Interleukin-8 and neutrophil activation in acute pancreatitis. Eur J Clin Invest 22:200–203
61. Browne GW, Pitchumoni CS (2006) Pathophysiology of pulmonary complications of acute pancreatitis. World J Gastroenterol 12:7087–7096
62. Zhang XP, Tian H (2007) Pathogenesis of pancreatic encephalopathy in severe acute pancreatitis. Hepatobiliary Pancreat Dis Int 6:134–140
63. Zhang XP, Wang L, Zhang J (2007) Study progress on mechanism of severe acute pancreatitis complicated with hepatic injury. J Zhejiang Univ Sci B 8(4):228–236
64. Schmid SW, Uhl W, Friess H et al (1999) The role of infection in acute pancreatitis. Gut 45:311–316
65. Clavien PA, Burgan S, Moossa AR (1989) Serum enzymes and other laboratory tests in acute pancreatitis. Br J Surg 76:1234–1243
66. Al-Bahrani AZ, Ammori BJ (2005) Clinical laboratory assessment of acute pancreatitis. Clin Chim Acta 362:26
67. Smotkin J, Tenner S (2002) Clinical reviews: pancreatic and biliary disease: laboratory diagnostic tests in acute pancreatitis. J Clin Gastroenterol 34:459–462
68. Yadav D, Agarwal N, Pitchumoni CS (2002) A critical evaluation of laboratory tests in acute pancreatitis. Am J Gastroenterol 97:1309–1318
69. Clavien PA, Robert J, Meyer P et al (1989) Acute pancreatitis and normoamylasemia. Not an uncommon combination. Ann Surg 210:614–620
70. Winslet M, Hall C, London NJ, Neoptolemos JP (1992) Relation of diagnostic serum amylase levels to aetiology and severity of acute pancreatitis. Gut 33:982–986
71. Matull WR, Pereira SP, O'Donohue JW (2006) Biochemical markers of acute pancreatitis. J Clin Pathol 59:340–344
72. American Gastroenterological Association (AGA) Institute on "Management of Acute Pancreatitis" Clinical Practice and Economics Committee; AGA Institute Governing Board. (2007) AGA Institute medical position statement on acute pancreatitis. Gastroenterology 132:2019–2021
73. Banks PA, Freeman ML (2006) Practice Parameters Committee of the American College of Gastroenterology. Practice guidelines in acute pancreatitis. Am J Gastroenterol 101:2379–2400
74. Schein M (2005) Acute pancreatitis. In: Shein M, Rogers PM (eds) Schein's common sense emergency abdominal surgery. Springer, pp 151–161
75. Baron TH, Morgan D (1999) Acute necrotizing pancreatitis. N Engl J Med 340:1412–1416
76. Ranson JH, Rifkind KM, Roses DF et al (1974) Prognostic signs and the role of operative management in acute pancreatitis. Surg Gynecol Obstet 139:69–81
77. Ranson JH (1982) Etiological and prognostic factors in human acute pancreatitis: a review. Am J Gastroenterol 77:633–638
78. Imrie CW, Benjamin IS, Ferguson JC et al (1978) A single-center double-blind trial of Trasylol therapy in primary acute pancreatitis. Br J Surg 65:337–341
79. Larvin M, McMahon MJ (1989) APACHE-II score for assessment and monitoring of acute pancreatitis. Lancet 2:201–205

80. Osvaldt AB, Viero P, Borges da Costa MS et al (2002) l. Evaluation of Ranson, Glasgow, APACHE II and APACHE 0 criteria to predict severity in acute pancreatitis. Int Surg 86(3):158–161

81. Gürleyik G, Emir S, Kiliçoglu G et al(2005) Computed Tomography Severity Index, APACHE II score and serum CRP concentration for predicting the severity of acute pancreatitis. JOP J Pancreas 6:562–567

82. Sandberg AA, Borgström A (2002) Early prediction of severity in acute pancreatitis. Is this possible? JOP J Pancreas (Online) 3(5):116–125

83. Wilson C, Heads A, Shenkin A, Imrie CW (1989) C-reactive protein, antiproteases and complement factors as objective markers of severity in acute pancreatitis. Br J Surg 76:177–181

84. Neoptolemos JP, Kemppainen EA, Mayer JM et al (2000) Early prediction of severity in acute pancreatitis by urinary trypsinogen activation peptide: a multicentre study. Lancet 355:1955–1960

85. Puolakkainen P, Valtonen V, Paananen A, Schröder T (1987) C-reactive protein (CRP) and serum phospholipase A2 in the assessment of acute pancreatitis. Gut 28:764–771

86. Assicot M, Gendrel D, Carsin H et al (1993) Serum pro-calcitonin and C-reactive protein levels as markers of bacterial infection. Lancet 341:515–518

87. Rau B, Steinbach G, Gansauge F et al (1997) The potential role of procalcitonin and interleukin 8 in the prediction of infected necrosis in acute pancreatitis. Gut 41:832–840

88. Rau BM, Kemppainen EA, Gumbs AA et al (2007) Early assessment of pancreatic infections and overall prognosis in severe acute pancreatitis by procalcitonin (PCT). A prospective international multicenter study. Ann Surg 245:745–754

89. Frossard JL, Hadengue A, Pastor CM (2001) New serum markers for the detection of severe acute pancreatitis in humans. Am J Respir Crit Care Med 164:162–170

Chapter 5

Imaging of Acute and Chronic Pancreatitis

Andrea Giovagnoni, Federico Crusco

Acute Pancreatitis

Acute pancreatitis (AP) is an acute inflammatory process of the pancreas that frequently involves peripancreatic tissues and even remote organ systems. The severity of the disease varies widely, from mild forms only affecting the pancreas to severe disease with multisystemic organ failure and death. The major pathobiological processes underlying AP are inflammation, edema, and necrosis of pancreatic tissue as well as inflammation and injury of extrapancreatic organs. Far more patients have interstitial pancreatitis than necrotizing pancreatitis (approximately 85% vs. 15%). Organ failure occurs more commonly in patients with necrotizing pancreatitis than in those with interstitial pancreatitis (approximately 50% vs. 5–10%). Mortality is higher in patients with necrotizing pancreatitis than in those with interstitial pancreatitis, in which there is little necrosis (approximately 17% vs. 3%). The prevalence of infected necrosis in patients with necrotizing pancreatitis is 15–20% and among this subgroup of patients mortality is greater than in those with sterile necrosis (approximately 30% vs. 12%). Although alcohol abuse and gallstone disease account for 70–80% of the cases of acute pancreatitis, the exact mechanisms by which these factors initiate the pathologic process are presently unknown.

The pathophysiology of AP is generally considered to proceed in three phases. In the first phase, there is premature activation of trypsin within pancreatic acinar cells. The enzyme then activates several injurious pancreatic digestive enzymes. The second phase is characterized by intrapancreatic inflammation, which occurs through a variety of mechanisms and pathways. The third phase consists of extrapancreatic inflammation, including acute respiratory syndrome (ARDS). In the majority of patients, AP is mild. In 10–20%, the pathways that contribute to increased intrapancreatic and extrapancreatic inflammation result in what is generally termed systemic inflammatory response syndrome (SIRS). In some instances, SIRS predisposes to multiple organ dysfunction and/or pancreatic necrosis. The factors that determine severity are not clearly understood, but appear to involve a balance between proinflammatory and anti-inflammatory factors.

W. Siquini (Ed.), *Surgical Treatment of Pancreatic Diseases.*
©Springer-Verlag Italia 2009

Most patients with AP experience abdominal pain that is located generally in the epigastrium and radiates to the back in approximately half the cases. The pain is notable for its swift onset, reaching maximum intensity within 30 min, is frequently unbearable, and characteristically persists for more than 24 h without relief. It is often associated with nausea and vomiting. Physical examination usually reveals severe upper abdominal tenderness. In severe pancreatitis, the patients have symptoms of toxicity and are quite ill. Relevant historical clues include any previous diagnosis of biliary tract disease or gallstones, cholecystectomy, other biliary or pancreatic surgery, acute or chronic pancreatitis or their complications, use of ethanol, medications and the timing of their initiation, recent abdominal trauma, weight loss or other symptoms suggesting a malignancy, or a family history of pancreatitis. Blood tests within the first 24 h should include liver chemistries, calcium, and triglycerides.

There is general acceptance that a diagnosis of AP requires two of the following three features: (1) abdominal pain characteristic of acute pancreatitis, (2) serum amylase and/or lipase ≥3 times the upper limit of normal, and (3) characteristic findings of AP on computed tomography (CT) scan. In a patient with abdominal pain characteristic of AP and serum enzyme levels that are lower than three times the upper limit of normal, a CT scan must be performed to confirm a diagnosis of acute pancreatitis. In general, both amylase and lipase are elevated during the course of acute pancreatitis; however, serum lipase is thought to be more sensitive and specific than serum amylase in the diagnosis of the disease.

The differential diagnosis of AP is broad and includes mesenteric ischemia or infarction, perforated gastric or duodenal ulcer, biliary colic, dissecting aortic aneurysm, intestinal obstruction, and possibly myocardial infarction involving the inferior wall.

Imaging Evaluation

Radiology plays an important role in the diagnosis and management of AP. In particular, the various imaging methods are used in the differentiation of acute edematous from acute necrotizing pancreatitis; staging the severity of the disease; determining its etiology (myeloproliferative disease abnormality, common bile duct stones); detecting complications; and guiding interventions (needle aspiration and catheter drainage of fluid collection; embolization for arterial bleeding or pseudoaneurysm).

Plain Radiographs

Conventional abdominal radiographs and barium studies, while occasionally useful in the diagnosis of pancreatitis and the detection of late complications (abscess, strictures, fistulas), have no role in the early evaluation of disease severity. Abnormal chest radiographs, however, can be useful in the prediction of severity. The reported incidence of pulmonary findings (infiltrates, effusions) in AP is 15–55%, mainly in patients with severe disease. The predictive value is increased with left-sided or bilateral pleural effusions. An isolated left pleural effusion, however, is seen in only 43% of patients with severe pancreatitis.

Abdominal Ultrasound

Abdominal ultrasound is usually performed at the time of admission to assess for gallstones as the etiology of AP rather than to establish diagnosis of this disease. Detection of common bile duct stones by ultrasound is limited by poor sensitivity, although specificity is quite high if they are identified. Dilation of the common bile duct alone is neither sensitive nor specific for the detection of stones at this site. Occasionally, the pancreas is visualized well enough by abdominal ultrasound to reveal features that are consistent with the diagnosis of AP, including diffuse glandular enlargement, hypoechoic texture of the pancreas reflective of edema, extrapancreatic fluid collections, and ascites. Nonetheless, the applications of ultrasound in early staging of the disease are limited. Visualization of the pancreas is often impaired because of overlying bowel gas, and the detection of intraparenchymal and retroperitoneal fluid collections correlates poorly with pancreatic necrosis. Abnormal ultrasound findings are seen in 33–90% of AP patients.

Overview of Computed Tomography

Contrast-enhanced CT scan is the modality of choice to confirm suspicions of AP, to exclude conditions that masquerade as AP, to distinguish interstitial from necrotizing pancreatitis, to diagnose the severity, and to identify complications. Moreover, CT is the best imaging technique for follow-up evaluation and to guide percutaneous and surgical interventions. It offers several advantages, such as easy accessibility, less cost, more favorable environment for severely ill patients, higher sensitivity in the detection of small gas bubbles (secondary infection, fistulous communication, or post-intervention) and calcifications (acute or chronic pancreatitis, biliary tract calculi). Contrast-enhanced CT scan may give clues as to the etiology of AP: for example, a pancreatic mass may suggest malignancy; a dilatation of the main branch of the common bile duct, an intraductal papillary mucinous neoplasia; a cystic lesion, a cystic neoplasia; a common bile duct stone, biliary pancreatitis; and pancreatic calcifications, alcohol-related pancreatitis. CT shows the morphologic changes in AP, ranging from minimal edema of the parenchyma in the interstitial inflammation of mild pancreatitis to the extensive fluid collections, necrosis, and hemorrhage that develop in fulminant severe pancreatitis. The diagnosis of mild AP generally is established by the clinical presentation and biochemical tests, without the need for diagnostic imaging; in this case, CT show a normal-appearing gland in one third or more of patients.

Morphologic changes detected by CT include diffuse or focal glandular enlargement, contour irregularity with blurring of the outline of a swollen-appearing pancreas, changes in the peripancreatic areolar tissues, fat and peritoneal planes. Because intestitial pancreatitis is characterized by an intact microcirculation, uniform enhancement of the gland is demonstrated after i.v. contrast medium.

Necrosis is the hallmark of severe AP. Necrotizing pancreatitis is characterized by disruption of the microcirculation such that devitalized areas do not enhance (Fig. 5.1).

Acute fluid collections arise from the exudation of fluid into the pancreatic interstitium and subsequent leakage of this fluid, which contains activated proteolytic enzymes, into the surrounding peripancreatic tissue spaces. Early changes caused by fluid dissection are recognizable in the anterior pararenal space, resulting in thickening of the anterior perinephric fascia of Gerota. As the inflammatory and the exudative processes continue, fluid extends posteriorly to a potential space between the laminae of the posterior renal and lateroconal fascia and subsequently to the lateral edge of the quadratus lumborum muscle (Gray-Turner sign of flank discoloration). Involvement of the true posterior pararenal and perirenal spaces is uncommon. Retroperitoneal pathways of fluid dissection commonly include the transverse mesocolon, mesenteric root, and the gastrohepatic, gastrosplenic, and gastrocolic ligaments. Following the pathways provided by the mesenteric root, collections can extend to and around the cecum and the ascending and discending colon as well as inferiorly into the lumbar, pelvic, and inguinal regions. Another direct pathway is extension to the round ligament and then to the properitoneal periumbilical fat (Cullen sign). Rarely, fluid collections extend superiorly into the mediastinum. In advanced forms of AP, the parietal peritoneum overlying the pancreas may be disrupted such that inflammatory fluid enters the lesser sac and then, through the foramen of Winslow, the peritoneal cavity.

Evolution of an acute fluid collection into a pseudocyst usually will occur over a period of 4 weeks or longer (Fig. 5.2); 50% of these pseudocysts sponta-

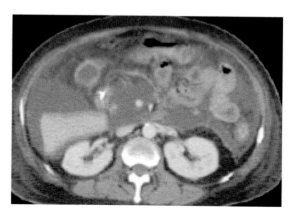

Fig. 5.1 Contrast-enhanced CT image showing extensive pancreatic and peripancreatic non-enhancing necrosis with large fluid collections

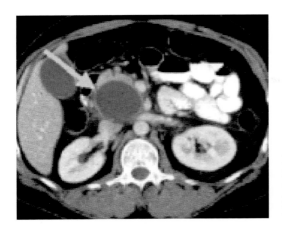

Fig. 5.2 Contrast-enhanced CT image show a pancreatic pseudocyst (*arrow*) as an ovoid, homogeneous, hypodense structure in the head of the pancreas

neously resolve. Unlike fluid collections, pseudocysts have a thick dense fibrous capsule and usually are round or oval in shape. Generally, the fluid in a pseudocyst is homogeneous with an attenuation value near that of water; heterogeneous or increased attenuation values suggest intracystic hemorrhage or infection. The wall of the pseudocyst typically shows delayed enhancement on contrast CT. While most pseudocysts are peripancreatic in location, intramural pseudocysts in the duodenum, stomach, and colon have been reported. CT features distinctive of the intramural location are a tubular shape conforming to the course of the intestine or abrupt flattening of tubular or spherical pseudocyst at the border of the duodenal lumen.

Infected necrosis (developing usually after the first week) and pancreatic abscess (developing later, generally after 5 weeks) must be suspected, as part of a precise clinical scenario, in the presence of gas bubbles in a fluid collection or pseudocyst. Other complications associated with pancreatitis, including arterial pseudoaneurysm, aneurysms and thrombosis of the splenic, mesenteric, or portal veins, and gastrointestinal and biliary complications (such as obstruction of the duodenum or stomach, inflammation of the transverse colon, and biliary obstruction) can be easily demonstrated by CT.

There have been concerns about possible aggravation of pancreatic injury through the use of iodinated contrast agents; however, recent studies have found no evidence of extension of necrosis on subsequent CT scans.

Predicting Severe Acute Pancreatitis

Older age (>55), obesity (BMI >30), organ failure, and pleural effusion and/or infiltrates are risk factors for severity that should be noted at admission. Patients with these traits may require treatment in a highly supervised area, such as an intensive care unit.

The two tests that are most helpful at admission in distinguishing mild from severe AP are the APACHE (Acute Physiology and Chronic Health Evaluation)-II score and serum hematocrit. The APACHE-II severity of disease classification system includes a variety of physiologic variables, age points, and long-term health points, which can be measured at admission and daily as needed to help identify patients with severe pancreatitis. Several reports have correlated a higher APACHE-II at admission and during the first 72 h with a higher mortality (<4% with an APACHE-II <8 and 11–18% with an APACHE-II >8). The advantage of the APACHE-II score is the availability of this information within the first 24 h and daily. In general, an APACHE-II score that increases during the first 48 h is strongly suggestive of the development of severe pancreatitis, whereas a score that decreases within the first 48 h strongly suggests mild pancreatitis. It is recommended that APACHE-II scores be generated during the first 3 days of hospitalization and thereafter as needed to help in making this distinction.

Ranson signs have been used for many years to assess the severity of AP but their disadvantage is that a full 48 h is required for a complete evaluation. In general, when Ranson signs are <3, mortality is 0–3%; when ≥3, 11–15%; and ≥6, 40%.

The reduction in intravascular volume, which can be detected by an increased serum hematocrit, can lead to decreased perfusion of the pancreatic microcirculation, resulting in pancreatic necrosis. As such, hemoconcentration has been proposed as a predictor of necrotizing pancreatitis. It is recommended that serum hematocrit be obtained at admission, 12 h after admission, and 24 h after admission.

C-reactive protein (CRP) is an acute-phase reactant. Plasma levels >150 mg/l within the first 72 h of disease correlate with the presence of necrosis with a sensitivity and specificity that are both >80%.

In addition to the clinical and physiologic evaluation methods described earlier, an important CT criterion is to determine whether pancreatic necrosis is present, as pancreatic necrosis and organ failure are the two most important markers of AP severity. The distinction between interstitial and necrotizing pancreatitis can be reliably made after 2–3 days of hospitalization by contrast-enhanced CT scan. Balthazar, in a study carried out in 1985, graded the severity of pancreatitis into five distinctive groups, from A to E (A: normal pancreas; B: pancreatic enlargement; C: pancreatic inflammation and/or peripancreatic fat; D: single peripancreatic fluid collection; E: two or more fluid collections and/or retroperitoneal air). Patients with grade D or E disease had a mortality of 14% and a morbidity of 54%, compared with no mortality and a morbidity of only 4% in patients with grade A, B, or C disease. This CT grading scale is easy to perform, fast, does not require intravenous administration of contrast material, and can be used to identify a subgroup of individuals (with grade D or E) at risk of death or with a high morbidity.

A major improvement in this early grading system was achieved with the introduction of the incremental dynamic bolus CT technique. As described above, patients with interstitial mild pancreatitis have an intact capillary network with vasodilation and, therefore, should exhibit uniform enhancement of the pancreatic gland. Areas of diminished or no enhancement indicate decreased blood flow and relate to pancreatic zones of ischemia or necrosis. Criteria for the CT diagnosis of pancreatic necrosis have been defined as focal or diffuse zones of nonenhanced pancreatic parenchyma depicted during an examination with intravenous bolus administration of contrast material. The extent of necrosis was further quantified to <30%, 30–50%, and >50% of the pancreatic gland. Patients with <30% necrosis exhibited no mortality and a morbidity of 48%, while larger areas of necrosis (30–50% and >50%) were associated with a morbidity of 75–100% and a mortality of 11–25%. The combined morbidity in patients with >30% necrosis was 94%, and mortality was 29% (Table 5.1).

The CT severity index was designed in an attempt to improve the early prognostic value of CT in cases of AP. Patients with grade A–E pancreatitis are assigned 0–4 points plus 2 points for necrosis of up to 30%, 4 points for necrosis of 30–50%, and 6 points for necrosis of >50%. Patients with a severity index of 0 or 1 exhibited 0% mortality and no morbidity, while those with a severity index of 2 had no mortality and 4% morbidity. In contrast, a severity index of 7–10 yielded a 17% mortality and a 92% complication rate (Table 5.2).

The determination that a patient has pancreatic necrosis has clinical implications because the morbidity and mortality of necrotizing pancreatitis is higher than that of interstitial pancreatitis. Nonetheless, clinicians should keep in mind that organ failure (and particularly multisystem organ failure) rather than the extent of necrosis appears to be a more important factor in the morbidity and mortality of AP.

Table 5.1 Bathazar-Ranson criteria for severity

CT grade	Score	Necrosis	Score
A	0	None	0
B	1	One-third	2
C	2	One-half	4
D	3	>One-half	6
E	4		

Table 5.2 CT severity index (CTSI)

CTSI	Complications (%)	Deaths (%)
0–3	8	3
4–6	35	6
7–10	92	17

Magnetic Resonance Imaging

In the care of patients with acute pancreatitis, MRI has not been widely used. While CT scan remains the primary imaging technique to evaluate patients with AP, recent reports have indicated that MRI has some advantages over CT: the lack of nephrotoxicity of gadolinium compared to iodinated preparations used for contrast-enhanced CT scan, potential concerns regarding radiation exposure, the greater ability of MRI to distinguish necrosis from fluid, and the overall higher reliability of MRI in staging the severity of AP and its complications. MRI is particularly useful in patients who cannot receive iodinated contrast material due to allergic reactions or renal insufficiency. Gadolinium-enhanced T1-weighted gradient-echo magnetic resonance images can depict pancreatic necrosis as areas of nonenhanced parenchyma (Fig. 5.3). Fat-suppression images are also helpful for defining subtle, diffuse, or focal parenchymal abnormalities. T2-weighted images can accurately depict fluid collections, pseudocysts, and areas of hemorrhage. MRI is sensitive for the detection of the subtle changes that occur in AP, particularly minor peripancreatic inflammatory changes even in the setting of a morphologically normal pancreas. CT imaging examinations are normal in 15–30% of patients with clinical features of acute pancreatitis; in this subgroup, the sensitivity of MRI exceeds that of CT imaging, suggesting a role for MRI in the setting of clinical suspicion and negative CT imaging examinations. Complications of AP, such as hemorrhage, pseudocyst formation, or abscess, are clearly shown by MRI. Hemorrhagic fluid collections are high in signal intensity on T1-weighted fat-suppressed images and depiction of hemorrhage is better on magnetic resonance images than on CT images.

The disadvantages of MRI include its lack of availability when urgently needed, variations in quality among centers, and the difficulty of supervising a critically ill patient undergoing MRI.

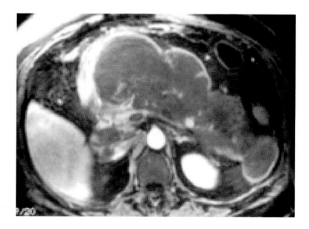

Fig. 5.3 Immediate post-gadolinium gradient-echo T1-weighted imaging shows a large heterogeneous non-enhancing necrotic fluid collection

Endoscopic Retrograde Cholangiography

In mild biliary pancreatitis, ERCP with removal of common bile duct stones has not been shown to improve the natural history of pancreatitis. In severe gallstone pancreatitis, the potential benefit of ERCP with sphincterotomy and stone extraction would be to prevent (or treat) ascending cholangitis and possibly also to prevent (or treat) organ failure. It is reasonable to perform ERCP when a retained common bile duct stone is highly suspected, such as by progressive abnormalities of liver function or evidence provided by abdominal ultrasound or CT scan. This approach makes sense because evidence of sepsis and/or organ failure could be directly attributable to ascending cholangitis caused by a retained gallstone. When there is inconclusive evidence that a stone is present in the common bile duct in severe gallstone pancreatitis, it is recommended that magnetic resonance cholangiopancreatography (MRCP) or endoscopic ultrasound (EUS) be employed to confirm the presence of the stone. Documentation of a stone would then be a reasonable indication for ERCP and stone removal.

Recommendations for Diagnosis

The three characteristic features upon which a diagnosis of AP is based were described above. In addition, the following should be noted:
– The diagnosis of AP should be established within 48 h of admission and is based on compatible clinical features together with elevations in amylase or lipase levels. Elevations in amylase or lipase levels greater than three times the upper limit of normal, in the absence of renal failure, are most consistent with AP, whereas elevations in the levels of these enzymes less than three times the upper limit of normal are of low specificity. Elevation of lipase levels is somewhat more specific and is thus preferred.
– AP should be considered among the differential diagnoses in patients admitted with unexplained multi-system organ failure or the SIRS.
– Confirmation of the diagnosis, if required, is best achieved by CT of the abdomen using intravenous contrast enhancement. Clinicians should be aware that an early CT (within 72 h of the onset of illness) might underestimate the extent of pancreatic necrosis. Many AP patients do not require a CT scan at admission or at any time during hospitalization. For example, a CT scan is usually not essential in patients with recurrent mild pancreatitis caused by alcohol. A reasonable indication for a CT scan at admission (but not necessarily a CT with i.v. contrast) is to distinguish AP from another serious intra-abdominal condition, such as a perforated ulcer.

Recommendations for Assessment of Severity

– Clinicians should define severe disease by mortality or by the presence of organ failure and/or local pancreatic complications, including pseudocyst, necrosis, or abscess. Multi-system organ failure and persistent or progressive organ failure are most closely predictive of mortality and are the most reliable markers of severe disease.

– The prediction of severe disease, before its onset, is best achieved by careful ongoing clinical assessment coupled with the use of a multiple factor scoring system and imaging studies. The APACHE-II system is preferred, with the cutoff set at ≥8. Those patients with predicted or actual severe disease and those with other severe comorbid medical conditions should be strongly considered for triage to an intensive care unit or intermediate medical care unit.

– Pancreatic necrosis and organ failure are the two most important markers of severity in AP. The distinction between interstitial and necrotizing pancreatitis can be reliably made after 2–3 days of hospitalization by contrast-enhanced CT scan. Rapid-bolus contrast-enhanced CT should be performed after 72 h of illness to assess the degree of pancreatic necrosis in patients with predicted severe disease (APACHE II score ≥8) and in those with evidence of organ failure during the initial 72 h. CT should be used selectively based on clinical features in those patients not satisfying these criteria. A reasonable indication for a contrast-enhanced CT scan acquired a few days after admission is to distinguish interstitial from necrotizing pancreatitis when there is clinical evidence of increased severity. The distinction between interstitial and necrotizing pancreatitis can be made much more readily when a contrast-enhanced CT scan is obtained on the second or third day after admission rather than at the time of admission. Additional contrast-enhanced CT scans may be required at intervals during the hospitalization to detect and monitor the course of intra-abdominal complications of AP, such as the development of organized necrosis, pseudocysts, and vascular complications including pseudoaneurysms.

– Laboratory tests may be used as an adjunct to clinical judgment, multiple-factor scoring systems, and CT to guide clinical triage decisions. A serum C-reactive protein level >150 mg/l at 48 h after disease onset is preferred.

Recommendations for the Determination of Etiology

– The initial history should particularly focus on previous symptoms or documentation of gallstones, alcohol use, history of hypertriglyceridemia or hypercalcemia, family history of pancreatic disease, prescription and nonprescription drug history, history of trauma, and the presence of concomitant autoimmune diseases.

– At admission, serum should be obtained from all patients for measurement of the levels of amylase or lipase, triglyceride, calcium, and liver enzymes (bilirubin, aspartate aminotransferase, alanine aminotransferase, and alkaline phosphatase). If triglyceride levels cannot be obtained at admission, fasting levels should be measured after recovery, when the patient has resumed normal intake of food.

- Abdominal ultrasonography should be obtained at admission to look for cholelithiasis or choledocholithiasis. If the initial ultrasound examination is inadequate or if gallstone pancreatitis is still suspected, repeat ultrasonography after recovery should be performed. Endoscopic ultrasonography (EUS) or MRCP can be used as an accurate alternative approach to screen for cholelithiasis and choledocholithiasis, either at admission or thereafter.
- CT or EUS should be performed in those patients with unexplained pancreatitis who are at risk for underlying pancreatic malignancy (age >40 years).
- Extensive or invasive evaluation is not recommended in those patients with a single episode of unexplained pancreatitis who are <40 years of age.
- In patients with recurrent episodes of pancreatitis, evaluation with EUS and/or endoscopic retrograde cholangiopancreatography (ERCP) should be considered. EUS is preferred as the initial test.

Management of Infected and Sterile Necrosis

Approximately 33% of patients with necrotizing pancreatitis develop infected necrosis, usually after 10 days of illness. The distinction between sterile and infected necrosis is an important concern throughout the course of necrotizing pancreatitis. CT-guided percutaneous aspiration with Gram's stain and culture is recommended when infected necrosis is suspected. The treatment of choice in infected necrosis is surgical debridement. Alternative, minimally invasive approaches may be used in selected circumstances; these techniques have generally been reserved for patients with infected pancreatic necrosis who are too ill to undergo prompt surgical debridement (such as those with organ failure and/or serious comorbid disease). The preferred technique is minimally invasive retroperitoneal necrosectomy; another is laparoscopic necrosectomy with placement of large-caliber drains under direct surgical inspection; a third is percutaneous catheter drainage under CT guidance in patients with infected necrosis.

Sterile necrosis is best managed medically during the first 2–3 weeks. Thereafter, if abdominal pain persists and prevents oral intake, debridement should be considered. This is usually accomplished surgically, but percutaneous or endoscopic debridement is a reasonable choice in selected circumstances with the appropriate expertise. Early fluid collections associated with pancreatic and peripancreatic necrosis may organize into a pancreatic pseudocyst, the management of which is also conservative because approximately 50% resolve spontaneously. In instances in which the patient is free from major symptoms, a "wait and see" policy of up to 12 weeks is justifiable.

Symptomatic pseudocysts can be treated by transmural drainage through the wall of the stomach using endoscopic ultrasound.

Transpapillary pancreatic duct stenting up to and/or across an area of duct disruption may require endoscopic or surgical therapy. External percutaneous drainage using imaging guidance is the least desirable option.

Chronic Pancreatitis

Chronic pancreatitis (CP) is characterized by progressive and irreversible pancreatic damage that eventually leads to impairment of both the exocrine and the endocrine functions of the pancreas. It is commonly accompanied by chronic disabling pain. Chronic alcohol abuse accounts for 70% of the cases of CP in adults, while genetic diseases and anatomic defects predominate in children. The TIGAR-O (toxic-metabolic, idiopathic, genetic, autoimmune; recurrent and severe acute pancreatitis, obstructive) classification system is based on the risk factors for CP.

Chronic pancreatitis can be classified into three categories: (1) chronic calcifying pancreatitis, (2) chronic obstructive pancreatitis, and (3) chronic inflammatory pancreatitis. Chronic calcifying pancreatitis is invariably related to alcoholism. The earliest finding is precipitation in the pancreatic ducts of proteinaceous material that forms protein plugs which subsequently calcify. The pancreatic ductal epithelium undergoes atrophy, hyperplasia, and metaplasia. The main pancreatic duct has a beaded appearance due to alternating stenoses and dilatation. In approximately 50% of patients with chronic calcific pancreatitis, the pancreatic parenchyma contains cysts of varying sizes (several millimeters to 5 cm) that are lined by cuboidal epithelium and contain pancreatic enzymes. Peripancreatic fibrosis is usually a late finding that involves the portal and/or splenic veins. In chronic obstructive pancreatitis, the prominent histologic changes are periductal fibrosis and subsequent ductal dilatation. These changes are much more focal than those in the other forms. Diffuse changes may occur, in which the main pancreatic duct or ampulla is obstructed. The pancreatic duct is dilated while the pancreas is normal in size, atrophic, or focally and/or globally enlarged. Numerous factors are implicated in chronic obstructive pancreatitis; these include ductal obstruction due to ampullary stenosis, inflammatory or neoplastic causes, surgical ductal ligation, and fibrosis due to a pseudocyst as a complication of an episode of AP. Chronic inflammatory pancreatitis is rare and can affect elderly persons without a previous history of alcohol excess.

Autoimmune-related CP is a distinct clinical entity that may present with signs of acute or chronic pancreatitis, sometimes associated with cholestatic jaundice. On imaging, this type of CP may appear as diffuse (duct destructive) or pseudotumoral lesions. Pancreatitis may be associated with Crohn disease and ulcerative colitis and thus provides justification to investigate those patients with idiopathic pancreatitis for underlying inflammatory bowel disease. Chronic autoimmune pancreatitis must always be considered in patients with a pancreatic mass that is atypical for carcinoma on imaging or based on clinical findings. Diagnosis depends on clinical and radiologic findings.

The most common presentation of CP is abdominal pain, which can be episodic, lasting hours to days, or persisting for months or even years. The pain is characteristically steady in the epigastrium and it frequently radiates to the back. Patients may also present with steatorrhea, malabsorption, vitamin deficiency, diabetes, or weight loss.

Pancreatic function tests (fasting serum glucose, fecal fat estimation, fecal elastase, secretin stimulation) are not diagnostic; they are most helpful when used in patients with suspected CP who have a normal CT scan. In addition, they are not specific for diagnosis and are difficult to perform; therefore, they are not routinely recommended.

Overview on Imaging Studies and Role of Radiology

Although ERCP is still used as the reference standard, it is rarely recommended for diagnosis because of the high risks of complications; instead, contrast-enhanced CT of the abdomen is the initial imaging modality of choice. Pathognomonic findings on CT are ductal dilatation and calcifications within the pancreatic ducts. For evaluation of the pancreatic parenchyma and ductal system, the diagnostic performance of MRI with MRCP and EUS is similar to that of ERCP. In general, the role of radiology is: to diagnose the chronic inflammatory damage (by detecting structural changes in the ducts and parenchyma and by assessing the functional integrity of the gland), to detect associated complications (biliary strictures, pseudocysts, vascular occlusion, pseudoaneurysm), and to assist in therapeutic decision-making. Most imaging procedures cannot depict early CP because the structural changes they rely on are only associated with moderate-to-advanced disease. Therefore, different imaging modalities depict only morphologic changes typical of advanced disease.

Plain Radiography

Pancreatic calcifications are a common finding in chronic calcific pancreatitis and are considered pathognomonic for alcoholic chronic pancreatitis. Calcification primarily represents intraductal calculi, either in the main pancreatic duct or in the smaller pancreatic ductal radicles. Calcification is punctate or coarse and may have a focal, segmental, or diffuse distribution. The sensitivity of plain abdominal radiography in the detection of pancreatic calcification is approximately 80%, which is higher than that of sonography but lower than that of CT. When seen, pancreatic calcification is pathognomonic for CP.

Upper GI-Tract Barium Series

An upper GI-tract barium series may provide information that is critical to the treatment of CP patients. Esophageal involvement rarely occurs in CP, and obstruction is usually the result of mediastinal extension of a pseudocyst. Pancreatic enlargement or a pseudocyst may compress the stomach. Peripancreatic fibrosis may involve the antrum of the stomach or the duodenum, resulting in stenosis. The anatomic proximity of the pancreatic head and stomach

antrum is constant, and enlargement of the pancreatic head usually causes efface-
ment of the antrum; this has been termed the pad sign. The C loop of the duodenum may be widened because of a mass effect from an enlarged pancreatic head,
or it may be present as an inverted *3* sign due to traction on the medial wall of the
duodenum. In the duodenum, concentric narrowing due to periduodenal fibrosis
can occur. Small-bowel changes are infrequently found in CP patients.

Ultrasonography

Primary findings on abdominal sonography include changes in the size, shape
contour, and echo texture of the pancreas. An irregular pancreatic contour is seen
in 45–60% of patients, focal enlargement is detected in 12–32%, and diffuse
enlargement in 27–45%. Peripancreatic fascial thickening and blurring of the
pancreatic margins are seen in approximately 15% of patients.

In early disease, the pancreas may be enlarged and hypoechoic, with ductal
dilatation. Later, the pancreas becomes heterogeneous, with areas of increased
echogenicity and focal or diffuse enlargement. Pseudocysts may occur, and focal
hypoechoic inflammatory masses can mimic pancreatic neoplasia. Calculi and
calcification in the gland result in densely echogenic foci, which may show
shadow. The pancreatic and common bile ducts may be dilated.

In late stages of the disease, the pancreas becomes atrophic and fibrotic, and
it shrinks. These changes result in a small echogenic pancreas with a heterogeneous echo texture. The pancreatic duct remains dilated and has a beaded
appearance because of multiple stenoses. When seen, biliary dilation is mild.
Other complications, such as arterial pseudoaneurysms, left-sided portal hypertension (i.e., splenic venous thrombosis), and pleural effusions are readily
detected on sonography.

Endoscopic Ultrasonography

The above-mentioned changes are best detected with EUS, which is more sensitive and detects the changes at an earlier stage of disease. The most characteristic EUS findings in CP are parenchymal changes presenting as oval hypoechoic
areas <1 mm and separated by hyperechoic fibrous septa. The sensitivity and
specificity of EUS for the diagnosis of CP are 97 and 60%, respectively. EUS can
be combined with fine-needle aspiration biopsy (FNAB) for histologic diagnosis.

Endoscopic Retrograde Cholangiopancreatography

The reference standard for the diagnosis of CP in many studies is ERCP, with a
reported sensitivity and specificity for the diagnosis of 75–95% and 90%, respectively. ECP is mainly used in the diagnosis of early CP in patients with normal CT

and pancreatic function tests. The disadvantages of the technique are its invasiveness and the high risks of complications. Therapeutic indications for ERCP include treatment of symptomatic stones, strictures, and pseudocysts. Ductal decompression by sphincterotomy or stent placement offers pain relief in most patients.

Computed Tomography

Currently, CT is regarded as the imaging modality of choice for the initial evaluation of suggested CP. CT is more sensitive than plain radiography and ultrasonography in the depiction of pancreatic calcification. Moreover, it depicts calcification in the pancreas, and confusion with non-pancreatic calcification is less likely. The sensitivity and specificity of CT for the diagnosis of CP are 75–90% and 85%, respectively. The diagnostic accuracy of CT is 75–90%; the variation is due to the wide discrepancy in the criteria used for diagnosis and in the quality of CT scanners. CT helps in the diagnosis of atrophy of the pancreas, providing better results than ultrasonography.

In a retrospective analysis of 56 patients with documented CP studied by CT, dilatation of the main pancreatic duct was seen in 68%, parenchymal atrophy in 54%, calcifications in 50%, fluid collections in 30%, focal pancreatic enlargement in 30%, biliary ductal dilatation in 29%, and alterations in peripancreatic fat or fascia in 16%. In only 7% of the patients were no abnormalities detected. Dilatation of the main pancreatic duct can be demonstrated by CT, with the width of the main pancreatic duct exceeding 5 mm in the head and 2 mm in the body and tail; smooth or beaded dilatation of the main pancreatic duct is most commonly associated with carcinoma, whereas irregular dilatation is more frequently seen in CP. Furthermore, a ratio of duct width to total gland width <0.5 favors the diagnosis of CP. CT is the most sensitive and specific modality for depicting pancreatic calcifications, which may be tiny and punctate or larger and coarse (Fig. 5.4). Focal enlargement or atrophy of the

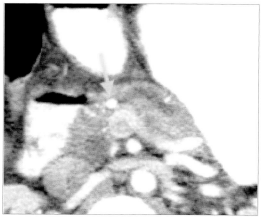

Fig. 5.4 Contrast-enhanced CT shows a punctate, single, intraductal calcification (*arrow*) at the level of the pancreatic neck. This feature is specific for chronic pancreatitis

pancreas is readily demonstrated on CT scans; focal enlargement associated with calcification or ductal dilatation in a mass is suggestive of CP. Pseudocysts can occur in acute or chronic pancreatitis; however, when they are found in association with ductal dilatation and intraductal calcifications CP is the underlying disease. Obliteration of the peripancreatic fat, which results in poor definition and an ill-defined pancreatic contour, is usually seen in acute exacerbations of CP. Obliteration of the fat sleeve around the superior mesenteric artery has been described in both CP and pancreatic carcinoma. Obstruction of the common bile duct may be visualized as a gradual tapering of the ductal lumen whereas a pancreatic carcinoma usually results in an abrupt transition of the common bile duct. Vascular complications of CP are best depicted by contrast-enhanced CT scans. In images of pseudoaneurysms, high-attenuation masses are seen during the arterial phase. Thrombosis of the portal and/or splenic vein and associated collateral venous channels is better delineated during the portal venous phase of contrast enhancement.

Pancreatic carcinoma and CP share many CT features; occasionally, differentiation between the two is impossible. Pseudotumoral enlargement around focal pancreatitis with extensive fibrous tissue proliferation usually fails to enhance after the administration of contrast material.

Magnetic Resonance Imaging with Magnetic Resonance Cholangiopancreatography

The changes of that occur in CP may be better visualized by MRI than by CT in that MRI detects not only morphologic findings but also the presence of fibrosis, which is shown by diminished signal intensity on T1-weighted fat-suppressed images, diminished heterogeneous enhancement on immediate post-gadolinium gradient-echo images, and delayed progressive enhancement on 5-min post-contrast images. This behavior reflects loss of soluble protein in the acini of the pancreas. Fibrosis is associated with decreased vascularity, which causes decreased gadolinium enhancement of the pancreas. Small punctate pancreatic calcification is difficult to detect using MRI, but larger calcifications may be seen as foci of a signal void. As a result of its ability to depict fluid, T2-weighted MRI may demonstrate irregularities in the pancreatic and common bile ducts and pseudocysts associated with CP.

As stated earlier, focal enlargement of the head of the pancreas due to CP may be difficult to distinguish from cancer on CT images whereas MRI permits distinction between these two entities with greater reliability. Both CP mass-like pseudotumor and carcinoma show focal enlargement (greater in the head), irregular dilatation of the main pancreatic duct, parenchymal atrophy, hypointensity on non-contrast fat-suppressed T1-weighted images, mild hyperintensity on T2-weighted images, and hypoenhancement on immediate post-gadolinium images (Fig. 5.5). However, heterogeneous enhancement with the presence of signal-

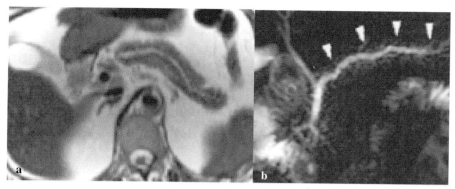

Fig. 5.5 Magnetic resonance imaging fast spin echo (FSE) (**a**) and single-shot FSE T2-weighted 2D thick-slab imaging (**b**) demonstrate irregular dilatation in the main pancreatic duct with evidence of a dilated side-branch duct (*arrowheads*)

void cysts, calcifications without evidence of a marginated definable mass, and the presence of the "duct penetrating sign" (i.e., penetration of a focal mass by a nonobstructed main pancreatic duct) add confidence to the diagnosis of CP. In contrast, in carcinoma the involved portion of the parenchyma loses its normal anatomic details, with disruption of the underlying architecture.

Acute or chronic pancreatitis is well-shown on MRI. Pseudocyst are also readily seen, appearing as signal-void oval structures on gadolinium-enhanced T1-weighted fat-suppressed images and high signal structures on T2-weighted images.

The global sensitivity and specificity of MRI and MRCP for the diagnosis of CP are 85 and 100%, respectively. MRCP is being increasingly employed as an effective noninvasive imaging technique for examining patients who are suspected of having pancreatic or biliary-tract disease. Its diagnostic accuracy is comparable to that of ERCP in the evaluation of disease and anatomic variants of the pancreatic duct. The diagnosis of CP is based on both the evaluation of the functional integrity of the gland and the typical morphologic changes in pancreatic ducts seen at ERCP; ductal abnormalities seen at ERCP, however, may not be closely related to the degree of pancreatic functional impairment and there is a discrepancy between morphology and function in 12–29% of cases. MRCP after secretin stimulation is potentially useful because it allows evaluation of morphologic and functional changes during a single noninvasive procedure, with combined enhancement of diagnostic accuracy. At MRCP after secretin stimulation, the exocrine functional reserve of the pancreas is derived by grading progressive duodenal filling on serial images. Compared to the biochemical intraductal secretin test for prediction of reduced exocrine function, duodenal filling seen at MRCP after secretin stimulation had a sensitivity of 72%, specificity of 76%, a positive predictive value of 76%, and a negative predictive value of 84%.

FDG-PET in the Detection of Pancreatic Carcinoma in Chronic Pancreatitis

Patients with CP are at risk of developing pancreatic cancer. Early detection is mandatory, as cure can only be achieved in nonadvanced disease; however, this is very difficult with conventional radiologic techniques. FDG-PET has been established as a tool for the diagnosis of pancreatic carcinoma in the presence of long-standing CP.

Approach to the Patient with Suspected Chronic Pancreatitis

Most cases of large-duct disease (pancreatic dilatation ≥7 mm) can be identified by CT, which is the initial diagnostic test of choice. When the test is positive for CP (presence of stones, strictures or dilatations of the main pancreatic duct, pseudocysts) MRCP or EUS can be performed to identify the ductal anatomy before ERCP or surgery. When CT is negative but there is a high degree of suspicion for CP, MRI with MRCP is the test of choice; EUS with FNAB and pancreatic function tests can be performed in patients with a negative MRI. These last tests are recommended when there is a cystic or mass lesion suspicious for malignancy.

Suggested Reading

Acute Pancreatitis

Balthazar EJ (2002) Acute pancreatitis: assessment of severity with clinical and CT evaluation. Radiology 223:603–613

Balthazar EJ (1985) Acute pancreatitis: prognostic value of CT. Radiology 156:767–772

Banks PA, Freeman ML; Practice Parameters Committee of the American College of Gastroenterology (2006) Practice guidelines in acute pancreatitis. Am J Gastroenterol 101:2379–2400

Forsmark CE, Baillie J; AGA Institute Clinical Practice and Economics Committee; AGA Institute Governing Board (2007) AGA Institute medical position statement on acute pancreatitis. Gastroenterology 132:2019–2021

Forsmark CE, Baillie J; AGA Institute Clinical Practice and Economics Committee; AGA Institute Governing Board (2007) AGA Institute technical review on acute pancreatitis. Gastroenterology 132:2022–2044

Frossard JL (2008) Acute pancreatitis. Lancet 371:143–152

Kalra MK, Maher MM, Sahani DV et al (2002) Current status of imaging in pancreatic disease. J Comput Assist Tomogr 26(5):661–675

Kingsnorth A, O'Reilly D (2006) Acute pancreatitis. BMJ 332:1072–1076

Pandol SJ, Saluja AK, Imrie CW, Banks PA (2007) Acute pancreatitis: bench to the bedside. Gastroenterology 132:1127–1151

Whitcomb DC (2006) Acute pancreatitis. N Engl J Med 354:2142–2150

Chronic Pancreatitis

Cappeliez O, Delhaye M, Devière J et al (2000) Chronic pancreatitis: evaluation of pancreatic exocrine function with MR pancreatography after secretin stimulation. Radiology 215:358–364

Etemad B, Whitcomb DC (2001) Chronic pancreatitis: diagnosis, classification, and new genetic developments. Gastroenterology 120:682–707

Kalra MK, Maher MM, Sahani DV et al (2002) Current status of imaging in pancreatic disease. J Comput Assist Tomogr 26(5):661–675

Nair RJ, Lawler L, Miller MR (2007) Chronic pancreatitis. Am Fam Phys 76:1679–1688

Remer EM, Baker ML (2002) Imaging of chronic pancreatitis. Radiol Clin N Am 40:1229–1242

Steer ML, Waxman I, Freedman S (1995) Chronic pancreatitis. N Engl J Med 332:1482–1490

Chapter 6

Medical Management of Acute Pancreatitis

Marco Romiti, Luciano Minestroni, Walter Siquini, Gabriele Corradini

Introduction

All cases of mild acute pancreatitis (AP) and the majority of the severe forms of the disease are treated conservatively. Medical therapy is therefore of fundamental importance in the management of this disease. However, apart from the common devices of cardiovascular and respiratory support, thanks to which the early mortality in severe AP has been greatly reduced, to this day we do not have a specific and effective drug capable of acting on the physiopathology of the disease and of leading to a positive outcome. Antibiotic prophylaxis, equally a cornerstone of medical therapy, has for the past few years come under critical scrutiny.

Mild Pancreatitis

Since mild AP is self-limiting, therapy is based on fasting, adequate fluid infusion, and analgesia (the use of opiates should be avoided because of the possibility of inducing spasm of the sphincter of Oddi, which could worsen the pancreatic inflammation). The benefits of antibiotics and gastric antisecretory drugs, in terms of accelerating healing and preventing complications, have not been demonstrated, although these drugs are in common use [1]. A nasogastric tube does not seem useful except in patients with recurrent vomiting. The treatment of mild AP is summarized in Table 6.1.

Patients with mild pancreatitis can be fed within 5–7 days, as soon as the bowel borborygmus reappears, the pain disappears, and the serum amylase concentration normalizes [1, 2]. Nutrition must be started with low-fat and low-protein meals.

Severe Pancreatitis

Severe pancreatitis represents 10%–20% of all cases of AP. It can cause local and generalized complications and is associated with a variable rate of mortali-

W. Siquini (Ed.), *Surgical Treatment of Pancreatic Diseases.*
©Springer-Verlag Italia 2009

Table 6.1 Medical management of mild acute pancreatitis

Monitoring
Fasting
Fluid/electrolytic support
Analgesia
Nasogastric tube only if patient vomiting

ty between 10 and 35%. This mortality is distributed, on a temporal axis starting at the beginning of the symptoms, in two peaks: the first peak develops within the 1st week and is associated with shock and with multiorgan failure secondary to the systemic inflammatory response syndrome; the second peak develops after the 2nd week and is related to sepsis caused by necrotic pancreatic infection. In accordance with this characteristic disease course, the medical strategy can be divided into:

1. Vital function support
2. Specific therapy aimed at counteracting the physiopathological mechanisms of AP
3. Prevention and treatment of the infective complications

Supportive Therapy

Monitoring

The patient affected by severe pancreatitis presents with a generalized compromised state of health that requires continues monitoring of the principal vital signs. This includes monitoring of the heart rate, blood pressure, urine production, and arterial oxygen saturation.

The central venous access is of fundamental importance because it provides a secure route for liquid infusion as well as the means to measure central venous pressure. A Swan–Ganz catheter is indicated in patients with severe conditions: this catheter provides precise measurement of the heart output and of the left ventricular filling pressure. The fluid balance must be calculated every day, or even at intervals of 8–12 h. The monitoring of vital functions allows clinicians not only to estimate the patient's general outcome, but also to verify the efficacy of treatment and to introduce necessary changes in real time.

The complex management of a patient in shock, the need for invasive monitoring such as with a Swan–Ganz catheter, and the onset of severe complications may require the patient to be transferred to an intensive care unit.

Cardiovascular Support

Severe AP is associated with very significant fluid collection in the third retroperitoneal space and in the bowel because of the paralytic ileus. Because of the retroperitoneal collection, which can be as much as several liters in volume, severe pancreatitis has been defined as the most feared abdominal "chemical burn." The resulting hypovolemia causes hypotension, acute renal failure, and pancreatic hypoperfusion, which aggravates the damage to the pancreas.

The first and most effective therapeutic step is therefore aggressive fluid infusion to maintain the normal intravascular volume. Several authors recommend daily infusion of 4–6 l of isotonic solutions; in some severe cases it may be as much as 10 l [1–3]. The efficacy of the infusion therapy must be checked by monitoring heart rate, blood pressure, and urine production. Fluid balance is also important.

Obviously this high-volume fluid infusion can itself cause congestive heart failure, in particular in patients with heart disease and in those who have developed pulmonary complications. The use of a central venous catheter or Swan–Ganz catheter allows infusions to be calibrated [1, 3].

If there is hypovolemic shock that is not responsive to isotonic fluids, crystalloid solutions and vasoactive drugs such as dopamine can be appropriate. Albumin infusion is indicated if the blood albumin level is less than 2 g/dl. When indicated, blood or coagulation factor transfusions are required [1]. If, in the state of shock, there is a cardiogenic component due to hypoxemia and myocardial depressant factors released during AP, vasoactive drugs may be employed. Several electrolytic disorders (hypochloremia, hypernatremia, hypomagnesemia, and hypocalcemia) can be found in the early phase and be corrected with fluid replacement and electrolytic infusion if necessary. The use of insulin is indicated in severe hyperglycemia [2].

Renal failure is generally corrected with fluid infusion, otherwise dialysis is required [1, 4].

Respiratory Support

Patients with severe AP can develop, usually between the 2nd and the 7th day, adult respiratory distress syndrome (ARDS). This syndrome is caused by alveolus–capillary degeneration due to the action of lipase or phospholipase, by the opening of arteriovenous shunt due to cytokines, by surfactant alteration due to lipolytic enzymes, and by the presence of shock lung factor. Atelectasis, pleural effusions, and pneumonia can also damage the respiratory function. Arterial oxygen saturation must be monitored and maintained above 90%. If oxygen therapy through a mask is not sufficient, assisted ventilation is required [4, 5].

In the presence of ARDS, fluid infusion must be accurately calibrated. These patients, who need invasive hemodynamic monitoring and respiratory support, are generally moved to the intensive care unit.

Analgesic Therapy

Severe AP is often characterized by considerable pain that must be controlled appropriately. Many authors consider the risk of spasm of the sphincter of Oddi to be only theoretical and use opiate drugs such as meperidine, pentazocine, and fentanyl [5, 6].

Specific Therapy

The main physiopathological mechanisms of AP are the damage caused by pancreatic enzymes and the subsequent proinflammatory cascade. Anything that can interfere with these mechanisms may be considered a specific therapy (Table 6.2).

Table 6.2 Specific therapy in acute pancreatitis

Suppression of pancreatic secretion:
    Fasting
    Nasogastric tube
    H_2 antagonists
    Antiacids
    Anticholinergics
    Glucagon
    Calcitonin
    Somatostatin
    Peptide YY
    Cholecystokinin receptor antagonists

Inhibition of pancreatic enzymes:
    Protease inhibitors (aprotinin, gabexate mesilate, camostat, fresh frozen plasma)
    Antifibrinolytics
    Phospholipase A_2 inhibitors

Anti-inflammatory activity:
    Lexipafant
    rh-ACP
    Peritoneal lavage
    Hemofiltration

Protection from oxygen free radicals:
    Xanthine oxidase inhibitors
    Free radical scavengers
    Isovolemic hemodilution

The oldest and most effective treatment is *fasting*, because nourishment is the principal stimulus of pancreatic secretion. Apart from fasting, no specific and really effective therapy has yet been discovered. In experimental pancreatitis, various devices and drugs studied show strong evidence and seem to improve some parameters if employed preventively. However, in clinical trials, none of them has proved to improve the outcome of patients with severe AP.

Pancreatic Secretion Inhibitors

H_2 receptor antagonists, proton pump inhibitors, antacids, and anticholinergic drugs reduce the volume of pancreatic secretion. They inhibit gastric secretion, reducing the passing of gastric acid into the duodenum (like the nasogastric tube). Duodenal acidification is a physiological stimulus for the release of secretin, a hormone that induces the production of pancreatic juice. Although they are employed daily, no trials have demonstrated that these devices can improve the outcome of AP [1, 3].

The use of a nasogastric tube in the case of a vomiting patient is justified, as are the use of H_2 antagonists or proton pump inhibitors to prevent gastritis and ulcers due to stress or to nonsteroidal anti-inflammatory drugs (NSAIDs).

Somatostatin and octreotide have been shown to inhibit gastric and pancreatic secretion in animals and in human subjects with pancreatic fistulas [7]. However, there is no certain evidence that they can be useful in AP [8, 9], except for a few isolated studies which showed a decrease of rate of sepsis, ARDS, and mortality [10, 11],

Among the cholecystokinin receptor antagonists (cholecystokinin is a hormone that induces pancreatic juice production), proglumide has been studied most: its effectiveness has been demonstrated in animals, although not yet tested in humans. The same goes for other molecules such as glucagon, calcitonin, and peptide YY [3].

Inhibitors of Pancreatic Enzyme Activation

Aprotinin, camostat, fresh frozen plasma, antifibrinolytics, and phospholipase A_2 inhibitors belong to the group of pancreatic enzyme activation inhibitors. Like the other treatments mentioned, they are strongly assumed to be therapeutic, but their real effectiveness is poor. Gabexate mesilate is the most studied inhibitor. It appears to have immunomodulating properties through the suppression of proinflammatory cytokines [12]. It has been proved to decrease amylase and phospholipase A_2 activity in the pancreatic juice. In addition, several authors have tested its efficacy in relation to abdominal pain, need for surgery, and mortality [13–15]. Other trials, however, and one meta-analysis did not confirm the effectiveness of gabexate mesilate [11, 16]. We may conclude that this drug, which is certainly useful in preventing AP after endoscopic retrograde cholangiopancreatography, seems to have a marginal role in the management of severe AP.

Techniques Employing Immunomodulating Activity

The abnormal inflammatory response of the body to damage caused by pancreatic enzymes is the basis of several complications of AP. There is a therapeutic window for the employment of anti-inflammatory drugs between the beginning of the symptoms and the development of systemic inflammatory response syndrome.

Several therapies that act against the activity of the proinflammatory mediators have been tested in animals, but not much data is available in humans. PAF (platelet activating factor) is one of the most important proinflammatory cytokines during multiorgan failure. Lexipafant, a PAF antagonist, initially appeared to decrease the rate of multiorgan failure and mortality if given within the first 48 h [17]; however a subsequent trial and a meta-analysis did not confirm its benefits [11, 17]. Use of rh-ACP (recombinant human activated C protein) was able to reduce mortality in patients with severe sepsis, and good results have been obtained in those with AP complicated by infections. However, further studies are necessary before its use can be recommended [17]. Finally, peritoneal lavage and hemofiltration, to remove toxic molecules that mediate several negative systemic effects (such as prostaglandins, histamine, and trypsin), have been proved to have no significant benefits and their use is not widespread nowadays [3, 18].

Protection from Oxygen Free Radicals

Radicals released during AP could contribute to tissue local damage. It has been demonstrated that some molecules such as superoxide dismutase and catalase (which are normally present in the body to protect from damage by radicals) can prevent experimental AP, but they are not effective if administered after the beginning of the pathophysiological process [3].

Prevention and Therapy of Infective Complications

The necrotic pancreatic areas developed in the 1st week of the disease can be colonized by different microorganisms. They are usually gram-negative bacteria that are part of the normal bowel flora, such as *Escherichia coli*, *Pseudomonas* spp., *Klebsiella* spp., *Proteus* spp., *Bacteroides* spp., *Enterococcus* spp., and *Clostridium* spp. More and more, however, nosocomial gram-positive bacteria and fungi are being isolated. Many studies suggest that colonization is possible through microbial translocation. According to this theory, the microorganisms pass through the intestinal mucosa (which is atrophic because it has been resting and because of ischemia) and penetrate into the blood and lymph stream, thus reaching the necrotic tissues.

Infections complicate 15–30% of cases of severe AP and cause sepsis and

multiorgan failure, with a high mortality rate (between 40 and 70%). Two important devices can be employed to prevent this terrible complication:
1. Early enteral feeding, to counteract microbial translocation (see Chapter 29)
2. Antibiotic prophylaxis, to prevent microbial colonization of the necrotic areas of the pancreas

Antibiotic and Antimycotic Prophylaxis

Several trials have demonstrated that i.v. imipenem, carbapenem, third-generation cephalosporin, piperacillin, mezlocillin, fluoroquinolones, and metronidazole penetrate effectively into the pancreatic tissue, whereas aminoglycoside, aminopenicillin, and first-generation cephalosporin do not [1]. The effectiveness and use of these antibiotics in severe AP are supported by clinical trials. Compared with results in an untreated control group, cefuroxime reduced infections and mortality (from 23 to 3%) [19], while a combination of ceftazidime, amikacin, and metronidazole brought sepsis down to zero versus 58% in the control group [20]. Ofloxacin and metronidazole have improved clinical outcome if used prophylactically rather than as treatment after necrosis infection has been demonstrated [21]. At least two trials have demonstrated that imipenem–cilastatin reduces morbidity in terms of multiple organ failure and infective complications [22, 23], and is more effective than pefloxacin [24]. The same results have been obtained with meropenem [25]. This molecule has been demonstrated to reduce the rate of pancreatic and extrapancreatic infection and to reduce the need for surgery if administered once severe AP has been diagnosed, rather than waiting for a diagnosis of pancreatic necrosis, confirming that early employment of the antibiotic is more effective [26]. Finally, at least six meta-analyses, two of them published in 2006, confirm that broad-spectrum antibiotic prophylaxis reduces the rate of sepsis and mortality in severe AP [11, 27–31].

These data, and the reduction of the prevalence of infections over the years from 60% to 15–30%, represent the basis of the assumptions about antibiotic prophylaxis that underlie several authors' opinions about their routine use [1]. Some more recent data, however, do not seem to confirm these conclusions. In 2004, the first randomized, double-blind, placebo-controlled study on this topic was published. No differences in terms of necrosis infection, systemic complications, or mortality were recorded between a patient group treated with ciprofloxacin/metronidazole and the placebo control group [32]. In a similar trial in 2007, it was observed that meropenem did not reduce the incidence of pancreatic and extrapancreatic infection, mortality, or the need for surgery [33]. Finally, a consensus statement concluded that routine use of systemic antibiotics in severe AP was unjustified [17]. What is more, these authors assert that prolonged antibiotic therapy increases the risk of infection from resistant microorganisms, and that it must be proven that the antibiotics can really reach the necrotic pancreatic tissues, since these areas are devascularized [4].

These last data are surely not sufficient basis on which to conclude that antibiotic prophylaxis is not useful: the present authors are convinced that antibiotic prophylaxis must be employed routinely in severe AP. Nevertheless, the inconsistency of the data (summarized in Table 6.3) suggests that, in the future, the use of antibiotic prophylaxis will probably be more selective.

Table 6.3 Main studies on antibiotic prophylaxis in severe acute pancreatitis

Trial	Patient group	Infected	Surgery necrosis %	Sepsis %	Mortality %	Results %
Sainio et al. [19]	30 Cefuroxime	30	23.3	3.3	3.3	Decrease in
	30 control	40	46.6	26.6	23.3	infections and mortality
Delcensire et al. [20]	11 Ceftazidime + amikacin + metronidazole	0	0	0	25	Decrease in infections
	12 control	33	25	58	9	
Schwarz et al. [21]	13 Ofloxacin + metronidazole as prophylaxis	62	–	31	0	"Better outcome"
	13 ofloxacin + metronidazole after diagnosis of infected necrosis	54	–	46	15	
Pederzoli et al. [22]	41 Imipenem	12.2	29.3	26.8	7.3	Decrease in
	33 control	30.3	33.3	78.8	12	MOF and infections
Nordback et al. [23]	25 Imipenem as prophylaxis	8	8	–	8	Decrease in
	33	42	36	–	15	MOF, infected necrosis and imipenem after diagnosis of infected necrosis
Manes et al. [26]	108 Meropenem as prophylaxis	13.3	–	16.6	–	Decrease in infections
	107 meropenem after diagnosis of necrosis	31	–	44.8	–	

continue →

Table 6.3 *continue*

Trial	Patient group	Infected	Surgery necrosis %	Sepsis %	Mortality %	Results %
Isenmann et al. [32]	58 Ciprofloxacin + metronidazole	12	24	–	5 differences	No
	56 placebo	9	17	–	7	
Dellinger et al. [33]	50 Meropenem	18	26	–	20	No differences
	50 placebo	12	20	–	18	

MOF, Multiple organ failure

The infusion of antibiotics into the locoregional arteries and oral antibiotic administration have also been tested. The interesting data obtained need further confirmation, however [3, 34].

More and more frequently – rates as high as 35–37% have been reported [35] – fungi are isolated in severe AP. Some data (not always confirmed) suggest that mycosis worsens mortality, behaving as a independent variable [36]. On this basis, several authors suggest the use of fluconazole, which has been proved to reduce the mycosis rate [35, 37]. At present there is insufficient evidence to support the routine use of antimycotic prophylaxis, but it could be useful in the presence of a high risk of mycotic dissemination (e.g., in patients with acute kidney failure, prolonged broad-spectrum antibiotic therapy, central venous catheters, and mechanical ventilation) [4, 17, 18].

Treatment of Infective Complications

The diagnosis of infected necrosis and pancreatic abscess, suspected on the basis of clinical, laboratory, and imaging data, must be confirmed by percutaneous aspiration of the infected areas. The presence of organisms can be demonstrated in a few minutes using the Gram stain on the specimen, and the culture will suggest which antibiotic will be effective. However, once infection has been demonstrated, the therapy of choice is surgical or percutaneous drainage of the infected areas. The main aspects of medical therapy in severe AP are summarized in Table 6.4.

Conclusions

All cases of mild AP can be cured in 1 week by fasting and e.v. fluid support. Severe AP is a much more complex form of the disease and is characterized by a mortality rate of 10–35%. The multiple organ failure caused by the systemic

Table 6.4 Medical management of severe acute pancreatitis

Close monitoring
Fasting

Cardiovascular support:
    Aggressive fluid/electrolytic replacement
    Vasoactive drugs, albumin, blood transfusions

Respiratory support:
    Oxygen therapy with mask
    Assisted ventilation

Analgesia
Antibiotic prophylaxis
Nutritional support
Antifungal prophylaxis (optional)
Gastric antisecretory drugs to prevent peptic complications
Nasogastric tube if patient vomiting

---

inflammatory response syndrome of the 1st week must be counteracted by supporting the vital functions and, in particular, with aggressive fluid replacement.

At the present date no drugs have been proved to interfere effectively with the inflammatory process. Although data in the literature are not uniform, early enteral feeding and e.v. antibiotic prophylaxis with molecules that are able to penetrate the pancreas are important techniques to prevent sepsis caused by infection of the necrotic pancreatic tissue, which is what causes the multiple organ failure and mortality in the 2nd week of the disease.

References

1. Feldman M, Friedman LS, Sleisenger MH (2004) Malattie dell'apparato gastrointestinale e del fegato: pancreas-vie biliari. Excerpta Medica, Milano
2. Frossard JL, Steer ML, Pastor CM (2008) Acute pancreatitis. Lancet 371 (9618):143–152
3. Sabiston (2003) Trattato di chirurgia: le basi biologiche della moderna pratica chirurgica. (1st italian edn, 16th American edn). Antonio Delfino Editore, Roma[
4. Chipman JG (2005) Acute pancreatitis in the surgical intensive care unit. In: Abrams JH, Druck P, Cerra FB (eds) Surgical critical care, 2nd edn. Taylor & Francis, London
5. Hayden P, Wyncoll D (2008) Severe acute pancreatitis. Curr Anaesth Crit Care 19:1
6. Whang EE (2006) Acute pancreatitis. In: Mulholland MW, Lillemoe KD, Doherty GM et al (eds) Greenfield's surgery: Scientific principles and practice, 4th edn. Lippincott Williams & Wilkins, Philadelphia
7. Caronna R, Diana L, Nofroni I et al (2005) Effects of gabexate mesilate (FOY) on amylase and phospholipase A2 in human serum and pancreatic juice. Dig Dis Sci 50:868–873
8. Uhl W, Büchler MW, Malfertheiner P et al (1999) A randomized, double blind, multicentre trial of octreotide in moderate to severe acute pancreatitis. Gut 45:97–104

9. Heinrich S, Schäfer M, Rousson V, Clavien PA (2006) Evidence-based treatment of acute pancreatitis. A look at established paradigms. Ann Surg 243:154–168

10. Paran H, Mayo A, Paran D et al (2000) Octreotide treatment in patients with severe acute pancreatitis. Dig Dis Sci 45:2247–2251

11. Andriulli A, Leandro G, Clemente R et al (1998) Meta-analysis of somatostatin, octreotide and gabexate mesilate in the therapy of acute pancreatitis. Aliment Pharmacol Ther 12:237–245

12. Pederzoli P, Cavallini G, Falconi M, Bassi C (1993) Gabexate mesilate vs aprotinin in human acute pancreatitis (GA.ME.P.A.). A prospective, randomized, double blind, multi-centre study. Int J Pancreatol 14:117–124

13. Chen HM, Chen JC, Hwang TL et al (2000) Prospective and randomized study of gabexate mesilate for the treatment of severe acute pancreatitis with organ dysfunction. Hepatogastroenterology 47:1147–1150

14. Pezzilli R, Miglioli M (2001) Multicentre comparative study of two schedules of gabexate mesilate treatment of acute pancreatitis. Italian Acute Pancreatitis Study Group. Dig Liver Dis 33:49–57

15. Messori A, Rampazzo R, Scroccaro G et al (1995) Effectiveness of gabexate mesilate in acute pancreatitis. A meta-analysis. Dig Dis Sci 40:734–738

16. Banfi R, Borselli G, Cappelletti S et al (2005) Gabexate mesilate and acute pancreatitis: an experience of evidence based drug information for improving rational drug use. Pharm World Sci 27:121–123

17. Nathens AB, Curtis JR, Beale RJ et al (2004) Management of the critically ill patient with severe acute pancreatitis. Crit Care Med 32:2524–2535

18. Schein M (2005) Acute pancreatitis. In: Schein's common sense emergency abdominal surgery. Springer, Berlin Heidelberg New York

19. Sanio V, Kemppainen E, Puolakkainen P et al (1995) Early antibiotic treatment in acute necrotizing pancreatitis. Lancet 346:663–667

20. Delcensire R, Yzet T, Ducroix JP et al (1996) Prophylactic antibiotics in treatment of severe acute alcoholic pancreatitis. Pancreas 13:198–201

21. Shwarz M, Isenmann R, Meyer H et al (1997) Antibiotic use in necrotizing pancreatitis: results of a controlled study. Dtsh Med Wochenschr 122:356–361

22. Pederzoli P, Bassi S, Vesentini S et al (1993) A randomized multicenter clinical trial of antibiotic prophylaxis of septic complications in acute necrotizing pancreatitis with imipenem. Surg Gynecol Obstet 176:480–483

23. Nordback I, Sand J, Saaristo R et al (2001) Early treatment with antibiotics reduces the need for surgery in acute necrotizing pancreatitis: a single-center randomized study. J Gastrointest Surg 5:113–119

24. Bassi C, Falconi M, Talamini G et al (1998) A controlled clinical trial of pefloxacin versus imipenem in severe acute pancreatitis. Gastroenterology 115:1513–1517

25. Manes G, Rabitti PG, Menchise A et al (2003) Prophylaxis with meropenem of septic complications in acute pancreatitis: a randomized, controlled trial versus imipenem. Pancreas 27:79–83

26. Manes G, Uomo I, Menchise A et al (2006) Timing of antibiotic prophylaxis in acute pancreatitis: a controlled randomized study with meropenem. Am J Gastroenterol 101:1348–1353

27. Golub R, Siddiqi F, Pohl D (1998) Role of antibiotics in acute pancreatitis: a meta-analysis. J Gastrointest Surg 2:496–503

28. Bassi C, Larvin M, Villatoro E (2003) Antibiotic therapy for prophylaxis against infection of pancreatic necrosis in acute pancreatitis. Cochrane Database Syst Rev 4:CD002941

29. Sharma VK, Howden CW (2001) Prophylactic antibiotic administration reduces sepsis and mortality in acute necrotizing pancreatitis: a meta-analysis. Pancreas 22:28–31

30. Zhou YM, Xue ZL, Li Ym et al (2005) Antibiotic prophylaxis in patients with severe acute pancreatitis. Hepatobiliary Pancreat Dis Int 4:23–27

31. Villatoro E, Bassi C, Larvin M (2006) Antibiotic therapy for prophylaxis against infection of pancreatic necrosis in acute pancreatitis. Cochrane Database Syst Rev 4:CD002941
32. Isenmann R, Runzi M, Kron M (2004) Prophylactic antibiotic treatment in patients with predicted severe acute pancreatitis: a placebo-controlled, double blind trial. Gastroenterology 126:997–1004
33. Dellinger EP, Tellado JM, Soto NE et al (2007) Early antibiotic treatment for severe acute necrotizing pancreatitis: a randomized, double blind, placebo-controlled study. Ann Surg 245:674–683
34. Luiten EJT, Hop WCJ, Lange JF et al (1995) Controlled clinical trial of selective decontamination for the treatment of severe acute pancreatitis. Ann Surg 222:57–65
35. De Waele JJ, Vogelaers D, Blot S et al (2003) Fungal infections in patients with severe acute pancreatitis and the use of prophylactic therapy. Clin Infect Dis 37:208–213
36. Grewe M, Tsiotos GG, Luque de Leon E et al (1999) Fungal infection in acute necrotizing pancreatitis. J Am Coll Surg 188:408–414
37. He YM, Lu XS, Ai ZL et al (2003) Prevention and therapy of fungal infection in severe acute pancreatitis: a prospective clinical study. World J Gastroenterol 9:2619–2621

Chapter 7

Endoscopic Retrograde Cholangiopancreatography and Endoscopic Sphincterotomy in Acute Pancreatitis: Indications and Technique

Emanuele Bendia, Marco Marzioni, Antonio Benedetti, Antonio Di Sario

Introduction

Acute pancreatitis is a disease of increasing annual incidence which is associated with significant morbidity and mortality. While many patients need only a general supportive care, about one out of five patients will develop severe acute pancreatitis, and 20% of these patients may die [1, 2].

The management of acute pancreatitis has evolved over several decades, and many treatments that were considered essential in the past have subsequently been abandoned on the basis of more recent findings from clinical trials. However, the proper management of patients with acute pancreatitis has not been fully established.

The prediction of severe disease before its onset is best achieved by careful ongoing clinical assessment coupled with the use of a multiple factor scoring system and imaging studies. The Acute Physiology and Chronic Health Evaluation II (APACHE II) system is preferred; patients with predicted or actual severe disease and those with other associated co-morbidities should be strongly considered for triage to an intensive care unit or intermediate medical care unit.

Usually the etiology of acute pancreatitis can be established in at least 75% of patients. Although gallstone pancreatitis is the most common cause of acute pancreatitis, other etiologies (alcohol intake, hypertriglyceridemia or hypercalcemia, family history of pancreatic disease, drugs, trauma, and autoimmune diseases) must be considered. A detailed history and careful physical examination are obviously the first step toward making the diagnosis.

Laboratory investigations are critical for diagnosis, as well as for predicting the prognosis. Documenting elevated serum amylase and/or lipase levels is helpful in diagnosing acute pancreatitis. Serum amylase, however, lacks specificity since it can be elevated in other disorders, such as ischemic or obstructed bowel and perforated gastric or duodenal ulcer [3]. Serum amylase can also be elevated in salivary disorders, renal insufficiency, ectopic pregnancy, and ovarian tumors. Serum lipase has a longer half-life than amylase and is more specific for acute pancreatitis [3]. Using a cut-off of three times the upper limit of normal,

W. Siquini (Ed.), *Surgical Treatment of Pancreatic Diseases.*
©Springer-Verlag Italia 2009

the sensitivity of serum lipase for pancreatitis approaches 90% in patients presenting with abdominal pain [4]. Several tests can help to differentiate biliary pancreatitis from other causes of pancreatitis. Aspartate aminotransferase (AST), alanine aminotransferase (ALT), alkaline phosphatase, and serum bilirubin are measures of liver function and should be reviewed before a confident diagnosis can be made. It has been shown that a serum ALT level greater than 150 IU/l has a 96% specificity for acute gallstone pancreatitis but only a 48% sensitivity [5]. Triglyceride and calcium levels should also be measured; if triglyceride levels cannot be obtained at admission, fasting triglyceride levels should be measured after recovery when the patient has resumed a normal diet.

Abdominal ultrasonography should be performed at admission to look for cholelithiasis or choledocholithiasis. The presence of choledocholithiasis on transabdominal ultrasound is relatively specific, although the sensitivity is low. If abdominal ultrasonography is not diagnostic for gallstone pancreatitis, endoscopic ultrasonography can be used as an accurate alternative approach to screen for cholelithiasis and choledocholithiasis, either at admission or thereafter.

Computed tomography (CT) may have a sensitivity as high as 80% for the detection of biliary stones [6]; however, sometimes CT can be less sensitive than abdominal ultrasound. Although CT scans can be normal in 15–20% of patients with mild acute pancreatitis, a CT scan obtained within the first 3–4 days of onset of symptoms has a 90% sensitivity for detecting pancreatic necrosis [7]. Anyway, CT should be reserved for those patients in whom the diagnosis is in doubt, or when severe pancreatitis is suspected or when conservative management fails.

The management of acute pancreatitis is usually conservative, including bowel rest and intravenous fluid replacement; the placement of a nasogastric tube should be reserved for those patients who present with intractable vomiting or severe nausea. Careful calculation of ongoing fluid losses is essential to ensure adequate replacement and to correct electrolyte and metabolic abnormalities. Strong analgesia is almost always required and usually consists of administration of morphine or meperidine. Nutritional support should be provided if patients remain on "nothing by mouth" for more than 7 days.

Endoscopic Treatment of Gallstone Pancreatitis

Urgent (within 24 h) endoscopic retrograde cholangiopancreatography (ERCP) should be performed in patients with gallstone pancreatitis who have concomitant cholangitis. Early ERCP (within 72 h) should be performed in those with a high suspicion of a persistent common bile duct stone (visible common bile duct stone on noninvasive imaging, persistently dilated common bile duct, jaundice). Endoscopic sphincterotomy in the absence of choledocholithiasis at the time of the procedure is a reasonable therapeutic option, but data supporting this practice are lacking.

Early ERCP in those with predicted or actual severe gallstone pancreatitis in the absence of cholangitis or a high suspicion of a persistent common bile duct stone is controversial; in addition, routine preoperative ERCP cannot be recommended, since the risk of complications might outweigh the potential benefits. In the presence of concomitant cholelithiasis, definitive surgical management (cholecystectomy) should be performed in the same hospital admission if possible, otherwise no later than 2–4 weeks after discharge.

Endoscopic Sphincterotomy

Endoscopic sphincterotomy (ES) has revolutionized the approach to patients with biliary tract and pancreatic diseases and can be performed on the biliary and pancreatic sphincters for a variety of indications, such as removal of stones, as part treatment of strictures, to facilitate placement of stents, for closure of ductal leaks, and so on [8]. Pancreatic sphincterotomy has been increasingly performed for the treatment of papillary stenosis, sphincter of Oddi dysfunction, and for chronic and acute recurrent pancreatitis. Minor papillotomy is most often performed for acute recurrent pancreatitis associated with pancreas divisum and for chronic pancreatitis [8]. Sometimes ES is also performed in order to obtain diagnosis, for example in patients in whom traditional noninvasive methods cannot identify a cause for their acute pancreatitis.

After biliary and/or pancreatic ducts are visualized, the sphincter is cut using a sphincterotome. The size of the incision is generally decided on the basis of the shape of the papilla, the size of stones, and the absence or presence of stones in the common bile duct, and may vary from 0.5 to 1 cm in length [9].

The main complications are acute pancreatitis (1.3–3.3%), bleeding (1.2–3.1%), cholangitis (0.9–2.7%), and perforation (0.4–2.1%). Usually most complications can be treated by a conservative therapy; surgery is necessary in less than 20–25% of cases, and death occurs in 0.2–1.3% of patients. Patient-related factors, such as age and underlying co-morbidities, are considerable determinants of complication risk. Complications are less frequent, but not fully eliminated, with an experienced endoscopist or an expert in the field.

When the access to the biliary duct is blocked in some manner (e.g., an impacted stone) a pre-cut biliary sphincterotomy can be performed to allow access to the biliary duct without prior deep cannulation. Once the biliary duct is accessed, conventional biliary sphincterotomy can be performed. Most endoscopists generally use a freehand needle-knife to perform the pre-cut, although there are several options for this technique [10].

The role of the different kinds of cut (pure cut vs. mixed cut) has been extensively studied, and results of three randomized trials have shown that the occurrence of acute pancreatitis is lower when the pure cut is used (3.5% vs. 11.9%). The new electrosurgical generators at present available in most endoscopic units allow better control of the endoscopic incision ("step by step cut").

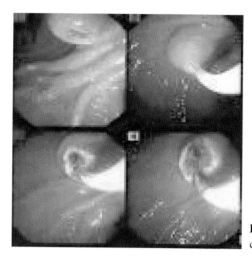

Fig. 7.1 Endoscopic sphincterotomy after cannulation of the papilla

Conclusions

ERCP is a useful tool in the evaluation and management of acute pancreatitis. The main role of ERCP in this clinical disorder is represented by the diagnosis and treatment of biliary tract stone disease and other potential causes of pancreatic duct obstruction. When endoscopic sphincterotomy is performed within 24 h in patients with severe acute pancreatitis, the morbidity and mortality rates (3 and 13%, respectively) are lower than those described in patients treated with a conservative medical therapy (28 and 54%, respectively) [11–14]. Therefore, with the advent of less invasive and safer diagnostic modalities, ERCP is becoming a therapeutic tool in the management of acute pancreatitis and its complications.

References

1. Lee SP, Maher K, Nicholls JF (1988) Origin and fate of biliary sludge. Gastroenterology 94:170–176
2. Lee SP, Nicholls JF, Park HZ (1992) Biliary sludge as a cause of acute pancreatitis. N Engl J Med 326:589–593
3. Agarwal N, Pitchumoni C, Sivaprasad A (1990) Evaluating tests for acute pancreatitis. Am J Gastroenterol 85:356–366
4. Clavien P, Burgan S, Moossa A (1989) Serum enzymes and other laboratory tests in acute pancreatitis. Br J Surg 76:1234–1238
5. Tenner S, Dubner H, Steinberg W (1994) Predicting gallstone pancreatitis with laboratory parameters: a meta-analysis. Am J Gastroenterol 89:1863–1866
6. Baron RL, Stanley RJ, Lee JK et al (1983) Computed tomography features of biliary obstruction. Am J Roentgenol 140:1173–1178
7. Balthazar E, Robinson D, Megibow A, Ranson JHC (1990) Acute pancreatitis: value of CT in establishing prognosis. Radiology 174:331–336

8. Freeman ML, Guda NM (2005) Endoscopic biliary and pancreatic sphincterotomy. Curr Treat Opin Gastroenterol 8:127–134
9. Li ZH, Chen M, Liu JK et al (2005) Endoscopic sphincterotomy in the treatment of cholangiopancreatic diseases. World J Gastroenterol 11:2678–2680
10. Freeman ML, Guda NM (2005) ERCP cannulation: a review of reported techniques. Gastrointest Endosc 61:112–125
11. Fan ST, Lai ECS, Mok FPT et al (1993) Early treatment of acute biliary pancreatitis by endoscopic papillotomy. N Engl J Med 328:228–232
12. Fan ST, Lai ECS, Mok FPT et al (1988) Controlled trial of urgent endoscopic retrograde cholangiopancreatography and endoscopic sphincterotomy versus conservative treatment for acute pancreatitis due to gallstones. Lancet 2:979–983
13. Van Steenbergen W (1996) Acute and chronic pancreatitis in the ederly patients. Tijdschr Gerontol Geriatr 27:191–196
14. Uomo G, Manes G, Laccetti M et al (1997) Endoscopic sphincterotomy and recurrence of acute pancreatitis in gallstone patients considered unfit for surgery. Pancreas 14:28–31

Chapter 8

Indications, Timing, and Techniques in the Surgical Treatment of Acute Pancreatitis

Walter Siquini, Gianluca Guercioni, Raffaella Ridolfo, Aroldo Fianchini

Introduction

Today acute pancreatitis still occupies one of the top positions among the so-called "benign" diseases which are, nevertheless, associated with high morbidity and mortality. Although 80–90% of cases of acute pancreatitis are of the *mild* type (MAP), i.e., they are self-limiting, spontaneously resolving within 5–7 days with minimal treatment ("a 1-week disease"), 10–20% of patients develop necrotizing *severe* acute pancreatitis (SAP), which carries a mortality of up to 30% [1, 2]. Treatment of SAP has been debated since the end of the 1800s, contrasting a conservative medical "wait and see" approach on the one hand against aggressive surgery on the other. At the end of the 1980s and for the first few years of the 1990s the following axiom ruled: "Edematous pancreatitis: medical therapy; necrotic pancreatitis: immediate surgery" [3, 4]. However, the unsettling results and high mortality rates that resulted from treatment following this paradigm soon led to debate about how appropriate it was. In the following years, the wider availability of CT scans with contrast and the Balthazar score made it possible to identify the extent of the necrosis and to apply a grading system to the severity of the illness [5]; furthermore, monoparametric prognostics (CRP, procalcitonin, IL-6) and multiparametric scores (Ranson, Glasgow, Apache II) were introduced, improving clinicians' ability to predict the severity of the illness.

In 1992, to solve the problem over terminology confusion which then existed, making comparison of the available results impossible, the Atlanta Consensus Meeting issued in unanimous agreement the classification of acute pancreatitis and a list of its possible complications, early and late, localized and systemic [6]. The conditions and parameters which make it possible to identify the severe forms of acute pancreatitis (Table 8.1) were also listed. In the last 20 years, therefore, tremendous developments have been achieved, with far better knowledge of the physiopathology, natural course, and complications of SAP [7], and a better understanding of the systemic inflammatory response syndrome (Table 8.2) and multiple organ dysfunction syndrome (Table 8.2), which, together with advances made in the intensive medical treatment of such conditions, have meant crucial progress in the planning of both conservative and surgical

W. Siquini (Ed.), *Surgical Treatment of Pancreatic Diseases.*
©Springer-Verlag Italia 2009

Table 8.1 Criteria by which to define *severe* acute pancreatitis

Acute pancreatitis is severe in the presence of one or more of the following:
Local complications
- Sterile pancreatic necrosis >30%
- Infected pancreatic necrosis
- Acute fluid collections
- Pseudocysts
- Pancreatic abscess
- Hemoperitoneum
- Pancreatic ascites
- Thrombosis of the splenic and portal vein
- Arterial pseudoaneurysms

Systemic complications
- Shock (systemic arterial pressure <90 mmHg)
- Respiratory failure (PaO_2 <60 mmHg)
- Renal failure(creatinine >2.9 mg/dl)
- Multiorgan dysfunction
- Septic shock
- Abdominal compartment syndrome

Multiparametric scores
- Ranson score ≥3
- Apache II score ≥8

Monoparametric score
- C-reactive protein >150 mg/dl

CT staging according to Balthazar
- Stage D–E

Table 8.2 Criteria by which to define systemic inflammatory response syndrome (SIRS) and multiorgan dysfunction syndrome (MODS)

SIRS: Presence of two or more of the following:
- Temperature >38 °C or <36 °C
- Heart rate >90 bpm
- Respiratory rate >20/min
- Pa_{CO_2} <32
- Leukocytes >12,000 or <4000/ml
- Immature neutrophils >10%

MODS: SIRS + one of the following:
- Acute respiratory distress syndrome
- Acute renal failure
- Hypotension
- Disseminated intravascular coagulation
- Acute hepatitis
- Metabolic encephalopathy
- Paralytic ileus

therapeutic strategies and in the production of well-defined diagnostic–therapeutic algorithms. It has been definitively established that in SAP the key prognostic factor with a negative influence on outcome is *superinfection of sterile pancreatic necrosis* [8, 9]. It is in this particular context that surgery plays a crucial role, and there is a unanimous view in literature that, given the presence of infected pancreatic necrosis, surgery is absolutely necessary [10–16]. Despite improvements in the definition of indications, timing, and the development of new surgical strategies over the past 30 years, however, a number of indications for surgical intervention are still debated today between different surgical schools: for instance, the controversy over the ideal timing, and over what operating strategy should represent the gold standard.

Natural History and Physiopathology of Acute Pancreatitis

The treatment of SAP requires in-depth knowledge of the natural history and physiopathology of the disease, which are indispensable to planning the correct therapeutic strategy, whether medical or surgical. Classically, pancreatologists divide SAP into two distinct physiopathological phases, each of which carries its own mortality risk [12].

Phase I or the *systemic inflammatory response syndrome* (SIRS) phase occurs during the 1st week from the beginning of the symptoms and is characterized by the presence of enzymes in the blood stream, acute inflammation, and hemodynamic instability. The early stage of acute pancreatitis is characterized by activation of a proteolytic enzyme cascade inside the pancreatic acinar cells. Activation of trypsin is followed by the activation of other zymogens (phospholipase, elastase, chymotrypsin, etc.), complement, the kinin-kallikrein system, coagulation, and the fibrinolytic cascade. Thus, a vicious circle begins in which the activated enzymes cause cell destruction, which is followed by recruitment and activation of inflammation cells (macrophages and polymorphonuclear cells) which, in their turn, release a wide range of proinflammatory cytokines (TNF, IL-1, IL-6, IL-8, PAF, prostaglandin, leukotrienes). This complex cytokine and enzymatic chain of events, which is still not completely understood in terms of molecular interactions, causes both self-digestion and necrosis of the pancreas, and the activation of a florid SIRS which can rapidly lead to multiorgan dysfunction and death [7]. The systemic consequences of the proinflammatory cytochemical SIRS-induced cascade can in fact cause renal, pulmonary, and cardiovascular failure, and correlate directly with the amount of "enzymatic and cytokine broth" released into the peritoneal cavity, the retroperitoneum, and systemic blood circulation.

The specific factors and molecular events which determine whether an acute pancreatitis episode will be self-limiting or whether it will progress into a necrotizing, perhaps fulminant form are as yet unknown. Unfortunately, neutralizing drugs able to counteract the inflammatory cascade induced by pancreatic necrosis and SIRS-induced multiorgan failure are not yet available, and in all randomized trials, both the pancreatic autodigestion inhibitors (aprotinin, gabexate mesilate), inhibitors of pancreatic secretions (somatostatin, octreotide), and inhibitors of the proinflammatory cytochemical cascade (PAF inhibitors) have been shown to be ineffective and virtually useless in reducing the mortality of SAP [11, 14, 16]. Today, however, thanks mainly to top-notch intensive care, the majority of patients get through phase I of SAP.

Phase II, or the *necrotizing infection* phase, takes place after the 2nd week from the beginning of symptoms (generally between the 2nd and the 4th weeks) and is characterized by deterioration of the patient's general condition combined with symptoms and signs of sepsis. Superinfection of the necrotic area is found in 30–70% of patients with necrotic acute pancreatitis, and the risk of infection increases depending on the intra- and extrapancreatic extent of the necrosis [2, 12–17]. Although large areas of necrosis can spontaneously self-heal, superinfection of necrotic areas does represents the single most important prognostic factor in SAP; it is the major risk factor for sepsis-related multiorgan failure, and also the main life-threatening risk factor in the second phase of the disease [8, 9]. The origins of the infective process can be traced to the microbial translocation. Hypotension, fasting, and the circulatory and inflammatory alterations during SAP lead to loss of the barrier function of the intestine, promoting the spreading of microorganisms (bacterial, fungal, and viral) from the enteric lumen into the systemic circulation and also into the areas of necrosis of the pancreas, with activation of a self-maintaining infective process [18]. It has been demonstrated during SAP that intestinal permeability is increased and can be related to endotoxinemia, multiorgan failure, and mortality [19]. The presence of gram-negative bacteria and intestinal anaerobes in pancreatic infections supports the assumption of such origins. Pancreatic necrosis develops within 4 days of the onset of symptoms; SIRS, however, usually develops in the absence of significant pancreatic necrosis and in fact is more commonly present in patients with noninfected pancreatic necrosis [12].

Mortality in SAP follows a two-phase trend and is attributable to different causes during those two phases. Early mortality (week 1) is mainly due to the systemic consequences of SIRS (multiple organ failure) following acute pancreatitis. The second peak, a few weeks after onset, also ends in multiorgan failure triggered by systemic sepsis secondary to the pancreatic necrosis infection. By different mechanisms, SIRS (early onset) and sepsis (later) can both lead to multiorgan failure, which is the common terminal stage before death. Treatment must be completely different in the two phases: conservative medical in phase I (except in rare exceptions which will be described later), whereas surgery must be considered in phase II [12–16].

Indications for Surgery

Indications for surgery in SAP have evolved considerably over the last 30 years. Up until the beginning of the early 1990s, the view held was that, once acute necrotic pancreatitis had been diagnosed (Fig. 8.1), immediate surgery should ensue if the patient was to have any chance of a cure [3, 4]. The rationale was to prevent the onset of superinfection of the necrosis by removing the source of the toxins and the chemical mediators of the inflammation. However, early peritoneal washing, performed with the aim of removing enzymes and cytokines from the peritoneal cavity and reducing their systemic absorption, did not lead to any reduction in mortality in clinical trials [20–22] (Table 8.3). Similarly, hemofiltration, despite undoubtedly removing the harmful chemical mediators released during SAP, still has to prove any efficacy. Following disappointing results obtained from early surgery (Table 8.4), attitudes changed, partly because it was also clearly seen that patients with sterile necrosis might actually get better without surgical intervention [1]. Currently there is a strong leaning towards

Table 8.3 Use of peritoneal lavage in severe acute pancreatitis

Study	Treatment	Number	Complications (%)	Mortality (%)
Teerenhovi et al. [20]	Control	12	50	17
	Lavage	12	73	36
Ihse et al. [21]	Control	20	30	5
	Lavage	19	42	21
Mayer [22]	Control	46	28	35
	Lavage	45	27	38

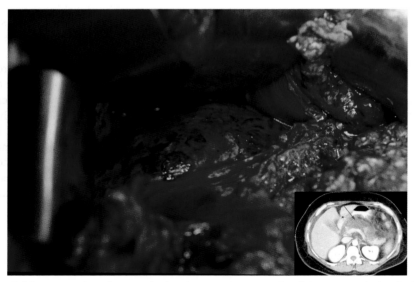

Fig. 8.1 Intraoperative photograph showing massive necrosis of the pancreatic head, also visible on CT scan with contrast (*arrow*)

Table 8.4 Results of conservative and surgical treatment in severe acute pancreatitis

	Indication for surgery	Group	No. of patients	Treatment	Mortality n	%
Open packing						
Bradley and Allen [1]	Infected necrosis	Infected necrosis	27	Surgery	4/27	14.8
		Sterile necrosis	11	Conservative	0/11	0
Tsiotos et al. [27]	Failure of medical treatment	Infected necrosis	57	Surgery	13/57	22.8
		Sterile necrosis	15	Surgery	5/15	33.3
Mier et al. [25]	Failure of medical treatment	Early	25	Surgery	14/25	56
		Late	11	Surgery	3/11	27.3
Nordback et al. [23]	Infected necrosis, multiple organ failure		22	Surgery	5/22	22.7
			11	Conservative	0/11	0
Kalfarentzos et al. [24]	Infected necrosis	Infected necrosis	7	Surgery	1/7	14.3
		Sterile necrosis	19	Conservative	1/19	5.3
Closed technique						
Büchler et al. [8]	Infected necrosis	Infected necrosis	27	Surgery	7/27	25.9
		Sterile necrosis	56	Conservative	1/56	1.8
Beger et al. [26]	Failure of medical treatment	Infected necrosis	37	Surgery	5/37	14
		Sterile necrosis	52	Surgery	3/52	6
Cumulative data						
Indications for surgery	Sterile necrosis		67	Surgery	8/67	11.9
			86	Conservative	2/86	2.3
Surgical technique	Infected necrosis		138	Open packing	37/138	26.8
			64	Closed technique	12/64	18.8

conservative treatment, given the better results demonstrated by this strategy [1, 8, 23, 24]. Heinrich et al. [11] carried out a recent review that included all the prospective studies available [1, 8, 23–28], although the lack of randomized studies does not allow statistically significant meta-analysis, and showed that in 153 patients with sterile necrosis, surgical treatment carried a higher mortality rate (11.9%) than conservative treatment (2.3%).

Nowadays all authors agree that the most common cause of mortality due to SAP is related to multiple organ failure secondary to the systemic sepsis triggered by the superinfection in pancreatic necrosis. Infection of pancreatic or peripancreatic tissue, or both, is in fact generally lethal if not operated on; historic data suggest a mortality approaching 100% in the presence of nonsurgically treated infection of the necrotic areas, whereas if surgery is carried out, mortality falls into a range somewhere between 14 and 30% [12, 16]. Since superinfection of pancreatic necrosis is the most important prognostic factor linked to an unfavorable outcome, it is now unanimously agreed that documented infected necrosis is an *absolute indication* for surgical necrosectomy [10–16].

Early recognition of infected pancreatic necrosis is the basic requirement for surgery which must be performed immediately [9]. Infected necrotic material, which is of a clayey texture, with necrotic foci and dense fluid collection areas, does not generally leave room for ultrasound- or CT-guided percutaneous drainage procedures. Infection of the necrotic tissue in SAP shows up generally (but not only) between the 2nd and 4th weeks after the beginning of symptoms; the appearance, after this sort of interval, of symptoms and clinical signs of sepsis and generalized deterioration (temperature >38 °C, pain, leukocytosis, and increased CRP levels) must raise the suspicion of necrosis infection [12, 13, 29, 30]. Since the occurrence of necrosis infection has a negative impact on the survival rate, it becomes critical to differentiate between sterile and infected necrosis and the patient must undergo an abdominal CT scan with contrast, which, apart from showing the extent of the necrosis, can also pick up the presence of small gas bubbles (Fig. 8.2) – a pathognomonic sign of superinfection from anaerobic germs [12–16, 31]. Unfortunately, anaerobic species account for only 15–33% of all cases of infection, and gas may not appear in the majority of the remaining cases. The only diagnostic procedure available is then ultrasound- or CT-guided fine-needle aspiration (FNA) of the necrotic areas suspected of infection, with subsequent microbiological culture and perhaps antibiotic sensitivity studies. This method is accurate, safe, complication-free, and has high sensitivity and specificity (88% and 90%, respectively) [32, 33]. The necrosis-superinfecting germs are generally gram-negative and anaerobes of intestinal origin, but recent research has also revealed an increase in the incidence of nosocomial and multiresistant gram-positive bacteria [34]. In the opinion of a few authors, needle aspiration is not always necessary: a septic state not linked to central line infection, pneumonia, or cystitis is in itself enough grounds to warrant a surgical approach [2, 8, 9]. After 2–3 weeks of aggressive medical therapy where SIRS has been controlled, the subsequent therapeutic strategy will depend on the presence or absence of infection. If the patient improves and there is no infec-

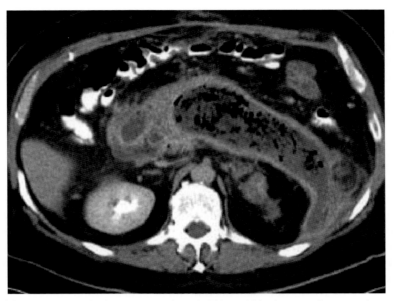

Fig. 8.2 CT scan reveals the presence of gas bubbles within the area of pancreatic necrosis, which is pathognomonic of superinfection

tion, the approach continues to be minimally invasive, whereas documented presence of infected necrosis dictates the surgical intervention route [11–16].

Another undisputed indication for surgery is the presence of hemoperitoneum (Fig. 8.3), a life-threatening complication which is found in 1–3% of cases of SAP [12]. Arterial pseudoaneurysms at high risk of bleeding complicate 10% of SAP cases. In these cases where early and curative treatment can be life-saving, arteriography with embolization is the gold standard of treatment. Generally, massive bleeding means there is no other option left but emergency laparotomy, which generally ends with packing and laparostomy, and a subsequent intervention to correct the hemostasis. Since infected necrosis can in itself be a cause of serious bleeding, some authors recommend arteriography, if necessary with embolization [12], after any necrosectomy for hemoperitoneum.

Other unquestionable indications for a surgical approach are *bacterial peritonitis due to intestinal perforation* and *pancreatic abscess*. For the latter, which is a later complication of SAP, the current accepted gold standard of treatment is ultrasound- or CT-guided percutaneous drainage. In fact, if an abscess forms after the 4th to 5th week, when the acute inflammation process has resolved, liquefaction has been well restrained, and the entire process seems less aggressive than infected necrosis, effective and curative drainage is generally possible with just a percutaneous approach [12–16].

These days, phase I of SAP is generally survived by the vast majority of patients thanks to vigorous rehydration and to modern techniques of intensive

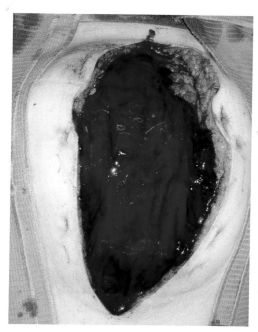

Fig. 8.3 Massive hemoperitoneum complicating severe acute pancreatitis

care. There are, however, rare cases of SIRS in which rapidly progressive multiple organ failure occurs in the first few days despite maximum intensive therapy. These are the "most seriously ill of the seriously ill" patients, and the speed with which the clinical picture can worsen is so awesome that it has become known as *fulminant acute pancreatitis* (Fig. 8.4). In these desperate cases, a surgical attempt is in principle justified, with the aim of removing the retroendoperitoneal enzymatic and cytokine broth that is causing the toxemia. Owing to the small number of cases in this subgroup of patients, it is impossible to obtain statistically significant data, though experience from nonrandomized studies indicates that there is no difference between the mortality of those who undergo surgery and those who do not [2]. Theoretically, peritoneal lavage, possibly combined with hemodialysis, should play a beneficial role, but its efficacy in reducing the risk of death is so far unproven [20–22]. Because of the poor results from both surgery and conservative treatment, the optimum treatment for this patient subgroup has not been defined and surgery is the last resort.

In fact, laparotomy has now been practically abandoned in stage 1 of SAP in favor of conservative treatment, with only two exceptions: fulminant acute pancreatitis and the *abdominal compartment syndrome* [11–14]. In the latter, the swelling of the pancreas, the fluid collections, the spread of fluids retro- and endoperitoneally, and the SIRS-induced edema of the intestines can create intra-abdominal hypertension. When *abdominal compartment syndrome,* combined with multiorgan failure, complicates a case of SAP, the abdomen must be quickly decompressed (laparostomy).

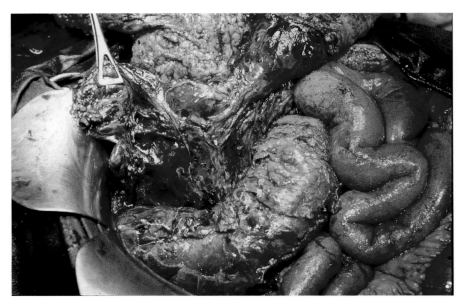

Fig. 8.4 Intraoperative photograph showing fulminant acute pancreatitis

Other indications for surgery are the subject of debate amongst the different schools of surgery. In particular, the role of surgery in patients with sterile necrosis continues to be controversial. Some authors maintain that *sterile pancreatic necrosis >50%* (Fig. 8.1) is an indication for early laparotomy, in that its removal would reduce the risk of infection and early necrosectomy would limit the release into the circulation of toxic substances and proinflammatory chemical mediators, with improvement in the SIRS [2]. In reality, with early surgical intervention, the risk of infecting sterile necrosis has been proven to be around 30%, and the release of proinflammatory cytokines in acute pancreatitis seem to occur so early that surgery cannot intervene in the various cytokine cascade systems which contribute to SIRS [12]. If, on the other hand, a patient with sterile necrosis is responding to medical treatment, surgery seems to worsen the prognosis compared with conservative treatment [11–16]. The majority of experts believe that the extent of the necrosis alone, in the absence of systemic complications (septic shock, hemodynamic instability), should not be considered an indication for surgery as it was in the early 1990s. Bradley and Allen [1] report that among 38 patients with sterile necrosis who were treated conservatively, the survival rate was 100%, and numerous other documented reviews demonstrate reduced mortality in the presence of sterile necrosis treated conservatively as opposed to surgically (2.3% vs. 11.9%) [11]. However, once sterile necrosis becomes complicated by organ failures, many authors do then support surgery. The occurrence of single or multiple organ failure in SAP is associated with a varying mortality rate between 23 and 75% [12]. In patients with *sterile necrosis and progressive systemic deterioration* despite intensive care, surgical treatment is accepted as the norm [11–16]. In any case, however, the patient who is not improving should be treated conservatively for as long as possible, at least 2 or 3 weeks, which should allow good demarcation of the necrotic area, making operation simpler should it become necessary.

Chemical peritonitis from cytokine–enzymatic irritation should also be carefully assessed, given that it generally tends to improve as the days go by. Peritoneal involvement alone, in the presence of firmly diagnosed SAP, is not an absolute indication to proceed with laparotomy. On the contrary, since laparotomy in SAP with sterile necrosis can have a negative impact on the natural course of the disease, increasing the risk of infection and death, laparotomy for peritonitis of uncertain etiology should not be performed until a diagnosis of acute pancreatitis has been ruled out.

For some authors, *complete rupture of the duct of Wirsung* is perceived as an indication for major surgery. In reality, trusting in the tremendous self-healing capacity of the pancreas, it is surely wiser to play the waiting game and drain a pancreatic pseudocyst some 2–3 months later (which represents the natural evolution of rupture of the duct when contained by reaction of the neighboring tissues), rather than treating the lesion in the acute stage, even more so if the proposed strategy includes extensive tissue demolition.

If the trigger of the acute pancreatitis is choledocholithiasis, in the presence of obstructive icterus, cholangitis, and either suspected or confirmed biliary origin, endoscopic retrograde cholangiopancreatography with endoscopic sphincterotomy to clear the main biliary system is mandatory within 48–72 h, in order to avoid the vicious circle of events that causes pancreatic damage to become independent from the primary etiological factor (see Chapter 7). Four randomized studies have demonstrated the efficacy of this treatment in terms of morbidity and mortality [35–38]. If endoscopic clearance of the papilla fails on two different attempts by two different operators (fortunately a very rare occurrence), and the gallstone remains trapped in the papilla, this is an indication for surgery with surgical clearance of the common bile duct and its external drainage by positioning a Kehr's T-tube with inferior choledochal branch nontranspapillary.

In all cases of acute pancreatitis of biliary origin, cholecystectomy should be considered to prevent relapse. In mild forms of the disease, this should be carried out via laparoscopy within the same hospital admission and possibly 4–6 days after the beginning of the symptoms; discharging the patient and delaying the cholecystectomy for 6 weeks runs a 50–70% risk of recurrence of the pancreatitis. On the other hand, in the severe, nonoperated forms, video-laparoscopic cholecystectomy should be carried out, without any increased risk, 6 weeks after discharge, which gives enough time for the inflammation to settle [11, 12, 14, 16]. Indications for surgery, both the accepted ones and those which are still the subject of debate, are listed in Table 8.5.

Table 8.5 Indications for surgery in severe acute pancreatitis

Unquestioned indications	Debated indications
Documented, infected necrosis	Sterile necrosis >30–50%
Sterile necrosis and irreversible clinical deterioration	SAP with biliary etiology and ERCP failure
Massive hemoperitoneum	Chemical peritonitis
Bacterial peritonitis from intestinal perforation	Complete rupture of the duct of Wirsung
Fulminant acute pancreatitis	Sterile necrosis with MODS without clinical improvement
Pancreatic abscess	
Abdominal compartment	

SAP, severe acute pancreatitis; *ERCP*, endoscopic retrograde cholangiopancreatography; *MODS*, multiple organ dysfunction

Surgical Timing

Although necrosectomy is crucial in the treatment of patients with SAP, ideal timing of the operation is equally important. In the 1980s the rule was early surgery in the presence of necrotizing acute pancreatitis. Mortality rates of up to 65% when early surgery was carried out as compared to 20–30% with medical treatment clearly negated the benefits of surgery within the first few days after the beginning of symptoms and ratified a nonsurgical strategy with intensive care as the best approach [11, 12]. Mier et al. randomly placed patients with indications for surgery (multiple organ failure with clinical deterioration) into two groups: early (surgery within 24–72 h) and late (surgery after 12 days), and recorded indisputably higher mortality in the early surgery group: 56% vs. 27% [25]. In fact, good progress in intensive care treatment means that the majority of patients now survive stage I of SAP, which then allows, even in cases of serious pancreatic necrosis, a waiting strategy and "maturation" of the necrotic process. As the days and weeks go by, necrotic tissue becomes more and more well demarcated and separates into well-circumscribed areas that are isolated from the blood circulation and also from the surrounding normal tissue. This means that the affected areas can be easily and safely removed with the surgical procedure of blunt-finger sequestrectomy. Such maneuvers carry markedly lower risks of bleeding and fistulas compared with necrosectomies carried out on "fresh" tissue when the surgeon is forced to perform urgent surgery in the early stages of the disease. Various studies demonstrate a reduction in the risk of death by some 37–69% in patients on whom necrosectomy has been carried out at least 2–3 weeks after the onset of symptoms [39–41]. Fernandez del Castillo et al. tried to identify the optimum timing for late necrosectomy and reported that the ideal moment would be 1 month from the beginning of the SAP; this timing seems to guarantee the best results [39]. Therefore, in stage I of SAP, surgery is relegated in favor of a conservative approach, except in the rare cases of fulminant acute pancreatitis, abdominal compartment syndrome, massive hemoperitoneum, and bacterial peritonitis.

Until a few years ago the diagnosis, generally late, between the 2nd and 4th week, of infected necrosis served as an absolute indication to proceed with immediate necrosectomy [11–16]. Even this dogma, however, has recently been called into question by two randomized studies [23, 42] which reported that patients with infected necrosis treated with specific antibiotic therapy can get better without surgery and, when surgery is performed, late intervention carries lower mortality and morbidity risk than early surgery. This algorithm might be able to spare many patients unnecessary surgery and postpone the operation for those patients who definitely need surgical treatment. Thus, even in the presence of infected necrosis, if the patient is hemodynamically stable and not showing signs of sepsis or systemic complications, it is acceptable to continue with noninvasive treatment, postponing surgery until the necrotic process has settled, vital tissue is demarcated, and the necrotic tissue is well confined. Only in cases of infected necrosis with systemic deterioration, bleeding, and perforation should immediate surgery be considered. Vast improvements in intensive care, more specific antibiotic therapy, and early enteral nutrition, although they cannot alone prevent superinfection of the necrotic areas, can delay its occurrence, allowing surgery to take place at a far later stage – which means a safer, more effective procedure, with fewer complications and greater possibilities for the pancreatic tissue to recuperate. Even with a lack of randomized studies indicating the optimum timing, there is general agreement amongst pancreatic surgeons that surgery in SAP should be carried out as late as possible and not before the 3rd–4th week after the onset of symptoms [11–16, 43–45]; the longer it is possible to wait, the better it is in terms of minimizing the difficulties associated with the operation and also minimizing postsurgical morbidity. Delayed surgery enables the identification of well-demarcated necrotic areas, in the context of the normal parenchyma, limits surgery to a single operation, and reduces risks of bleeding and fistulas.

Surgical Strategies

Surgeons have a range of necrosectomy procedures at their disposal which aim, albeit via different times and methods, to remove all the necrotic pancreatic and infected peripancreatic tissue and to drain and prevent the accumulation of toxic substances, avoiding intestinal and vascular damage. Despite the commonly held view that necrosectomy is essential in infected SAP, unanimous consensus on the optimum treatment for the pancreatic area and the peripancreatic tissue after necrosectomy is still lacking [46]. Since recurrent intra-abdominal sepsis

remains a problem peculiar to necrosectomy, the most modern surgical procedures combine the operation with postoperative strategies to maximize the subsequent evacuation and washing out of residual necrotic infection and pus secretions. Ample demolition techniques, quite fashionable in past times, have now
been abandoned [11–13, 47]. Furthermore, in many cases of SAP, only the external portion of the gland is necrotic whilst the central parenchyma is unharmed,
and *resections* (pancreatoduodenectomy and distal pancreatectomy) which also
remove a vast portion of normal pancreatic tissue are associated with prohibitive
mortality and very high incidences of pancreatic failure, both endocrine and
exocrine, compared to necrosectomy; for these reasons they are theoretically
incorrect and are now blacklisted.

Surgeons have three different surgical strategies at their disposal:
– Closed technique with postoperative peritoneal lavage
– Open packing technique
– Mixed technique with a zip

The *closed technique with postoperative peritoneal lavage* (Fig. 8.5) proposed by Beger et al. [26, 28] involves full exposure of the pancreatic area, glandular and peripancreatic necrosectomy, cleansing of the peritoneal cavity, and
closure of the abdominal walls with prior positioning of multiple abdominal
large drainage tubes with multiple windows; they allow continuous washing and
active drainage of the necrotic areas with efficient evacuation of the secretions,
necrotic residual tissue, and any loss of pancreatic secretion. Anything between
5 and 20–30 l/day of physiological solution or standard fluid for peritoneal dialysis is infused until the outflow solution is completely clear, which then permits
removal of the tubes.

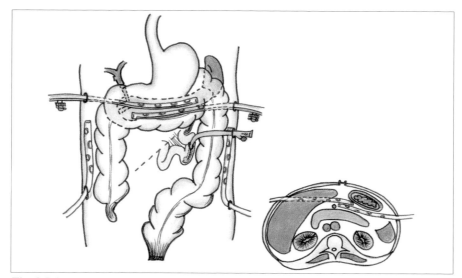

Fig. 8.5 Closed technique with postoperative peritoneal lavage

The *open technique* or *open packing technique* (Fig. 8.6) described by Bradley and Allen [1] consists of the necrosectomy exactly as described in the aforementioned technique, but at the end the abdomen is filled with laparotomy packing strips and left open (laparostomy); a series of further operations are then planned 24–72 h apart from one another, with repeated necrosectomies. On successive explorations, areas of necrosis which escaped in the previous operation or were not yet fully outlined become more obvious. Finally, when the necrosectomy is believed to be complete, drainage is left in place and the abdomen is closed.

The *mixed technique with zip* (Fig. 8.7) proposed by Sarr and colleagues [27] sees multiple laparotomies planned every 48 h (staged laparotomy). This technique represents a sort of mixture of the two previously described procedures. At the end of the necrosectomy, the areas of necrosis are plugged with gauze tampons and the abdomen is closed with a zip, bringing the edges of the incision together. This permits quick and easy reopening of the abdomen for repeated necrosectomies until such time as the surgeon is sure that the necrotizing process is fully under control. At this point the zip is removed and the abdomen closed, but with abdominal drainage in place.

With the growing knowledge that it is best to delay necrosectomy as much as possible, disagreement on how to treat the pancreatic "bed" and surrounding tissue has become less crucial; with surgery at 3–4 weeks after presentation of symptoms, the necrosis is well demarcated and a complete sequestrectomy by "digitoclasia" can be executed in one single operation using the closed tech-

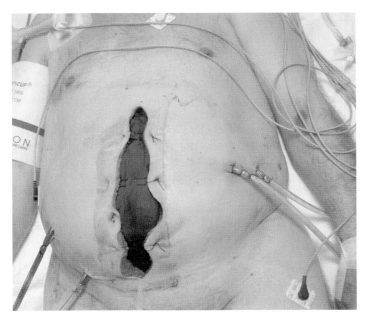

Fig. 8.6 Open packing technique

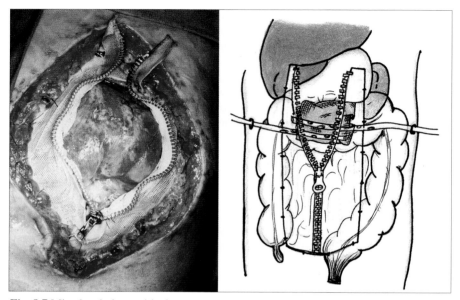

Fig. 8.7 Mixed technique with zip

nique, avoiding the need for a series of repeated laparotomies with their associated increase in general morbidity. Two recent reviews [11, 48] seem to show weak evidence in favor of necrosectomy followed by continuous postoperative lavage as being possibly the superior technique. A Dutch multicenter study on 106 patients who underwent surgery reports mortality of 70% with the open packing technique as compared to 25% with the closed technique and ongoing postoperative lavage [49]. It also indicates the latter as being the preferred method, but concludes that randomized studies are needed for confirmation of which would be the optimum surgical strategy. The comparison between open packing (138 patients in 5 prospective trials) and the closed technique with lavage (64 patients in 2 trials) recorded higher mortality for the first technique (26.8% vs. 18.8%), although it was not a statistically significant sample; and also a higher level of fistulas, bleeding, and disembowelments [11]. Unfortunately, the meager number of prospective studies and the absence of randomized studies for comparison do not make it possible to specify which would be the best surgical approach. That said, nevertheless, reasonable criteria for making a choice can be suggested (Table 8.6). In late operations with "mature" necrosis the more favorable technique seems to be the "closed" option, given that it is technically and logistically easier and has fewer complications than the others, even though it is sometimes complicated by recurrent intra-abdominal abscesses requiring repeated laparotomies. In patients undergoing early surgery, in whom the necrotizing areas are not yet well demarcated, it is preferable to use the mixed technique with a zip which makes re-entry to the pancreatic cavity possible, in order to repeat the necrosectomy whilst keeping the abdomen still

Table 8.6 Criteria for the choice of surgical strategy in severe acute pancreatitis

Conditions	Strategy to choose
Late surgery (3rd–4th week) with mature necrosis	Closed technique with continuous postoperative lavage
Abdominal compartment syndrome or massive bleeding	Open packing
Early surgery (1st–2nd week) with immature necrosis	Mixed technique with zip

closed. Lastly, the open packing technique would be a choice for SAP complicated by massive abdominal bleeding and in abdominal compartment syndrome, where closure of the abdomen, apart from being technically extremely difficult, is also contraindicated because of high mortality.

The open and mixed techniques grant lower incidence of recurrent abdominal sepsis compared with single necrosectomy performed with closed technique, but their morbidity, on the other hand, is much higher [11, 12]. The incidence of pancreatic and intestinal fistulas (duodenal, ileal, and colonic), bleeding, and disembowelments increases in proportion to the number of surgical operations performed. Generally, a duodenal fistula is treated via drainage and enteral or total parenteral nutrition via the jejunostomy, whilst colic and ileal fistulas are corrected with segmental resection and anastomosis, and, if required, protected by an upstream enterostomy. On the other hand, external pancreatic fistulas, if well drained and peripheral, are left to self-heal spontaneously. Centrally located external pancreatic fistulas, should the self-healing process be problematic (perhaps because of difficult evacuation of the duct of Wirsung into the duodenum) may require caudal resection if distal; those located on the pancreatic head might require internalizing of the fistulous segment into an intestinal loop using the Roux-en-Y technique. Despite the necrosectomy, unlike in resective surgery, the capacity of the pancreas to secrete is preserved; long-term follow-up of patients who have undergone the operation has shown that around 25% develop exocrine pancreatic failure and around 30% endocrine failure [12]. Recently, laparoscopic and percutaneous approaches to necrosectomy have been published, but with these methods complete debridement of the necrotic tissue becomes very difficult and these options should only be considered in rare, very well selected cases.

Surgical Techniques

Surgical incision can be *longitudinal midline-transperitoneal* or *bilateral subcostal* or *monolateral lumbar retroperitoneal* (Fig. 8.8). The choice will depend on the surgeon's preferences and on the type of strategy used. Many authors prefer a midline laparotomy as opposed to incision under the ribs, given that it allows a better view of the entire abdominal cavity, easier postoperative management of

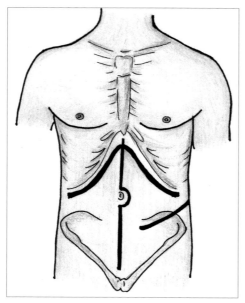

Fig. 8.8 Surgical incisions for pancreatic necrosectomy

drainage and of the jejunostomy, and easier correction of evisceration. Others prefer an incision under the ribs, claiming that in the case of the open packing technique it will limit contamination of the submesocolic area and reduce the risk of fistulas of the intestine. If opting for the closed technique, the majority of surgeons are generally in favor of midline laparotomy, whilst in the open packing and mixed techniques, both incisions are used equally. Monolateral lumbar incision, while having the advantage of avoiding contamination of the peritoneal cavity, does not allow adequate exploration and necrosectomy; moreover, it is not complication-free, and problems such as bleeding and colic fistulas are still possible. It is generally reserved in cases of repeated surgery, for those rare cases with demarcated areas of confined necrosis of the pancreatic head (right lobotomy) or the tail (left lombotomy).

The first step of the operation involves access to the pancreatic area and exposure of the anterior aspect of the gland by *opening the gastrocolic ligament*, preserving the gastroepiploic arch (Fig. 8.9). In truth, this maneuver can be extremely difficult given that the necrotic–inflammatory process may obliterate this space and create firm adhesion between the gastrocolic ligament and mesocolon, transverse colon, pancreas, and posterior stomach wall. If the rear cavity is obliterated and the stomach and transverse colon cannot be separated, it is possible to take a transmesocolic route; this route, however, only offers suboptimal access, is quite tricky because of the risk of damaging the right and mid colic vessels or the vessels of Riolan's arch, and can put the posterior infected peritoneal necrosis in direct communication with the submesocolic compartment of the abdomen. A third access route to the pancreatic area would be by passing through the superior margin of the stomach, undermining throughout the poste-

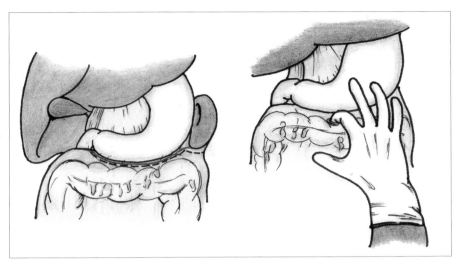

Fig. 8.9 Opening of the gastrocolic ligament. Manual probing of the rear cavity through the the gastrocolic ligament and identification of the area of necrosis

rior gastric wall by blunt dissection all the way down, and then opening a little gap on the gastrocolic ligament. Usually the pancreatic cavity is probed with a finger penetrating through the gastrocolic ligament to identify the area of necrosis (Fig. 8.9). Subsequently the gastrocolic ligament is carefully opened up, taking care not to damage the gastroepiploic arch, the colon, and the vessels of the transverse colon. The surgeon must, therefore, enter the pancreatic space via the easiest route to then completely expose it, taking care not to worsen the danger.

Next a *systematic exploration* of the whole pancreas and the peritoneum must be carried out, both visually and manually, covering the two paracolic spaces, the mesenteric root below the transverse mesocolon and the retroperitoneal space above the pancreas. Retroperitoneal necrosis can spread along these routes (Fig. 8.10); if this is found, opening the peritoneum and carrying out necrosectomy of those areas is mandatory. Careful evaluation of the preoperative CT scan is an essential step in this context, since it makes it possible to map all the areas of necrosis – even those far away from the pancreas (retroperitoneal, paracolic, perirenal, and also the mesenteric root) – and guide the surgeon in conducting the necrosectomy, helping him or her nor to miss any areas of necrosis, neither to access others which would make a future laparotomy necessary. If the necrosis extends from the root of the mesocolon to inside the mesenteric root in close proximity to the mesenteric vessels and is not well delimited, a deep necrosectomy into that location runs the risk of serious bleeding; for these reasons, in such circumstances it is preferable to carry out packing and reoperate 48 h later.

All necrotic pancreatic and peripancreatic tissues must be located, debrided, and removed with delicate digital dissection via an undermining technique

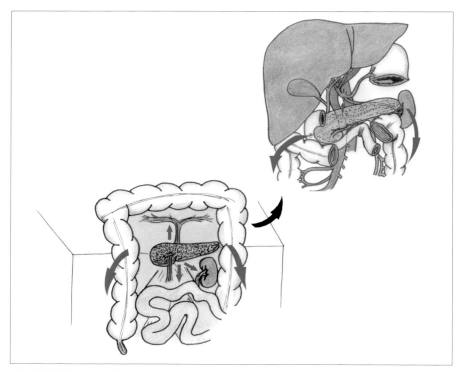

Fig. 8.10 Direction of pancreatic necrosis spread: parietocolic cavity, transverse mesocolon, mesenteric root, renal space, and suprapancreatic retroperitoneal space

which has been termed *necrosectomy by blunt-finger dissection*, avoiding cutting and the use of sharp instruments. The objective of necrosectomy is, in fact, the removal of all the areas of necrosis but avoiding bleeding. In the presence of areas where there are doubts about the extent of the necrotic tissue, which might not be well demarcated and is tenaciously adherent to normal tissue, aggressive removal by undermining and the use of scalpels can damage normal tissue, causing bleeds which are difficult to control; in these circumstances it is preferable to use packing and perhaps return to the focus 48 h later. If there is a section of apparently normal tissue crossing the necrotic cavity, despite the temptation to remove it, it is better to leave it alone, because it usually carries blood vessels (Fig. 8.11).

After performing the necrosectomy, *meticulous washing of the retroperitoneal cavity and of the debrided areas* is carried out using many liters of sterile saline solution to remove the necrotic debris, inflammatory secretions, and residual bacteria. In the closed technique, generally *four or more multiwindowed drains are positioned*, two with double lumens and two or more Silastic types of 28 or 32 Fr, to ensure continuous postoperative washing (Fig. 8.5). The two double-lumen drains, providing the washing flow, cross one another in the epiploic

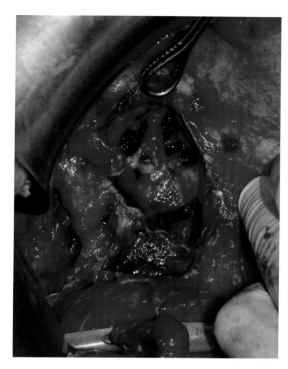

Fig. 8.11 Intraoperative photograph showing partial destruction of the pancreatic head with residual parenchymal links containing pancreaticoduodenal vessels

retrocavity. The first, entering via the right flank, has its extremity on the pancreatic tail; the other, which enters via the left flank, ends close to the pancreatic head. These drains must exit the abdomen at a downward slant to facilitate the evacuation of the washing solution. They are positioned far away from blood vessels and also avoid direct contact with the small intestine and the colon; for this reason, the right drain must pass below the liver and behind the hepatic flexure, the left under the spleen and behind the splenic flexure. The other two or more, Silastic drains are placed inside the parietocolic spaces (ascending and descending colon) if open, and in any other areas subjected to necrosectomy.

If the etiology is biliary and preoperative endoscopic clearance of the common bile duct has not been carried out, a Kehr T-tube is positioned in the duct and a cholecystectomy is carried out.

At the end of the operation *a jejunostomy is performed* to begin early enteral feeding which, in contrast to the bacterial translocation responsible for superinfection of sterile pancreatic necrosis, represents a basic protective treatment to improve the outcome for these patients. Finally, the *gastrocolic ligament is sutured* to create a closed retroperitoneal space for continuous lavage and *the abdominal wall is finally closed layer by layer*. Twelve to twenty-four hours later, continuous lavage is started using a physiological solution or standard fluid for peritoneal dialysis (perhaps diluted with 2–4% iodine polyvinylpyrrolidone or with gabexate mesilate), which is intended to complete the cleansing of the areas of necrotic infection. The amount of washing can vary from a little to 30–40 l/day, depending upon the extent of the area to be cleansed. Importantly, the times are not set in stone but dictated by the clinical evolution as documented by CT scans confirming the progressive self-resolution of the disease process. After surgery, a temporary deterioration of the hemodynamic parameters is quite common, due to the transitory bacteremia caused by mobilizing the septic debris from the pancreatic space, but it improves within 72 h. When the hemodynamics have improved, the enteral and total parenteral nutritioncan begin.

Should the necrosectomy be incomplete, due to immature necrosis (early surgery), and the decision be made to proceed with a mixed zip technique, packing of all the areas of necrosis with damp gauze ensues, followed by the positioning of two aspiration tubes above the packing to drain the secretions which unless evacuated would cause an increase in abdominal pressure. The abdominal wall is closed with a zip attached to the fascia, avoiding excessive retraction; the zip permits quick opening and shutting of the abdomen, keeps the abdominal compartment isolated, and offers the possibility of deferring closure. At 48-h intervals the zip is reopened and the necrosectomy repeated until the necrotizing process stops. The abdomen can then be closed, with prior positioning of soft drainage which reduces the risk of ulceration. If open packing has to be performed (massive bleeding and/or abdominal compartment syndrome, early surgery with incomplete necrosis and unavailability of the zip), a Bogotà bag is placed over the packing strips or a piece of Steri-Drape under the fascia and the laparotomy is left open, simply covered by strips and a cutaneous Steri-Drape. In the event of bleeding of the area which has undergone necrosectomy, some authors advise that the omental sac be mobilized and placed between the area of necrosis and the laparotomy strips, so that the latter do not come into direct contact with the areas of surgical trauma. When reoperating, the surgeon must take great care not to use hard drainage and must be particularly gentle, working delicately around the colon, duodenum, small intestine, and spleen, which are more vulnerable to the corrosive action of the activated enzymes. Rechecks with repacking are performed at 48-h intervals, until evidence of recovery of the necrosis becomes obvious, at which time the decision is made to close the abdominal walls leaving only soft drainage in place.

Conclusions

Much more in-depth knowledge of the physiopathology, natural course, and complications of SAP have led, in the last 20 years, to an improvement in treatment strategies and results, with global mortality being reduced to 5%, and to 10–20% for the most severe forms [12]. Although the presence of infected necrosis is considered by everyone to be an indication for surgery, the choice of treatment in the presence of *sterile* necrosis with systemic complications remains the subject of controversy. With regard to the timing, despite a general consensus as to the usefulness of delaying surgery to the 3rd–4th week from the onset of the symptoms, no randomized controlled studies exist that would pinpoint the ideal timing. Similarly, there is no clear scientific evidence in favor of a particular surgical strategy. Finally, in such a complex and evolving field, where there is little robust scientific evidence and numerous uncertainties, it is prudent to keep an open mind and not to exclude, through prejudice, any approach. Further randomized controlled studies are mandatory to clearly define the indications, timing, and optimum procedures for the treatment of SAP.

References

1. Bradley EL, Allen K (1991) A prospective longitudinal study of observation versus surgical intervention in the management of necrotizing pancreatitis. Am J Surg 161:19
2. Baron TH, Morgan DE (1999) Acute necrotizing pancreatitis. N Engl J Med 340:1412
3. Ranson JH (1984) Acute pancreatitis: pathogenesis, outcome and treatment. Clin Gastroenterol 13:843
4. Steinberg W, Tenner S (1994) Acute pancreatitis. N Engl J Med 330:1198
5. Balthazar EJ, Ranson JH, Naidich DP et al (1985) Acute pancreatitis: prognostic value of CT. Radiology 156:767
6. Bradley EL (1993) A clinical based classification system for acute pancreatitis: Summary of the International Symposium on Acute Pancreatitis, Atlanta, Georgia, 1992. Arch Surg 128:586
7. Ratary MG, Connor S, Criddle DN et al (2004) Acute pancreatitis and organ failure: pathophysiology, natural history and management strategies. Curr Gastroenterol Rep 6:99
8. Büchler MW, Gloor B, Müller CA et al (2000) Acute necrotizing pancreatitis: treatment strategy according to the status of infection. Ann Surg 232:619
9. Bassi C (1994) Infected pancreatic necrosis. Int J Pancreatol 16:1
10. Fernandez del Castillo C, Rattner DW, Herferth C et al (1993) Acute pancreatitis. Lancet 342:475
11. Heinrich S, Schäfer M, Rousson V et al (2006) Evidence-based treatment of acute pancreatitis: a look at established paradigms. Ann Surg 243:154
12. Werner J, Uhl W, Büchler MW (2004) Acute pancreatitis. In: Cameron JL (ed) Current surgical therapy. Mosby, St Louis, p 459
13. Whang EE (2006) Acute pancreatitis. In: Greenfield's surgery: scientific principles and practice, 4th edn. Lippincott Williams & Wilkins, Philadelphia, p 840
14. Nathens AB, Curtis JR, Beale RJ et al (2004) Management of the critically ill patient with severe acute pancreatitis. Crit Care Med ;32:2524
15. Mayumi T, Takada T, Kawarada Y et al (2006) Management strategy for acute pancreatitis in the Japan Guidelines. J Hepatobiliary Pancreat Surg 13:61
16. Banks PA, Freeman LM (2006) Practice guidelines in acute pancreatitis. Am J Gastroenterol 101:2379
17. Beger HG, Bittner R, Block S et al (1986) Bacterial contamination of pancreatic necrosis: a prospective clinical study: Gastroenterology 91:433
18. Gianotti L, Munda R, Alexander JW (1992) Pancreatitis-induced microbial translocation: a study of the mechanism. Res Surg 4:87
19. Ammori BJ, Leeder PC, King RF et al (1999) Early increase in intestinal permeability in patients with severe acute pancreatitis: correlation with endotoxemia, organ failure, and mortality. J Gastrointest Surg 3:252
20. Teerenhovi O, Nordback I, Eskola J (1989) High volume lesser sac lavage in acute necrotizing pancreatitis. Br J Surg 76:370

21. Ihse I, Evander A, Gustafson I et al (1986) Influence of peritoneal lavage on objective prognostic signs in acute pancreatitis. Ann Surg 204:122

22. Mayer AD (1985) Controlled clinical trial of peritoneal lavage for the treatment of severe acute pancreatitis. N Engl J Med 312:399

23. Nordback I, Paajanet H, Sand J (1997) Prospective evaluation of a treatment protocol in patients with severe acute necrotizing pancreatitis. Eur J Surg 163:357

24. Kalfarentzos FE, Kehagias J, Kakkos SK et al (1999) Treatment of patients with severe acute necrotizing pancreatitis based on prospective evaluation. Hepatogastroenterology 46:3249

25. Mier J, Leon EL, Castillo A et al (1997) Early versus late necrosectomy in severe necrotizing pancreatitis. Am J Surg 173:71

26. Beger HG, Büchler M, Bittner R et al (1988) Necrosectomy and postoperative local lavage in necrotizing pancreatitis. Br J Surg 75:207

27. Tsiotos GG, Luque-de Leon E, Soreide JA et al (1998) Management of necrotizing pancreatitis by repeated operative necrosectomy using a zipper technique. Am J Surg 175:91

28. Beger HG (1991) Operative management of necrotizing pancreatitis and continous closed postoperative lavage of the lesser sac. Hepatogastroenterology 38:129

29. Draganov P, Forsmark CE (2005) Disease of the pancreas. In: ACP Medicine. Gastroenterology 5. WebMB, p 689. Available at: www.acponline.com

30. Schein M (2005) Acute pancreatitis. In: Schein M, Rogers PM (eds) Schein's common sense emergency abdominal surgery. Springer, Berlin Heidelberg New York, p 154

31. Banks PA (1997) Practice guidelines in acute pancreatitis. Am J Gastroenterol 92:377

32. Gerzof SG, Banks BA, Robbins AH et al (1987) Early diagnosis of pancreatic infection by computed tomography-guided aspiration. Gastroenterology 93:1315

33. Rau B, Pralle U, Mayer JM et al (1998) Role of ultrasonographically guided fine-needle aspiration cytology in the diagnosis of infected pancreatic necrosis. Br J Surg 85:179

34. Garg PK, Khanna S, Bohidar NP et al (2001) Incidence, spectrum and antibiotic sensitivity pattern of bacterial infection among patients with acute pancreatitis. J Gastroenterol Hepatol 16:1055

35. Neoptolemos JP, Carr-Locke DL, London NJ et al (1988) Controlled trial of urgent endoscopic retrograde cholangiopancreatography and endoscopic sphincterotomy versus conservative treatment for acute pancreatitis due to gallstones. Lancet 2:979

36. Novak A, Nowakowska E, Marek TA et al (1995) Final results of the prospective, randomized, controlled study on endoscopic sphincterotomy versus conventional management in acute biliary pancreatitis. Gastroenterology 108:A380

37. Fan ST, Lai EC, Mok FP et al (1993) Early treatment of acute biliary pancreatitis by endoscopic papillotomy. N Engl J Med 328:228

38. Folsch UR, Nitsche R, Ludtke R et al (1997) Early ERCP and papillotomy compared with conservative treatment for acute biliary pancreatitis. N Engl J Med 336:237

39. Fernandez del Castillo C, Rattner DW, Makary MA et al (1998) Debridement and closed packing for the treatment of necrotizing pancreatitis. Ann Surg 228:676

40. Hungness ES, Robb BW, Seeskin C et al (2002) Early debridement for necrotizing pancreatitis: is it worthwhile? J Am Coll Surg 194:740

41. Hartwig W, Maksan S, Foitzik T et al (2002) Reduction in mortality with delayed surgical therapy of severe pancreatitis. J Gastrointestinal Surg 6:481

42. Nordback I, Sand J, Saaristo R et al (2001) Early treatment with antibiotics reduces the need for surgery in acute necrotizing pancreatitis: a single center randomized study. J Gastrointest Surg 5:113

43. Besselink MG, Verwer TJ, Schoenmaeckers EJ et al (2007) Timing of surgical intervention in necrotizing pancreatitis. Arch Surg 142:1194

44. Mofidi R, Lee AC, Madhavan KK et al (2007) Prognostic factors in patients undergoing surgery for severe necrotizing pancreatitis. World J Surg 31: 2002

45. Rodriguez JR, Razao AO, Targarona J et al (2008) Debridement and closed packing for sterile or infected necrotizing pancreatitis: insights into indications and outcomes in 167 patients. Ann Surg 274:294

46. Sarr MG, Tsiotos GG (2004) Necrosectomia per pancreatite acuta necrotica. In: Baker RJ, Fischer JE (eds) Mastery in chirurgia. Verduci, Roma, p 1305
47. Teerenhovi O, Nordback I, Isolauri J (1988) Influence of pancreatic resection on systemic complication in acute pancreatitis. Br J Surg 75:793
48. Kingsnorth A, O'Reilly D (2006) Acute pancreatitis. BMJ 332:1072
49. Besselink MG, De Brujin MT, Rutten JP et al (2006) Dutch Acute Pancreatitis Study Group. Surgical intervention in patients with necrotizing pancreatitis. Br J Surg 93:593

Chapter 9

Indications for Surgery and Surgical Procedures for Chronic Pancreatitis

Francesca Gavazzi, Alessandro Zerbi, Valerio Di Carlo

Indications for Surgery

In the management of chronic pancreatitis, pain has remained the main indication for surgical treatment over the years, but for a long time the high morbidity and mortality associated with pancreatic operations limited the use of this procedure for benign disease.

In 1998 the American Gastroenterological Association (AGA) produced treatment guidelines. The AGA guidelines advocate a four-phase concept of: (1) primary noninterventional, supportive treatment (nonnarcotic analgesics, low-fat diet, alcohol abstinence); (2) medical therapy, including pancreatic enzymes and acid suppression; (3) endoscopic therapy: pancreatic sphincterotomy (the first in 1985), lithotripsy for stones, and placement of stents to treat ductal strictures; and (4) surgery. The AGA guidelines promote conservative treatment on the basis that the duration of pain is unpredictable and it eventually subsides as a consequence of "burn-out" of the pancreas.

Conservative treatment has become obsolete as a result of significant progress made in surgical and interventional techniques. Besides, these guidelines ignore two important aspects: first, the typical pancreatic pain is preceded by a long history of "nonspecific" pain, and when the patient is finally visited by an expert, his gland already has severe pathological changes; second, early operation is able to prevent further organ impairment, suggesting that the timing of intervention has an impact not only on functional derangement but also on pain control and quality of life [1].

Pancreatic pain often does not respond to analgesics, persisting in 85% of conservatively managed patients 5 years after diagnosis and in 55% 10 years after diagnosis. Surgical intervention is indicated if long-lasting, persistent pain is not adequately relieved by analgesic drugs and when intraglandular complications develop, such as pseudocysts, a possible source of further complications like bleeding, infection, and internal fistula. Other indications for surgery are complications involving organs around the pancreas, such as common bile duct stenosis and duodenal obstruction; endoscopic or surgical treatment of these complications is still debated. The solution of this problem as such does not con-

W. Siquini (Ed.), *Surgical Treatment of Pancreatic Diseases.*
©Springer-Verlag Italia 2009

cern this chapter; however, the reader is reminded of the recent publication of a randomized study in which surgery proved to be quite superior to endoscopy [2].

There are other reasons for using surgery to treat patients suffering from chronic pancreatitis, such as suspicion of the presence of a pancreatic cancer. In recent years, too, new pathological entities have been identified: cystic dystrophy of the duodenal wall and pancreas divisum, both of which could benefit from surgery [3].

Surgical Procedures

Surgical treatment of chronic pancreatitis is traditionally divided into drainage and resective procedures, although some belong to both groups. The physiopathological interpretation of the pancreatic pain – ductal hypertension and/or increased parenchymal pressure (compartment syndrome) versus neural damage from inflammation and fibrosis – underlies the choice between a drainagee and a resective procedure [4].

The drainage operations, the Partington–Rochelle longitudinal pancreaticojejunostomy in particular, are usually used when the pancreatic duct is mildly dilated (diameter 4–5 mm), to preserve pancreatic endocrine and exocrine function. If an inflammatory mass is present at any location in the pancreas, a resection procedure is indicated.

The supporters of resection of the head of the pancreas believe that, even in the case of duct dilatation, the Partington–Rochelle operation or endoscopic procedures cannot relieve pain because they ignore the morphological change to the head of the pancreas, which is considered the pacemaker of the disease. Moreover, resection can be performed in any patient, regardless of the presence of pseudocysts and/or dilatation of the pancreatic duct. The main resective operation is the pancreaticoduodenectomy, which removes, together with the head, the organs neighboring the pancreas. Recently, a new surgical procedure has been developed to avoid this wide demolition.

Pancreaticoduodenectomy

Pancreaticoduodenectomy for chronic pancreatitis is the same as that performed for malignancy. *Surgical technique:* A wide opening of the lesser sac is made. The gastrocolic ligament is separated off the superior edge of the transverse colon; the right gastroepiploic vessels are divided and ligated as they emerge from the head of the pancreas. These surgical maneuvers allow exposure of the head and neck of the pancreas. Next comes a complete Kocher maneuver all the way to the superior mesenteric vein, moving the right colic flexure caudally to expose the duodenum completely and to feel the thickness and consistency of the head between the thumb and fingers. The inferior border of the neck of the pancreas is mobilized and the superior mesenteric vein is identified and mobilized along the anterior surface from the gland, up to the superior border of the neck. This is followed by cholecystectomy, section of the common hepatic duct, and division and ligation of the gastroduodenal artery at its origin on the common hepatic artery.

Gastric resection is carried out, or, if a pylorus-preserving technique is preferred, section of the duodenum 2 cm from the pylorus. The duodenum is divided 20–30 cm distal to the ligament of Treitz with a linear stapler. The body of the pancreas is resected. The draining veins of the uncinate process and of the head into the superior mesenteric vein and portal vein are freed up. At this point the surgical specimen is excised. The free jejunum is passed through an opening in the transverse mesocolon (Roux limb) to carry out the three anastomoses. Reconstruction can be accomplished in a variety of ways, but the most common involves a pancreaticojejunostomy (end-to-side), a hepaticojejunostomy (end-to-side), and then an antecolic end-to-side gastro-jejunostomy (standard Whipple) or duodenojejunostomy (pylorus-preserving Whipple), in that order, sutured on the same loop.

Pylorus-preserving pancreaticoduodenectomy is to be preferred: by preserving the stomach, the pylorus, and the first part of the duodenum, this surgical procedure protects against gastric dumping, marginal ulceration, and bile-reflux gastritis. Pancreaticoduodenectomy is mandatory when duodenal stenosis is irreversible, even if inflammatory cephalic mass is removed (for example, cystic dystrophy of the duodenal wall in which the cause of the disease is excised); when duodenal wall could be freed from inflamed and fibrotic surrounding tissue, but only by risking the integrity of its blood supply; when the pain recurs after a duodenum-preserving operation (10% –40%); and, finally, when the presence of pancreatic cancer cannot be ruled out.

Duodenum-Preserving Resection of the Pancreatic Head

The operation of a duodenum-preserving pancreatic head resection (DPPHR), introduced by Beger in 1972, includes a subtotal resection of the pancreatic head, preserving a thin rim of the pancreas dorsal and close to the duodenum, to protect its blood supply; the duodenum together with the stomach, the common bile duct, and the body and the tail of the pancreas are not excised. This surgical procedure safely removes the inflammatory mass in the head of the pancreas and thereby leads to decompression and/or drainage of the duct of Wirsung (main pancreatic duct), the common bile duct, the duodenum, and major retropancreatic vessels, preserving endocrine and exocrine function of the gland.

Surgical technique: The first phase involves opening the gastrocolic ligament, wide kocherization, and dissection of the pancreatic neck by tunneling under the pancreas; then the neck is gently lifted up, away from the superior mesenteric vein and portal vein. In the second phase, multiple stay sutures are made in the gland parenchyma, all along the periphery of the head; they provide excellent hemostasis and serve as reference point for the resection so as to prevent the surgeon from injuring the C-loop of the duodenum and ensure that a cuff of pancreatic tissue (5 mm, up to a maximum of 10 mm) along the duodenal wall is left behind. The pancreas is resected from the right border of the portal vein towards the prepapillary common bile duct, with meticulous hemostasis of the left pancreas (Fig. 9.1). In the third phase, an end-to-side or end-to-end pancreaticojejunostomy (Roux limb) is created, and a side-to-side anastomosis between the remaining pancreatic head along the duodenum and the interposed jejunal loop (Fig. 9.2).

In cases of stenosis of the common bile duct in the intrapancreatic segment which cannot be decompressed by resection of the surrounding pancreatic head, or if the common bile duct is accidentally opened during subtotal pancreatic head resection, a biliary anastomosis with cholecystectomy can easily be added. In patients with multiple stenoses and dilatations in the left-side main pancreatic duct, a longitudinal incision of the duct of Wirsung can be performed with reconstruction by a side-to-side pancreaticojejunostomy, similar to the Frey operation.

The main indications for DPPHR are abdominal pain, inflammatory enlargement of the pancreatic head, common bile duct stenosis, pancreatic duct obstruction, compression of the peripancreatic vessels, and duodenal obstruction. In a randomized prospective single-center controlled study, DPPHR, compared to pylorus-preserving pancreaticoduodenectomy, was associated 6 months postoperatively with less recurrence of pain and greater weight gain (statistically significant); in addition, earlier return to work, better glucose tolerance, and fewer rehospitalization episodes were registered in the DPPHR group [5]. In comparison to pancreaticoduodenectomy, Beger's operation offers the advantage of preserving the normal biliary–duodenal anatomy, including ampulla of Vater function, and a normal upper digestive route, allowing normal food passage. The complexity of neurohumoral regulation of digestion and absorption and physiological passage is best preserved by a DPPHR. Delayed gastric emptying, observed in patients after a pylorus-preserving Whipple procedure, is not report-

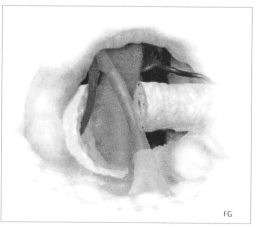

Fig. 9.1 Duodenum-preserving pancreatic head resection (Beger procedure): surgical field after removal of the specimen

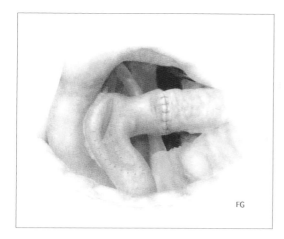

FG

Fig. 9.2 Duodenum-preserving pancreatic head resection (Beger procedure): an end-to-side pancreaticojejunostomy (Roux limb) and a side-to-side anastomosis between the remaining pancreatic head and the interposed jejunal loop

ed after Beger's procedure. Furthermore, DPPHR is associated with a low incidence of surgically induced diabetes mellitus, due to the presence of the duodenum, which plays a central role in the enteroinsular axis, and above all to the preservation of pancreatic parenchyma.

Exocrine function too undergoes less deterioration after DPPHR than after a Whipple operation [6]. However, the Beger procedure is technically highly demanding and only a few centers have enough experience of it.

Frey Operation (Local Resection of the Pancreatic Head with Lateral Pancreaticojejunostomy)

This operation, introduced by Frey and Smith in 1987 [7], combines derivative and resective elements: it is composed of a pancreaticojejunostomy and local resection of the pancreatic head (LR-LPJ), without tunneling under the neck of the parenchyma and sectioning it. The goals of this surgical procedure are: drainage of the secondary ducts in addition to the main duct and freeing the Wirsung duct from compression by the inflamed tissue, avoiding disruption of the biliary system. During the operation the surgeon excises 4–12 g of pathological pancreatic tissue (including nervous structures inside the head of the gland) and opens the main duct into the neck, body, and tail. All three ducts of the pancreas are decompressed or resected, together with the tributary ones, coring that amount of cephalic parenchyma out (Fig. 9.3); the duct of Wirsung and that of the uncinate process, which pass near the posterior surface of the head, are decompressed and the accessory pancreatic duct (duct of Santorini), which crosses the head anteriorly and superiorly, is excised [8, 9]. This type of resection theoretically relieves pain caused by either ductal hypertension or by neural injury. The posterior shell of the head of the pancreas is intact and so it is pos-

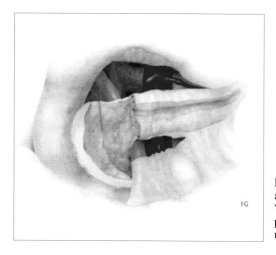

FG

Fig. 9.3 Frey procedure: surgical field after opening the whole of the duct of Wirsung and removal of tissue of the pancreatic head, preserving the posterior shell

sible to carry out the anastomoses with the remaining head and the left portion of the pancreas with the same jejunal loop (Fig. 9.4). The pancreaticojejunostomy drains the duct of the neck, body, and tail, and both stenoses and stones are cured; the pancreatic tissue preserved (60–65%) prevents the occurrence of endocrine and exocrine insufficiency. LR-LPJ can be used in patients in whom the main pancreatic duct of the left pancreas is only 2–3 mm wide, because the anastomosis is made with the capsule of the gland. DPPHR requires dividing the pancreas at its neck: this maneuver may be technically difficult in the event of inflammatory changes and extrahepatic or intrahepatic portal hypertension, because of the increase of blood supply and the adhesion of the gland to the mesenteric and portal veins. Besides, DPPHR does not preserve the posterior

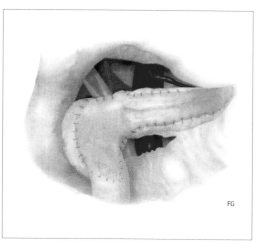

FG

Fig. 9.4 Frey procedure: wide side to side pancreatico-jejunostomy

capsule of the head of the pancreas, necessitating two anastomoses: a pancreaticojejunostomy with the body of the divided pancreas and another with the remnant of the pancreas on the inner aspect of the duodenum. In a randomized controlled prospective trial comparing pancreatic head resection according to Beger and limited pancreatic head excision combined with lateral pancreaticojejunostomy according to Frey, there were no notable differences within the two groups. This result is not surprising because the operations are similar: the Frey operation appears to be a modification of the Beger one rather than a new intervention, and the decision which to choose should be based on the surgeon's experience [10].

Both these surgical procedures are useful to relieve the pain and resolve the obstruction of the common bile duct and the stenosis of the duodenum caused by pseudocysts. Neither the LR-LPJ nor the DPPHR is useful in patients with gastric bleeding varices from left-sided portal hypertension or pseudoaneurysms of the pancreatic blood vessels. Likewise, when there is a strong suspicion of an underlying malignancy, both these operations are contraindicated.

Distal Pancreatectomy

Surgical technique: The anterior surface of the pancreas is exposed and explored after division of the gastrocolic ligament to open the lesser sac. The parenchyma is tunneled under at the pancreatic neck; the peritoneum is opened all along the inferior border of the gland to its tail, gently separating off the posterior wall of the pancreas, beginning to the left of the superior mesenteric vein to reach the superior border of the neck. This may be performed with splenectomy (distal splenopancreatectomy): the spleen is mobilized after ligation and section of short gastric vessels. The splenophrenic and splenocolic ligaments are incised. The splenic pedicle is dissected and the artery and the vein divided at their origins. If the spleen is being preserved, the posterior aspect of the pancreas is separated from the splenic vessels after ligation of the multiple vascular branches supplying the parenchyma. The operation ends with section of the pancreas and closure of the main pancreatic duct with a double suture approximating the superior and inferior borders of the pancreatic stump.

This surgical procedure is rarely performed in patients with chronic pancreatitis: only when the disease is limited to the body and tail of the gland, without dilatation of the main duct (<5 mm). At a mean follow-up of 5 years adequate pain relief is present in 50–95% of patients. An increasing number of patients with chronic pancreatitis are diagnosed with splenic vein thrombosis and secondary left-sided portal hypertension: in such cases splenectomy is the treatment of choice with distal pancreatectomy. Asymptomatic patients with splenic vein thrombosis should be treated expectantly; a prophylactic splenectomy is not indicated [11].

Total Pancreatectomy

This intervention is exceptional in patients with chronic pancreatitis. The surgical technique is described in Chapter 25.

Longitudinal Pancreaticojejunostomy According to Partington-Rochelle

Surgical technique: The anterior aspect of the pancreas is widely exposed. The duct of Wirsung is incised and opened from the point on the neck/body of the gland where it is superficial and can be palpated, all along towards the edge of the duodenum and the tail. Stones impacted inside the duct are removed. A one-layer, side-to-side pancreaticojejunostomy consisting of interrupted sutures is performed on a Roux limb.

Puestow and Gillesby technique [12]: distal pancreatic tail resection with splenectomy and invagination of the body of the gland into the end of a Roux-en-Y jejunal limb. The Partington-Rochelle operation [13] is indicated when the Wirsung duct is obstructed in the head of the pancreas and dilated to a diameter greater than 5 mm, without inflammatory cephalic enlargement of the gland ("mass-forming-like"). Longitudinal pancreaticojejunostomy initially achieves pain relief in 75–80% of the patients, but after 3–5 years only 50% of patients or fewer continue to have pain relief [14]. Possible reasons for this are incomplete decompression of the duct within the head of the pancreas (the opening of the duct is to be extended to the edge of the duodenum as described by the authors); lack of decompression of the other two ducts of the head of the gland (Santorini and that of the uncinate process) or of their tributary ducts, located deep within the head; and progressive obstruction of the anastomosis. The Puestow and Gillesby procedure is now confined to patients presenting problems of differential diagnosis from intraductal tumors or when dealing with a sectorial pancreatitis limited to the tail or with a pseudocyst involving the spleen; its fault is that it does not drain the cephalic portion of the duct.

Cystojejunostomy/Cystogastrostomy

In this intervention a pseudocyst is anastomized to the stomach or to a jejunal loop, using a defunctionalized Roux-en-Y limb. Pseudocysts complicate chronic pancreatitis in 30–40% of patients. Treatment is reserved for patients with symptomatic pseudocysts (pain, early satiety, compression of the duodenum or stomach causing obstruction and compression of the main bile duct causing jaundice), rapidly enlarging pseudocysts, and complicated pseudocysts (rupture, infection, or pseudoaneurysm). If the pseudocyst is adherent to the posterior wall of the stomach, the preferred operation is a cystogastrostomy; in other cases, particularly if the pseudocyst is in the head of the pancreas or plunges under the transverse colon, a Roux-en-Y cystojejunostomy is advisable. The wall of the cyst must be sufficiently thick to allow safe performance of the anastomosis.

Surgical technique: A median or subcostal incision is used. A cephalad pseudocyst is approached by opening the gastrocolic ligament, while to drain the pseudocyst that is plunged under the transverse colon, the peritoneum of the mesocolon has to be incised, paying attention to the middle colic artery and the arch of Riolan. An incision is made in the wall of the pseudocyst in its caudal part, at least 4–5 cm long; the cyst is emptied and the internal septa manually disrupted to remove the matter entirely. A biopsy specimen is taken from the wall and histologic examination carried out intraoperatively to rule out a cystic neoplasm. This is followed by hemostasis of parietal cyst vessels and the anastomosis is performed with a jejunal loop or with the posterior wall of the stomach.

Laparoscopic Surgery

Laparoscopic surgery is not widely developed in the surgical treatment of chronic pancreatitis. All types of pancreatic surgical procedures have been carried out laparoscopically. In 1994 Gagner and Pomp successfully first performed a laparoscopic pylorus-preserving pancreaticoduodenectomy [15]. In pancreaticoduodenectomy the access trauma comprises only a small component of the total operative insult to the patient; therefore, this operation should be done via the laparoscopic approach only when the postoperative course shows a better outcome than could be obtained with the current open approach. By contrast, spleen-preserving distal pancreatectomy is a good indication for laparoscopic technique and this has been successfully carried out at several centers of pancreatic surgery. The magnified view afforded by the laparoscopic approach facilitates the separation of the splenic artery and vein from the pancreatic parenchyma and the identification of the small arteries and veins, which are then easily controlled by laparoscopic instruments [16]. Pancreatic pseudocysts can also be managed by laparoscopy: since 1994 laparoscopic anterior or posterior cystogastrostomy has been described.

Conclusions

About 50% of patients with chronic pancreatitis are operated on [17]. The key points are two: what type of surgery to use and the timing. Patients with chronic pancreatitis who require operative intervention include those with severe pain, those with complications of chronic pancreatitis, and those in whom cancer cannot be ruled out. Ideally, the operation for the patient experiencing "pancreatic pain" should have low associated mortality and morbidity, be easy to perform, provide long-lasting pain relief, cure the complications of this disease, and not worsen exocrine and endocrine pancreatic function. No single operation so far introduced fulfills this ideal, including the LR-LPJ (Frey procedure) and the DPPHR (Beger operation), because none of these addresses all the structural abnormalities and the complications associated with chronic pancreatitis. Both drainage of the Wirsung duct and pancreatic resection have been shown to provide longer-lasting, more complete pain relief than sensory denervation of the pancreas or reduction of pancreatic secretion. All the operative procedures that provide long-lasting pain relief in about 75–80% of cases resect all or a portion of the head (duodenopancreatectomy, DPPHR, LR-LPJ, and total pancreatectomy) [18]. The type of surgical intervention and its long-term results have to be carefully analyzed and individualized for every patient, for whom the best operative strategy has to be tailored. Regarding the timetable of surgical approach, the best approach relies upon clinical balance and consists of performing surgery only after the failure of medical and endoscopic treatment.

References

1. Izbicki JR, Yekebas EF (2005) Chronic pancreatitis – lessons learned. Br J Surg 92:185–1186
2. Cahen DL, Gouma DJ, Nio Y, et al (2007) Endoscopic versus surgical drainage of the pancreatic duct in chronic pancreatitis. N Engl J Med 356:676–684
3. Falconi M, Valerio A, Caldiron E, et al (2000) Changes in pancreatic resection for chronic pancreatitis over 28 years in a single institution. Br J Surg 87:428–433
4. Devière J, Bell RH Jr, Beger HG, Traverso LW (2008) Treatment of chronic pancreatitis with endotherapy or surgery: critical review of randomized control trials. J Gastrointest Surg 12:640–644
5. Büchler MW, Friess H, Müller MW et al (1995) Randomized trial of duodenum-preserving pancreatic head resection versus pylorus-preserving Whipple in chronic pancreatitis. Am J Surg 169(1):65–69; discussion 69–70
6. Ozawa F, Friess H, Kondo Y, et al (2000) Duodenum-preserving pancreatic head resection (DPPHR) in chronic pancreatitis: its rationale and results. J Hepatobiliary Pancreat Surg 7:456–465
7. Frey CF, Smith GJ (1987) Description and rationale of a new operation for chronic pancreatitis. Pancreas 2(6):701–707
8. Ho HS, Frey CF (2001) The Frey procedure. Local resection of pancreatic head combined with lateral pancreaticojejunostomy. Arch Surg 136:1353–1358
9. Frey CF, Reber HA (2005) Local resection of the head of the pancreas with pancreaticojejunostomy. J Gastrointest Surg 9:863–868
10. Frey CF, Mayer KL (2003) Comparison of local resection of the head of the pancreas combined with longitudinal pancreaticojejunostomy (Frey procedure) and duodenum-preserving resection of the pancreatic head (Beger procedure). World J Surg 27:1217–1230
11. Gourgiotis S, Germanos S, Ridolfini MP (2007) Surgical management of chronic pancreatitis. Hepatobiliary Pancreat Dis Int 6:121–133
12. Puestow CB, Gillesby WJ (1958) Retrograde surgical drainage of pancreas for chronic relapsing pancreatitis. AMA Arch Surg 76(6):898–907
13. Partington PF, Rochelle RE (1960) Modified Puestow procedure for retrograde drainage of the pancreatic duct. Ann Surg 152:1037–1043
14. Hartel M, Tempia-Caliera AA, Wente MN, et al (2003) Evidence-based surgery in chronic pancreatitis. Langenbecks Arch Surg 388:132–139

15. Gagner M, Pomp A (1994) Laparoscopic pylorus-preserving pancreatoduodenectomy.Surg Endosc 8(5):408–410
16. Fernández-Cruz L, Cesar-Borges G, López-Boado MA, et al (2005) Minimally invasive surgery of the pancreas in progress. Langenbecks Arch Surg 390:342–354
17. Witt H, Apte MV, Keim V, Wilson JS (2007) Chronic pancreatitis: challenges and advances in pathogenesis, genetics, diagnosis, and therapy. Gastroenterology 132:1557–1573
18. Thuluvath PJ, Imperio D, Nair S, Cameron JL (2003) Chronic pancreatitis. Long-term pain relief with or without surgery, cancer risk, and mortality. J Clin Gastroenterol 36:159–165

Chapter 10

Pancreatic Pseudocyst

Franco Roviello, Corrado Pedrazzani, Daniele Marrelli, Enrico Pinto

Definition

Pancreatic pseudocyst is defined as a cystic cavity bound to the pancreas by inflammatory tissue and containing pancreatic juice or amylase-rich fluid. Typically, the wall of the pancreatic pseudocyst is fibrous and lacks an epithelial lining, making it different from a true pancreatic cyst. Pseudocyst is the most frequently observed cystic lesion of the pancreas (80–85%) and it is usually related to an acute or chronic inflammatory process of the pancreas [1].

Classification

Several clinical definitions and classification systems have been proposed in the past in order to define and characterize all aspects of pancreatic pseudocyst. At present, the classification system most used is the one proposed at the International Symposium on Acute Pancreatitis held in Atlanta in 1992:
- *Acute fluid collections* occur early in the course of acute pancreatitis. They are located in or near the pancreas, and always lack a wall of granulation or fibrous tissue.
- *Acute pseudocysts* are constituted by pancreatic juice enclosed by a wall of fibrous or granulation tissue, arising as a consequence of acute pancreatitis or pancreatic trauma.
- *Chronic pseudocysts* are constituted by pancreatic juice enclosed by a wall of fibrous or granulation tissue, arising as a consequence of chronic pancreatitis and lacking an antecedent episode of acute pancreatitis.
- *Pancreatic abscess* is a circumscribed intra-abdominal collection of pus, usually in proximity with the pancreas, containing little or no pancreatic necrosis, arising as a consequence of acute pancreatitis, trauma, or chronic pancreatitis [2].

The differentiation between acute fluid collection, pseudocyst, and abscess well defines the natural history of peripancreatic fluid collections, but it is confusing in the use of terms "acute" and "chronic" to define the pseudocyst since they relate to the underlying pancreatic disease, not to the mode of presentation of the pseudocyst itself.

Recently, Nealon and Walser proposed a new classification based on the pancreatic ductal anatomy seen in patients with pseudocysts as a tool to guide treatment (Fig. 10.1):

- *Type I*: Normal duct and no communication with cyst
- *Type II*: Normal duct with duct–cyst communication
- *Type III*: Otherwise normal duct with stricture and no duct–cyst communication
- *Type IV*: Otherwise normal duct with stricture and duct–cyst communication
- *Type V*: Otherwise normal duct with complete cut-off
- *Type VI*: Chronic pancreatitis, no duct–cyst communication
- *Type VII*: Chronic pancreatitis with duct–cyst communication [3]

Pathogenesis

Acute pseudocyst

Acute pancreatic pseudocyst usually derives from the spreading of pancreatic juice into the peripancreatic tissue, which subsequently leads to the organization of fluid in a walled-off collection. The spreading of pancreatic fluid is typically

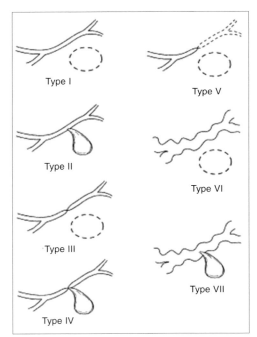

Fig. 10.1 Classification proposed by Nealon and Walser. *Type I*: Normal duct and no communication with cyst. *Type II*: Normal duct with duct–cyst communication. *Type III*: Otherwise normal duct with stricture and no duct–cyst communication. *Type IV*: Otherwise normal duct with stricture and duct–cyst communication. *Type V*: Otherwise normal duct with complete cut-off. *Type VI*: Chronic pancreatitis, no duct–cyst communication. *Type VII*: Chronic pancreatitis with duct–cyst communication [3]

due to the rupture of a pancreatic duct secondary to acute inflammation or trauma of the pancreas. Mostly, even if the pancreatic capsule undergoes opening, fluid remains confined within the peripancreatic tissue; otherwise, it spreads along the pararenal anterior fascia to the lesser omental sac. At first, the collection is not well circumscribed and lacks a definite wall; this is called an acute fluid collection. Most acute fluid collections undergo natural absorption or else, if the collection persists for more than 4–6 weeks, a wall of fibrous or granulation tissue develops, creating a true pancreatic pseudocyst, rich in pancreatic enzymes and containing necrotic debris.

Chronic pseudocyst

Pancreatic pseudocysts are more commonly associated with chronic pancreatitis. The underlying mechanisms are: first, (as in acute pseudocyst), a sequela of limited pancreatic necrosis that produces a pancreatic ductal leak in a case of acute-on-chronic pancreatitis. Second, a sequela of chronic pancreatitis due to blockage of a major branch of a pancreatic duct by a protein plug, calculus, or localized fibrosis that leads to pancreatic cyst or pseudocyst formation. When there is blockage of the major branch of the main pancreatic duct, the ongoing pancreatic secretion proximal to the obstruction leads to a saccular dilatation of the duct, which is filled with pancreatic juice. Such cysts are truly retention cysts and they do not contain solid debris. The microcysts formed can eventually coalesce and lose their epithelial lining as they enlarge. Initially, cysts are intrapancreatic fluid collections, but they can reach the capsule of the pancreas when they grow. If the capsule ruptures, then pancreatic fistula may develop. The rupture of the capsule can occur in one, two, or even multiple sites, resulting in pancreatic juice entering the retroperitoneal space or peritoneal cavity. Pancreatic juice may migrate from the pancreas, its limits being the adjacent organs or a fibrous layer. If the ductal disruption persists, however, then a pancreatic pseudocyst may develop. The pseudocyst is, in fact, a longstanding peripancreatic or intrapancreatic fluid collection which develops a significant wall, as defined by imaging studies. This process develops insidiously, although the cyst itself can become the source of pain once it reaches sufficient size.

The location of pancreatic fluid collections can be explained by the location of the disruption in the ductal system. A ductal disruption ventrally results in fluid accumulation in the lesser sac or in the peritoneal cavity. Therefore, the location of the fluid collection is the key to the location of the pancreatic duct disruption. Ductal disruption is more frequently located in the head of the pancreas (50% of the cases) than in the body (30%) or tail (20%) [4]. This is due to the anatomy of the main pancreatic duct, which turns cranially and ventrally forming an angle as it passes from the head to body ("genu blow-out" theory).

Macroscopic Anatomy, Size, and Location of Pseudocysts

A pancreatic pseudocyst is commonly a round or oval lesion and its wall is composed of fibrous and granulation tissue without well-defined cleavage between the adjacent viscera. A pseudocyst of the pancreas may, on occasion, have a blue appearance on external inspection, hence the appellation "blue dome" pseudocyst. The wall is friable, shaggy, and discolored (Fig. 10.2). The formation of a pseudocyst usually takes 4–6 weeks. The size and volume of a pseudocyst are variable. In the literature, the size of pseudocysts varies from 2 to 35 cm, and estimated volumes range between 10 and 6000 ml.

Pseudocyst fluid is sterile, rich in pancreatic enzymes, and most often blood-tinged or frankly hemorrhagic. Following the removal of the fluid from the cavity, there may be gritty, mud-like material remaining. In the literature, bacterial cultures of cyst fluid are usually positive in 20–50% of patients cultured [5]. However, these figures probably overestimate the incidence of positive bacterial growth since asymptomatic patients and pancreatic pseudocysts with clear fluid are excluded [6]. Pancreatic pseudocysts are often single (about 90% of cases), but sometimes there are two or more (10–20%). Multiple pseudocysts have been diagnosed in both chronic and acute alcoholic pancreatitis. This might be explained by the fact that alcohol is more likely to cause widespread, diffuse injuries to the pancreatic ducts and it may result in the increased incidence of multiple pseudocysts [7].

Like their size, the location of pseudocysts is important in the management and often terms of the symptoms caused. Most pancreatic pseudocysts are retrogastric. However, the location of pseudocysts is different in acute and in chronic pancreatitis. According to some authors [8], acute pancreatic pseudocysts are frequently located in the tail of the gland, whereas others have found nearly equal distribution of the pseudocysts in the head and body, with only 7% appear-

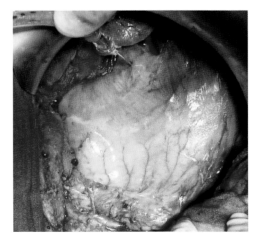

Fig. 10.2 Intraoperative view of an acute pancreatic pseudocyst located in the lesser sac

ing in the tail [9]. Chronic pseudocysts are frequently located in the head of gland (50% of cases), in agreement with the theory of "genu blow-out" of the duct of Wirsung [4]. Pancreatic pseudocysts located in the body of the pancreas may extend between the stomach and colon, into the gastrocolic ligament. Sometimes the cysts may extend into the upper space, between the liver and stomach; rarely into the transverse mesocolon. Pseudocysts located in the tail of the gland tend to remain in the retroperitoneum and may extend to the diaphragmatic space or the abdominal cavity, so cysts dislocate the stomach anteriorly and tend to extend into the retrogastric space. In a few cases pseudocysts are located in the splenopancreatic ligament, near the splenic hilum. Mediastinal pancreatic pseudocysts are a rare complication of the diffusion of pancreatic fluid through the aortic and esophageal hiatus. Very rarely, a pseudocyst is located in the pleural space.

Clinical History and Symptoms

The symptoms of pancreatic pseudocysts are related to underlying pancreatic disease (e.g., chronic pancreatitis) or the mass effect of a pseudocyst on adjacent viscera (e.g., gastric compression, obstruction of the Wirsung duct). The most frequent symptoms are pain, especially epigastric pain with radiation to the back, early satiety, and dyspeptic disease. Acute pancreatitis is possible if the duct of Wirsung is obstructed. Gross pancreatic pseudocysts may extend into adjacent viscera, obstructing or compressing them. In these cases frequent symptoms are vomiting and delayed gastric emptying secondary to stomach compression and jaundice secondary to compression of the bile duct system. Acute pancreatic pseudocysts should be excluded in patients with a previous history of acute pancreatitis and recurrent pain or increase in pancreatic enzymes (amylase and lipase). In some cases, the diagnosis of a pancreatic pseudocyst is incidental, usually in asymptomatic patients without a history of acute pancreatitis. In such cases, potential risk factors for pancreatitis such as recent abdominal trauma – even low-energy trauma – and alcoholic abuse should be considered.

Diagnostic Work-up

Radiologic imaging alone has limited accuracy in diagnosing and defining pancreatic pseudocysts because the imaging findings are similar to those of other, non-pseudocystic lesions. The currently available tools are: abdominal ultrasound, computed tomography, magnetic resonance imaging, and magnetic resonance cholangiopancreatography.

Abdominal ultrasound (US) is the first-level examination, used to confirm the presence of an intrapancreatic or extrapancreatic cystic lesion. At US, a pancreatic pseudocyst resembles a hypoechoic round or oval-shaped mass with a hyperechoic external wall (Fig. 10.3). Typically, no septum or vegetation is pres-

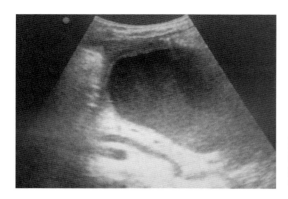

Fig. 10.3 Abdominal ultrasound image of an acute pancreatic pseudocyst of the body of the pancreas

ent inside. Furthermore, US may demonstrate associated pancreatic parenchymal changes related to recent acute pancreatitis, or it may show main duct dilatation or pancreatic calcifications related to chronic pancreatitis. US has emerged as a useful tool in monitoring acute fluid collections and pseudocysts. It suffers from the limitations of the technique and from the retroperitoneal location of the pancreas.

Computed tomography (CT) is the most useful method in defining pancreatic pseudocysts and parenchyma (Fig. 10.4). The cystic lesion is demonstrated in different regions of the abdominal cavity, pelvis, and mediastinum, in relation to the diffusion and organization of pancreatic juice collections. The pseudocyst appears as a hypodense round or oval intrapancreatic or peripancreatic fluid collection within a hyperdense wall. The wall may vary very much in thickness; sometimes it is a thin, barely perceptible wall, sometimes a thick wall that shows

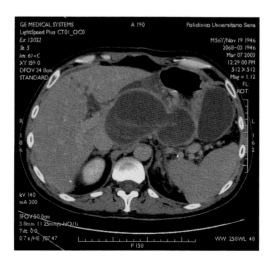

Fig. 10.4 CT of multiple large acute pancreatic pseudocysts involving the whole pancreatic parenchyma

evidence of contrast enhancement. It is interesting to note that no correlation exists between wall thickness, enhancement of the wall after contrast administration, and the stage of the pseudocyst. At present thin-section CT (multislice CT) has gained popularity because of the potential advantage of visualizing communication between the main pancreatic duct and cystic lesions noninvasively. An accurate evaluation of surrounding pancreatic parenchyma is also possible with CT and multislice CT.

Magnetic resonance imaging (MRI) is usually combined with CT in studying and defining cystic lesions of the pancreas. MR cholangiopancreatography is particularly useful in showing the pancreatic excretory system, defining the presence of stenosis, dilatation, or communication with the cystic lesion. An involvement of the bile duct system may also be demonstrated. Particularly in young patients, MR should be preferred to CT in monitoring pancreatic pseudocyst evolution when US is not sufficient.

When patient history and noninvasive radiologic imaging are not sufficient to allow diagnosis and accurate definition of a cystic lesion, endoscopic tools and fine-needle aspiration are indicated.

Endoscopic ultrasound (EUS) is usually performed in cases of chronic pancreatic pseudocyst to better define the underlying parenchyma. The accuracy of EUS in defining chronic pancreatitis is around 80% due to its high sensitivity in detecting initial ductal changes characteristically related to chronic inflammation. EUS is also indicated for defining the anatomy of a pseudocyst prior to endoscopic drainage.

Endoscopic retrograde cholangiopancreatography (ERCP) is usually indicated in cases of chronic pancreatitis or post-traumatic lesion of the main duct. ERCP clearly shows the ductal anatomy and changes and the possible communication with the cystic lesion. ERCP is essential in the planning of endoscopic stenting.

Imaging-guided *fine-needle aspiration (FNA)* is indicated in all cases where the diagnosis is uncertain, for example, when a history of chronic pancreatitis, previous acute pancreatitis, or pancreatic trauma is absent. FNA consists in the aspiration of a small amount of cyst content in order to perform a cytological examination, to analyze the presence of mucin, and to determine tumor markers (CEA and CA 19–9) and assay pancreatic enzymes (amylase and lipase).

Differential Diagnosis

Usually, a previous clinical history of acute pancreatitis or pancreatic trauma or else coexistent chronic pancreatitis helps in defining a cystic lesion of the pancreas with typical imaging findings as a pseudocyst. However, sometimes differentiating pseudocysts from true cysts and from cystic tumors may be difficult.

True cysts of the pancreas are infrequent. They may be congenital (simple cyst, polycystic disease, lymphoepithelial cyst, duodenal enteric cyst, dysontogenetic cyst) or acquired (retention cyst, hydatid cyst).

Serous cystic neoplasms usually appear as expanding masses composed of multiple cysts varying in size from 0.2 to 2 cm, with an overall diameter ranging from 1 to 12 cm or even more. Typically, serous cystic neoplasms have a honeycombed appearance with multiple thin septations and a central stellate scar, sometimes with irregular calcifications. On US, the lesion may appear as a solid echogenic mass due to the interfaces produced by the numerous cysts. It may appear as a solid mass on CT, depending on the size of the cysts and the amount of fibrous tissue. Usually these cysts show marked contrast enhancement. Serous cystic neoplasms are most frequently located in the head of the pancreas and they have lobulated margins. They are typically found in women over the age of 60 years with nonspecific complaints of abdominal pain or weight loss or, more commonly, as an incidental finding. Less frequently, serous cystic neoplasms present as macrocystic or oligocystic variants that are more difficult to differentiate from mucinous cystic neoplasms or pseudocysts.

Mucinous cystic neoplasms are the most common cystic tumors of the pancreas. They are usually large and located in the body or tail of the pancreas. Mucinous cystic neoplasms may be unilocular or multilocular, always more than 2 cm in size. The wall thickness varies and sometimes presents calcifications; the epithelial lining produces mucin. Solid papillary excrescences and septations may protrude from the wall into the intracystic space, but absence of these does not exclude malignancy. There is a spectrum of mucinous cystic neoplasms from benign to malignant, but it is rarely possibly confidently to exclude malignancy on the basis of imaging findings alone. The cysts are usually diagnosed in women during two age spans: between 30 and 35 years of age for benign or borderline lesions and between 65 and 70 for malignant lesions.

Mucinous cystic tumors should always be resected because they are all potentially malignant. When the cyst is small in an asymptomatic patient, cyst aspiration and analysis of the cyst fluid can be helpful in the differential diagnosis.

Owing to partial volume averaging with the hypoattenuating cyst fluid, the fine internal septa and small intramural nodules may not be visible on conventional contrast-enhanced CT. This is why mucinous cystic neoplasm is sometimes misdiagnosed as pseudocysts. Thin-section CT has been known to depict internal anatomic details more clearly, which may help to avoid misdiagnosis. The large size of unilocular cysts excludes the diagnosis of intraductal papillary mucinous tumor.

Intraductal papillary mucinous tumor is characterized by the papillary proliferation of pancreatic ductal epithelium and production of mucin. It is characterized by cystic dilatation of the main or a side branch duct that contains thick mucoid secretions. Intraductal papillary mucinous tumor typically has a grape-like appearance and is located in the uncinate process (lesser pancreas). It is usually diagnosed in men aged 65–70 years.

The side branch duct type is the most commonly mistaken for mucinous cystic tumor or pseudocyst. Its typical location (uncinate process), typical appearance (grape-like locular appearance), and communication with the duct as seen on ERCP or MR cholangiopancreatography usually distinguish it from other lesions in the pancreas. A markedly dilated uncinate branch filled with mucus is a typical feature of a side branch intraductal papillary mucinous tumor.

Solid and papillary epithelial neoplasms, also known as solid and pseudopapillary tumors, papillary and cystic tumors, or solid–cystic tumors, are histologically distinctive neoplasms of low malignant potential with a favorable prognosis. Solid and papillary epithelial neoplasms are typically found in young women. The tumor tends to be a large, well-circumscribed, and slowly growing mass. It may have a variety of internal appearances, from purely cystic to completely solid, but is usually surrounded by a thick, well-defined rim. The appearance of the internal architecture typically depends on the degree of hemorrhage and necrosis of the tumor.

Complications

The majority of acute pancreatic pseudocysts undergo spontaneous resolution; 20–70% of pseudocysts resolve within a period of not more than 6 weeks [10, 11]. Recent studies demonstrate that 38% of acute pseudocysts may undergo absorption even after 6 months. Otherwise, both acute and chronic pancreatic pseudocysts may undergo complications.

Hemorrhage

Hemorrhage is one of the most fatal complications of pancreatic pseudocyst. It may be intracystic or secondary to portal hypertension due to a thrombosis involving the splenic vein or, less frequently, the portal vein. Arterial intracystic hemorrhage is the most frequently observed, taking place in 2–13% of cases. The splenic, pancreaticoduodenal, and gastroduodenal arteries are generally the vessels involved. Less frequently, the common hepatic artery, superior mesenteric artery or one of its proximal branches (Fig. 10.5), and left renal arteries are involved.

Intracystic hemorrhage may lead to hemoperitoneum due to rupture of the cyst into the abdominal cavity or to gastrointestinal bleeding when rupture occurs into the gastrointestinal tract. Rarely, gastrointestinal bleeding may be secondary to intracystic hemorrhage with passage of blood into the pancreatic duct or, theoretically, due to erosion of the bile duct system. Pseudoaneurysm of the splenic artery or other splanchnic arteries related to the inflammatory process of pseudocyst formation may similarly lead to intra-abdominal hemorrhage. Occasionally, perisplenitis secondary to pseudocyst of the pancreatic tail leads to intra-abdominal bleeding. Thrombosis of the splenic vein is associated with pancreatic pseudocysts in 7–20% of cases and leads to the formation of esophageal and gastric varices due to left-side portal hypertension. Portal vein thrombosis is less frequent and usually secondary to large pseudocysts of the pancreatic head.

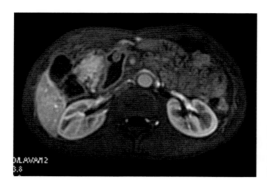

Fig. 10.5 MRI of a pancreatic pseudo-cyst. A proximal branch of the superior mesenteric artery is embraced by the cystic lesion

Rupture and Fistulization

Pancreatic pseudocysts may rupture into the abdominal cavity or retroperitoneal space. Leakage of pseudocyst content into the peritoneal cavity leads to pancreatic ascites with evolution to peritonitis. Retroperitoneal rupture may lead to the formation of collections in the retroperitoneal space that occasionally spread to the mediastinum with secondary mediastinitis. Rupture may also occur into the gastrointestinal tract: stomach, duodenum, colon, and small intestine. Fistulization into the gastrointestinal tract may result in resolution of the pseudocyst if it occurs into the stomach or duodenum. On the other hand, if the colon or the distal tract of the small intestine is involved, superinfection of the pancreatic pseudocyst frequently occurs. Occasionally fistulization into the pleural cavity or the skin may happen.

Infection

Infection may result from colonization of the pseudocyst by micro-organisms from the gastrointestinal tract or may be iatrogenic, secondary to diagnostic and therapeutic procedures (e.g., ERCP, FNA, etc.). Previous operations for the treatment of acute pancreatitis may also be the cause. It is important to note that positive microbiologic results are not considered to represent infection if no symptoms are present. It is also important to differentiate a pancreatic abscess from an abscess pseudocyst as defined by the Atlanta classification.

Treatment

Management options of pancreatic pseudocysts include conservative, percutaneous, endoscopic, and surgical treatment.

Conservative Treatment

Life-threatening complications related to conservative, noninterventional treatment of pancreatic pseudocysts have been frequently reported in the literature. On the other hand, spontaneous resolution of pancreatic pseudocysts has been reported in 20–70% of cases. On this point, it should be noted that the real percentage may be much lower because many studies do not distinguish between pseudocyst and acute fluid collection [12]. It should also be noted that chronic pseudocysts rarely undergo spontaneous resolution [13]. Several authors have demonstrated that spontaneous resolution is related to the type and severity of the inflammatory process and to the size of lesion. Acute pancreatic pseudocysts measuring 6 cm or more in diameter are usually related to severe pancreatitis and rarely resolve spontaneously. Pseudocysts equal to or less than 4 cm in diameter are a consequence of mild to moderate pancreatitis and usually resolve without treatment [14].

Absolute indications for treatment are the presence of symptoms, enlargement of the cystic lesion, especially in chronic pancreatitis, suspicion of cystic neoplasms, and complications. Potential indications for treatment are a diameter equal to or greater than 6 cm, persistence for 6 weeks or more, changes in ductal anatomy, and multiple pseudocysts if suggestive of intraductal papillary mucinous tumor.

Percutaneous Treatment

Percutaneous drainage of acute and chronic pancreatic pseudocysts should be reserved for symptomatic cases, especially when infection/abscess is present. US-guided drainage of acute pancreatic pseudocysts has been recently proposed as the first option in high-risk patients, especially those with pseudocysts that do not communicate with the ductal system. The most frequently observed complications after percutaneous drainage are infection and fistulization. Furthermore, complete emptying of the cystic lesion is infrequent even with large-caliber catheters. Percutaneous drainage has rarely demonstrated its utility in chronic pancreatic pseudocysts.

Endoscopic Treatment

Endoscopic management of pancreatic pseudocysts consists in transpapillary and transmural drainage. Transpapillary drainage consists of stent placement in the main duct, after sphincterotomy if this is performed. This procedure has shown itself to be very useful for a ruptured duct of Wirsung or for pseudocysts that communicate directly with the ductal system. Stent placement should be also considered in chronic pancreatic pseudocysts in the presence of changes in the ductal anatomy (e.g., stenosis, fibrosis) or stones.

Transmural drainage consists in the placement of one or more stents through the gastric or duodenal wall into the pseudocyst. Usually preoperative staging includes EUS. Sometimes transmural and transpapillary drainage are used together. The main adverse events with transmural drainage are incomplete drainage of the pseudocyst and infection of the pseudocyst secondary to communication with the gastrointestinal tract.

Surgical Treatment

Surgical treatment should treat both the pancreatic pseudocyst and the underlying disease. Actually, surgical treatment remains the first option for low-risk patients affected by a large cystic lesion with high debris content. Recurrence after percutaneous or endoscopic treatment represents an absolute indication. Surgical treatment for pancreatic pseudocyst includes resection and derivative procedures. Derivative procedures use the stomach, duodenum, or small bowel. Jejunal Roux-en-Y loop seems to be the preferred procedure in order to reduce the possibility of infection of the cystic cavity.

Resection is the preferred procedure for complex or multiple pseudocysts if easily resectable or if cystic neoplasm is suspected. Distal splenopancreatectomy is the preferred option for pseudocysts of the body and tail with associated thrombosis of the splenic vein. Duodenopancreatectomy is rarely performed, usually in cases of multiple intrapancreatic pseudocysts of the head related to chronic pancreatitis.

Treatment of Complications

Hemorrhage, rupture, or abscess formation requires urgent treatment. Intracystic and pseudoaneurysm hemorrhage are usually treated by angiographic embolization. If radiologic embolization fails, surgical intervention is needed, with ligation of the vessel concerned, pancreatic resection, and derivation of the pseudocyst. The type of procedure depends on the type and site of the hemorrhage as well as on the patient's general condition. Packing is even indicated in extremely severely ill patients.

With regard to infection, percutaneous drainage is the first option in high-risk patients, but it may also be considered in low-risk patients as a bridge treatment for acute noncommunicating pseudocysts, allowing definitive surgical intervention to be postponed. In low-risk patients, derivative or resective treatment should be considered as the first option.

Rupture usually requires resection. In patients with pseudocysts that are complex or located in the pancreatic head, a derivative procedure should be preferred. Some authors propose stent placement together with surgical operation [12] (Fig. 10.6).

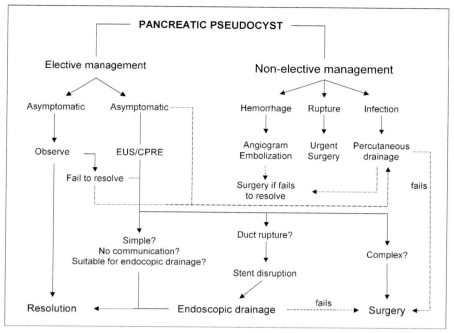

Fig. 10.6 Algorithm for elective and urgent treatment of pancreatic pseudocysts. Modified from Baillie [12]

References

1. Singhal D, Kakodkar R, Sud R, Chaudhary A (2006) Issues in management of pancreatic pseudocysts. JOP 7:502–507
2. Bradley EL 3rd (1993) A clinically based classification system for acute pancreatitis. Summary of the International Symposium on Acute Pancreatitis. Arch Surg 128:586–590
3. Nealon WH, Walser E (2002) Main pancreatic ductal anatomy can direct choice of modality for treating pancreatic pseudocysts (surgery versus percutaneous drainage). Ann Surg 235:751–758
4. Traverso LW, Newman RM, Kozarek RA (1998) The management of pancreatic ductal disruption leading to pancreatic fistula, pancreatic ascites, or pleural effusion. In: Cameron JL (ed) Current surgical therapy, 6th edn. Philadelphia: Mosby-Year Book, pp 510–514
5. Baillie J (2004) Pancreatic pseudocysts (Part I). Gastrointest Endosc 59:873–878
6. Kane MG, Guenter JK (1984) Pancreatic pseudocyst. Adv Intern Med 29:271–300
7. Nguyen BL, Thompson JS, Edney JA, et al (1991) Influence of the etiology of pancreatitis on the natural history of pancreatic pseudocysts. Am J Surg 162:527–530
8. Bradley EL 3rd (1984) Cystoduodenostomy. New perspectives. Ann Surg 200:698–701
9. Sanfey H, Aguilar M, Jones RS (1994) Pseudocysts of the pancreas: a review of 97 cases. Am Surg 60:661–668
10. Andren-Sandberg A, Dervis C (2004) Pancreatic pseudocysts in the 21st century. Part I: classification, pathophysiology, anatomic considerations and therapy. JOP 5:8–24
11. Warshaw AL, Rattner DW (1985) Timing of surgical drainage for pancreatic pseudocyst. Clinical and chemical criteria. Ann Surg 202:720–724

12. Baillie J (2004) Pancreatic pseudocysts (Part II). Gastrointest Endosc 60:105–113
13. Soliani P, Ziegler S, Franzini C, et al (2004) The size of pancreatic pseudocyst does not influence the outcome of invasive treatments. Dig Liver Dis 36:135–140
14. Yeo CJ, Lynch-Nyhan A, Fishman EK, et al (1990) The natural history of pancreatic pseudocysts documented by computed tomography. Surg Gynecol Obstet 170:411–447

Chapter 11

Cystic Neoplasms of the Pancreas

Pierfilippo Crucitti, Sergio Valeri, Andrea Garberini, Roberto Coppola

Cystic neoplasms of the pancreas are a particular category of pancreatic tumor. They are commonly classified into serous types, mucinous types, and intraductal papillary mucinous neoplasms (IPMNs). The serous types account for 35% of cystic neoplasms and 1–2% of all neoplasms of the exocrine pancreas [1]. The mucinous types account for 1% of all exocrine pancreatic tumors and 27% of cystic neoplasms of the pancreas (20.1% cystadenoma and 7.0% cystadenocarcinoma) [2]. Then there are the IPMNs, which account for 0.5–9.8% of all tumors of the pancreatic parenchyma [3, 4].

Serous Cystic Tumors

The serous type of pancreatic cystic tumor mainly consists of cystadenoma; the malignant form (serous cystadenocarcinoma) is of low incidence. These tumors are generally characterized by lesions of small size (≤2 cm) containing clear or brownish liquid, having a capsule, and made up of multiple loculations, which give it a typical spongy or honeycombed look. The capsule, like the covering tissue of the internal chamber, is made up of a single layer of flat or cubical epithelium. There can also be small calcifications, which are important for the differential diagnosis. Patients affected by serous cystic tumors have symptoms that are often vague and nonspecific. The forms range from the nonsymptomatic to those that cause abdominal pain associated with nausea, vomiting, and, more rarely, obstructive jaundice.

Mucinous Cystic Tumors

Mucinous cystic tumors are classified into benign neoplasms (cystoadenoma, 60% of cases) and malignant neoplasms (cystadenocarcinoma, 40% of cases) [5]. These tumors mainly affect women (more than 95% of cases) in their 40s and 50s; they are rarely found in men or in postmenopausal women [6]. They

W. Siquini (Ed.), *Surgical Treatment of Pancreatic Diseases.*
©Springer-Verlag Italia 2009

generally appear as single lesions, capsuled, multiloculated, with mucinous content and, rarely, with calcifications inside. They are often larger than serous cystic tumors. In 95% of cases they are located in the body or tail of the pancreas [7], and communication with the main pancreatic duct (duct of Wirsung) is very rare; the latter appears normal at radiological investigation. Histologically the "ovarian-like stroma" is typical of this tumor and allows a definite diagnosis [8]. The "ovarian-like stroma" is a typical multilayered tissue made of fusiform cells with an oval nucleus that express receptors for estrogen and progesterone. The clinical presentation of a patient affected by mucinous cystic neoplasm is basically comparable to the serous forms [9].

Over the years, given the incidence of the malignant type, several factors predictive of malignancy have been studied in order to select patients for surgical resection.

Intraductal Papillary Mucinous Neoplasms

Intraductal papillary mucinous neoplasms of the pancreas were described by Ohashi et al. for the first time in 1982 [10]. They reported four cases of "mucin-producing cancer" involving the main pancreatic duct. These neoplasms were characterized by the endoscopic triad of mucin production, dilatation of the pancreatic duct, and a swollen papilla (Fig. 11.1). Only in 2000 did the World Health Organization rename these lesions "intraductal papillary mucinous neo-

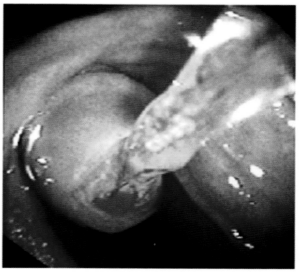

Fig. 11.1 Endoscopic retrograde cholangiopancreatography (ERCP): swollen papilla with hypersecretion of mucus

plasm." The median age at diagnosis ranges from 60 to 70 years, and these neo-plasms develop most frequently in the head of the pancreas (61.1%). They are found in the body or tail in only 28.9% of cases, while 10% of cases involve the whole gland [11]. Compared to the more common pancreatic adenocarcinoma, for which the mean 5-year survival after surgery is 5%, IPMNs allow a decided-ly better prognosis after radical surgical resection, with an average patient sur-vival rate of 5 years after surgery varying from 75 to 78% [3–12]. The natural history of this disease is not yet clear, however, which often makes it difficult to determine the best therapeutic strategy [13].

Macroscopically, IPMNs appear as cystic multiloculated villous neoplasms. They can be classified as *main duct type*, affecting the main pancreatic duct; *branch duct type*, affecting only branch ducts; or *combined type*, in which both main and branch ducts are involved. Unlike the main duct and the combined types, branch duct IPMNs seem to be benign in most cases; only rarely are they associated with an invasive carcinoma (57– 92% in main duct IPMNs, compared to 6–46% in branch duct IPMNs) [14]. Histologically, IPMNs are characterized by an intraductal papillary proliferation of neoplastic cells with dilatation of the main and/or branch ducts. On the basis of histological characteristics and the presence or absence of dysplasia, IPMNs can be classified as benign (adenoma, 10.4%, and borderline form, 17.6%) or malignant (carcinoma in situ, 33.8%, and invasive carcinoma, 38.2%) [15] (Fig. 11.2). A salient characteristic of IPMNs is their multifocality, which according to some researchers is responsible for recurrence of the disease even in patients who have undergone radical surgical resection [13, 16, 17].

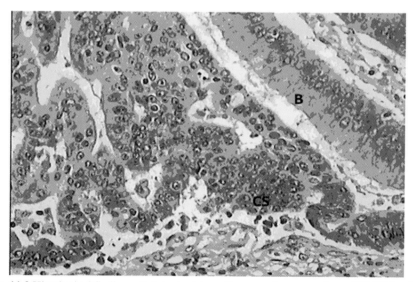

Fig. 11.2 Histological findings. *B*, Intraductal papillary mucinous neoplasm (IPMN) border-line; *CS*, IPMN with carcinoma in situ

Most patients affected by IPMN present symptoms at the time of diagnosis, with percentages varying in different studies from 70 to 81% [3, 11, 17]. Abdominal pain is the most common symptom (70–80%) [18] and is usually caused by partial or complete obstruction of the pancreatic ducts by mucin and/or intraductal growth of the neoplasm itself, with a mechanism similar therefore to that of obstructive chronic pancreatitis. Jaundice, on the other hand, is a less common symptom in these patients (18%) [14] than it is in pancreatic adenocarcinoma.

As we have seen previously, IPMNs of the pancreas can be subdivided into benign and malignant forms, with 5-year survival rates varying, respectively, from 77 to 100% and from 43 to 80% [10, 11, 18, 19].

Unlike the situation for ductal adenocarcinoma, there continues to be debate as to the best course of therapy for patients affected by IPMN, and in particular as to which patients can benefit most from surgical resection. This is due to a number of factors, such as the limited current knowledge of the natural history of these neoplasms, the great variability of histotype, and the difficulty of obtaining a preoperative diagnosis of malignancy. For these reasons, the attention of researchers has been increasingly focused on the identification of predictive factors of malignancy, in order to classify patients with malignant IPMNs more accurately and select those who could truly benefit from surgical treatment. In order to establish unequivocal criteria, in 2006 the International Association of Pancreatology carried out a meta-analysis from which there emerged five predictive factors for malignancy in patients affected by IPMNs [20]:

1. Clinical presentation
2. Type of ductal involvement (main duct vs. branch duct)
3. Size of the neoplasm
4. Mural nodules
5. Dilatation of the main pancreatic duct

In addition to those mentioned above, a number of researchers are working to identify further factors in order to improve the prediction of malignancy for these neoplasms. Among the aspects under study are the cytological characteristics of the lesion, production of mucus and the type of mucin expressed, and the value of neoplastic markers in the pancreatic juice (CEA and CA 19-9).

Differential Diagnosis

Serous Cystic Tumors

When a serous cystic tumor is suspected, the first diagnostic step consists in an ultrasonography (US) and/or computed tomography (CT), given the aspecific symptomatology and absence of specific laboratory signs. The typical radiological report shows the presence of small calcifications in the capsule that encloses the neoformation.

Mucinous Cystic Tumors

The presurgical diagnosis and differential diagnosis between benign and malignant neoplasms may be done both on anamnestic-clinical data and on the basis of an instrumental work-up such as by CT, magnetic resonance imaging (MRI), endoscopic retrograde cholangiopancreatography (ERCP), and fine-needle aspiration under endoscopic ultrasound guidance (EUS-FNA), by which it is possible to take intracystic liquid for cytologic examination or to measure neoplastic markers.

Intraductal Papillary Mucinous Neoplasms

The presence or absence of neoplastic markers (CEA, CA 19-9, and CA 125) in the cystic fluid is important for diagnosis, especially because they help to differentiate malignant from benign lesions. However, the imaging tests are the preferred tests to differentiate benign from malignant IPMNs and to distinguish IPMNs from other cystic formations found in the pancreatic parenchyma. Abdominal US is often the first step in diagnosing patients with an IPMN, even though its specificity and sensitivity are low [21]. CT (Fig. 11.3) is now the test of choice for suspected pancreatic neoplasms, with a sensitivity of 92%, a speci-

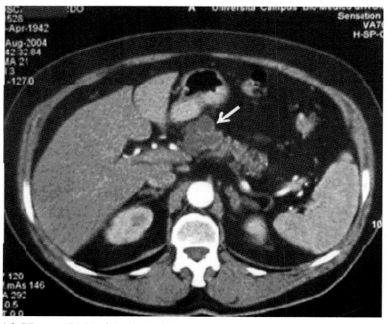

Fig. 11.3 CT scan: IPMN of the head of the pancreas

ficity of 85%, and an accuracy of 89% in differentiating benign from malignant lesions [21]. Using CT it is possible to evaluate multifocal involvement and the presence of mural nodules (sensitivity 73%) [22] or intraluminal calcifications. MRI, especially MR cholangiopancreatography (MRCP) (Fig. 11.4), is very useful in the study of IPMNs [23]. EUS is a very effective method for evaluating IPMNs, with 91% sensitivity, 64% specificity, and 78% accuracy in differentiating benign from malignant lesions [15] (Fig. 11.5). Moreover, with EUS it is pos-

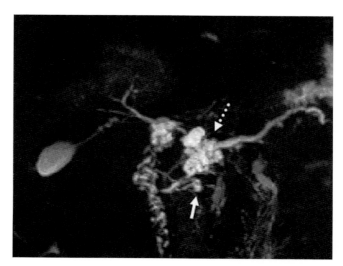

Fig. 11.4 Magnetic resonance cholangiopancreatography (MRCP): IPMN of the head of the pancreas. *Full white arrow:* tumor of a branch duct (uncinate process); *dotted arrow:* tumor of the main pancreatic duct

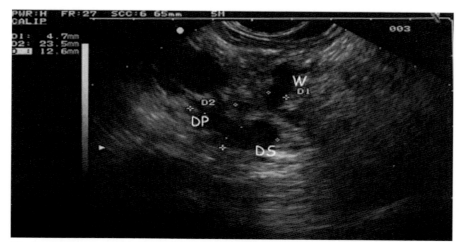

Fig 11.5 Endoscopic ultrasonography (EUS): IPMN of the head of the pancreas. *W* main pancreatic duct (duct of Wirsung); *DP,* tumor of the main pancreatic duct; *DS,* tumor of a branch duct (uncinate process)

sible to take cytological samples of the lesion, which are essential for a differential diagnosis from other cystic lesions, and for an evaluation of the malignancy of the neoplasm. Finally, ERCP is a technique that is being used less and less for the diagnosis of pancreatic lesions, having been replaced in part by noninvasive techniques such as CT, MRCP, and EUS. This test does, however, allow mucus samples to be obtained for chemical-physical and cytological examination.

Surgical Treatment

Serous Cystic Tumors

Surgical therapy of serous cystic tumors of the pancreas is determined by the characteristics of the lesion. Given a benign lesion of small size (≤ 2 cm) in an asymptomatic patient, it is acceptable to decide not to operate and to start a protocol of observation in time. Simple enucleation could also be suggested. Larger cystadenomas must be treated with a minimal pancreatic resection including the tumor. In the rare cases of cystadenocarcinoma, on the other hand, a radical operation such as pancreaticoduodenectomy or distal pancreatectomy (depending on its location) is necessary.

Mucinous Cystic Tumors

For mucinous cystic tumors, surgery is the answer (if there are no comorbidities) [24]. It is important to remember that all cystadenomas can evolve (although only a few do) into an invasive form with a prognosis as bad as that of ductal adenocarcinoma [25]. Moreover, in 40% of cases an adenocarcinoma can be found. This is why surgical treatment must be correct from the oncological point of view, with complete excision of the tumor combined with a peripancreatic lymphadenectomy [26–28].

Intraductal Papillary Mucinous Neoplasms

Indications for surgical treatment in patients affected by an IPMN are dictated by the criteria we have mentioned as predictive of malignancy. However, controversy remains over the type and especially the extent of the surgical resection. Depending on the site of the lesion, the treatments of choice are pancreaticoduodenectomy (Whipple procedure or pylorus-preserving pancreaticoduodenectomy) for neoplasms of the pancreatic head; distal pancreatectomy for neoplasms of the body and tail; central pancreatectomy for neoplasms limited to the body of the pancreas; and total pancreatectomy in the case of lesions diffused throughout the parenchyma. In cases of benign lesions of limited extent, atypical surgical resections have been proposed in order to preserve endocrine and exocrine pancreatic function as much as possible, despite the technical difficulties and the greater incidence of postoperative complications [29–32]. The aspect of surgical treatment of IPMNs most discussed at present concerns the extent of the resection, due to the fact that the incidence of local recurrence is as high as 11% in some studies, even though the prognosis is better than that of ductal adenocarcinoma [15, 18, 19, 14]. A crucial role in deciding the extent of the surgical resection – both in patients with invasive IPMNs and, perhaps more clearly, in patients with noninvasive IPMNs – is played by the frozen section of the resection margin. Nevertheless, it must be noted that finding negative margins does not indicate with absolute certainty that the disease has been definitively cured. In fact, it is well known that IPMNs can be multifocal, and therefore it is not uncommon to find skip lesions within healthy pancreatic tissue [20]. If a positive resection margin is found, the surgical approach differs sharply depending on the degree of histological malignancy encountered. In the presence of an IPMN adenoma, the tendency now is not to further extend the surgical resection, but in a case of IPMN with carcinoma in situ and invasive carcinoma there is an indication for extending the surgical resection right up to total pancreatectomy. The real problem is the presence of a borderline IPMN at frozen section, where the decision whether or not to extend the surgical resection should be guided more by the condition of the patient than by the histological examination alone [20].

Follow-up

Serous Cystic and Mucinous Cystic Tumors

Patients who have undergone resection of either serous or mucinous cystoadenomas do not need follow-up, according to studies that demonstrated a relapse rate equal to zero [7]. Meanwhile, patients who have undergone resection of either serous or mucinous cystoadenocarcinomas are at significant risk of relapse. In these patients a follow-up with MRI is necessary every 6 months in order to rule out local recurrence of the disease and/or the presence of metastasis.

Intraductal Papillary Mucinous Neoplasms

Follow-up for patients who have undergone surgery for an IPMN is essential both because of our uncertain knowledge of the natural history of these neoplasms, the risk of local recurrence, and the possibility of a second surgical procedure. The frequency of follow-up must be determined individually in each case, depending on the histotype and thus on the risk of recurrence. Patients with an IPMN adenoma, with negative resection margin and normal pancreatic stump, require annual follow-ups. For those with a borderline IPMN or IPMN with carcinoma in situ with a positive resection margin or with an indeterminate cystic lesion in the pancreatic parenchyma, frequent follow-ups are necessary for the first 2–3 years [33]. As for patients who do not require surgical treatment, they must be given a strict follow-up program (as often as every 3–6 months). It seems reasonable to perform follow-up annually in cases of lesions smaller than 10 mm; every 6–12 months for lesions between 10 mm and 20 mm; and every 3–6 months for lesions larger than 20 mm [20]. During these check-ups, the appearance of symptoms (such as recurring pancreatitis), an increase in size of the cyst (>30 mm), or increased dilatation of the main pancreatic duct (>6 mm) is an indication for surgical treatment [20].

References

1. Hamilton SR, Aaltonen LA (eds) (2002) WHO histological classification of tumors of the exocrine pancreas. IARC Press, Lyon, pp 219–251
2. Sheehan MK, Beck K, Pickleman J, Aranha GV (2003) Spectrum of cystic neoplasms of the pancreas and their surgical management. Arch Surg 138:657–662
3. Adsay NV, Conlon KC, Zee SY et al (2002) Intraductal papillary-mucinous neoplasms of the pancreas: an analysis of in situ and invasive carcinomas in 28 patients. Cancer 94:62–77
4. Tanaka M, Kobayashi K, Mizumoto K, Yamaguchi K (2005) Clinical aspects of intraductal papillary mucinous neoplasm of the pancreas. J Gastroenterol 40:669–675
5. Thompson LD, Becker RC, Przygodzki RM et al (1999) Mucinous cystic neoplasm (mucinous cystadenocarcinoma of lowgrade malignant potential) of the pancreas: a clinicopathologic study of 130 cases. Am J Surg Pathol 23:1–16
6. Reddy RP, Smyrk TC, Zapiach M et al (2004) Pancreatic mucinous cystic neoplasm defined by ovarian stroma: demographics, clinical features, and prevalence of cancer. Clin Gastroenterol Hepatol 2:1026–1031
7. Zamboni G, Scarpa A, Bogina G et al (1999) Mucinous cystic tumors of the pancreas: clinicopathological features, prognosis, and relationship to other mucinous cystic tumors. Am J Surg Pathol 23:410–422
8. Izumo A, Yamaguchi K, Eguchi T et al (2003) Mucinous cystic tumor of the pancreas: immunohistochemical assessment of "ovarian-type stroma". Oncol Rep 10:515–525
9. Wilentz RE, Albores-Saavedra J, Zahurak M et al (1999) Pathologic examination accurately predicts prognosis in mucinous cystic neoplasms of the pancreas. Am J Surg Pathol 23:1320–1327
10. Ohashi K, Murakami Y, Maruyama M et al (1982) Four cases of mucin-producing cancer of the pancreas on specific findings of the papilla of Vater. Prog Dig Endoscopy 20:348–351
11. Jang JY, Kim SW, Ahn YJ et al (2005) Multicenter analysis of clinicopathologic features of intraductal papillary mucinous tumor of the pancreas: is it possible to predict the malignancy before surgery? Ann Surg Oncol 12:124–132
12. Conlon KC (2005) Intraductal papillary mucinous tumors of the pancreas. J Clin Oncol 23:4518–4523
13. Wang S, Shyr YM, Chen TH et al (2005) Comparison of resected and non-resected intraductal papillary mucinous neoplasms of the pancreas. World J Surg; 29:1650–1657
14. Wada K, Kozarek RA, Traverso LW et al (2005) Outcomes following resection of invasive and noninvasive intraductal papillary mucinous neoplasms of the pancreas. Am J Surg 189:632–637
15. Sohn TA, Yeo CJ, Cameron JL et al (2004) Intraductal papillary mucinous neoplasm of the pancreas: an updated experience. Ann Surg 239:788–799
16. Azar C, Van de Stadt J, Rickaert F et al (1996) Intraductal papillary mucinous neoplasms of the pancreas: clinical and therapeutic issues in 32 patients. Gut 39:457–464

17. Nagai E, Ueki T, Chijiiwa K et al (1995) Intraductal papillary mucinous neoplasms of the pancreas associated with so-called "mucinous ductal ectasia": histochemical and immunoistochemical analysis of 29 cases. Am J Surg Pathol 19:576–589

18. D'Angelica M, Brennan MF, Suriawinata AA et al (2004) Intraductal papillary mucinous neoplasm of the pancreas: an analysis of clinicopathologic features and outcome. Ann Surg 239:400–408

19. Salvia R, Fernández-del Castillo C, Bassi C et al (2004) Main-duct intraductal papillary mucinous neoplasms of the pancreas: clinical predictors of malignancy and long-term survival following resection. Ann Surg 239:678–687

20. Tanaka M, Chari S, Adsay V et al (2006) International consensus guidelines for management of intraductal papillary mucinous neoplasms and mucinous cystic neoplasms of the pancreas. Pancreatology 6:17–32

21. Kawai M, Uchiyama K, Tani M et al (2004) Clinicopathological features of malignant intraductal papillary mucinous tumors of the pancreas: the differential diagnosis from benign entities. Arch Surg 139:188–192

22. Sugiyama M, Atomi Y (1998) Intraductal papillary mucinous tumors of the pancreas. Imaging studies and treatment strategies. Ann Surg 228:685–691

23. Cellier C, Cuillerier E, Palazzo L et al (1998) Intraductal papillary and mucinous tumors of the pancreas: accuracy of preoperative computer tomography, endoscopic retrograde pancreatography and endoscopic ultrasonography, and long term outcome in a large surgical series. Gastrointest Endosc 47:42–49

24. Lillemoe KD, Kaushal S, Cameron JL et al (1999) Distal pancreatectomy: indications and outcomes in 235 patients. Ann Surg 229:693–698

25. Sarr MG, Carpenter HA, Prabhakar LP et al (2000) Clinical and pathologic correlation of 84 mucinous cystic neoplasms of the pancreas: can one reliably differentiate benign from malignant (or premalignant) neoplasms? Ann Surg 231:205–212

26. Shoup M, Brennan MF, McWhite K et al (2002) The value of splenic preservation with distal pancreatectomy. Arch Surg 137:164–168

27. Warshaw AL (1988) Conservation of the spleen with distal pancreatectomy. Arch Surg 123:550–553

28. Lukish JR, Rothstein JH, Petruzziello M et al (1999) Spleen-preserving pancreatectomy for cystic pancreatic neoplasms. Am Surg 65:596–599

29. Imaizumi T, Hanyu F, Suzuki M et al (1995) Clinical experience with duodenum-preserving total resection of the head of the pancreas with pancreatico-choledochoduodenectomy. J Hepatobiliary Pancreat Surg 2:38–44

30. Nakao A (2004)Pancreatic head resection with segmental duodenectomy and preservation of the gastroduodenal artery. Hepatogastroenterology 145:533–535

31. Takada T, Amano H, Amori BJ et al (2000) A novel technique for multiple ancreatectomies: removal of uncinate process of the pancreas combined with medial pancreatectomy. J Hepatobiliary Pancreat Surg 7:49–52

32. Shoup M, Brennan ME, McWhite K et al (2002) The value of splenic preservation with distal pancreatectomy. Arch Surg 137:164–168

33. White R, D'Angelica M, Katabi N et al (2007) Fate of the remnant pancreas after resection of noninvasive intraductal papillary mucinous neoplasm. J Am Coll Surg 7:664–671

Chapter 12

Pancreatic Endocrine Tumors

Letizia Boninsegna, Massimo Falconi, Rossella Bettini, Paolo Pederzoli

Epidemiology and Classification

Precise epidemiological data on pancreatic endocrine tumors (PETs) are lacking, even though increased knowledge of the clinical symptoms, pathological characteristics (in particular immunohistochemical), and improved radiological studies and laboratory tests have made detection of these tumors both easier and more frequent [1]. In general, PETs can be considered rare, with an incidence of less than 1 case per 100,000 inhabitants [1, 2], although autopsy data have suggested an incidence of up to 1.5% in the general population [3]. PETs represent about 8–10% of all pancreatic neoplasms [2, 4]. To date, there is no general agreement regarding their cytohistological origin: an early hypothesis was that they derive from islet cells, although the possibility that they arise from pluripotential (neuroendocrine) stem cells in the epithelial duct is another plausible alternative [5]. The study of transgenic mice, moreover, has demonstrated that both cells destined for endocrine differentiation and differentiated adult endocrine cells can give rise to endocrine tumors [6, 7]. In any case, PETs and the entire gastrointestinal tract express a phenotype similar to cells of the so-called diffuse endocrine system (DES) [8], a fact that has facilitated their study from pathological/histological and immunohistochemical standpoints. The World Health Organization (WHO) [9] proposed a classification system in 2000 that uses the term "endocrine," recognizing the histogenic relationship of these neoplasms with endocrine organs and/or cells of the DES. The term "neuroendocrine" is also used interchangeably with "endocrine."

In particular, the classification system takes account of the potential biological aggressiveness of neuroendocrine tumors by distinguishing:
- Well-differentiated endocrine tumors: (a) nonaggressive behavior; (b) uncertain biological behavior
- Well-differentiated endocrine carcinomas
- Poorly differentiated endocrine carcinomas

Endocrine tumors are also frequently classified on the basis of their clinical/biological characteristics [1]:

W. Siquini (Ed.), *Surgical Treatment of Pancreatic Diseases.*
©Springer-Verlag Italia 2009

- Functioning PETs (F-PETs), which give rise to specific clinical symptoms as they secrete functional hormones. These include insulinomas, gastrinomas, glucagonomas, VIPomas, somatostatinomas, and carcinoids.
- Nonfunctioning PETs (NF-PETs), which do not cause any endocrine-related clinical symptoms, since no functional hormones able to interact with peripheral cellular receptors are secreted.

Moreover, PETs may be associated with several neoplastic syndromes, in particular with the multiple endocrine neoplasia type 1 (MEN1) and von Hippel–Lindau syndromes. Patients affected with MEN1 develop PETs in 40–90% of cases [10], while 12–20% of patients with von Hippel–Lindau syndrome develop endocrine tumors [11].

Diagnosis

Diagnosis can usually take place in one of three ways:
1. The presence of a clinical endocrine syndrome, which forces the patient to seek medical attention. In this case, diagnosis is considered "early" and permits the identification of the endocrine neoplasm when it is still small. For this reason, F-PETs are usually found to be nonaggressive according to the WHO classification [8], and only a small number of functioning tumors are biologically aggressive (well-differentiated endocrine carcinomas according to the WHO). During preoperative assessment of F-PETs, it should be kept in mind that, even if the patient has been completely studied from the clinical and endocrinological standpoints, the neoplasm will still be too small to be located by diagnostic radiology.
2. The presence of clinical symptoms related to growth of the neoplasm or the presence of pain related to retroperitoneal infiltration [12–14]. Such cases usually involve a NF-PET and do not lead to early symptoms, and are diagnosed by symptoms caused by the increase in tumoral mass. NF-PETs do not necessarily show aggressive biological behavior; however, in the absence of certainty as to their benign nature, surgical intervention must always be planned with radical intent.
3. Incidental diagnosis. In this case the patient has undergone diagnostic radiological evaluation for other reasons. In these patients, decisions about surgical intervention must be balanced, taking into consideration not only the pancreatic lesion(s), which may be of variable aggressiveness, but also the age of the patient and his or her overall clinical condition.

Laboratory Evaluations

There are generally two types of laboratory analysis:
- In the case of F-PETs, concentration of specific hormones, which include glucagon, somatostatin, serotonin, gastrin, insulin, etc., under baseline con-

ditions and after stimulation by means of the respective clinical laboratory tests [15, 16]
– Concentration of generic neuroendocrine markers
  In addition to assessment of plasma levels of pancreatic markers, including CEA and CA 19-9, two markers specific for neuroendocrine neoplasms are chromogranin A (CgA) and neuron-specific enolase (NSE). The former is a glycoprotein located inside secretory vesicles of endocrine cells as well as neuronal cells of the central and peripheral nervous system; it is the most important generic neuroendocrine marker, with a sensitivity between 60 and 90% [17]. It is worth mentioning that plasma levels can be falsely positive in the presence of altered renal function, atrophic chronic gastritis, and during therapy with proton pump inhibitors. NSE is found at the cytoplasmic level in endocrine cells and neurons. From a strictly surgical standpoint, the evaluation of these markers is important for postoperative follow-up. In particular, the plasma level of CgA is lowered after surgery and/or following administration of somatostatin analogs, independently of the efficacy of treatment. Increased values of CgA after each therapy during follow-up can be indicative of recurrence of disease [17].

Instrumental Diagnostic Methods

Instrumental assessment is valuable not only to localize the pancreatic neoplasm and any metastases and/or retroperitoneal lymphadenopathies, but also permits evaluation of the relationship of the tumor with nearby organs and vascular structures. Such information is essential for the planning of surgical intervention. Nevertheless, it should be kept in mind that small endocrine neoplasms will not be visible on instrumental studies, thus forcing a surgical approach that, as will be seen later, will be both diagnostic and therapeutic.

Radiological examinations such as abdominal CT and ultrasound, especially using contrast medium, are able to locate the neoplasm and deliver a complete preoperative assessment in about 60% of cases [18]. Hypervascularization of endocrine tumors, present in 60–70% of patients [19, 20], can be observed by both CT and ultrasound with contrast medium, and can localize the lesion and provide other information regarding its nature. Due to the excellent quality of these methods, angiographic studies are needed less often than previously. While MRI is necessary for the study of other types of pancreatic neoplasm, such as intraductal tumors, in the case of endocrine pathologies it does not appear to provide any advantages over CT or ultrasound with contrast medium. Endoscopic ultrasound (EUS) can be useful when it is difficult to localize the neoplasm, as can other techniques [21] such as venous sampling during angiography [15, 22, 23].

Scintigraphy using radiolabeled octreotide (Octreoscan) is a useful only for endocrine neoplasms in which receptors are present and relies on the density of receptors on the membrane of neoplastic cells. Positivity, reported in 40–90% of cases, is lowest for insulinomas and highest for gastrinomas. As for other instrumental exams, the results of scintigraphy are also influenced by the dimensions of the tumor. Scintigraphy is less specific than CT in the identification of both primary and secondary neoplasms [24]. An Octreoscan study is, however, an important exam that should be considered necessary when somatostatin analogs are to be administered.

Cytological and Histological Characterization

In the case of locally advanced disease with or without metastasis, which is therefore not a candidate for surgical therapy, characterization of the tumor by fine-needle biopsy or percutaneous biopsy is needed for planning the most appropriate course of treatment. When palliative surgical intervention is deemed necessary to reduce the tumoral mass, histological characterization can be carried out intraoperatively. If an endocrine tumor is suspected, fine-needle biopsy is preferred over fine-needle aspirate to permit the evaluation of cellular patterns and the correct differential diagnosis from other forms of tumor, such as papillary cystic and acinar tumors and lymphomas with a pancreatic location (in the case of poorly differentiated endocrine carcinomas) [25]. Moreover, immunohistochemical studies can be performed on biopsy specimens for evaluation of the Ki-67 proliferative index [26].

Surgical Treatment

Surgical intervention for PETs requires ample operator experience, not only in regard to the skill in pancreatic surgery, but also in regard to the correct preoperative planning that will make the surgery valid and efficacious. Surgical evaluation of PETs must take into account that, in comparison to pancreatic neoplasms with an exocrine component, the prognosis is much more favorable, and patients may have a lengthy clinical history even when they have hepatic metastases. Surgical approaches can be quite variable, from the attempt to preserve as much parenchymal tissue as possible in the benign forms, up to massive demolition not only of the pancreas but also of adjacent organs, including hepatic resection in the more aggressive forms. Table 12.1 details the general principles to follow depending on the indication and choice of surgical intervention, which will be discussed in the next section.

Insulinoma

Insulinomas are the most frequent form of F-PET, with an incidence of 1–6 per 1,000,000 in the general population [27, 28]. In 90% of cases, insulinomas are benign neoplasms, and surgery is the only definitive treatment [29–31]. Diagnosis is generally reached from a clinical standpoint and the patient is sur-

Table 12.1 Suggested surgical procedures for endocrine tumors of the pancreas

	Type of resection	
	Typical[a]	Atypical[b]
Insulinoma		Preferred
Sporadic gastrinoma	Preferred	
Gastrinoma in MEN1	Preferred (for lesions ≥3 cm)	
Nonfunctioning tumors	>2 cm	≤2 cm
Other functioning tumors	Preferred	
Nonfunctioning tumor in MEN1		
≤2 cm	No	No
>2 cm	Preferred	

MEN1, multiple endocrine neoplasia type 1

[a]Typical resection: pancreaticoduodenectomy and left pancreatectomy for head and body-tail localizations, respectively

[b]Atypical resection: enucleation and middle pancreatectomy, according to the distance of the lesion from the main pancreatic duct; spleen-preserving distal pancreatectomy for localization at the tail

gically evaluated after having undergone clinical, radiological, and laboratory exams (hormone concentrations, fasting glucose tolerance test, etc.). While these exams may be sufficient for diagnosis of disease, they may not necessarily be sufficient for localization of the tumor exactly. Insulinomas usually present as small neoplasms and are less than 1 cm in size in about 85% of cases [32, 33]; in 10–20% of cases they cannot be localized. In the majority of cases, however, ultrasound with contrast medium, abdominal CT [34], and EUS [35, 36] are sufficient to localize the neoplasm. In any case, intraoperative assessment is an integral and fundamental part of the diagnostic routine.

1. *Surgical exploration:* must be performed whenever the lesion has not been localized. A laparotomic approach is to be preferred as it permits meticulous manual exploration of the pancreas [37, 38]. Complete palpation of the pancreatic head and partial visualization of the posterior wall of the organ is achieved by opening the gastrocolic ligament using a Kocher maneuver. Mobilization and visualization of the pancreatic body and tail are obtained by sectioning the superior and inferior margins as well as the splenic ligament. Insulinomas have a very similar consistency to the surrounding parenchyma, and, when visible, are red-violet in color. In cases in which the lesion is neither visible nor palpable, intraoperative ultrasonography must be carried out using a probe with a frequency of 8–10 MHz [37]. The lesion is hypoechogenic with respect to the surrounding parenchyma.

2. *"Blind resection":* is warranted when the insulinoma is localized with equal probability to pancreatic head, body, or tail [39]. Blind resection should be performed only if it is combined with intra-arterial calcium stimulation and if sampling of the hepatic vein for insulin is indisputably positive to the extent that it will permit regional localization of the insulinoma [22, 40].

3. *Atypical resection* (enucleation and middle pancreatectomy): should be preferred for small, benign tumors as it allows for the greatest preservation of pancreatic parenchyma. In middle pancreatectomy, drainage of the pancreatic stump is restored using pancreaticojejunal anastomosis to minimize the risk of complications (Fig. 12.1). Even though enucleation is an apparently simple procedure, when not performed by an expert surgeon it can be associated with severe complications such as postoperative pancreatitis and pancreatic fistula. For this reason, evaluation with intraoperative ultrasound is fundamental, which permits both precise localization of the lesion and definition of its relationship with the main pancreatic duct, in addition to verification that the neoplasm has been excised in its entirety. In fact, when intraoperative ultrasound is used, complete recovery after excision of insulinomas is seen in almost all patients [30, 31]. It should be kept in mind that even when an atypical resection is performed, the residual pancreatic parenchyma should always be protected by appropriate drainage.

4. *Typical resection* (pancreaticoduodenectomy, distal pancreatectomy with or without splenic preservation): these procedures are used for particularly large neoplasms or in the case of a malignant insulinoma. This type of intervention is performed for endocrine carcinomas (or suspicious lesions) and is combined with accurate lymphadenectomy and excision of any eventual secondary hepatic lesions.

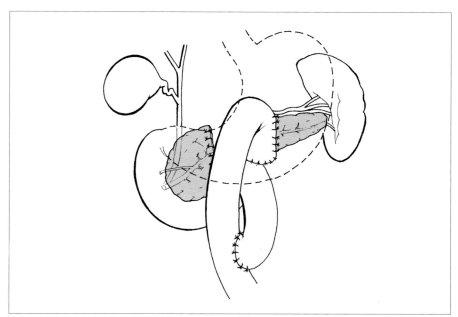

Fig. 12.1 Reconstruction of the pancreas after middle pancreatectomy. The proximal stump is sutured, while a Roux-en-Y jejunal loop is used for pancreaticojejunostomy at the level of the distal stump

Gastrinoma

Gastrinomas are the second most frequent functioning endocrine tumor of the pancreatic area, with an incidence of less than 10 per 1,000,000 in the general population [28, 41]. In 20% of cases, gastrinomas are associated with MEN1 syndrome. Gastrinomas are malignant in 60–90% of cases and have a very aggressive behavior in about 25% of cases. Like other malignant lesions, around one-half of gastrinomas present at diagnosis with metastases, which are localized to the liver in 30% of cases [39]. Gastrinomas are most frequently localized to the duodenum (49% of cases), although they are also found in the pancreas (24%) and lymph nodes (11%). Similar to other functioning endocrine neoplasms, the suspicion of a gastrinoma is based on a set of clinical symptoms, known in the case of gastrinoma as Zollinger–Ellison syndrome, and diagnosis is confirmed based on laboratory tests of acid secretion and gastrin levels before and after secretin stimulation. As with insulinomas, gastrinomas are often diagnosed when small, with a diameter less than 1 cm in 49% of cases [42], and therefore are difficult to localize using preoperative investigations.

1. *Surgical exploration:* as for insulinomas, laparotomy should include thorough exploration of the pancreas using Kocher's maneuver associated with careful exploration of the stomach and mesentery. To determine whether a small gastrinoma is localized to the submucosa of the duodenal wall requires transillumination and longitudinal duodenotomy (about 3 cm) for correct palpation of the medial surface of the duodenal wall [39]. Even in this case, the use of intraoperative ultrasonography is important to evaluate the parenchyma of the pancreas and liver.

2. *Typical resection* (pancreaticoduodenectomy, left pancreatectomy): although some authors recommend atypical resection for small gastrinomas (enucleation whenever possible) [42], it should be kept in mind that gastrinomas are generally malignant tumors and are often associated with unrecognized nodal metastases. Thus, whenever possible intervention with radical intent should be performed, which includes typical pancreatic resection (depending on the tumor site) with lymphadenectomy and may include hepatic metastasectomy. When a radical surgical procedure is not possible, debulking (excision of at least 90% of disease) can nonetheless be performed, which will allow easier control of the clinical syndrome with medical therapy [43].

Other Functioning Endocrine Tumors of the Pancreas

Among other pancreatic neoplasms associated with a clinical syndrome, VIPomas, glucagonomas, and somatostatinomas are worthy of mention. These are very rare tumors that are generally malignant and associated with hepatic metastases at diagnosis. One-year survival rates are not usually more than 50% [44–48]. Given the severe symptoms associated with these neoplasms, a radical operation is justified even in cases in which it can be obtained only through extensive pancreatic resection or in the presence of hepatic metastasis. Surgical procedure usually consists in major pancreatic resection, such as pancreatico-duodenectomy, in particular in somatostatinomas (frequently in a periampullary site), or with left pancreatectomy, in particular in glucagonomas (frequently in the body/tail of the pancreas) [43]. The results of surgical therapy are often only temporary, and in many cases debulking and reintervention are needed in the attempt to control clinical symptoms.

Nonfunctioning Endocrine Tumors of the Pancreas

More than one-half of pancreatic neuroendocrine tumors are nonfunctioning, and of these about 50% are malignant. They may remain asymptomatic until they reach a size that causes clinical symptoms related to the tumoral mass and/or infiltration of the nerve plexus (in the case of malignant tumors).

Surgical Treatment

The following approaches are recognized:
1. *Atypical resections:* enucleation and middle pancreatectomy (Fig. 12.1) are reserved for neoplasms in which there is almost certain evidence of nonaggressive biological behavior. During the preoperative assessment, criteria for malignancy include the presence of metastasis, tumor dimensions larger than 2 cm, and infiltration of adjacent organs or vascular structures [8].
2. *Typical resections:* in the case of a localized lesion, but with a strong suspicion of a well and/or poorly differentiated carcinoma, the surgeon should consider radical intervention in relation to the localization of the tumor: pancreaticoduodenectomy for lesions involving the head, the uncinate process, and/or periampullary region; distal pancreatectomy for lesions involving the body/tail [49, 50].
3. *Extended resections:* the slow growth of endocrine carcinomas and the good survival prospects are such that, even in the case of locally advanced lesions, surgical radicality should be achieved even if neighboring organs must be sacrificed (stomach, colon, adrenal glands, kidney) or if resection of major vessels is required. An intervention that is extensive will thus be preceded by preoperative or intraoperative histological characterization of the lesion. Such a surgical approach is justified even in the presence of hepatic metastases as long as the lesion can be radically excised at a local level. In these cases, in fact, compartmentalization of the disease is permitted at the hepatic level, allowing not only for improvements in clinical conditions, but also for a subsequent therapeutic approach aimed only at the hepatic metastases. In all other cases, or when the only aim of surgical intervention is debulking with residual, local macroscopic disease, surgery is not indicated. Cytoreduction would lead to fragmentation of the tumor in the abdominal

cavity, in addition to a high risk of postoperative bleeding as these neoplasms are highly vascularized.

4. *Palliative intervention* (biliary bypass, gastric bypass, double bypass): this type of surgical intervention is indicated in patients with tumors that are not resectable, and who have symptoms related to the tumoral mass , such as jaundice and/or obstruction of the upper intestinal tract. Nonsurgical pallia- tion of jaundice (positioning an endoprosthesis) should be avoided as the life expectancy of the patient is high, and would thus require repeated substitu- tion of the endoprosthesis, which is associated with procedural risk and sub- stantial patient discomfort.

Prognostic Factors at Diagnosis

The good medium- to long-term survival of patients with NF-PETs is well known, with survival rates of 67, 49, and 33% at 5, 10, and 15 years, respective- ly [51]. In particular, survival rates are also significantly increased when patients are subjected to surgery with radical intent, thus confirming the value of extend- ed resections, with 5, 10, and 15 year survival rates of 93, 80, and 65%, respec- tively. The WHO classification system provides good prognostic parameters, which include the presence of hepatic metastases, the grade of differentiation, and the proliferative index (Ki-67). In addition to the more common prognostic factors, other important prognostic parameters are weight loss greater than 10% at diagnosis and the presence of lymph node metastases. In particular, the find- ing of positive lymph nodes at histological exam appears to have a prognostic value similar to that of hepatic metastases [51].

MEN1 and Von Hippel-Lindau Syndrome

These multiendocrine pathologies, genetically transmitted in an autosomal dom- inant manner, can give rise to pancreatic localizations of an endocrine nature, and may be either functioning or nonfunctioning. In both syndromes, there may be multiple lesions, disseminated in the pancreatic parenchyma, or individual lesions that can appear at later times. About 10% of insulinomas and 25% of gas- trinomas are associated with MEN1. The most frequent sites of localization are pancreatic (68%) and duodenal (57%), while lymph nodes (4%) and undeter- mined sites (7%) are found in only a small proportion of cases (7%).

Surgical therapy should be immediately evaluated both in the case of multi- ple and of single localizations, with the knowledge that the patient will almost undoubtedly have recurrent lesions. For the functioning subtypes, therefore, the correct surgical balance should be evaluated on a case-by-case basis even for eventual treatment of clinical symptoms that may be difficult to control. In the case of NF-PETs associated with MEN1, surgical resection is indicated if the lesion is greater than 2 cm; this can range from simple enucleation to total pancreatectomy for multiple lesions in patients with a family history of death related to disease. Nonfunctioning lesions that are less than 2 cm in diameter can be kept under strict surveillance; surgery is indicated only if the mass increases in volume [52].

Treatment of Synchronous and Metachronous Hepatic Metastases

It has been amply demonstrated that treatment of hepatic metastases, either surgically or with radiofrequency, prolongs survival [39, 53–56]. Surgical treatment may vary according to the specific situation: metastasectomy, "wedge resection," lobectomy, and/or segmentectomy combined with ipsilateral or contralateral "wedge resection" [57–59]. In the case of poorly differentiated carcinomas, an aggressive surgical approach involving the liver is not recommended; in these cases treatment with radiofrequency, radiometabolic therapy, and/or somatostatin analogs is preferred, whenever possible. In general, however, synchronous hepatic metastases have a poorer prognosis than metachronous metastases, which is directly proportional to the disease-free interval before their appearance [39, 49–50].

Conclusions

PETs tumors are rare neoplasms, and even when they show aggressive biological behavior, the prognosis is favorable and the patient has a good life expectancy. F-PETs (in particular, insulinomas) are often small at diagnosis and are usually amenable to atypical pancreatic resection. When the tumor cannot be localized preoperatively, intraoperative ultrasonography can be used to find it. In the case of a tumor with aggressive biological behavior, surgical therapy should incline towards typical pancreatic resections (pancreaticoduodenectomy, left pancreatectomy, total pancreatectomy), and if necessary extend to neighboring organs and/or hepatic metastases. NF-PETs are malignant in about 50% of cases. In these tumors, radical resection can be achieved only by using typical and/or extended resections, which will ensure good medium- to long-term survival. Treatment of synchronous and/or metachronous metastases with either medical or surgical therapy can also provide good survival outcomes.

References

1. Modlin I, Zikusoka M, Kidd M et al (2006) The history and epidemiology of neuroendocrine tumours. In: Caplin M, Kvols L (eds) Handbook of neuroendocrine tumors, their current and future management. Bioscientifica, Bristol, p 9
2. Eriksson B, Oberg K (2000) Neuroendocrine tumours of the pancreas. Br J Surg 87:129–131

3. Grimelius L, Hultquist G, Stenkvist B (1975) Cytological differentiation of asymptomatic pancreatic islet cell tumours in autopsy material. Virchows Arch [A] Pathol Anat Histopathol 365:275–288

4. Norton JA (1994) Neuroendocrine tumours of the pancreas and duodenum. Curr Probl Surg 31:77–156

5. Andrew A, Kramer B, Rawdon B (1983) Gut and pancreatic amine precursor uptake and decarboxylation cells are not neural crest derivatives. Gastroenterology 84:429–431

6. Efrat S, Teitelman G, Anwar M et al (1988) Glucagon gene regulatory region directs oncoprotein expression to neurons and pancreatic alpha cells. Neuron 1:605–613

7. Rindi G, Grant AG, Yiangou Y et al (1990) Development of neuroendocrine tumours in the gastrointestinal tract of transgenic mice. Heterogeneity of hormone expression. Am J Pathol 136:1349–1363

8. Rindi G, Bordi C (2006) Classification of neuroendocrine tumours. In: Caplin M, Kvols L(eds) Handbook of neuroendocrine tumours, their current and future management. Bioscientifica, Bristol, p 39

9. Solcia E, Kloppel G, Sobin LH (2000) Histological typing of endocrine tumours. Springer, New York

10. Trump D, Farren B, Wooding C et al (1996) Clinical studies of multiple endocrine neoplasia type 1 (MEN I). Q J Med 89:653–669

11. Hammel PR, Vilgrain V, Terris B et al (2000) Pancreatic involvement in Von Hippel Lindau disease. The Groupe Francophone d'Etude de la Maladie de von Hippel Lindau. Gastroenterology 119:1087–1095

12. Dial PF, Braasch JW, Rossi RL et al (1985) Management of nonfunctioning islet cell tumours of the pancreas. Surg Clin North Am 65:291–299

13. Madura JA, Cummings OW, Wiebke EA et al (1997) Nonfunctioning islet cell tumours of the pancreas: a difficult diagnosis but one worth the effort. Am Surg 63:573–578

14. Evans DB, Skibber JM, Lee JE et al (1993) Nonfunctioning islet cell carcinoma of the pancreas. Surgery 114:1175–1182

15. Thom AK, Norton JA, Doppman JL et al (1992) Prospective study of the use of intraarterial secretin injection and portal venous sampling to localize duodenal gastrinomas. Surgery 112(6):1002–1009

16. Doppman JL, Miller DL, Chang R et al (1993) Intraarterial calcium stimulation test for detection of insulinomas. World J Surg 17:439–443

17. Oberg K (2006) Diagnostic pathways. In: Caplin M, Kvols L (eds) Handbook of neuroendocrine tumours, their current and future management. Bioscientifica, Bristol, p 103

18. Rothmund M (1994) Localization of endocrine pancreatic tumours. Br J Surg 81:164–166

19. Nojima T, Kojima T, Kato H et al (1991) Cystic endocrine tumour of the pancreas. Int J Pancreatol 10:65–72

20. Modlin IM, Tang LH (1997) Approaches to the diagnosis of the gut neuroendocrine tumours: the last word. Gastroenterology 112:583–590

21. Lightdale CJ, Botet JF, Woodruff JM et al (1991) Localization of endocrine tumours of the pancreas with endoscopic ultrasonography. Cancer 68(8):1815–1820

22. Gunther RW, Klose KJ, Ruckert K et al (1985) Localization of small islet-cell tumours. Preoperative and intraoperative ultrasound, computed tomography, arteriography, digital subtraction angiography, and pancreatic venous sampling. Gastrointest Radiol 10:145–152

23. Miller DL (1993) Endocrine angiography and venous sampling. Radiol Clin North Am 31:1051–1067

24. Corleto VD, Scopinaro F, Angeletti S et al (1996) Somatostatin receptor localization of pancreatic endocrine tumours. World J Surg 20:241–244

25. Klimstra DS, Rosai J, Heffess CS (1994) Mixed acinar-endocrine carcinomas of the pancreas. Am J Surg Pathol 18:765–778

26. von Herbay A, Sieg B, Schurmann G et al (1991) Proliferative activity of neuroendocrine tumours of the gastroenteropancreatic endocrine system: DANN flow cytometric and immunohistological investigations. Gut 32:949–953

27. Lairmore TC, Moley JF (2004) Endocrine pancreatic tumours. Scan J Surg 93:311–315
28. Taal BG, Visser O (2004) Epidemiology of neuroendocrine tumours. Neuroendocrinology 80(Suppl 1):3–7
29. Dolan JP, Norton JA (2000) Occult insulinoma. Br J Surg 87:385–387
30. Hiramoto JS, Feldstein VA, LaBerge JM et al (2001) Intraoperative ultrasound and preoperative localization detects all occult insulinomas. Arch Surg 136:1020–1026
31. Fendrich V, Bartsch DK, Langer P et al (2004) Diagnosis and surgical treatment of insulinoma – experiences in 40 cases. Dtsch Med Wochenschr 129:941–946
32. Masayuki I (2008) Surgical treatment of endocrine tumors. In: Beger HG, Warshaw AL et al (eds) The pancreas, an integrated textbook of basic science, medicine and surgery, 2nd edn. Blackwell Sciences, Oxford, pp 826–834
33. Peplinski G, Skinner M, Norton J (1998) Insulinoma and nesidioblastosis. In: Howard J, Idezuki Y, Ihse I et al (eds) Surgical disease of the pancreas, 3rd edition. Williams and Wilkins, Baltimore, vol II, pp 717–732
34. Ba-ssalamah A, Schima W (2003) Imaging of endocrine tumours of the pancreas [in German]. Wien Klin Wochenschr 115(Suppl 2):50–55
35. Fritscher-Ravens A (2004) Endoscopic ultrasound and neuroendocrine tumours of the pancreas. J Pancreas 5:273–281
36. Espana-Gomez MN, Pantoja JP, Herrera MF (2004) Laparoscopic surgery of pancreas [in Spanish]. Rev Gastroenterol Mex 69(Suppl 1):84–90
37. Norton JA (1999) Intraoperative methods to stage and localize pancreatic and duodenal tumours. Ann Oncol 10(Suppl 4):182–184
38. Stabile BE, Morrow DJ, Passaro E (1984) The gastrinoma triangle: operative implications. Am J Surg 147:25–31
39. Norton J (2006) Surgical management of neuroendocrine tumours: pancreas and intestine. In: Caplin M, Kvols L (eds) Handbook of neuroendocrine tumours, their current and future management. Bioscientifica, Bristol, p 159
40. Jackson JE (2005) Angiography and arterial stimulation venous sampling in the localization of pancreatic neuroendocrine tumours. Best Pract Res Clin Endocrinol Metab 19:229–239
41. Kloppel G, Perren A, Heitz PU (2004) The gastroenteropancreatic neuroendocrine cell system and its tumours: the WHO classification. Ann NY Acad Sci 1014:13–27
42. Norton JA, Fraker DL, Alexander HR et al (1999) Surgery to cure the Zollinger Ellison syndrome. N Engl J Med 341(9):635–644
43. Falconi M, Bettini R, Boninsegna L et al (2006) Surgical strategy in the treatment of pancreatic neuroendocrine tumours. JOP 7:150–156
44. Nikou GC, Toubanakis C, Nikolaou P et al (2005) VIPomas: an update in diagnosis and management in a series of 11 patients. Hepatogastroenterology 52:1259–1265
45. Anlauf M, Sipos B, Kloppel G (2005) Tumours of the endocrine pancreas. Pathologe 26:46–51
46. Burgos L, Burgos ME (2004) Pancreatic endocrine tumours. Rev Med Chil 132:627–634
47. McLoughlin JM, Kuhn JA, Lamont JT (2004) Neuroendocrine tumours of the pancreas. Curr Treat Options Gastroenterol 7:355–364
48. Oberg K (2004) Management of neuroendocrine tumours. Ann Oncol 15(Suppl 4):iv293–iv298
49. Falconi M, Plockinger U, Kwekkeboom DJ et al (2006) Well-differentiated pancreatic nonfunctioning tumours/carcinoma. Neuroendocrinology 84:196–211
50. Gullo L, Migliori M, Falconi M et al (2003) Nonfunctioning pancreatic endocrine tumours: a multicenter clinical study. Am J Gastroenterol 98:2435–2439
51. Bettini R, Boninsegna L, Mantovani W et al (2008) Prognostic factors at diagnosis and value of WHO classification in a mono-insitutional series of 180 non-functioning pancreatic endocrine tumours. Ann Oncol 19:903–908
52. Triponez F, Goudet P, Dosseh D et al; French Endocrine Tumor Study Group (2006) Is surgery beneficial for MEN 1 patients with small (< or = 2 cm), non-functioning pancreaticoduodenal endocrine tumor? An analysis of 65 patients from the GTE. World J Surg 30:654–662

53. Sutcliffe R, Maguire D, Ramage J et al (2004) Management of neuroendocrine liver metastases. Am J Surg 187:39–46
54. Norton JA, Warren RS, Kelly MG et al (2003) Aggressive surgery for metastatic liver neuroendocrine tumours. Surgery 134:1057–1065
55. Norton JA (2005) Surgical treatment of neuroendocrine metastases. Best Pract Res Clin Gastroenterol 19:577–583
56. Gillams AR (2004) Liver ablation therapy. Br J Radiol 77:713–723
57. Sarmiento JM, Que FG (2003) Hepatic surgery for metastases from neuroendocrine tumours. Surg Oncol Clin North Am 12:231–242
58. Sarmiento JM, Heywood G, Rubin J et al (2003) Surgical treatment of neuroendocrine metastases to the liver: a plea for resection to increase survival. J Am Coll Surg 197:29–37
59. Vyhnanek F, Denemark L, Duchac V et al (2003) What are indications for hepatic resection in metastases? [In Czech.] Rozhl Chir 82:570–576

Chapter 13

Epidemiology, Risk Factors, and Prevention of Pancreatic Cancer

Federico Mocchegiani, Roberto Ghiselli, Michela Cappelletti, Vittorio Saba

Epidemiology

Cancer of the pancreas is a neoplasm which occurs infrequently, although cases are increasing and the death rate is very high death. The incidence of this neoplasm in the United States is around 11 cases per 100,000 inhabitants, equating to around 30,000 new cases per year [1, 2]. In Europe, the incidence is around 5.2–8.7 cases per 100,000 inhabitants, with a lot of variations among the different nations [3, 4]. The lowest incidences have been recorded in Africa and in Asia, at 2 cases per 100,000 inhabitants, although over the last 40 years a large increase in the number of cases in Japan has been noticed, with 19,700 new cases per year (15 per 100,000 inhabitants) [2, 5] (Table 13.1). The growing trend appears to be mainly related to two factors: the rise in average age, which is the main risk factor for all the principal gastroenteric neoplasms, and the spread of tobacco-smoking habits.

The epidemiology of pancreatic cancer presents significant variability attributable to sex, age, geographic area, and race. Incidences of pancreatic cancer are greater in men than in women, by 40% in the United States and by 70% in Japan [2]. This is a disease that affects mainly the elderly. According to the US National Reports, the average age at which this disease occurs is 69.2 years in men and 69.5 years in women. In the United States only 13% of patients are less than 60 years old, while half are over 75 years old [2]. For this neoplasm, the fastest manifestation process is generally related to genetic factors or genetic anomalies.

Table 13.1 Incidence of pancreatic carcinoma worldwide [1, 2, 5]

Nations	Incidence (cases per 100,000 persons)
USA	11
Europe	5.2/8.7
Africa	2
Asia	2
Japan	15

W. Siquini (Ed.), *Surgical Treatment of Pancreatic Diseases.*
©Springer-Verlag Italia 2009

The epidemiology of pancreatic cancer presents a significant geographic variability, showing the important role of environmental carcinogenic factors for this as for other neoplasms of the gastroenteric tract. The USA and Japan are the countries at greatest risk from this disease, with an incidence 5–7 times higher than in Spain, Singapore, and Hong Kong [6]. There are racial differences among the cases of this neoplasm. The Maoris of New Zealand and members of the Ashkenazi Jewish ethnic group are the populations with the highest presence of pancreatic carcinomas and also of all the other types of neoplasms related to tobacco [7–10]. The African–American population have an increased risk due to a mutation of the K-*ras* gene which is more frequent than in the white population. Less aggressive pancreatic neoplasms are seen in Asiatic than in white or African–American populations [11].

The most dramatic epidemiologic aspect of this disease is certainly the mortality rate, which is almost 100%. Data updated to 2002 identify pancreatic cancer as the eighth most common cause of death by neoplasm in the world [12] (Table 13.2). In the United States pancreatic cancer represents the fourth most common cause of death from neoplasms: in men after cancer of the lungs, prostate, and colon; in women after cancer of the lungs, breast, and colon [1, 2]. In Japan it is the fifth-ranking cause of death from neoplasms: in men after cancer of the lungs, stomach, liver, and colon; in women after cancer of the stomach, colon, lungs, and breast [1, 2]. In Europe, the mortality rate is highest in Austria and Sweden at around 11 cases per 100,000 inhabitants each year, while Spain, Portugal, and Greece have the lowest rates [13].

Table 13.2 Global statistics for the year 2002 demonstrating that pancreatic cancer is the eighth commonest cause of cancer mortality in the world [12]

Cancer	Number of deaths
Lung	1,178,900
Stomach	700,300
Liver	598,300
Bowel	529,000
Breast	410,700
Esophagus	385,900
Cervix	273,500
Pancreas	227,000
Leukemia	222,500
Prostate	221,000
Bladder	145,000
Ovary	124,900
Kidney	101,900

The survival rate of people with a pancreatic carcinoma is low, and it is barely influenced by surgical resection and by adjuvant chemotherapy. The average survival rate of patients with nonresectable forms is around 4 months: 7–9 months if the superior mesenteric vessels are not involved at the time of diagnosis [14]. Between 0.4 and 5% of patients can survive for 5 years after developing pancreatic carcinoma [15–18].

At diagnosis only 10–15% of patients undergo surgical resection, and surgical resection only increases the average survival rate to 13–15 months. Of these patients, 10% are alive after 5 years [15–18]. A tumor size less than 1 cm at diagnosis and an absence of lymph-node metastasis positively influence survival rates at 1–5 years [19, 20]. Adjuvant chemotherapy improves the survival rate by up to some weeks or months [15–18].

Risk Factors

Environmental and hereditary risk factors along with conditions for the development of pancreatic cancer have been identified [21] (Table 13.3).

Table 13.3 Risk factors for sporadic (nonhereditary) pancreatic cancer [21]

Definite risk factors	Possible risk factors	Unclear risk
Increasing age	High intake of fat	Diabetes mellitus type 1
Tobacco smoking	Low intake of fresh fruit	Obesity
Chronic pancreatitis	Low intake of vegetable	Alcohol intake
Hereditary pancreatitis	Occupational exposure	Coffee intake
Familial pancreatic cancer	Diabetes mellitus type 2	
	Genetic polymorphisms	
	Hereditary syndromes	

Environmental Risk Factors

Tobacco smoking, diet, and also occupation have relevance as risk factors for the development of pancreatic cancer.

Smoking is the most important environmental risk factor for pancreatic cancer. The carcinogens deriving from tobacco can spread to the pancreas by direct oropharyngeal absorption but also through the circulatory apparatus, and can indirectly damage the pancreas, facilitating duodenopancreatic reflux. The major part of this research shows a significantly higher risk in smokers than in nonsmokers, highlighting a direct connection with tobacco smoking especially in the 15 years before evaluation [22–26]. An important English study published in 1994 and conducted over 40 years revealed an annual mortality for pancreatic cancer that was progressively higher in nonsmokers, exsmokers, and then smokers: respectively 16, 23, and 35 deaths per 100,000 persons per year [27]. Only 15 years after a person stops smoking is the risk of developing this neoplasm significantly reduced [26].

Diet also influences the risk of pancreatic neoplasms and is a major factor in gastrointestinal cancers. A high-calorie diet, especially one which is high in fats, is associated with various types of neoplasm, one of which is carcinoma of the pancreas. The risk of developing this cancer is further increased by a high consumption of red meat cooked at high temperatures and grilled [28]. On the other hand, the consumption of fruit and vegetables seems to reduce this risk [29–35]. In Japan, the traditional diet comprised of tofu and fish presents a lower risk than the Western diet introduced to Japan in the second half of the 20th century, rich in meat and animal fats [36].

With regard to occupation, occupational exposure to carcinogens contributes only a small part of the risk for pancreatic neoplasm. However, some occupational carcinogens are strongly associated with the risk of neoplasm, such as hydrofluorocarbons, formaldehyde, pesticides, and all substances containing cadmium, chromium, and radon [21, 37–44]. For many other factors the correlation with pancreatic cancer has been evaluated, but without irrefutable proof and with conflicting evidence.

Obesity, too, has a connection with the risk of developing pancreatic neoplasms; in particular, the risk increases in direct proportion to body mass index [45]. However, this association is strongly linked to the consumption of fats in the diet [35].

Alcohol represents one of the main risk factors for pancreatitis. Alcohol does not seem to have a direct correlation to the development of tumors; however it could increase the inflammatory response to other carcinogens [46].

A high consumption of coffee is not a clear risk factor for this tumor, although there is a link to suggest this for decaffeinated coffee – or, more precisely, for the chemical substances used in its production [47–49].

Hereditary Diseases

Around 5–10% of all pancreatic neoplasms have a genetic background [50]. A neoplasm with hereditary characteristics occurs a decade before a sporadic neoplasm. The hereditary genetic disorder which is strongly linked to the onset of familiar pancreatic cancer is a mutation of the BRCA2 gene. This mutation is present in 7–10% of patients with sporadic tumors and in 15–20% of persons with a clear family history [51, 52]. Mutation of chromosome 4q32–34 is associated with a high risk of cancer, pancreatitis, and diabetes mellitus, thus showing the complete picture of *familial pancreatic cancer*. A person is at risk if there are two or more first-degree relatives or three relatives of any other degree within their family tree who are affected with cancer of the pancreas [53].

Hereditary syndromes transmitted with an autosomal dominant pattern with incomplete penetrance or autosomal recessive forms confer an increased risk of developing pancreatic cancer. In cystic fibrosis, mutation of chromosome 7q31 is linked to an increased risk of digestive neoplasms including pancreatic carcinoma, and in Peutz–Jeghers syndrome the mutation of chromosome 19p is linked to both sporadic and familial forms of neoplasia [54–56].

With respect to the general population, persons with *familial atypical multiple mole–melanoma* [57, 58] are at a double risk of developing pancreatic neoplasms; this is linked to inactivation of the oncosuppressor gene *p16* [INK4A]. Cases of pancreatic tumors are also seen in ataxia–telangiectasia, in Li–Fraumeni syndrome, in familial adenomatous polyposis, in familial breast and ovarian cancer, and in extracolic forms of nonpolyposis colorectal carcinoma [59, 60] (Table 13.4).

Table 13.4 Hereditary cancer syndromes associated with increased pancreatic cancer risk [60]

Syndrome	Comments
Hereditary pancreatitis	Significantly increased risk of pancreatic cancer after 20–30 years from pancreatitis onset
Peutz–Jeghers syndrome	High risk of pancreatic cancer
Familial pancreatic cancer/site	
Specific familial pancreatic cancer	Linked to autosomal dominant mutation of palladin gene (proto-oncogene)
Familial atypical multiple mole–melanoma	Increased risk of endometrial, lung, and breast cancer
Hereditary breast–ovarian cancer	BRCA2 mutations are common in familial pancreatic cancer
Familial adenomatous polyposis (FAP)	PanIN lesions in FAP kindred
Hereditary nonpolyposis colorectal cancer	High risk of biliary tract and papilla of Vater tumors

PanIN, Pancreatic intraepithelial neoplasia

The incidence of sporadic neoplasms is also affected by genetic factors. The carriers of genetic polymorphisms have a higher risk of developing the cancer. "Genetic polymorphisms" is a term that covers the onset of mutations in more than 1% of the population and altered individual susceptibility to environmental carcinogens [61]. For example, mutations of the cytochrome P_{450} gene are linked in an undefined way to the risk of pancreatic carcinomas. The effect of the mutation of the gene may reduce the organism's ability to detoxify some carcinogens taken in food [62, 63]. In the same way, the scientific evidences regarding the alterations of the N-acetyltransferase are poor [64].

A stronger link with pancreatic cancer is present in other genetic polymorphisms. For example, in smokers the presence of a deletion of the gene for glutathione *S*-transferase (GSTT1) significantly increases the risk of developing the disease [63], as does the presence of the allele UGT1A7*3 for uridine 5'-diphosphate glucuronosyltransferase (UGT) [65].

Preneoplastic Conditions

Carcinoma of the pancreas is also linked to pre-existent pathological conditions. All the types of chronic pancreatitis (alcoholic, nonalcoholic, hereditary, and tropical) are associated with development of the neoplasm [66–68]. In particular, patients affected with alcoholic and nonalcoholic types of chronic pathology have a risk of pancreatic cancer that is 10–20 times greater than that of the normal population; those with a hereditary pathology have a risk 50–60 times greater than the general population [8]. Furthermore, in smokers the risk increases and the age of onset decreases to around 20 years [69].

Type 2 and possible type 1 diabetes mellitus are linked to the development of pancreatic cancer. An important meta-analysis published in 1995 indicates that people with diabetes have a doubled risk of developing pancreatic cancer [70]. We have found that this risk is higher if the diabetes is of recent onset or if it has been diagnosed within less than 5 years [71, 72]. This evidence alone suggests that is possible for diabetes not to be the only predispositioning factor, but that it may be one of the primary symptoms of pancreatic tumor onset [73–75].

Currently there is no scientific agreement on the consequentiality of these pathologies.

Prevention and Screening

All in all, the pathogenesis of pancreatic carcinoma occurs more or less like that of all digestive tumors: a combination of genetic mutations more or less known and the impact of different environmental carcinogens.

Primary prevention of pancreatic carcinoma is not possible because of the lack of adequately sensitive and specific tests. Research into the K-*ras* [76] mutation, the BRCA2 mutation, and *p16* [INK4A] inactivity promises to result in genetic tests that will be able to identify persons at higher risk of developing the neoplasm [77]. Meanwhile, the only feasible strategy is to reduce exposure to well-known risk factors, the main priority being the fight against tobacco smoke.

In the USA, it is plausible that the reduction in the incidence of pancreatic cancer observed in men but not in women is predominantly due to changes in the smoking habits in those observed. In Japan the incidence of the disease is increasing progressively at the same rate as the spread of tobacco smoking. Today, the reduction of smoking is the most important measure for the prevention of pancreatic cancer.

Diet represents another risk factor, although it is not as strong as smoking. Reduced consumption of animal fats and increased consumption of fruit and vegetables, in particular citrus fruits and carrots, together with regular moderate physical exercise should have an extremely positive impact in reducing the onset of obesity, diabetes, and hence exocrine pancreatic neoplasms [78].

The role of chemoprevention is widely debated, but there is no significant evidence because of the lack of randomized controlled trials. It has been hypothesized that the use of some inhibitors of COX2 and of aspirin reduces the risk of the disease because of the action which inhibits chronic inflammation [79–81]. Extracts of green tea, polyphenol, and other substances such as vitamins A, C, and E and selenium seem to prevent the onset of the cancer by acting as an antioxidant [82].

Secondary prevention, with screening of the general population, cannot currently be done due to the relatively low incidence of pancreatic cancer, especially given the lack of clinical symptoms, biohumoral markers, and sensitive, specific and low-cost imaging techniques that could be used in order to identify the neoplasms in the initial stages. Anorexia, jaundice, hyperchromic stools, acholic urine, weight loss, and abdominal ache are nonspecific symptoms and often first arise when the neoplasia is no longer confined to the pancreas [83]. CA19-9 is the most frequent tumoral marker associated with pancreatic tumors, but a raised level is also seen in persons affected by neoplasms of the colon, stomach, and bile ducts and in benign conditions such as chronic pancreatitis, hepatitis, and obstructive jaundice. Its concentration in the pancreatic juice is not specifically affected. Furthermore, some persons do not have the necessary enzyme to synthesize the CA19-9, further reducing its sensitivity as a marker [84, 85].

Ultrasonography, computed tomography, and magnetic resonance imaging are imaging techniques frequently used to diagnose pancreatic cancer; their major limitation is their inability to identify lesions smaller than 1 cm in size [86]. The endoscopic retrograde cholangiopancreatography and endoscopic ultrasonography appear to be more sensitive, although they are invasive and more expensive [87].

However, in light of the genetic predisposition of this neoplasm, it is useful to do screening in selected populations, in other words, in persons with a family history of pancreatic cancer, starting from a decade before the youngest age at diagnosis in the family, and in persons with hereditary pancreatitis age who are aged 40 years or over [88–91].

In conclusion, the social impact of pancreatic cancer, despite its relatively low frequency, is dramatic because of the high mortality rate of this disease. Regarding genetic disorders, greater knowledge of patients with familial forms will be useful to have and will help fight it in the wider population of those affected by sporadic forms.

Further research is necessary to evaluate the real benefit of screening programs in persons at higher risk of pancreatic cancer.

References

1. Ries LAG, Melbert D, Krapcho M et al (eds) (2008) SEER Cancer Statistics Review, 1975–2005, National Cancer Institute. Bethesda, MD. http://seer.cancer.gov/csr/1975_2005/, based on November 2007 SEER data submission, posted to the SEER web site, 2008
2. Japan National Cancer Center (2007) Cancer Statistic in Japan 2007. http://ncc.go.jp/
3. Moossa AR (1991) Tumours of the pancreas. In: Moossa AR, Schimpf SC, Rabson MC (eds) Comprehensive textbook of oncology, vol 1, 2nd edn. Williams and Wilkins, Baltimore, pp 958–988
4. Mori K, Ikei S, Yamane T et al (1990) Pathological factors influencing survival of carcinoma of the ampulla of Vater. Eur J Surg Oncol 16(3):183–188
5. Lin Y, Tamakoshi A, Wakai K et al (1998) Descriptive epidemiology of pancreatic cancer in Japan. J Epidemiol 8(1):52–59
6. Parkin DM, Muir C, Whelan SL et al (1992) Cancer incidence in five continents. IARC Scientific Publications, Lyon 120:1–1033
7. Fraumeni JF Jr (1975) Cancers of the pancreas and biliary tract: epidemiological considerations. Cancer Res 35(11 Pt 2):3437–3446
8. Phillips AR, Lawes CM, Cooper GJ, Windsor JA (2002) Ethnic disparity of pancreatic cancer in New Zealand. Int J Gastrointest Cancer 31(1–3):137–145
9. McCredie M, Cox B, Stewart JH (2000) Smoking-related cancers in Maori and non-Maori in New Zealand, 1974–1993: fewer bladder cancers among Maori. Asian Pac J Cancer Prev 1(3):221–225
10. Gold EB, Goldin SB (1998) Epidemiology of and risk factors for pancreatic cancer [review]. Surg Oncol Clin N Am 7(1):67–91
11. Pernick NL, Sarkar FH, Philip PA et al (2003) Clinicopathologic analysis of pancreatic adenocarcinoma in African Americans and Caucasians. Pancreas 26:28–32
12. Parkin DM, Bray F, Ferlay F, Pisani P (2005) Global cancer statistics. CA Cancer J Clin 55(2):74–108
13. Pisani P, Parkin DM, Bray F, Ferlay J (1999) Estimates of the worldwide mortality from 25 cancers in 1990. Int J Cancer 83(1):18–29. Erratum in: Int J Cancer 83(6):870–873
14. Phoa SS, Tilleman EH, van Delden OM et al (2005) Value of CT criteria in predicting survival in patients with potentially resectable pancreatic head carcinoma. J Surg Oncol 91(1):33–40
15. Andren-Sandberg A, Neoptolemos JP (2002) Resection for pancreatic cancer in the new millennium. Pancreatology 2:431–439
16. Bramhall SR, Allum WH, Jones AG et al (1995) Treatment and survival in 13,560 patients with pancreatic cancer, and incidence of the disease in the West Midlands: an epidemiological study. Br J Surg 82:111–115
17. Shore S, Raraty M, Ghaneh P et al (2003) Chemotherapy for pancreatic cancer. Aliment Pharmacol Ther 18:1049–1069
18. Neoptolemos JP, Dunn JA, Stocken DD et al (2001) Adjuvant chemoradiotherapy and chemotherapy in respectable pancreatic cancer: a randomized controlled trial. Lancet 358:1576–1585
19. Yeo CJ, Cameron JL, Lillemoe KD et al (1995) Pancreaticoduodenectomy for cancer of the head of the pancreas. 201 patients. Ann Surg 221(6):721–731
20. Ariyama J, Suyama M, Satoh K, Wakabayashi K (1998) Endoscopic ultrasound and intraductal ultrasound in the diagnosis of small pancreatic tumors. Abdom Imaging 23(4):380–386
21. Lochan R, Daly AK, Reeves HL, Charnley RM (2008) Genetic susceptibility in pancreatic ductal adenocarcinoma. Br J Surg 95(1):22–32
22. Silverman DT, Dunn JA, Hoover RN et al (1994) Cigarette smoking and pancreas cancer: a case-control study based on direct interviews. J Natl Cancer Inst 86:1510–1516
23. Mack TM, Yu MC, Hanisch R et al (1986) Pancreas cancer and smoking, beverage consumption, and past medical history. J Natl Cancer Inst 76:49–60

24. Lin Y, Tamakoshi A, Kawamura T et al (2002) A prospective cohort study of cigarette smoking and pancreatic cancer in Japan. Cancer Causes Control 13:249–254
25. Akiba S, Hirayama T (1990) Cigarette smoking and cancer mortality risk in Japanese men and women – results from reanalysis of the six-prefecture cohort study data. Environ Health Perspect 87:19–26
26. Fuchs CS, Colditz GA, Stampfer MJ et al (1996) A prospective study of cigarette smoking and the risk of pancreatic cancer. Arch Intern Med 156(19):2255–2260
27. Doll R, Peto R, Wheatley K et al (1994) Mortality in relation to smoking: 40 years' observations on male British doctors. Br Med J 309:901–911
28. Stolzenberg-Solomon RZ, Cross AJ, Silverman DT et al (2007) Meat and meat-mutagen intake and pancreatic cancer risk in the NIH-AARP cohort. Cancer Epidemiol Biomarkers Prev 16(12):2664–2675
29. Baghurst PA, McMichael AJ, Slavotinek AH et al (1991) A case-control study of diet and cancer of the pancreas. Am J Epidemiol 134:167–179
30. Bueno de Mesquita HB, Maisonneuve P, Moerman CJ et al (1991) Intake of foods and nutrients and cancer of the exocrine pancreas: a population-based case-control study in the Netherlands. Int J Cancer 48:540–549
31. Ghadirian P, Simard A, Baillargeon J et al (1991–1992) Nutritional factors and pancreatic cancer in the francophone community in Montreal, Canada. Int J Cancer 47:1–6; 52:17–23
32. Ghadirian P, Thouez JP, PetitClerc C (1991) International comparisons of nutrition and mortality from pancreatic cancer. Cancer Detect Prev 15:357–362
33. Zatonski W, Przewozniak K, Howe GR et al (1991) Nutritional factors and pancreatic cancer: a case-control study from south-west Poland. Int J Cancer 48:390–394
34. Howe GR, Ghadirian P, Bueno de Mesquita HB et al (1992) A collaborative case-control study of nutrient intake and pancreatic cancer within the SEARCH programme. Int J Cancer 51:365–372
35. Stolzenberg-Solomon RZ, Pietinen P, Taylor PR et al (2002) Prospective study of diet and pancreatic cancer in male smokers. Am J Epidemiol 155:783–792
36. Ohba S, Nishi M, Miyake H (1996) Eating habits and pancreas cancer. Int J Pancreatol 20:37–42
37. Ojajarvi A, Partanen T, Ahlbom A et al (2001) Risk of pancreatic cancer in workers exposed to chlorinated hydrocarbon solvents and related compounds: a meta-analysis. Am J Epidemiol 153:841–850
38. Collins JJ, Esmen NA, Hall TA (2001) A review and meta-analysis of formaldehyde exposure and pancreatic cancer. Am J Ind Med 39:336–345
39. McCallion K, Mitchell RM, Wilson RH, Kee F et al (2001) Flexible sigmoidoscopy and the changing distribution of colorectal cancer: implications for screening. Gut 48:522–525
40. Kauppinen T, Partanen T, Degerth R et al (1995) Pancreatic cancer and occupational exposures. Epidemiology 6:498–502
41. Alguacil J, Kauppinen T, Porta M et al (2000) Risk of pancreatic cancer and occupational exposures in Spain. PANKRAS II Study Group. Ann Occup Hyg 44:391–403
42. Hoppin JA, Tolbert PE, Holly EA et al (2000) Pancreatic cancer and serum organochlorine levels. Cancer Epidemiol Biomarkers Prev 9:199–205
43. Porta M, Malats N, Jariod M et al (1999) Serum concentrations of organochlorine compounds and K-ras mutations in exocrine pancreatic cancer. PANKRAS II Study Group. Lancet 354:2125–2129
44. Fryzek JP, Garabrant DH, Harlow SD et al (1997) A case-control study of self-reported exposures to pesticides and pancreas cancer in southeastern Michigan. Int J Cancer 72:62–67
45. Michaud DS, Giovannucci E, Willett WC et al (2001) Physical activity, obesity, height, and the risk of pancreatic cancer. JAMA 286(8):921–929
46. Ye W, Lagergren J, Weiderpass E et al (2002) Alcohol abuse and the risk of pancreatic cancer. Gut 51:236–239
47. Partanen T, Hemminki K, Vainio H, Kauppinen T (1995) Coffee consumption not associated with risk of pancreas cancer in Finland. Prev Med 24(2):213–216

48. Stensvold I, Jacobsen BK (1994) Coffee and cancer: a prospective study of 43,000 Norwegian men and women. Cancer Causes Control 5(5):401–408

49. Michaud DS, Giovannucci E, Willett WC et al (2001) Coffee and alcohol consumption and the risk of pancreatic cancer in two prospective United States cohorts. Cancer Epidemiol Biomarkers Prev 10(5):429–437

50. Brand RE, Lynch HT (2006) Genotype/phenotype of familial pancreatic cancer [review]. Endocrinol Metab Clin North Am 35(2):405–415, xi

51. Lal G, Liu G, Schmocker B et al (2000) Inherited predisposition to pancreatic adenocarcinoma: role of family history and germ-line p16, BRCA1, and BRCA2 mutations. Cancer Res 60: 409–416

52. Kern SE, Hruban RH, Hidalgo M et al (2002) An introduction to pancreatic adenocarcinoma genetics, pathology and therapy. Cancer Biol Ther 1:607–613

53. Rulyak SJ, Lowenfels AB, Maisonneuve P et al (2003) Risk factors for the development of pancreatic cancer in familial pancreatic cancer kindreds. Gastroenterology 124:1292–1299

54. Maisonneuve P, FitzSimmons SC, Neglia JP et al (2003) Cancer risk in nontransplanted and transplanted cystic fibrosis patients: a 10-year study. J Natl Cancer Inst 95:381–387

55. Neglia JP, FitzSimmons SC, Maisonneuve P et al (1995) The risk of cancer among patients with cystic fibrosis. N Engl J Med 332:494–499

56. Su GH, Hruban RH, Bansal RK et al (1999) Germline and somatic mutations of the STK11/LKB1 Peutz–Jeghers gene in pancreatic and biliary cancers. Am J Pathol 154:1835–1840

57. Efthimiou E, Crnogorac-Jurcevic T, Lemoine NR (2001) Inherited predisposition to pancreatic cancer. Gut 48:143–147

58. Goldstein AM, Fraser MC, Streuwing JP et al (1995) Increased risk of pancreatic cancer in melanoma-prone kindreds with p16INK4 mutations. N Engl J Med 333:970–974

59. Hahn SA, Bartsch DK (2005) Genetics of hereditary pancreatic carcinoma. Clin Lab Med 25(1):117–133

60. Greer JB, Whitcomb DC, Brand RE (2007) Genetic predisposition to pancreatic cancer: a brief review. Am J Gastroenterol 102(11):2564–2569

61. Harris CC (1989) Interindividual variation among humans in carcinogen metabolism, DNA adduct formation and DNA repair. Carcinogenesis 10(9):1563–1566

62. Foster JR, Idle JR, Hardwick JP et al (1993) Induction of drug-metabolizing enzymes in human pancreatic cancer and chronic pancreatitis. J Pathol 169:457–463

63. Duell EJ, Holly EA, Bracci PM et al (2002) A population-based case-control study of polymorphisms in carcinogen-metabolizing genes, smoking and pancreatic adenocarcinoma risk. J Natl Cancer Inst 94:297–306

64. Bartsch H, Malaveille C, Lowenfels AB et al (1998) Genetic polymorphism of N-acetyl-transferases, glutathione S transferase M1 and NAD(P)H:quinone oxidoreductase in relation to malignant and benign pancreatic disease risk. The International Pancreatic Disease Study Group. Eur J Cancer Prev 7:215–223

65. Ockenga J, Vogel A, Teich N et al (2003) UDP glucuronosyltransferase (UGT1A7) gene polymorphisms increase the risk of chronic pancreatitis and pancreatic cancer. Gastroenterology 124:1802–1808

66. Lowenfels AB, Maisonneuve P, Cavallini G et al (1993) Pancreatitis and the risk of pancreatic cancer. International Pancreatitis Study Group. N Engl J Med 328:1433–1437

67. Lowenfels AB, Maisonneuve P, DiMagno EP et al (1997) Hereditary pancreatitis and the risk of pancreatic cancer. International Hereditary Pancreatitis Study Group. J Natl Cancer Inst 89:442–446

68. Chari ST, Mohan V, Pitchumoni CS et al (1994) Risk of pancreatic carcinoma in tropical calcifying pancreatitis: an epidemiologic study. Pancreas 9:62–66

69. Lowenfels AB, Maisonneuve P, Whitcomb DC et al (2001) Cigarette smoking as a risk factor for pancreatic cancer in patients with hereditary pancreatitis. JAMA 286(2):169–170

70. Everhart J, Wright D (1995) Diabetes mellitus as a risk factor for pancreatic cancer. A meta-analysis. JAMA 273:1605–1609

71. Chari ST, Leibson CL, Rabe KG et al (2005) Probability of pancreatic cancer following diabetes: a population-based study. Gastroenterology 129(2):504–511

72. Huxley R, Ansary-Moghaddam A, Berrington de González A et al (2005) Type-II diabetes and pancreatic cancer: a meta-analysis of 36 studies. Br J Cancer 92(11):2076–2083

73. Karmody AJ, Kyle J (1969) The association between carcinoma of the pancreas and diabetes mellitus. Br J Surg 56:362–364

74. Permert J, Adrian TE, Jacobsson P et al (1993) Is profound peripheral insulin resistance in patients with pancreatic cancer caused by a tumor-associated factor? Am J Surg 165:61–66

75. Permert J, Ihse I, Jorfeldt L et al (1993) Pancreatic cancer is associated with impaired glucose metabolism. Eur J Surg 159:101–107

76. Chu TM (1997) Molecular diagnosis of pancreas carcinoma. J Clin Lab Anal 11:225–231

77. Vimalachandran D, Ghaneh P, Costello E, Neoptolemos JP (2004) Genetics and prevention of pancreatic cancer. Cancer Control 11(1):6–14

78. Norell SE, Ahlbom A, Erwald R et al (1986) Diet and pancreatic cancer: a case-control study. Am J Epidemiol 124:894–902

79. Kokawa A, Kondo H, Gotoda T et al (2001) Increased expression of cyclooxygenase-2 in human pancreatic neoplasms and potential for chemoprevention by cyclooxygenase inhibitors. Cancer 91:333–338

80. Anderson KE, Johnson TW, Lazovich D et al (2002) Association between nonsteroidal anti-inflammatory drug use and the incidence of pancreatic cancer. J Natl Cancer Inst 94:1168–1171

81. Larsson SC, Giovannucci E, Bergkvist L, Wolk A (2006) Aspirin and nonsteroidal anti-inflammatory drug use and risk of pancreatic cancer: a meta-analysis. Cancer Epidemiol Biomarkers Prev 15(12):2561–2564

82. Doucas H, Garcea G, Neal CP et al (2006) Chemoprevention of pancreatic cancer: a review of the molecular pathways involved, and evidence for the potential for chemoprevention [review]. Pancreatology 6(5):429–439

83. Holly EA, Chaliha I, Bracci PM, Gautam M (2004) Signs and symptoms of pancreatic cancer: a population-based case-control study in the San Francisco Bay area. Clin Gastroenterol Hepatol 2(6):510–517

84. Niederau C, Grendell JH (1992) Diagnosis of pancreatic carcinoma. Imaging techniques and tumor markers. Pancreas 7(1):66–86

85. Steinberg W (1990) The clinical utility of the CA 19–9 tumor-associated antigen [review]. Am J Gastroenterol 85(4):350–355

86. Saisho H, Yamaguchi T (2004) Diagnostic imaging for pancreatic cancer: computed tomography, magnetic resonance imaging, and positron emission tomography. Pancreas 28(3):273–278

87. Yasuda K, Mukai H, Nakajima M (1995) Endoscopic ultrasonography diagnosis of pancreatic cancer. Gastrointest Endosc Clin North Am 5(4):699–712

88. Durie P, Lerch MM, Lowenfels AB et al (2002) Genetic disorders of the exocrine pancreas. An overview and update. Karger, Basel

89. McFaul CD, Greenhalf W, Earl J et al (2006) Anticipation in familial pancreatic cancer. Gut 55:252–258

90. Brentnall TA, Bronner MP, Byrd DR et al (1999) Early diagnosis and treatment of pancreatic dysplasia in patients with a family history of pancreatic cancer. Ann Intern Med 131:247–255

91. Brentnall TA (2000) Cancer surveillance of patients from familial pancreatic cancer kindreds. Med Clin North Am 84:707–718

Chapter 14

Imaging of Pancreatic Neoplasms

Sara Cecchini, Linda Cacciamani, Arianna Lorenzoni, Giancarlo Fabrizzi

Introduction

Computed tomography (CT), magnetic resonance imaging (MRI), and ultra-sonography are the most commonly used modalities for pancreatic imaging. Recent breakthroughs in imaging technologies have had a significant impact on the accuracy and use of pancreatic imaging in the diagnosis and staging of malignant and benign pancreatic diseases.

With the introduction of multidetector row spiral computed tomography (MDCT) technology, the speed and quality of CT imaging has significantly improved. The pancreas can be imaged at a very high spatial and temporal resolution and the study can be performed within a short breath-hold. The data sets obtained with MDCT allow considerable postprocessing to be performed. Postprocessed images maximize the diagnostic yield of the scan and improve the visualization of the pancreatic vasculature and biliary tree. CT is now considered to be the imaging modality of choice for the detection and presurgical staging of pancreatic cancer.

Technical advances in MRI, such as higher magnetic field strengths, phased-array coils, and ultrafast imaging, have yielded excellent results in the evaluation of solid pancreatic masses. Magnetic resonance cholangiopancreatography (MRCP) is as sensitive as endoscopic retrograde cholangiopancreatography (ERCP) in detecting pancreatic cancers, but, unlike conventional ERCP, does not require injection of contrast material into the ducts, thus avoiding the morbidity associated with endoscopic procedures. A magnetic resonance (MR) multi-imaging protocol, which includes MR cross-sectional imaging, MRCP, and dynamic contrast-enhanced MR angiography, integrates the advantages of various special imaging techniques.

Because of its ready availability, repeatability, and low cost, ultrasound (US) imaging retains an important role in identifying pancreatic masses, and echo-enhanced ultrasound may have an emerging role in evaluating them.

W. Siquini (Ed.), *Surgical Treatment of Pancreatic Diseases.*
©Springer-Verlag Italia 2009

Solid Pancreatic Neoplasms: Adenocarcinoma

Pancreatic adenocarcinoma is the most common exocrine pancreatic neoplasm and accounts for 90–95% of all pancreatic malignancies. It originates from ductal epithelial cells and is mainly localized in the head of the pancreas. Although it has an unfavorable prognosis, in the case of tumors less than 2 cm, 5-year survival rates up to 30% have been reported [1]. Surgical resection is the only strategy that can guarantee the possibility of long-term survival, although fewer than 10–20% of tumors are resectable at the time of initial diagnosis [2]; the response to chemotherapy as the only therapeutic modality is in most cases poor.

Detection of pancreatic carcinoma is invariably based on imaging methods. Transabdominal ultrasonography often serves as the first imaging method, with a diagnostic sensitivity currently ranging from 67 to 85% (it varies according to the patient's constitution, the site of the lesion, and the operator's experience) and rising to 90–95% when color Doppler imaging is used [3, 4]. US imaging is used to identify the lesion, whereas staging is still mainly performed using CT or MR, although in this regard the validity of color Doppler and contrast-enhanced ultrasonography are recognized. On US examination, the carcinoma appears as a ill-defined hypoechoic mass with shaded margins, and in the case of larger forms shows coarse echoes or anechoic areas of necrosis (Fig. 14.1). In rare cases, a global and diffuse increase in the volume of the gland (secondary to chronic pancreatitis resulting from the neoplasm itself) or, even more rarely, disseminated calcifications can be detected, which can mislead the clinician into a diagnosis of chronic pancreatitis or a neuroendocrine tumor [5].

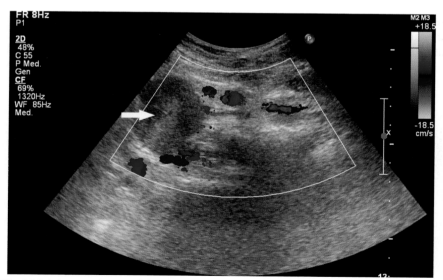

Fig. 14.1 Adenocarcinoma of the head of the pancreas. Ultrasound (US) examination shows a hypoechoic mass with shaded margins and multilobulated contours in the pancreatic head

CT is currently considered the imaging technique of choice for preoperative diagnosis and staging of pancreatic adenocarcinoma, since it allows the identification of even small tumors and provides useful data for the assessment of resectability, which has a significant effect on patient survival [6].

With the advent of MDCT, the pancreas can be imaged at a very high spatial and temporal resolution and the study can be performed within a short breathhold. Short volume acquisitions and faster scan times allow the acquisition of images in multiple phases of enhancement without concerns for tube heating, with narrow slice thickness, 2.5 mm or less. Due to the thinner slice collimation and multiphase imaging, MDCT identifies small focal lesions, showing a tumor-to-gland attenuation difference of at least 10 Hounsfield units (HU) [7].

The use of a near-isotropic voxel (data set with a similar spatial resolution in each dimension) allows multiplanar and curvilinear reconstruction, which are useful for the representation of ductal and vascular structures and the evaluation of their involvement in the neoplastic process [8]. Findings at CT in the evaluation of a pancreatic adenocarcinoma vary according to the extent of the neoplasm and to the possible presence of intralesional necrotic degeneration. On routine examination, tumor more frequently shows a density similar to that of normal parenchyma (Fig. 14.2a). Sometimes it shows diffuse necrosis or causes a contour deformity of the gland.

Following intravenous contrast injection, the most frequent appearance is of a focal mass that is hypodense compared with the surrounding healthy pancreatic parenchyma (Fig.14.2b). In the case of advanced lesions, even technically nonoptimal CT studies may allow the diagnosis of pancreatic neoplasm and determination of its unresectability, but only the use of optimal scanning parameters and contrast technique allows detection of potentially resectable small lesions. Their identification after intravenous contrast injection depends on maximization of the tumor-to-pancreas attenuation differences rather than on the absolute degree of tumoral enhancement.

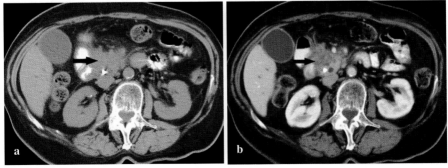

Fig. 14.2 Pancreatic adenocarcinoma. **a** Isodense lesion on routine computed tomography (CT). **b** Hypodense mass after intravenous contrast injection

The tumor-to-gland attenuation differences are greatest on images obtained in the "pancreatic phase," which is intermediate between the early arterial phase and the portal venous phase (40–70 s after infusion of intravenous contrast material at 3 ml/s) [7]. This pancreatic phase is influenced by the concentration, quantity, and injection rate of the contrast material. Different study protocols [8–11] have been proposed, including thin-section, two-phase, and three-phase studies, with an early arterial phase for documenting vessels (15–20 s after intravenous contrast injection), a pancreatic parenchymal phase for optimal identification of adenocarcinoma (35 s following contrast injection), and an early portal venous phase for optimal opacification of the veins and the liver. Other authors demonstrate the possibility of combining angiographic and parenchymal studies into a single thin-section acquisition phase (1 mm) at 60 s after contrast injection, in a caudocranial direction from the inferior hepatic margin to the diaphragm.

According to these authors single-phase helical CT is equivalent to dual- or multiphase techniques in terms of diagnostic effectiveness and assessment of resectability, and has the advantages of a lower radiation dose to the patient and a smaller number of images to film and store [11]. In the diagnosis of pancreatic neoplasms, MRI shows diagnostic accuracy values that are equivalent to those of MDCT when performed with high intensity magnetic field equipment (>1 T) providing a high signal-to-noise ratio, multichannel surface coils, and powerful gradients. The development of fast sequences with the acquisition of breath-hold images free from breathing artefacts, the use of an automatic injector, and fat signal saturation also allow a dynamic study of the upper abdomen during administration of gadolinium chelate contrast agent. Currently MRI is used as a "problem-solving" tool in patients with an inconclusive CT diagnosis or for small pancreatic masses that do not deform the profile of the gland [12]. This justifies the use of MRI as a method of second choice for identifying or excluding pancreatic neoplasms in those patients in whom US and/or CT have only demonstrated a volumetric increase of the pancreatic head or of the uncinate process and in the case of small suspected masses without contour deformity of the pancreas [8]. On MRI, pancreatic adenocarcinoma appears hypointense on T1-weighted unenhanced images and has a variable signal on T2-weighted sequences, depending on the amount of desmoplastic response associated with the tumor. It appears better distinguishable on GRE T1-weighted sequences with fat saturation, in particular during the pancreatic phase of the dynamic study. On dynamic imaging following a gadolinium contrast injection, an adenocarcinoma enhances relatively less than the background pancreatic parenchyma in the pancreatic phase and then reveals progressive enhancement in the subsequent phases (Fig. 14.3).

The sensitivity of MRI in the diagnosis of pancreatic tumors can be further increased by intravenous injection of a tissue-specific contrast agent, mangafodipir trisodium, which is taken up by normal pancreatic parenchyma [8]. Furthermore, the most recent studies with diffusion-weighed sequences and MR spectrography provide additional possibilities for using this method in the iden-

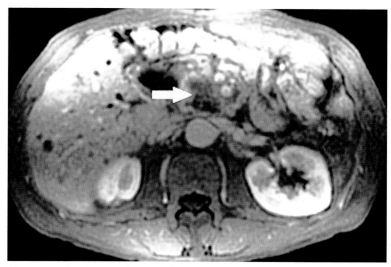

Fig. 14.3 Pancreatic adenocarcinoma. The tumor is typically hypointense in the pancreatic phase (*arrow*)

tification and follow-up of lesions [13–15]. The appreciation of some secondary signs can help the identification and diagnosis of pancreatic adenocarcinoma in the case of neoplastic masses that are not easily distinguishable. US examination can demonstrate dilatation of the common bile duct and secondary dilatation of the intrahepatic biliary tract and gallbladder in tumors of the head of the pancreas (even small ones) and in body/tail tumors, where obstruction generally results from lymph node metastases in the hepatic hilum. The main pancreatic duct upstream of the neoplasm may appear dilated with regular margins. This dilatation may be associated with concomitant dilatation of the common bile duct ("double duct" sign) and tumor of the head of the pancreas or ampulla may be suspected if there is an increased distance between the two dilated ducts [16].

On CT examination, the identification of obstruction of the main pancreatic duct in the absence of an obstructing calculus allows suspicion of a neoplastic process, in spite of the isodensity to the surrounding parenchyma that makes it poorly distinguishable (Fig. 14.4a). The use of curved multiplanar reconstructions, which allow visualization of the main pancreatic duct along its whole course, may highlight the sudden interruption of its distal end and a smooth rather than irregular profile of its walls, associated with an irregular and multilobulated profile of the gland, atrophy, and/or the presence of obstructing cysts of the distal pancreatic parenchyma, providing additional elements for the differential diagnosis between a neoplastic and an inflammatory pathology [17, 18].

MRCP has proven to be very useful for identifying tumor according to the site of ductal obstruction [8]. It is an MR technique for noninvasive assessment of the bile and pancreatic ducts, without the use of contrast media, by means of T2-dependent sequences with very long TE, so that only stationary fluids present in the ducts (bile and pancreatic juice) are able to provide signals (parenchymatous organs are completely relaxed and are unable to emit a signal) (Fig. 14.4b).

Once a tumor has been identified, surgical resection is the only treatment in patients without evident metastases at the time of diagnosis. In such patients the task of imaging methods is to assess the resectability of the tumor, which will be conditioned by findings of local tumor spread including infiltration of vascular structures. Appropriate selection of patients whose tumors are unresectable would reduce the mortality and morbidity from nontherapeutic laparotomies, and symptoms could be better treated with nonsurgical procedures without significant modifications of the survival curve. US imaging tends to understage the local diffusion of the tumor, that appear as hypoechoic tissue protruding from the gland and coming into contact with neighboring organs. In the evaluation of vascular infiltration, some reports consider US and color Doppler US imaging as having a diagnostic accuracy superior to that of angiography – especially in the evaluation of arterial involvement – although inferior to that of CT [19]. In general, US visualization of a cleavage plane maintained between tumor and peripancreatic vessels and an intact appearance of the echogenic vessel wall are signs of vascular integrity; conversely, substantial contiguity between lesion and vessel, widespread perivascular presence of neoplastic tissue, and an irregular or unrecognizable vascular wall are signs of infiltration.

Besides facilitating the demonstration of the abovementioned findings, the use of color Doppler imaging allows demonstration of flow turbulences and possible endoluminal neoplastic thromboses, with a sensitivity and specificity for venous infiltration of 72% and 45% respectively, increasing to 83% and 100% respectively with the use of echo-enhancing contrast agent [20].

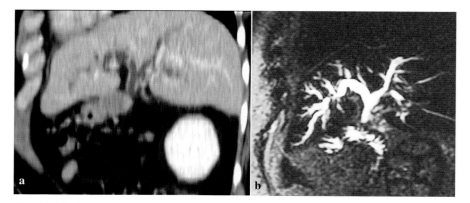

Fig. 14.4 Isodense pancreatic adenocarcinoma. On multiplanar reformation (MPR) of a CT study (**a**) the presence of tumor may be suspected on the evidence of dilatation of the common bile duct and intrahepatic bile ducts, in the absence of obstructing calculi. MRCP (**b**) strengthens the suspicion of a tumoral mass, showing discrete ectasia of the right and left intrahepatic ducts and common bile duct, with sudden interruption of its most distal tract

The identification of hepatic and lymph node metastases through US examination, which are specific signs of unresectability of a pancreatic tumor, may render any further diagnostic investigations useless, or, in those patients undergoing nonadjuvant therapies, definition of the site and number of hepatic localizations, together with other criteria, allows assessment of the response to therapy and the identification of operable cases. US imaging of hepatic metastases includes all US patterns, mostly hypoechoic in exocrine tumors and hyperechoic in islet cell (endocrine) tumors. In this regard, the importance of combining US imaging and echo-enhancing contrast agent has been recently stressed, the latter demonstrably improving the ability of US to detect hepatic metastases (even small ones) and visualize peritoneal carcinosis nodules, which along with ascitic effusion are signs of advanced tumor. Regarding the involvement of lymph nodes – lymph nodes in the hepatoduodenal ligament, retroperitoneal lymph nodes (particularly pancreatic), and mesenteric lymph nodes are the most frequently involved – they appear as ovoid, multilobulated, hypoechoic masses, well-defined compared with the surrounding tissues and structures. It should be borne in mind, however, that small adenopathies may go undetected by US, and that failure to identify normal-sized lymph nodes harboring micrometastases is also frequent [5].

MDCT, using multiphase study protocols, allows hepatic metastases and peritoneal carcinosis nodules to be visualized and a preoperative vascular map to be obtained for patients who are candidates for surgery. Arterial opacification is maximal in the early arterial and pancreatic parenchymal phases, whereas venous opacification is optimal in the portal venous phase. In general, criteria of unresectability include neoplastic infiltration ("encasement") of any vessel, especially arterial vessels, extended to over 50% or 180° in circumference, altered shape of the venous lumen, thrombosis with nonopacification of the vessel, and dilatation of the small superior pancreaticoduodenal veins and visualization of the inferior pancreaticoduodenal veins, a sign of infiltration of the central splanchnic veins [6, 7, 21, 22] (Fig.14.5).

CT imaging has a high diagnostic accuracy in assessing unresectability, but it does not have the same level of accuracy in assessing resectability: in a significant number of cases patients who are judged to be potentially operable on CT are then found to be inoperable at laparotomy. However, the introduction of the multilayer spiral technique with the possible use of CT-angiography and multiplanar reconstructions has increased the diagnostic accuracy of CT imaging in assessing tumor resectability. The high spatial resolution along the z-axis allows high-quality images to be obtained of vascular profiles and small-caliber peripancreatic vessels. Multiplanar reconstructions and VR (volume rendering) allow the vessel to be followed along its whole course. Maximum intensity projection (MIP) reconstructions provide a general overview in cases of vascular obstruction with development of collateral circles [8]. Moreover, postprocessing images are easier for nonradiologist physicians to read [23].

Currently, the most advanced breath-hold MR acquisition techniques, integrated with images from MR-angiography, allow an accurate noninvasive study for the assessment of unresectability. Considering the threshold for circumferen-

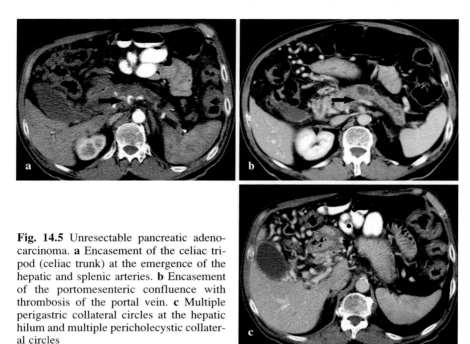

Fig. 14.5 Unresectable pancreatic adeno-carcinoma. **a** Encasement of the celiac tripod (celiac trunk) at the emergence of the hepatic and splenic arteries. **b** Encasement of the portomesenteric confluence with thrombosis of the portal vein. **c** Multiple perigastric collateral circles at the hepatic hilum and multiple pericholecystic collateral circles

tial vascular involvement of 180° as the limit of resectability, MR appears to be more accurate than CT in predicting operability [8, 13]. Although some authors consider MR to be superior to CT in detecting small hepatic metastases, the difficulty in identifying small peripancreatic lymph nodes and peritoneal implants represents a limitation of MR as an evaluation technique.

In neoplastic differential diagnoses, or more simply in identifying the nature of tumor lesions, US-guided biopsy is resorted to less and less frequently due both to the difficulty in reaching the lesion and to the high risk of neoplastic cell contamination, and, not least, to its poor diagnostic sensitivity and specificity.

A separate matter is EUS-FNAB (endoscopic ultrasonography-guided fine-needle aspiration biopsy) by the transduodenal approach, which can be very useful in the histological diagnosis of tumor in the head of the pancreas, drastically reducing the risk of peritoneal dissemination. For a few years now, endoscopic ultrasonography (EUS) has been playing a significant role in the locoregional staging of pancreatic neoplasms, combining the advantages of both methods. Many studies have demonstrated its importance in assessing tumor stage and signs of vascular and lymph node involvement, with diagnostic accuracy data that were found to be superior to those of CT [8]. Although an evaluation of its costs and invasiveness do not make it a routine method for all patients, EUS can and must be proposed in cases of strong clinical suspicion but nonidentification of tumor by other diagnostic imaging techniques, or in those cases in which these techniques are unable to give a certain diagnosis [24–26].

Neuroendocrine Tumors

Neuroendocrine tumors of the pancreas, or gastroenteropancreatic tumors, are very rare types of tumor, although highly malignant. They are classified into functioning (secreting various hormones) and nonfunctioning tumors. The latter are clinically silent until they cause symptoms due to their size or to the presence of metastases. The most common are insulinomas and gastrinomas. Differential diagnosis between nonfunctioning neuroendocrine pancreatic tumors and ductal adenocarcinomas is important, because the former have a better prognosis owing to their good response to surgery and specific chemotherapy. A diagnosis of nonfunctioning neuroendocrine tumor must be suspected when a considerably large pancreatic lesion is found, with calcifications visible on US and CT scans and inhomogeneous contrast enhancement, in the absence of cystic areas [27]. Functioning neuroendocrine tumors show onset symptoms that depend on the hormone secreted; they are small in size and rarely modify the profile of the pancreatic gland. Characteristically, they show greater contrast impregnation than that of normal pancreatic parenchyma (Fig. 14.6).

On precontrast MRI functioning neuroendocrine tumors appear hypointense on T1-weighted sequences with fat suppression and, unlike adenocarcinomas, they appear hyperintense on T2-weighted sequences, characteristically showing early and homogeneous contrast enhancement [28] (Fig. 14.7). Hypervascular hepatic metastases are often demonstrated, whereas signs of circumferential vascular infiltration and central necrosis are always absent.

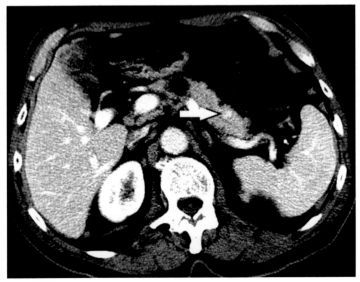

Fig. 14.6 Neuroendocrine tumor of the pancreas. CT scan shows a small hypervascular nodule of the tail of the pancreas in a patient with a cystic-type lesion of the isthmus

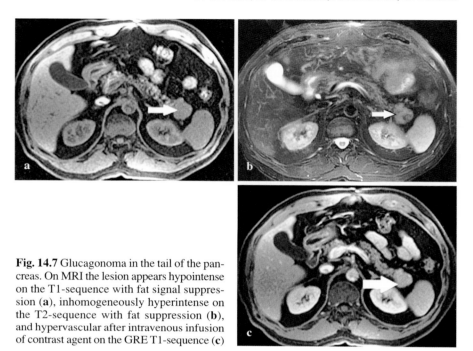

Fig. 14.7 Glucagonoma in the tail of the pancreas. On MRI the lesion appears hypointense on the T1-sequence with fat signal suppression (**a**), inhomogeneously hyperintense on the T2-sequence with fat suppression (**b**), and hypervascular after intravenous infusion of contrast agent on the GRE T1-sequence (**c**)

Recently, EUS has established itself as a technique for visualizing small functioning neuroendocrine tumors not detectable using traditional imaging methods, in cases of high clinical suspicion, and for diagnosing multiple tumor localizations. This technique has proven to be extremely accurate for identifying these tumors, allowing their visualization within the gastroduodenal wall or within the pancreatic parenchyma with reported sensitivity values up to 94%, although it is not equally valid for diagnosing extrapancreatic localizations. EUS-FNAB also allows cytological confirmation of the nature of the lesions to be obtained [29, 30].

Cystic Neoplasms of the Pancreas

The increased availability of imaging techniques has caused cystic pancreatic lesions to be found more and more frequently in asymptomatic patients. Although only 5–15% of these lesions are neoplastic in nature, and inflammatory pseudocyst is the most frequent cystic lesion of the pancreas, the hypothesis of cystic neoplasm has to be taken into consideration in the absence of clinical and laboratory evidence of pancreatitis [31]. Among the various histological types of pancreatic cystic neoplasm, serous cystadenomas, mucinous cystic neoplasms, and intraductal papillary mucinous tumors (IPMTs) account for 90% of cases [32]. The first are benign tumors, whereas most mucin-producing lesions are potentially malignancies and require surgical treatment. Occasionally also some solid tumors of the pancreas, such as adenocarcinomas and endocrine tumors, may show a liquid component, mimicking a cystic neoplasm. In these cases differential diagnosis is important since cystic neoplasms have a better prognosis than adenocarcinoma. Although US, CT, and MRI allow characterization of cysts in a large number of patients, overlapping of different morphological characteristics sometimes makes the differential diagnosis difficult. In these cases EUS-FNAB can provide additional diagnostic information.

Microcystic Adenoma

This benign cystic neoplasm of the pancreas, also known as serous cystadenoma or glycogen-rich adenoma, is more prevalent in women of middle to advanced age and is generally asymptomatic. It is a large well-defined cystic lesion, composed of innumerable tiny cysts (<2 cm in diameter), separated by thin septa, sometimes converging towards a central stellate fibrous or fibrocalcific scar. It is more frequently localized in the head of the pancreas. On US examination the lesion may appear as a cribrate mass or as a formation having a paradoxically solid, hyperechoic appearance due to the multitude of interfaces produced by the numerous cysts [33]. On CT examination the classic appearance is of a hypodense mass, with the same density as water or soft tissues, or of a mixed mass, composed of multiple small cysts with a "honeycomb" appearance. Cyst walls and internal septations may show a variable degree of enhancement after contrast administration [34] (Fig.14.8). On MRI, microcystic adenoma appears

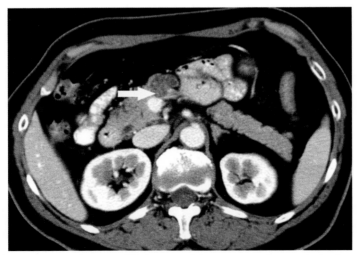

Fig. 14.8 Microcystic adenoma. CT shows an inhomogeneously vascularized mass at the pancreatic isthmus: the thin hyperdense internal septations are visible

hypointense on T1-weighted images and hyperintense on T2-weighted images, with evidence of septations and central scar. There is a unilocular macrocystic variant of microcystic adenoma that is a rarer form and can be erroneously interpreted as a mucinous cystic tumor. Lobulated contours, localization in the pancreatic head, absence of wall enhancement, and the presence of a thin capsule are characteristic of the macrocystic serous form, and the presence of two or three of these morphological characteristics generally allows a correct diagnosis with a specificity of 83% or 100%, respectively [35, 36]. In doubtful cases, percutaneous needle aspiration biopsy can contribute to the diagnosis, identifying the presence of cytoplasmic glycogen and the absence of mucin.

Mucinous Cystic Tumor

Mucinous cystic tumor, also referred to as macrocystic adenoma or cystadenoma, mucinous cystadenocarcinoma, or mucin-hypersecreting carcinoma, is considered potentially malignant and therefore a candidate for surgical excision. It is more frequent in women between the 5th and 6th decades of life, and is more frequently localized in the body and tail of the pancreas. On US examination it appears as a uni- or multilocular cystic formation, with loculations greater than 2 cm in diameter and less than six in number, with thick walls and internal hyperechoic septa [37]. On CT examination the cystic mass shows a density close to that of water (Fig. 14.9a), a thick wall, with possible nodular excrescences and septa, which are better visualized after contrast agent injection. On MRI the appearance of the lesion may vary, since it can occasionally appear hyperintense on both T1- and T2-weighted images, although the mucin content generally causes high signal intensity on T2-weighted images and low signal intensity on T1-weighted images (Fig. 14.9b).

In fact, the signal intensity depends on the mucin protein content. The presence of curvilinear calcifications in the peripheral capsule or in the cyst wall,

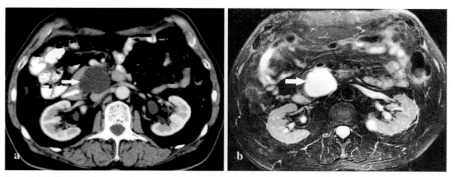

Fig. 14.9 Unilocular mucinous cystic tumor. CT (**a**) shows a nodule with liquid content in the cephalopancreatic region. MRI (**b**) shows a hyperintense nodule on T2-weighted sequence with fat suppression

which are better shown by CT scanning, has proved to be a characteristic morphological feature allowing differential diagnosis from other cystic lesions of the pancreas. The lack of relationship with the main pancreatic duct allows its differentiation from pseudocysts [38–42].

Intraductal Papillary Mucinous Tumor

IPMT, also known as ductectatic tumor or ductectatic cystadenoma, is a slow-growing and potentially malignant neoplasm. It is characterized by intraductal papillary growth of mucin-producing columnar cells. Most patients are men who have pancreatitis-like symptoms, which can be due to ductal obstruction resulting from papillary proliferations and/or mucin with subsequent atrophy of the pancreatic parenchyma. IPMT must be treated by surgical resection and have the same favorable prognosis as mucinous cystic tumor.

On US examination it appears as a septated cystic formation of varying size, depending on its origin, with segmentary or diffuse dilatation of the main pancreatic duct. These aspects, which are like those of pseudocystic obstructive chronic pancreatitis, make US diagnosis difficult. On CT examination, too, IPMT of the main pancreatic duct, appearing as a diffuse dilatation of the same, often associated with atrophy of the gland and intraductal dystrophic calcifications, may mimic the pattern of chronic pancreatitis. Unlike typical chronic pancreatitis, however, IPMT shows dilatation of the distal pancreatic duct due to mucin and an enlarged papilla protruding into the duodenal lumen. The evidence of mural nodules in the duct are suggestive of malignancy.

The CT appearance of IPMT originating from the secondary ducts is different: it appears as a uni- or multilocular cystic lesion with a "grape-like" appearance, localized in the uncinate process and in the pancreatic head [43]. The main pancreatic duct may be dilated due to mucin production (Fig. 14.10a). MDCT, through multiplanar reconstructions, or, even better, MRCP in the individual coronal partitions, can demonstrate communication between the cystic lesion and the main pancreatic duct (Fig. 14.10b). In particular, MRCP is currently considered the method of choice for demonstrating the morphological characteristics of cysts (including septa and intramural nodules), for establishing the presence of communication between the cystic lesion and the pancreatic duct, and for evaluating the extent of ductal dilatation [44–47].

Solid Pseudopapillary Tumor

Among the pancreatic cystic tumors, a progressive increase in the incidence of solid pseudopapillary tumor (SPPT) has been reported in the new millennium, and currently this tumor accounts for 6% of all exocrine neoplasms of the pancreas. It mainly affects young women, in whom it is generally an incidental finding on US examination performed for other indications. It is slow growing, often

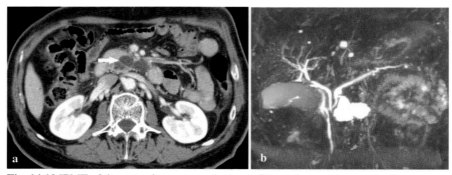

Fig. 14.10 IPMT of the secondary pancreatic ducts. CT (**a**) shows a "grape-like" hypodense cystic mass of the pancreatic isthmus and body. MRCP (**b**) shows communication between the mass and the main pancreatic duct

reaching a large size, and in most cases it has a low degree of malignancy. US and CT show a well-defined round lesion, characteristically including solid and cystic areas and occasionally calcifications. MRI can further characterize the lesion, demonstrating its hemorrhagic content. Furthermore, MRCP allows the relationship between lesion, biliary tract, and the main pancreatic duct to be established. After intravenous administration of contrast agent, the lesion shows early centripetal peripheral enhancement.

FNAB can allow a correct preoperative diagnosis, demonstrating epithelial cells organized in papillary structures [48].

References

1. Fontham ET, Correa P (1989) Epidemiology of pancreatic cancer. Surg Clin North Am 69:551–567
2. Tsuchiya R, Noda T, Harada N et al (1986) Collective review of small carcinoma of the pancreas. Ann Surg 203:77–81
3. Angeli E, Venturini M, Vanzulli A et al (1997) Color-Doppler imaging in the assessment of vascular involvement by pancreatic carcinoma. AJR Am J Roentgenol 168: 193–197
4. Gorelick AB, Scheimann JM, Fendrick AM (1998) Identification of patients with resectable pancreatic cancer: at what stage are we? Am J Gastroenterol 93:1995–1996
5. Di Candio G et al (2006) Le neoplasie del pancreas. In: Busilacchi , Rapaccini GL (eds) Ecografia clinica. Idelson-Gnocchi, Napoli, p 849
6. Megibow AJ, Zhou XH, Rotterdam H et al (1995) Pancreatic adenocarcinoma: CT versus MR imaging in the evaluation of resectability – report of the Radiology Diagnostic Oncology Group. Radiology 195:327–332
7. Lu DSK, Vedantham S, Krasny RM et al (1996) Two-phase helical CT for pancreatic tumors: pancreatic versus hepatic phase enhancement of tumor, pancreas and vascular structures. Radiology 199:697–701
8. Sahani DV, Shah ZK, Catalano OA et al (2008) Radiology of pancreatic adenocarcinoma: current status of imaging. J Gastroenterol Hepatol 23:23–33
9. McNulty NJ, Francis IR, Platt JF et al (2001) Multi-detector row helical CT of the pancreas: effect of contrast-enhanced multiphasic imaging on enhancement of the pancreas, peripancreatic vasculature, and pancreatic adenocarcinoma. Radiology 220:97–102

10. Fletcher JG, Wiersema MJ, Farrell MA et al (2003) Pancreatic malignancy: value of arterial, pancreatic, and hepatic phase imaging with multi-detector row CT. Radiology 229:81–90

11. Massimo I, Megibow AJ, Ragozzino A et al (2005) Value of the single-phase technique in MDCT assessment of pancreatic tumors. AJR Am J Roentgenol 184:1111–1117

12. Schima W (2006) MRI of the pancreas: tumours and tumour-simulating processes. Cancer Imaging 6:199–203

13. Schima W, Ba-Ssalamah A, Kölblinger C et al (2007) Pancreatic adenocarcinoma. Eur Radiol 17:638–49

14. Miller FH, Rini NJ, Keppke et al (2006) MRI of adenocarcinoma of the pancreas. AJR Am J Roentgenol 187:W365-W374

15. Takeuchi M, Matsuzaki K, Kubo H et al (2008) High-b-value diffusion-weighted magnetic resonance imaging of pancreatic cancer and mass-forming chronic pancreatitis: preliminary results. Acta Radiol 49:383–386

16. Gibson RN, Yeung E, Thompson JN et al (1986) Bile duct obstruction: radiologic evaluation of level, cause, and tumor resectability. Radiology 160:43–47

17. Prokesch RW, Chow LC, Beaulieu CF et al (2002) Local staging of pancreatic carcinoma with multi-detector row CT: use of curved planar reformations – initial experience. Radiology 225:759–765

18. Ichikawa T, Erturk SM, Sou H et al (2006) MDCT of pancreatic adenocarcinoma: optimal imaging phases and multiplanar reformatted imaging. AJR Am J Roentgenol 187:1513–1520

19. Ahmad NA, Kochman ML, Lewis JD et al (2001) Endosonography is superior to angiography in the preoperative assessment of vascular involvment among patients with pancreatic carcinoma. J Clin Gastroenterol 32:54–58

20. Candiani F (2006) Tumori pancreatici. In: Rabbia C, De. Lucchi R, Cirillo R (eds) Eco color-Doppler vascolare, 3rd edn. Minerva Medica, Torino, pp 1021–1024

21. Valls C, Andia E, Sanchez A et al (2002) Dual phase helical CT of pancreatic adenocarcinoma: assessment of resectability bifore surgery. AJR Am J Roentgenol 178:821–826

22. Yamada Y, Mori H, Kiyosue H et al (2000) CT assessment of the inferior peripancreatic veins: clinical significance. AJR Am J Roentgenol 174:677–684

23. Brennan DD, Zamboni G, Sosna J et al (2007) Virtual Whipple: preoperative surgical planning with volume-rendered MDCT images to identify arterial variants relevant to the Whipple procedure. AJR Am J Roentgenol 188:W451-W455

24. Latronico A, Crosta C, De Fiori E et al (2005) Ecografia endoscopica e tomografia computerizzata nella diagnosi, stadiazione loco-regionale ed infiltrazione vascolare del carcinoma del pancreas. Radiol Med (Torino) 109:508–509

25. Kulig J, Popiela T, Zajac A et al (2005) The value of imaging techniques in the staging of pancreatic cancer. Surg Endosc 19:361–365

26. Midwinter MJ, Beveridge CJ, Wilsdon JB et al (1999) Correlation between spiral computed tomography, endoscopic ultrasonography and findings at operation in pancreatic and ampullary tumors. Br J Surg 86:189–193

27. Eelkema EA, Stephens DH, Ward EM et al (1984) CT features of nonfunctioning islet cell carcinoma. AJR Am J Roentgenol 143:943–948

28. Buetow PC, Parrino TV, Buck JL et al (1995) Islet cell tumors of the pancreas: pathologic-imaging correlation among size, necrosis and cysts, calcification, malignant behavior, and functional status. AJR Am J Roentgenol 165:1175–1179

29. Rockall AG, Reznek RH (2007) Imaging of neuroendocrine tumours (CT/MR/US). Best Pract Res Clin Endocrinol Metab 21:43–68

30. Ruszniewski PH, Amouyal P, Amouyal G et al (1995) Localization of gastrinomas by endoscopic ultrasonography in patients with Zollinger-Ellison syndrome. Surgery 117:629–635

31. Chaudhari VV, Raman SS, Vuong NG et al (2007) Pancreatic cystic lesions: discrimination accuracy based on clinical data and high resolution CT features. J Comput Assist Tomogr 31:860–867

32. Francis IR (2003) Cystic pancreatic neoplasm. Cancer Imaging 3:111–116

33. Gandolfi L , Torresan F, Solmi L, Puccetti A (2003) The role of ultrasound in biliary and pancreatic disease. Eur J Ultrasound 16:141–159

34. Procacci C, Graziani R, Bicego E et al (1997) Serous cystadenoma of the pancreas: report of 30 cases with emphasis on imaging findings. J Comput Assist Tomogr 21:373–382

35. Cohen-Scali F, Vilgrain V, Brancatelli B et al (2003) Discrimination of unilocular macrocystic serous cystadenoma from pancreatic pseudocyst and mucinous cystadenoma with CT: initial observations. Radiology 228:727–733

36. Hyoung JK, Dong HL, Young TK et al (2008) CT of serous cystadenoma of the pancreas and mimicking masses. AJR Am J Roentgenol 190:406–412

37. Grogan J, Saeian K, Taylor AJ et al (2001) Making sense of mucin-producing pancreatic tumors. AJR Am J Roentgenol 176:921–929

38. Demos TC, Posniak HV, Harmath C et al (2002) Cystic lesions of the pancreas. AJR Am J Roentgenol 179:1375–1388

39. Curry CA, Eng J, Horton KM et al (2000) CT of primary cystic pancreatic neoplasms: can CT be used for patient triage and treatment? AJR Am J Roentgenol 175:99–103

40. Sarr MG, Kendrick ML, Nagorney DM et al (2001) Cystic neoplasms of the pancreas: benign to malignant epithelial neoplasms. Surg Clin North Am 81:497–509

41. Adsay NV, Longnecker DS, Klimstra DS (2000) Pancreatic tumors with cystic dilatation of the ducts: intraductal papillary mucinous neoplasms and intraductal oncocytic papillary neoplasms. Semin Diagn Pathol 17:16–30

42. Visser BC, Yeh BM, Qayyum A et al (2007) Characterization of cystic pancreatic masses: relative accuracy of CT and MRI. AJR Am J Roentgenol 189:648–656

43. Takeshita K, Kutomi K, Takada K et al (2008) Differential diagnosis of benign or malignant intraductal papillary mucinous neoplasm of the pancreas by multidetector row helical computed tomography: evaluation of predictive factors by logistic regression analysis J Comput Assist Tomogr 32:191–197

44. Silas AM, Morrin MM, Raptopoulos V et al (2001) Intraductal papillary mucinous tumors of the pancreas. AJR Am J Roentgenol 176:179–185

45. Lim JH, Lee G, Oh YL (2001) Radiologic spectrum of intraductal papillary mucinous tumor of the pancreas. Radiographics 21:323–337

46. Fukukura Y, Fujiyoshi F, Sasaki M et al (2000) Intraductal papillary mucinous tumors of the pancreas: thin-section helical CT findings. AJR Am J Roentgenol 174:441–447

47. Sahani DV, Kadavigere R, Blake M et al (2006) Intraductal papillary mucinous neoplasm of pancreas: multi-detector row CT with 2D curved reformations – correlation with MRCP. Radiology 238:560–569

48. Siquini W, Marmorale C, Guercioni G et al (2006) Tumore solido pseudopapillare del pancreas: a proposito di tre casi e revisione della letteratura. Chir Ital; 58:235–245

Chapter 15

Pancreatic Cancer: Pathological Factors and TNM Staging

Angelo de Sanctis, Massimiliano Rimini, Mario Guerrieri

Introduction

Ductal adenocarcinoma, a solid, exocrine epithelial neoplasm, represents with its variations the large majority of primitive malignant tumors of the pancreas (about 90% of cases) [1]. It is typically characterized by insidious growth with a generally unfavorable prognosis. At the time of diagnosis in most cases there are already peripancreatic lymph node metastases, and at post mortem, liver (80%), peritoneal (60%), pulmonary (50–70%), and suprarenal metastases (25%) are also frequently found [2]. Despite the recent knowledge acquired in the biomolecular genetics of this neoplasm and the progress made in instrumental diagnostic technology, the prognosis of this tumor is still poor, with an average survival of 19% at 1 year after diagnosis and 2–4% after 5 years: pancreatic cancer still has the worst prognosis of the solid neoplasms [3].

Anatomicopathological Findings

Histological Types

Presently, the most commonly adopted classification system is that proposed in 1997 by the AFIP (Armed Forces Institute of Pathology) of Rockville, Washington DC (Table 15.1) [4]. In this classification, the lesions are not distinguished as solid, cystic, or mixed, as in that proposed by the World Health Organization (WHO classification), whose last edition was in 1996, although the latter did already make the distinction between benign, malignant, and borderline [5].

In the AFIP classification, the classic form of ductal adenocarcinoma (80–85% of cases) has five rarer variations, with differing degrees of cellular atypia and malignancies, which together constitute about 7–10% of cases of pancreatic adenocarcinoma. These are: mucinous noncystic carcinoma (1–3%), signet-ring cell carcinoma, adenosquamous carcinoma (3–4%), undifferentiated (anaplastic) carcinoma (2–7%), and mixed ductal-endocrine carcinoma (rare).

W. Siquini (Ed.), *Surgical Treatment of Pancreatic Diseases.*
©Springer-Verlag Italia 2009

Table 15.1 US Armed Forces Institute of Pathology classification of primary pancreatic tumors (adapted from [4])

Tumors of the exocrine pancreas
Benign
Serous cystadenoma
Mucinous cystadenoma
Intraductal papillary-mucinous adenoma
Mature cystic teratoma)

Borderline (uncertain malignant potential)
Mucinous cystic tumor with moderate dysplasia
Intraductal papillary-mucinous tumor with moderate dysplasia
Solid-pseudopapillary tumor

Malignant
Ductal adenocarcinoma
    Mucinous noncystic carcinoma
    Signet-ring cell carcinoma
    Adenosquamous carcinoma
    Undifferentiated (anaplastic) carcinoma
    Mixed ductal-endocrine carcinoma
Osteoclast-like giant cell tumor
    Serous cystadenocarcinoma
    Mucinous   cystadenocarcinoma: noninvasive; invasive
    Intraductal papillary-mucinous carcinoma: noninvasive; invasive
    Acinar cell carcinoma
        Acinar cell cystadenocarcinoma
        Mixed acinar-endocrine carcinoma
    Pancreatoblastoma
    Solid-pseudopapillary carcinoma
    Miscellaneous carcinomas

Tumors of the endocrine pancreas
Benign
Well-differentiated adenoma
    Insulinoma
    Nonfunctioning adenoma

Borderline (uncertain malignant potential)
Well-differentiated nonangioinvasive tumor
    Insulinoma
    Gastrinoma, VIPoma, glucagonoma, somatostatinoma, others
    Nonfunctioning tumor

Low-grade malignant
Well to moderately differentiated carcinoma
    Insulinoma

continue →

continue **Table 15.1**

Gastrinoma, vipoma, glucagonoma, somatostatinoma, others
Nonfunctioning carcinoma

High-grade malignant
Poorly differentiated carcinoma (i.e., small cell carcinoma)
Functioning or nonfunctioning

Nonepithelial tumors
Benign soft tissue tumors
Malignant soft tissue tumors
Malignant lymphomas

Of these, adenosquamous carcinoma is defined by a predominantly squamous differentiation and by a particularly poor prognosis, as is the undifferentiated variation (anaplastic, also known as giant-cell carcinoma), which is characterized by cells whose shape is extremely pleomorphic, with nuclei of bizarre shapes and eosinophilic cytoplasm; it can often be characterized only on the basis of cytokeratin immunohistochemical study [4]. The other malignant variations are less frequent, but the prognosis is always severe. Acinar cell carcinoma, which is often remarkably large at the time of diagnosis, has a better prognosis than ductal carcinoma. Histologically, the formation if acinar cells with eosinophilic granular cytoplasm cells is typical.

Ductal Adenocarcinoma

Ductal adenocarcinoma originates in 65% of cases in the head of the pancreas, in the isthmus, or in the uncinate process in 15% it is in the body and tail, while in 20% it can diffusely affect the whole gland [6]. At diagnosis, tumors in the head, isthmus, or uncinate process are generally smaller (2.5–3 cm) than those found in the body or tail (5–7 cm) [4].

Macroscopically it appears as a white-yellowish hard mass, with poorly defined borders, scirrhous texture, and containing possible microcystic areas; hemorrhagic or necrotic areas are rarer. Carcinoma of the head of the pancreas early forms an intimate relationship with the duct of Wirsung, causing its obstruction (in the majority of cases the tumor develops in close proximity to the knee of the main pancreatic duct): this implies upstream dilatation, combined with parenchymal fibrosis and subsequent atrophy of the acinar component (expression of obstructive chronic pancreatitis). Moreover, from the initial stages, tumors that originate from the head and the uncinate process have an aggressive course, with early involvement of the common bile duct, the retroperitoneal adipose tissue, and the vascular structures (particularly the celiac tripod or trunk, the superior mesenteric artery, the portal vein, and the superior mesenteric vein) [4]. If located in the body and the tail, the tumor soon involves the near organs (stomach, spleen, colon) [6].

On microscopic examination, it is seen to be constituted by infiltrating glandular structures of varying shapes and dimensions (whose epithelial cells have differing degrees of atypia), surrounded by a thick reagent and fibrous reaction which is responsible for the hard consistency of the tumor; in many cases there is infiltration of the vascular, lymphatic, or perineural areas [7]. In the immediate proximity of ductal adenocarcinoma, it is possible to observe intraductal proliferative lesions, with varying degrees of mucin-secreting cytological and structural atypia. It has been demonstrated that before reaching the invasive carcinoma stage, numerous genetic alterations occur in the tumor cells, (K-*ras* gene, *p16*, *p53*, *BRCA2* and *DPC4* genetic mutations) [8]. To concretize a malignant lesion of the pancreatic ductal epithelium, there thus has to be a series of mutations, not a single event, and the epithelial malignant transformation is what results from the DNA mutations that take place in the following phases. This hypothesis is supported by the detection of associated lesions, precursors of ductal adenocarcinoma defined as pancreatic intraductal neoplasms (PanINs) [9–11]. These are precancerous forms in the pancreatic duct epithelium. A PanIN can be flat (PanIN-1A), papillary without atypia (PanIN-1B), papillary with atypia (PanIN-2), or it can have the features of carcinoma in situ (PanIN-3). During observations of the genetic mutations in these lesions, it has been remarked that K-*ras* activation and *p16* inactivation appear in the PanIN-1 and 2 lesions and that subsequent mutation of *DCP4* causes progression to PanIN-3; on the basis of these genetic modifications, a progression model of PanIN-1 lesions to pancreatic ductal adenocarcinoma has recently been proposed [12–18].

Other biological aspects of this tumor are little known, such as the role of stromal reaction. It is well known that the interaction between tumor cells and the surrounding stroma is identified as responsible for the growth, invasion, and neoplastic metastasization, as it plays a central role in angiogenesis and chemoresistance [19–23]. While physiologically the normal interaction between neoplastic cells and the surrounding stroma maintains tissue integrity, in cancer, through signals such as transforming growth factor-β (TGFβ) and platelet-derived growth factor (PDGF), an abnormal, anomalous interaction ends in desmoplastic reaction, invasion, and metastasis formation [24]. Histologically, the primary invasion area of ductal adenocarcinoma is therefore almost uniformly characterized by a marked widespread desmoplastic reaction. The interaction between tumor and stroma could explain the aggressive behavior of the pancreatic carcinoma, a hypothesis supported by the experimental evidence that the neoplastic cell invasive potential can be notably increased by stromal fibroblast culture [25]. The concept is further confirmed by the observation that mucinous adenocarcinoma, which is less aggressive, is associated with a minimal stromal reaction around the tumor [26]. The neoplastic cells can stimulate the "tumoral stroma" formation due to the aberrant growth factor production and/or to the constitutive induction of the relative receptors in the stromal compartment.

The continuous interaction between tumor cells and the stromal environment (mutual regulation and modulation) is a fundamental precondition for the development and progression of the carcinoma, promoting the invasiveness and angiogenesis of the tumoral cells. It has been remarked how targeted blocking of hepatocyte growth factor (HGF; a pleiotropic cytokine mainly produced by the stromal fibroblasts inhibits the growth, invasion, and metastasization of various types of tumors including pancreatic carcinoma [27, 28].

Many studies have shown the connection between cancer and the endocrine component of the pancreas. In fact the presence of islands appears to be a prerequisite for the induction of pancreatic carcinoma in murine experimental models [29–33]. Although pancreatic adenocarcinoma shows a ductal morphology, at the moment the cells from which it arises have not been identified, and some authors have suggested that it could arise from pancreatic islands. In experimental models using guinea-pigs, most adenocarcinomas begin their development inside the islands, in all probability through resident stem cells; moreover some observations have suggested a relationship between carcinoma of the pancreas and the development of diabetes [34–36].

However it is the stromal "fibroblasts" and the extracellular matrix proteins that they produce that are to be considered as key components of the desmoplastic response to tumors. Circulating fibroblasts are potentially the precursors of this cellular component, and there is some evidence that, under appropriate conditions, fibroblast differentiation can be modulated toward a myofibroblastic phenotype [37, 38]. The spinal origin of both tumoral myofibroblasts and fibroblasts has recently been confirmed, in turn confirming previous evidence of cells of spinal derivation both inside and around the pancreatic tumor in the RIPTag mouse model [39]. Other authors have, however, demonstrated that even same epithelial cells can act as myofibroblast precursors (epithelium–mesenchymal transition) [40]. It has also been assumed that they can protect neoplastic cells from the immune system in such a way as to increase their invasive ability [41]. On the other hand, there is also some evidence that patients with hepatocellular encapsulated carcinoma survive longer than those with nonencapsulated tumors [42].

The presence of significant hypoxia in cancer of the pancreas has been recently supported by Koong et al., who directly measured the oxygen inside the tumor in seven patients [43]. The carcinomatous area showed a mean P_{O2} of 0–5.3 mmHg, while the nearby areas of normal pancreatic tissue had mean P_{O2} measurements of 24–92.7 mmHg. Studies on the effects of a hypoxic environment are being carried out on the molecular mechanisms of carcinomatous cells in relation to the expression of hypoxia-inducible factor 1α (HIF-1α) that, induced by hypoxia, contributes to the survival and proliferation of cancerous cells [44]. The effects of a hypoxic environment on the tumor–stroma interactions are as yet absolutely unknown.

Among the most recent additions to the understanding of present alterations in the pancreatic carcinoma we mention the multidimensional protein identification technology (MuDPIT), which is used for the analysis of secreted proteins in the overfloating cell culture, based on bidimensional capillary chromatography combined with tandem mass spectrometry (2DC-MS/MS) [45].

Lately, Moniaux reported that neutrophil gelatinase-associated lipocalin (NGAL), a serum 24-kDa glycoprotein, is highly expressed in early dysplastic lesions in the pancreas, as early as the PanIN-1 stage, suggesting a possible role as a diagnostic marker of the earliest premalignant changes in the pancreas [46].

Staging System

Classifications

The two classifications most used at present, both published in 2002, are those of the Union International Contre le Cancer (UICC, 6th edition) (Table 15.2) and that of the Japan Pancreas Society (JPS, 5th edition) (Table 15.3) [47, 48]. Both of these classifications are based on the TNM international system.

Table 15.2 TNM classification of pancreatic tumors (from [47])

Primary tumor (T)

TX:	Primary tumor cannot be assessed
T0:	No evidence of primary tumor
Tis:	In situ carcinoma
T1:	Tumor limited to the pancreas 2 cm or less in greatest dimension
T2:	Tumor limited to the pancreas more than 2 cm in greatest dimension
T3:	Tumor extends directly into any of the following: duodenum, bile duct, or peripancreatic tissues
T4:	Tumor extends directly into any of the following: stomach, spleen, colon, or adjacent large vessels

Regional lymph nodes (N)

NX:	Regional lymph nodes cannot be assessed
N0:	No regional lymph node metastasis
N1:	Regional lymph node metastasis

Distant metastasis (M)

MX:	Distant metastasis cannot be assessed
M0:	No distant metastasis
M1:	Distant metastasis

Stage

0	Tis	N0	M0
I A	T1	N0	M0
I B	T2	N0	M0
II A	T3	N0	M0
II B	T1–2–3	N1	M0
III	T 4	N0–N1	M0
IV	Any T	N0–N1	M1

Table 15.3 Pancreatic tumor staging of the Japan Pancreas Society (from [48])

	T	S	RP	PV	N	M
Stage I	T1	S0	RP0	PV0	N0	M0
Stage II	T2	S1	RP1	PV1	N1	M0
Stage III	T3	S2	RP2	PV2	N2	M0
Stage IV	T4	S3	RP3	PV3	N3	M1

T1 = <2 cm; *T2* = 2–4 cm; *T3* = 4–6 cm; *T4* = >6 cm

S, serosal invasion; *RP*, retropancreatic tissue invasion; *PV*, portal venous system invasion; *0*, absence of invasion; *1*, suspected invasion; *2*, definite invasion; *3*, severe invasion;

N0, no involvement; *N1*, involvement of primary group of lymph nodes; *N2*, involvement of secondary group of lymph nodes; *N3*, involvement of tertiary lymph nodes regarded as juxtaregional lymph nodes

Distant metastasis including hepatic metastasis or peritoneal dissemination is allocated to stage IV

Within the classification proposed by the UICC, compared to the 1998 previous version, the T3 and T4 definition has changed: in the current version those tumors which do not involve the celiac axis or the superior mesenteric artery are considered T3, and invasion of these structures characterizes T4. In this way venous invasion is distinguished from arterial invasion, this latter being considered a worse prognostic factor.

Although the classification proposed by the UICC is easier to understand and is therefore the most used in Western countries, the one proposed by the JPS is more detailed and accurate; particularly, for the definition of locoregional tumor extent, it also takes into consideration infiltration of the portal venous axis and possible infiltration of retroperitoneal tissue.

Instrumental Methods of Staging

Ultrasonography

Ultrasonography is usually the first diagnostic investigation when a pancreatic neoplastic lesion is suspected clinically. When the neoplastic lesion is visible, most ductal adenocarcinomas appear as solid, hypoechogenic lesions with undefined and irregular borders [49–51], like endocrine neoplasms [52], while mucinous neoplasms look like fluid-filled lesions, uni- or multilocular, with septa which can look thickened and which, in malignant forms, show vegetations; serious cystic neoplasias on the other hand are characterized instead by the typical "beehive" appearance [51]. In some cases only indirect signs of the presence of neoplasia can be identified, such as dilatation of the duct of Wirsung and/or bile duct [52]. Ultrasonography can identify the presence of locoregional lymphadenopathies, hepatic metastases, or ascitic fluid, this latter the exteriorization of possible peritoneal carcinosis [52]. The biggest limitation of the technique is its poor sensitivity to vascular invasion, although color Doppler imaging seems to increase the accuracy of ultrasonography, reaching unsteady values between 84 and 87% [51].

In recent years the introduction of contrast ultrasonography has made it possible to identify more accurately both the neoplasms and their relationship with peripancreatic arterial and venous vessels[53, 54]. The endoscopic ultrasonography (ultrasound transducer mounted onto a modified gastroscope) appears to be reliable in identifying the lesion and also in predicting its unresectability (sensitivity and specificity 80%) [51, 55, 56].

Magnetic Resonance Imaging

The recent use of fast sequences (fast imaging) has allowed certain limitations of MRI to be overcome, such as the movement artifacts (respiratory, vascular, and peristaltic) and the low spatial resolution which previously limited the use of this method of studying the pancreatic gland [57, 58].

Pancreatic adenocarcinoma appears as a hypointense lesion in T1-weighted sequences with low dynamic image enhancement after vascular interstitial distribution of injected contrast medium (gadolinium chelates), which is related to its hypovascular nature and to the perilesional desmoplastic reaction [51]. Endocrine neoplasms also show a low-resonance signal intensity in T1-weighted sequences where they appear iso- or hypointense, while they are hyperintense in T2-weighted sequences [58]. Recently, organ-specific contrast media have been used for the study of pancreas, as for example manganese compounds which are caught by healthy pancreatic parenchyma and not by the neoplastic lesion [59]. By using particular sequences which raise the signal of static fluids (highly T2-weighted) or through the biliary excretion of injected contrast medium (gadolinium BOPTA), MRI enables the acquisition of a panoramic map of the biliary tree and of the pancreatic excretory system (MR cholangiopancreatography) with a diagnostic accuracy very similar to that of endoscopic retrograde cholangiopancreatography (ERCP) [60]. In addition, administration of secretin can improve the visualization and characterization of any endoluminal irregularities [61]. It is also possible to process angiographic sequences (MR angiography), which give information on the relationship between the neoplasm and vessels with 94% diagnostic accuracy in the vascular detection [62].

Computed Tomography

CT is currently the reference method for the staging of pancreatic neoplasms, particularly multidetector CT, because of its excellent spatial resolution, making it a first-quality method [60, 63].

Direct signs of neoplasia are considered: focal alteration of the globular structure, focal volume growth or pancreatic spread, alteration of the profile of the gland, and deformation of the uncinate process. Indirect signs are expansion of the common bile duct, expansion of the duct of Wirsung], atrophy of pancreatic parenchyma above the lesion, and the presence of retention cysts [64].

According to the different kinds of growth (expansive or infiltrative) and to the patterns of contrast enhancement, CT can also indicate the nature of the neoplasm (solid ductal, cystic, neuroendocrine). The peculiar CT characteristic of pancreatic adenocarcinoma is its constant hypodense appearance after contrast administration. This is related to its predominant desmoplastic component [49, 60, 65]. The venous acquisition phase becomes important in the definition of the relationship between the mass with the vascular structures and in the search for secondary hepatic lesions. In the case of suspicious lesions of a neuroendocrine nature it is necessary to perform an early arterial study, since such lesions typically show hypervascularization [66]. Cystic lesions are characterized by a constant hypodensity caused by the presence of a fluid component.

As regards the evaluation of lymph node invasion, CT is not very reliable; the most commonly used criterion is to consider a lymph node pathological when its short axis is longer than 1 cm [67]. The limitation of CT is still that it cannot be used to exclude the presence of micrometastases in lymph nodes of normal size. A 75% specificity has been reported in the detection of metastatic lymph nodes, but only a 24% sensitivity and a positive predictive value of 17% [68].

The liver represents the most common area of pancreatic neoplastic metastasization, and the secondary lesions in general reproduce the characteristics of the primary. In ductal carcinoma they are recognized in the venous acquisition phase and constantly appear hypodense, sometimes umbilical, often with undefined borders, without a capsule, often with a subglissonian area [65]. Secondary lesions of a neuroendocrine nature, on the other hand, typically appear hypervascularized [69]. The diagnostic sensitivity of spiral CT in the individualization of hepatic lesions is very high when the lesions are smaller than 1 cm (as more than 90% of them are); its specificity is lower because of the possibility of false positives [57]. Now MRI with organ-specific contrast media and the contact intraoperative ultrasonography play the role of completing the diagnostic work-up [64]. In the evaluation of peritoneal carcinosis, too, CT has low accuracy: the suspect appearance is often related to the presence of ascites [64].

The evaluation of the invasion of surrounding structures is of fundamental importance to determining the resectability of a tumor. If the duodenal wall and the common bile duct are involved, the neoplasm (T1–T2) is considered to be resectable, while if there is invasion of surrounding organs, vascular infiltration, or infiltration of the retroperitoneal tissue (T3–T4), the tumor is considered to be locally advanced [70–72].

Angiography was the method most used for the evaluation of vascular infiltration in the past; the angiographic classification of vascular involvement proposed by Nakao et al., which distinguished four types of increasingly threatening relationship between the neoplasm and the portal mesenteric venous axle

[73], was related to the histological stage of the vascular infiltration of the wall [64]. At present it is recommended that vascular staging be done by CT instead. Signs suggestive of vascular invasion that can be detected by CT are: the presence of hypodense neoplastic tissue connecting the tumor with the vessel [51]; the presence of a coupling that leads to obliteration of the perivascular adipose cleavage plane (encasement) and which surrounds the tumor for a more or less complete portion of its circumference [74]; caliber reduction or complete obstruction of the vessel; the presence of thrombotic material in the vessel lumen [75].

With the intention of defining a correct CT grading of vascular infiltration, in 1997 Lu et al. proposed a classification in which the relationship of contiguity between the neoplasm and vessel is expressed as follows: grade 0: no contiguity between neoplasm and vessel; grade 1: tumor is adjacent to the vessel, but for less than 25% of its circumference; grade 2: the contiguity between neoplasm and vessel is between 25 and 50%; grade 3: contiguity is between 50 and 75% of the vessel circumference; grade 4: tumor surrounds the vessel for more than 75% of its circumference and causes a reduction of its lumen [76]. According to these authors, the tumor–vessel contiguity is not a sure sign of vascular invasion; the probability of infiltration is very high in grade 3 (88% of the cases), in grade 2 it goes down to 57%, and it is 0% in grade 1. Grade 3 represents the cut-off for resectability of the neoplasm.

Another aspect of great importance for staging purposes is the evaluation of any infiltration of the peripancreatic adipose tissue (T3–T4 tumor), and particularly, in cases of carcinoma of the head and uncinate process, of the retroportal lamina [77]. On CT the signs of possible infiltration are: increased density of the adipose tissue; irregularity of the adipose tissue corresponding to the medial area of the uncinate process; complete obliteration of the adipose tissue itself [57].

Intraoperative Staging

Intraoperative Ultrasonography or Contact Ultrasonography

Intraoperative ultrasonography (IOUS, using high-frequency probes (5–10 MHz) equipped with color Doppler processing with a resolution power up to 2 mm, must be done before every surgical dissection maneuver which can obstruct ultrasound exploration by the interposition of microbubbles of air in the different anatomical dissected levels [64]. Even though the preoperative diagnosis allows a diagnosis of unresectability in over 90% of cases and with an 80% accuracy, routine IOUS should be done to confirm the preoperative reports and to correct possible errors of understaging [64]. Intraoperative ultrasound staging allows evaluation of the same parameters as were examined at preoperative CT: signs of vascular infiltration from the tumor or metastatic lymph nodes and the presence of small underestimated focal hepatic lesions at the transparietal diagnosis [78].

Laparoscopic Staging

Laparoscopic staging can be done before the resection or before a neoadjuvant treatment. Peritoneal metastases and hepatic micrometastases can easily be visualized and confirmed by a video-guided biopsy. It is possible to inspect suspicious lymph nodes like those of the hepatic pedicle. White stated that unresectable disease was identified laparoscopically in 145 of 1045 radiographically resectable patients (14%) [79].

References

1. Yeo CJ (1998) Pancreatic cancer: 1998 Update. Am J Coll Surg; 187:429
2. Cotran RS, Kumar V, Collins T (2000) Robbins: le basi patologiche delle malattie. Piccin Editore, Padova
3. Sohn TA, Yeo CJ, Cameron JL et al (2000) Resected adenocarcinoma of the pancreas – 616 patients: results, outcomes and prognostic indicators. J Gastrointest Surg 4:567
4. Solcia E, Capella C, Kloppel G (1997) Tumor of the pancreas. In: Atlas of Tumor Pathology. Armed Forces Institute of Pathology, Washington DC, USA, p 26
5. Kloppel G, Solcia E, Longnecker DS et al (1998) Histological typing of tumors of the exocrine pancreas. In: WHO, International Histological Classification of Tumors. Springer, Berlin Heidelberg New York, p 24
6. Zamboni G, Capelli P, Pesci A et al (2000) Pancreatic head mass: what can be done? Classification: the pathological point of view. JOP 1:77
7. Li D, Xie K, Wolff R et al (2004) Pancreatic cancer. Lancet 363:1049
8. Kloppel G (1984) Pancreatic, non-endocrine tumors. In: Kloppel G, Heitz PH (eds) Pancreatic pathology. Churchill Livingstone, New York, p 79
9. Takaori K, Hruban RH, Maitra A et al (2006) Current topics on precursors to pancreatic cancer. Adv Med Sci 51:23
10. Takaori K (2007) Current understanding of precursors to pancreatic cancer. J Hepatobiliary Pancreat Surg 14:217
11. Hruban RH, Fukushima N (2007) Pancreatic adenocarcinoma: update on the surgical pathology of carcinomas of ductal origin and PanINs. Mod Pathol 20:61
12. Brat DJ, Lillemoe KD, Yeo CJ et al (1998) Progression of pancreatic intraductal neoplasias to infiltrating adenocarcinoma of the pancreas. Am J Surg Pathol 22:163
13. Wilentz RE, Iacobuzio-Donahue CA, Argani P et al (2000) Loss of expression of Dpc4 in pancreatic intraepithelial neoplasia: evidence that DPC4 inactivation occurs late in neoplastic progression. Cancer Res 60:2002
14. Hruban RH, Adsay NV, Albores-Saavedra J et al (2001) Pancreatic intraepithelial neoplasia: a new nomenclature and classification system for pancreatic duct lesions. Am J Surg Pathos 25:579
15. Bianco AR (2003) Manuale di oncologia clinica. McGraw-Hill, Milan
16. Zhang L, Sanderson SO, Lloyd RV et al (2007) Pancreatic intraepithelial neoplasia in heterotopic pancreas: evidence for the progression model of pancreatic ductal adenocarcinoma. Am J Surg Pathol 31:1191
17. Sanada Y, Yoshida (2007) Immunohistochemical analyses in intraductal gradually transitional components is useful for evaluation of stepwise progression of pancreatic intraepithelial neoplasia. Pancreas 35:101
18. Koorstra JB, Feldmann G, Habbe N et al (2008) Morphogenesis of pancreatic cancer: role of pancreatic intraepithelial neoplasia (PanINs). Langenbecks Arch Surg 393:561
19. Gleave M, Hsieh JT, Gao CA et al (1991) Acceleration of human prostate cancer growth in vivo by factors produced by prostate and bone fibroblasts. Cancer Res 51:375

20. Nakamura T, Matsumoto K, Kiritoshi A et al (1997) Induction of hepatocyte growth factor in fibroblasts by tumor-derived factors affects invasive growth of tumor cells: in vitro analysis of tumor-stromal interactions. Cancer Res 57:3305

21. Janvier R, Sourla A, Koutsilieris M et al (1997) Stromal fibroblasts are required for PC-3 human prostate cancer cells to produce capillary-like formation of endothelial cells in a three-dimensional co-culture system. Anticancer Res 17:1551

22. Anderson IC, Mari SE, Broderick RJ et al (2000) The angiogenic factor interleukin 8 is induced in non-small cell lung cancer/pulmonary fibroblast co-cultures. Cancer Res 60:269

23. Bhowmick NA, Chytil A, Plieth D et al (2004) TGF-beta signaling in fibroblasts modulates the oncogenic potential of adjacent epithelia. Science 303:848

24. De Wever O, Mareel M (2003) Role of tissue stroma in cancer cell invasion. J Pathol 200:429

25. Maehara N, Matsumoto K, Kuba K et al (2001) NK4, a four-kringle antagonist of HGF, inhibits spreading and invasion of human pancreatic cancer cells. Br J Cancer 84:864

26. Kimura W, Kuroda A, Makuuchi M (1998) Problems in the diagnosis and treatment of so-called mucin-producing tumor of the pancreas. Pancreas 16:363

27. Kuba K, Matsumoto K, Date K et al (2000) HGF/NK4, a four-kringle antagonist of hepatocyte growth factor, is an angiogenesis inhibitor that suppresses tumor growth and metastasis in mice. Cancer Res 60:6737

28. Tomioka D, Maehara N, Kuba K et al (2001) Inhibition of growth, invasion, and metastasis of human pancreatic carcinoma cells by NK4 in an orthotopic mouse model. Cancer Res 61:7518

29. Pour PM (1995) The role of Langerhans islets in exocrine pancreatic cancer. Int J Pancreatol 17:217

30. Pour PM, Schmied B (1999) The link between exocrine pancreatic cancer and the endocrine pancreas. Int J Pancreatol 25:77

31. Schmied B, Liu G, Moyer MP et al: Induction of adenocarcinoma from hamster pancreatic islet cells treated with N-nitrosobis(2-oxopropyl)amine in vitro. Carcinogenesis 1999; 20:317

32. Pour PM, Pandey KK, Batra SK (2003) What is the origin of pancreatic adenocarcinoma? Mol Cancer 2:13

33. Hennig R, Ding XZ, Adrian TE (2004) On the role of the islets of Langerhans in pancreatic cancer. Histol Histopathol 19:999

34. Batty GD, Shipley MJ, Marmot MG et al (2004) Diabetes status and post-load glucose concentration in relation to site-specific cancer mortality: findings from the original Whitehall study. Cancer Causes Control 15:873

35. Michaud DS (2004) Epidemiology of pancreatic cancer Minerva Chir 59:99

36. Coughlin SS, Calle EE, Teras LR et al (2004) Diabetes mellitus as a predictor of cancer mortality in a large cohort of US adults. Am J Epidemiol 159:1160

37. Abe R, Donnelly SC, Peng T et al (2001) Peripheral blood fibrocytes: differentiation pathway and migration to wound sites. J Immunol 166:7556

38. Gabbiani G (2003) The myofibroblast in wound healing and. fibrocontractive diseases. J Pathol 200:500

39. Direkze NC, Forbes SJ, Brittan M et al (2003) Multiple organ engraftment by bone-marrow-derived myofibroblasts and fibroblasts in bone-marrow-transplanted mice. Stem Cells 21:514

40. Kalluri R, Neilson EG (2003) Epithelial-mesenchymal transition and its implications for fibrosis. J Clin Investig 112:1776

41. Lieubeau B, Heymann MF, Henry F et al (1999) Immunomodulatory effects of tumor-associated fibroblasts in colorectal-tumor development. Int J Cancer 81:629

42. Ng IO, Lai EC, Ng MM et al (1992) Tumor encapsulation in hepatocellular carcinoma. A pathologic study of 189 cases. Cancer 70:45

43. Koong AC, Mehta VK, Le QT et al (2000) Pancreatic tumors show high levels of hypoxia. Int J Radiat Oncol Biol Phys 48:919

44. Büchler P, Reber HA, Büchler M et al (2003) Hypoxia-inducible factor 1 regulates vascular endothelial growth factor expression in human pancreatic cancer. Pancreas 26:56
45. Mauri P, Scarpa A, Nascimbeni AC et al (2005) Identification of proteins released by pancreatic cancer cells by multidimensional protein identification technology: a strategy for identification of novel cancer markers. FASEB J 19:1125
46. Moniaux N, Chakraborty S, Yalniz M et al (2008) Early diagnosis of pancreatic cancer: neutrophil gelatinase-associated lipocalin as a marker of pancreatic intraepithelial neoplasia. Br J Cancer 98:1540
47. Sobin LH, Wittekind C (2002) TNM classification of malignant tumors. Wiley-Liss, New York
48. Isaji S, Kawarada Y, Uemoto S (2004) Classification of pancreatic cancer. Comparison of Japanese and UICC classifications. Pancreas 28:231
49. Balci NC, Semelka RC (2001) Radiologic diagnosis and staging of pancreatic ductal adenocarcinoma. Eur J Radiol 38:113
50. Furukawa H, Mukai K, Kosugeet T et al (1998) Non functioning islet cell tumors of the pancreas: clinical aspects in 16 patients. Jpn J Clin Oncol 28:255
51. D'Onofrio M, Zamboni G, Malagò R et al (2005) Pancreatic pathology. In: Quaia E (ed) Contrast media in ultrasonography. Springer, Berlin Heidelberg New York, p 335
52. Yeo CJ, Cameron JL (2003) Pancreas esocrino. In: Sabiston (ed) Trattato di Chirurgia. Antonio Delfino Editore, Rome, p 112
53. D'Onofrio M, Mansueto G, Vasori S et al (2003) Contrast enhanced ultrasonographic detection of small pancreatic insulinoma. J Ultrasound Med 22:4413
54. Akahoshi K, Chijiiwa Y, Nakano I et al (1998) Diagnosis and staging of pancreatic cancer by endoscopic ultrasound. Br J Radiol 71:492
55. Rosch T, Dittler HJ, Strobel K et al (2000) Endoscopic ultrasound criteria for vascular invasion in the staging of cancer of the head of the pancreas: a blind reevaluation of videotapes. Gastrointest Endosc 52:469
56. Nishiharu T, Yamashita Y, Abe Y et al (1999) Local extension of pancreatic carcinoma: assessment with thin section helical CT versus breath-hold fast MR imaging-ROC analysis. Radiology 212:445
57. Ragozzino A, Scaglione M (2000) Pancreatic head mass: what can be done? Diagnosis: magnetic resonance imaging. JOP 1:100
58. Schima W, Fugger R Schober E et al (2002) Diagnosis and staging of pancreatic cancer: comparison of mangafodipir trisodium-enhanced MR imaging and contrast-enhanced helical hydro CT. AJR Am J Roentgenol 179:717
59. Di Cesare E, Puglielli E, Nichelini O et al (2003) Malignant obstructive jaundice: comparison of MRCP and ERCP in the evaluation of distal lesions. Radiol Med 105:445
60. McNulty N, Francis I, Platt J et al (2001) Multi-detector row helical CT of the pancreas: effect of contrast-enhanced multiphasic imaging on enhancement of the pancreas, peripancreatic vasculature and pancreatic adenocarcinoma. Radiology 220:97
61. Yoshihiko F, Fumito F, Michiro S et al (2002) Pancreatic duct: morphologic evaluation with MR cholangiopancreatography after secretin stimulation. Radiology 222:674
62. Hänninen E, Amthauer H, Hosten N et al (2002) Prospective evaluation of pancreatic tumors: accuracy of MR imaging with MR cholangiopancreatography and MR angiography. Radiology 224:34
63. Horton KM (2002) Multidetector CT and three dimensional imaging of the pancreas: state of the art. J Gastrointest Surg 6:126
64. Di Candio G, Giulianotti PC (1997) Pancreas: imaging diagnostico e interventistico. Paletto, Milan
65. Boland GW, O'Malley ME, Saez M et al (1999) Pancreatic-phase versus portal vein-phase helical CT of the pancreas: optimal temporal window for evaluation of pancreatic adenocarcinoma. AJR Am J Roentgenol 172:605
66. Tabuchi T, Itoh K, Ohshio G et al (1999) Tumor staging of pancreatic adenocarcinoma using early and latephase helical CT. AJR Am J Roentgenol 173:375

67. Lee JKT, Sagel SS (1998) Computed body tomography with MRI correlation. Lippincott-Raven, Philadelphia

68. Roche C, Hughes M, Garvey CJ et al (2003) CT and pathologic assessment of prospective nodal staging in patients with ductal adenocarcinoma of the head of the pancreas. AJR Am J Roentgenol 180:475

69. Winternitz T, Habib H, Kiss K et al (2000) Pancreatic head mass: what can be done? diagnosis: computed tomography scan. JOP 1:95

70. Scaglione M, Pinto A, Romano S et al (2005) Using multidetector row computer tomography to diagnose and stage pancreatic carcinoma: the problems and possibilities. JOP 6:1

71. Prokesch RW, Chow LC, Beaulieu CF et al (2002) Local staging of pancreatic carcinoma with multi-detector row CT: use of curved planar reformations – initial experience. Radiology 225:759

72. Klauss M, Mohr A, von Tengg-Kobligk H et al (2008) A new invasion score for determining the resectability of pancreatic carcinomas with contrast-enhanced multidetector computed tomography. Pancreatology 23:204

73. Nakao A, Harada A, Nonami T et al (1995) Clinical significance of portal invasion by pancreatic head carcinoma. Surgery 117:50

74. Lepanto L, Arzoumanian Y, Gianfelice D et al (2002) Helical CT with CT angiography in assessing periampullary neoplasm: identification of vascular invasion. Radiology 222:347

75. Loyer EM, David CL, Dubrow RA et al (1996) Vascular involvement in pancreatic adenocarcinoma: reassessment by thin-section CT. Abdom Imaging 21:202

76. Lu DSK, Reber HA, Krasny RM et al (1997) Local staging of pancreatic cancer: criteria for unresectability of major vessels as revealed by pancreatic-phase, thin section helical CT. AJR Am J Roentgenol 168:1439

77. Lüttges J, Vogel I, Menke M et al (1998) The retroperitoneal resection margin and vessel involvement are important factors determining survival after pancreaticoduodenectomy for ductal adenocarcinoma of the head of the pancreas. Virchows Arch 433:237

78. Di Candio G, Giulianotti PC, Pietrabissa A et al: Ecografia intraoperatoria del pancreas. In: Ecografia in chirurgia. Modalità diagnostiche e terapeutiche. Paletto, Milano, 1997

79. White R, Winston C, Gonen M et al (2008) Current utility of staging laparoscopy for pancreatic and peripancreatic neoplasms. J Am Coll Surg 206:445

Chapter 16

Preoperative Staging and Resectability Assessment of Pancreatic Cancer

Roberto Persiani, Alberto Biondi, Marco Zoccali, Domenico D'Ugo

Introduction

Surgical resection is the most important aspect of therapy for pancreatic carcinoma. However, surgery is increasingly considered as a therapeutic option to be combined with other treatments such as chemotherapy and radiotherapy. This is especially true for locally advanced tumors, where surgical treatment alone does not typically result in a satisfactory rate of overall survival. For pancreatic carcinoma, as for other solid tumors, the therapeutic strategy depends on the stage of the disease, and accurate staging is mandatory before starting treatment. In the last 20 years, this strategy has promoted the development of more accurate and sophisticated staging techniques; historically, exploratory laparotomies accounted for up to 50% of the patients considered to be resectable at preoperative staging [1–4], and modern multimodal treatments are diversified regardless of whether the tumor is resectable, locally advanced, or metastatic [5, 6].

Preoperative staging and evaluation of resection has two fundamental purposes:

– *Reduction* of exploratory laparotomy through the identification of patients with nonresectable tumors [7–11]
– *Selection* of patients with locally advanced tumors to undergo neoadjuvant and chemo(radio)therapeutic treatments, while patients with metastatic tumors undergo palliative chemotherapeutic treatments [5, 6]

However, clinical staging through the coding of T-N-M parameters does not always give a clear indication regarding the resectability of tumors in patients with a pancreatic neoplasm. For this purpose, a more reliable tumor staging assessment is the result of various procedures in which the preoperative diagnostic results are combined with surgical exploration (laparoscopic and laparotomic) to establish whether the tumor should be surgically removed (*resectable tumor*), if it is resectable but has a high risk of microscopic or macroscopic residual margins (*borderline resectable tumor*) or, finally, if it is *nonresectable*, because of metastasis or locally advanced disease.

To date, there have been no unequivocal definitions of these three categories, which depend on several elements such as the technical experience of the sur-

geon, the availability of a multidisciplinary staff able to schedule tailored multimodal treatments, and last, though not least, patient compliance. For the above
reasons, the references for resectability criteria should be determined by international guidelines or set by the world's leading centers for pancreatic cancer
care (Tables 16.1 and 16.2) [12, 13].

Table 16.1 Criteria defining resectability status of pancreatic tumors (National
Comprehensive Cancer Network, 2008) [12]

Tumor status	Tumor site	Resectability criteria
Resectable	Head/body/tail	No distant metastases Clear fat plane around celiac and SMA Patent SMV/PV
Borderline resectable	Head/body	Severe unilateral SMV/PV impingement Tumor abutment on SMA GA encasement up to origin at hepatic artery Tumors with limited involvement of the IVC SMV occlusion, if of a short segment, with open vein both proximally and distally (if the proximal SMV were occluded up to the portal vein branches then it would be unresectable) Colon or mesocolon invasion
	Tail	Adrenal, colon or mesocolon, or kidney invasion Preoperative evidence of biopsy-positive common hepatic artery or hepatoduodenal lymph node
Unresectable	Head	Distant metastases (includes celiac and/or para-aortic) SMA, celiac encasement SMV/PV occlusion Aortic, IVC invasion or encasement Invasion of SMV below transverse mesocolon
	Body	Distant metastases (includes celiac and/or para-aortic. Body and tail lesions that have positive celiac and/or para-aortic nodes in close vicinity to the primary may be borderline rather than unresectable) SMA, celiac, hepatic encasement SMV/PV occlusion Aortic invasion
	Tail	Distant metastases (includes celiac and/or para-aortic. Body and tail lesions that have positive celiac and/or para-aortic nodes in close vicinity to the primary may be borderline rather than unresectable) SMA, celiac encasement Rib, vertebral invasion

SMA, Superior mesenteric arteries; *PV*, portal vein; *SMV*, superior mesenteric vein; *GA*, gastroduodenal artery; *IVC*, inferior vena cava

Table 16.2 M. D. Anderson Cancer Center anatomical CT-based criteria for resectability of pancreatic cancer [13]

Vessels	Resectable	Borderline resectable	Locally advanced
SMA	No tumor extension	Tumor abutment <180° (one-half or less) of the circumference of the artery; periarterial stranding and tumor points of contact forming a convexity against the vessel improve chances of resection	Vessel encased (>180°)
Celiac axis/ hepatic artery	No tumor extension	Short-segment encasement/abutment of the common hepatic artery (typically at the gastroduodenal origin); the surgeon should be prepared for vascular resection/ interposition grafting	Vessel(s) encased and no technical option for reconstruction, usually because of tumor extension to the celiac axis/ splenic/ left gastric junction or the celiac origin
SMV/PV	Vessel(s) patent	Short-segment occlusion with suitable vessel above and below; segmental venous occlusion alone without SMA involvement is rare and should be apparent on CT images	Vessel(s) occluded and no technical option for reconstruction

SMA, Superior mesenteric artery; *SMV/PV*, superior mesenteric vein/portal vein; *CT*, computed tomography

This chapter will report reliable data on the accuracy of several recent radiological, endoscopic, and surgical staging procedures introduced into clinical practice in the last 20 years. It will present a diagnostic–therapeutic algorithm that may be considered as a suitable model for the proper preoperative assessment of patients affected by pancreatic tumors.

Clinical Staging

Abdominal Ultrasonography

Ultrasonography, considered the first choice of imaging study before the introduction of computed tomography (CT) [14, 15], currently has a high diagnostic accuracy only in jaundiced patients with a new pancreatic formation more than 3 cm in diameter [16, 17]. However, according to sensitivity data (67–90%) reported by some authors [14–17], ultrasonography is still the first study to perform in cases of suspected pancreatic tumor within diagnostic algorithms [18, 19], because it is noninvasive and inexpensive.

Although ultrasonography has a limited role in the first-stage assessment of a pancreatic tumor, it is strongly recommended for use when searching for hepatic metastases. Sometimes it can even be used as a supplementary methodology and integrated with CT, because of its high negative predictive value (71%). However,, it provides limited visualization of the posterior segments of the liver [14–17].

Finally, color Doppler analysis is recommended by experts for the evaluation of neoplastic vascular infiltration, such as in the celiac axis, the superior mesenteric artery, the common hepatic artery, the gastroduodenal artery, and the splenic artery, with sensitivity and specificity values of 90 and 96%, respectively [20, 21].

Endoscopic Ultrasonography

Endoscopic ultrasonography (EUS) is a diagnostic procedure that combines endoscopy and ultrasonography. It uses an acoustic window to produce extremely detailed anatomical ultrasound images of the wall of the stomach and the duodenum. This mode of imaging was introduced for pancreatic carcinomas at the end of the 1980s [22]. In most reports published to date, EUS yields sensitivity and positive predictive values equal to or even higher than 90% [4, 23–28], revealing itself as superior to CT and MRI in the study of lesions of less than 3 cm diameter [29, 30].

As a staging technique, EUS provides increased accuracy in the evaluation of early-stage tumor progression (74–95%) and of lymph node involvement (74–87%) [4, 18, 19, 23–28]. Above all, in terms of predicting resectability, EUS is the most accurate method for the assessment of portal vein infiltration (sensitivity 81%, specificity 86%); however, it has poor accuracy in the evaluation of arterial involvement (sensitivity 17%, specificity 67%) [31] (Fig. 16.1). In general, EUS allows the resectability of a pancreatic neoplasm to be estimated with an overall accuracy of 80%, for which a curative (R0) resection rate of up to 78% is correlated with a strong improvement in therapeutic results [4, 18, 19, 31–34].

An important drawback of this endoscopic procedure is its low specificity (70%) in differentiating pancreatic cancer from mass-forming chronic pancreatitis [35]. However, EUS-guided fine needle aspiration (EUS-FNA) seems to overcome this limitation [36] and is a valid tool for diagnostic work-up. It provides histological or cytopathological assessment of the main lesion as well as the peripancreatic lymph nodes. This method can be practiced with low complication rates (1.9%). Conversely, ultrasound -or CT-guided percutaneous needle aspiration produces poor results for small lesions, and also expose the patient to a hypothetical risk of neoplastic dissemination along the line of penetration of the needle [37]. The overall accuracy of EUS-FNA in ruling out a diagnosis of pancreatic cancer is 88%, with a reported sensitivity of 73–90%, specificity of 94–100%, positive predictive value of 100%, and negative predictive value of 86%, as reported in the literature [37, 38].

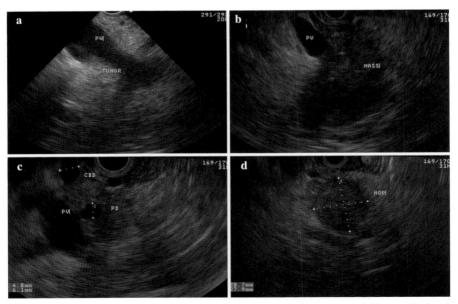

Fig. 16.1 Endoscopic ultrasonography. **a, b** Portal vein infiltration. **c, d** Pancreatic head tumor (*HOP*) with dilation of the common bile duct (*CBD*) and main pancreatic duct (*PD*). The ultrasonographic pattern of the tumor appears mixed, and more hypoechoic than the pancreatic gland

Computed Tomography

CT, and in particular spiral CT, is a more commonly used imaging technique for the diagnosis and staging of pancreatic carcinoma. The development of spiral CT is an important technological evolution for conventional CT and is currently considered to be the "gold standard" in the diagnosis and preoperative evaluation of pancreatic tumors [4, 39–42]. Compared to standard CT, the introduction of spiral CT has led to a remarkable improvement in the study of early-stage tumors and the assessment of local vascular invasion (portal vein, celiac axis, and mesenteric vein and artery), with a positive predictive value of 100%, a negative predictive value of 56%, and an overall accuracy of 70% [3, 40–43].

Further technological evolution of spiral CT has occurred with the development of multidetector CT (MDCT), in which different transducers are used at the same time. Each transducer has a different orientation and acquires the same number of projections, which are subsequently integrated and processed using a computer [44, 45], leading to multiplanar reconstructions of images which are of great benefit not only for tumor studies, but also for studies of veins and arteries. Moreover, MDCT has a sensitivity of 75% and a specificity of 100% in the diagnosis of small pancreatic masses (<2 cm) [46], and in larger tumors it is able to define the involvement of the vascular wall as greater than (so-called tumor encasement) or less than (tumor abutment) 50% of the circumference of the vessel, with a sensitivity and specificity of over 90% [47–49] (Fig. 16.2).

However, although MDCT is useful for evaluating resectability, it is not able to provide a global and accurate staging of disease. Staging of lymph node involvement relies on the morphological evaluation of lymph nodes (volume enlargement, irregular shape, lack of peri-lymph-node adipose tissue, peri-lymph-node and central necrosis). The accuracy of these parameters has not been fully proven yet [50]. Moreover, for metastatic disease, several studies have shown that almost 20% of all tumors initially thought to be resectable on the basis of CT were found to be unresectable at the time of surgical exploration (laparoscopic or laparotomic) [18, 19, 51].

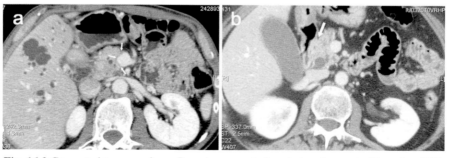

Fig. 16.2 Computed tomography. **a** Superior mesenteric vein involvement of less than 50% of the circumference: tumor abutment (*arrows*); **b** duodenal infiltration (*arrow*)

Abdominal Magnetic Resonance Imaging

Until the 1990s, magnetic resonance imaging (MRI) was considered an optional imaging technique and had not yet replaced the CT scan in the routine work-up for pancreatic cancer diagnosis.

For a diagnosis of pancreatic cancer, MR is mostly suitable after CT has proved nondiagnostic or in the event of patient allergy to the contrast medium. Since the introduction of new techniques for image acquisition (turbo spin-echo sequence, gradient echo, inversion recovery), the use of this imaging mode has increased [52–55]. All of these improvements have been shown to reduce acquisition times and motion artifacts from respiration.

With the availability of paramagnetic contrast media (gadolinium-DTPA) that have a pharmacokinetic distribution pattern analogous to the iodine solution used for CT, MRI achieves a sensitivity equal to that of spiral CT in the identification of small pancreatic tumors. Moreover, the high resolution of soft-tissue contrast between the pancreatic gland and the surrounding adipose tissue leads to a superior diagnostic accuracy to that of CT in the evaluation of peripancreatic infiltration and vascular involvement (MR angiography) [56].

As concerns lymph node involvement, MRI does not overcome the limitations of CT, mostly because it is based on morphological criteria; that is to say, upon nonsignificant values of sensitivity [57] (Fig. 16.3).

When evaluating the "M" parameter, MR offers a sensitivity equal to that of spiral CT, although it is considered by many authors to be useful for the characterization of doubtful hepatic lesions, mostly after the introduction of a liver-specific contrast medium that is exclusively taken up by hepatocytes or by cells of the reticuloendothelial system of the liver and not by neoplastic tissue [56].

Magnetic Resonance Cholangiopancreatography

Since 1991 [58, 59], magnetic resonance cholangiopancreatography (MRCP) has been fully used for the diagnosis of biliary tract and pancreatic diseases, and for this reason it has become a direct part of the preoperative staging of pancreatic cancer.

MRCP is a noninvasive diagnostic method (it does not use any contrast medium) which studies the biliopancreatic system even when it is inaccessible to endoscopic retrograde cholangiopancreatography (ERCP). MRCP offers detailed images of the pancreaticobiliary tract, and suppresses the visibility of adipose tissue using sophisticated acquisition sequences [58, 59]. This method, in the case of pancreatic neoplasms, can emphasize the expansion of the intrahepatic biliary tree, the confluence of the liver duct, common bile duct, and duct of Wirsung (the "double duct sign"), and detects both the level of obstruction and morphological peculiarities of the obstruction itself [58, 59] (Fig. 16.3).

It has been proved that cholangiopancreatographic images obtained by MR always provide a good comparison both with transhepatic transcutaneous

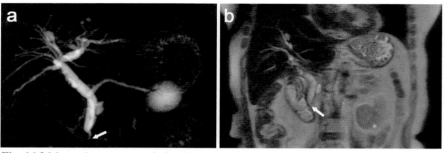

Fig. 16.3 Magnetic resonance cholangiopancreatography (**a**) and abdominal magnetic resonance imaging (**b**). The common bile duct is interrupted by a pancreatic mass, which is visible

cholangiography and with ERCP. These methods are considered the "gold standards" of reference for the study of the pancreaticobiliary duct system, in terms of image quality as well as anatomical definition [60, 61].

Endoscopic Retrograde Cholangiopancreatography

ERCP, introduced into clinical use for the first time in 1958 [62], is a combined endoscopic and fluoroscopic technique that uses a side-viewing duodenoscope in the second portion of the duodenum, which aids the incannulation of the ampulla of Vater. Contrast medium is injected into the bile ducts and/or the biliary pancreatic duct through the probe. At this point, fluoroscopy allows visualization of the two ducts, the cystic duct, the gallbladder, and the intrahepatic biliary system [63].

ERCP may be particularly helpful for evaluating patients with obstructive jaundice without a detectable mass by CT or MRI. It can identify nonmalignant causes of obstructive jaundice, define the location of the bile duct obstruction, identify ampullary and periampullary lesions, and establish the diagnosis of intraductal papillary mucinous neoplasm (IPMN) if mucus is seen extruding through a fish-mouth papillary opening. Observations of superimposable bile duct and pancreatic duct strictures (i.e., "double duct sign") by ERCP are highly suggestive of pancreatic head cancer [64].

However, the role of ERCP in the management of patients with a mass observed by CT is more controversial. Many authors think that ERCP is not a useful procedure for staging pancreatic carcinoma, and that it therefore has limited value in the assessment of resectability [63–66].

The future of ERCP is in its therapeutic forms for palliation of biliary obstruction of malignancy, although the outcomes of surgical bypass and stent placement by ERCP are similar. More major complications are associated with surgery, but recurrent jaundice due to stent occlusion can occur with ERCP.

Preoperative stent placement is associated with more overall complications than surgery alone and does not appear to improve the surgical outcome [64–67].

Positron Emission Tomography

Positron emission tomography (PET) was applied for the first time to diagnosing pancreatic cancer in 1990 [68]. The use of this scintigraphic method was introduced because of the insufficient reliability of the diagnostic methods used up until then to locate small pancreatic tumors and to detect small, distant metastases [68–70].

PET is a not an invasive exam and has a high sensitivity in searching for distant metastases in many neoplasms. It usually uses a radiolabeled compound (18-fluorodeoxyglucose, ^{18}FDG) which is taken up by neoplastic tissues (which rapidly metabolize glucose) when injected, thus allowing the location of neoplastic tissue to be visualized through a gamma camera.

In the literature, the sensitivity and the specificity of PET for the diagnosis of pancreatic neoplasms, with wide oscillations, are as follows: sensitivity 71–92%, specificity 64–94% [69–71]. The variability is mostly due to a high number of false negatives, especially in diabetic patients (diabetes is often associated with pancreatic carcinoma), and poor specificity in differentiating neoplastic disease from inflammatory disease. Considering these issues, together with the increased costs, the PET scan currently does not have a defined role in the diagnosis and staging of patients affected with pancreatic carcinoma [72–74].

Laparoscopic Staging

Laparoscopy, which was introduced into clinical use in 1911 by Bernheim [75], has assumed a large role in the staging of many abdominal neoplasms, including pancreatic carcinomas. Due to the work of Cuschieri and his colleagues in 1978 [76], laparoscopy became a valid method for the identification of peritoneal and hepatic metastases whose clinical staging was unknown. In combination with laparoscopic ultrasonography (LUS), this method of evaluating the potential for resective surgery of abdominal neoplasms [51, 77] has helped to achieve a remarkable reduction in exploratory laparotomies [5, 77].

In the published literature, the diagnostic accuracy in assessing the resectability of early-stage tumors is up to 90%, and at specialized institutes with the addition of LUS the procedure can achieve up to 98% accuracy [77].

According to these data, laparoscopic staging should be used on a routine basis, but at the moment the role of this method remains controversial. Recent studies have suggested that the routine employment of staging laparoscopy does not affect the management of the majority of patients and also is not cost-effective. Conversely, selective use of laparoscopy is recommended for patients whose preoperative staging is uncertain or highly predictive of a nonresectable tumor. In fact, an emerging indication for staging laparoscopy occurs in patients with locally advanced pancreatic cancer and no evidence of distant disease who are being considered for chemoradiation. In this subgroup of patients, staging laparoscopy may effectively identify up to 37% of patients with imaging-occult stage IV disease [5, 6, 51, 77, 78], as well as prevent the morbidity and cost associated with unnecessary treatment [5].

Surgical Technique

From a technical point of view, we refer to the staging laparoscopy procedure described by Conlon et al. in 1996 and in 1998 [7, 79], which includes an extended multiport laparoscopy and uses, in addition to the periumbilical trocar of Hasson and three other trocars, two 10-mm trocars in the left hypochondrium and right side, and one 5-mm trocar in the right hypochondrium.

The first step in laparoscopic exploration, as for other gastrointestinal neoplasms, aims to evaluate the "M" parameter through the study of peritoneal carcinomatosis and/or hepatic metastases. The second aim is to visualize lymph node involvement ("N" parameter), and finally, to evaluate the degree of tumor infiltration ("T" parameter).

Before any manipulation of the viscera in the presence of ascitic fluid, a peritoneal fluid sample is taken to be sent for immediate and definitive cytological study. In the absence of ascitic fluid, samples can be obtained from peritoneal washing with approximately 200 ml of physiological solution and successive aspiration from the pelvis via Morison's pouch and the splenic lodge. A number of studies have addressed the role of peritoneal washing in the staging of pancreatic cancer patients, because patients with positive peritoneal cytology have similar outcomes to patients with metastatic disease. This is reflected in the sixth edition of The American Joint Commission on Cancer (AJCC) Cancer Staging Manual, which designates positive peritoneal cytology as M1 disease.

Although malignant cells can be identified in 3–53% of peritoneal washing samples from patients with pancreatic cancer [77], the clinical significance of their presence has yet to be determined. Earlier studies have suggested that positive peritoneal cytology may be a marker of advanced disease, predictive of early metastasis and shortened survival, and should therefore be considered a contraindication to attempts at curative resection [80, 81]. In contrast to this, several authors have found no correlation between positive peritoneal cytology and the postoperative development of peritoneal metastasis [82–84]. Consequently, these investigators claim that this parameter is not a contraindication to radical surgery in the absence of macroscopic peritoneal metastasis.

We must therefore proceed to completely explore the supramesocolic and submesocolic peritoneal walls, using the slope of the operating table to search for peritoneal carcinomatosis implants in order to perform a biopsy (Fig. 16.4). During this exploration, the presence of subglissonian hepatic metastasis (Fig.

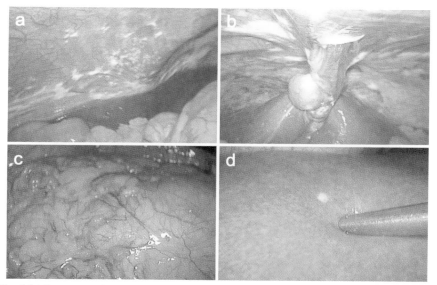

Fig. 16.4 Laparoscopic staging: **a** peritoneal carcinomatosis and malignant ascites; **b** peritoneal carcinomatosis implant along falciform ligament; **c** omental carcinomatosis; **d** small subglissonian metastasis of left liver lobe

16.4) is also evaluated. In this case, it is necessary to make an incision in the lesser omentum to expose the caudal lobe.

To evaluate the "M" parameter, we may use a LUS to explore the hepatic parenchyma. The ultrasound probe is generally inserted through the periumbilical trocar and the optical probe through the trocar in the left hypochondrium. The insertion of the instruments can also be done the other way around, inserting the probe for the LUS through the trocar in the left hypochondrium, or, if it is possible, inserting a third trocar in the right hypochondrium.

There are two methods used for hepatic laparoscopic ultrasound exploration: geographical and systematic. In the first, ultrasonography is performed with a medial-to-lateral movement from the falciform ligament to the right and left hepatic margins. Starting from the dome of the liver and drawing back from time to time, the ultrasound probe covers the entire surface of the organ. In the second method, the scanning follows Couinaud segments to reveal the suprahepatic veins and the portal segment peduncles [85]. During this phase, in cases where there are suspicious lesions, biopsy of the lesion can always be performed under ultrasound guidance. The ultrasound and laparoscopic images are viewed simultaneously using standard video-mixing electronics (Fig. 16.5).

To evaluate the "N" parameter, identification of the hilum of the liver, the foramen of Winslow, and the hepatoduodenal ligament is needed, and periportal lymph nodes are biopsied if required. In addition, the Kocher maneuver can be useful in pancreatic head neoplasms in order to visualize retropancreatic lym-

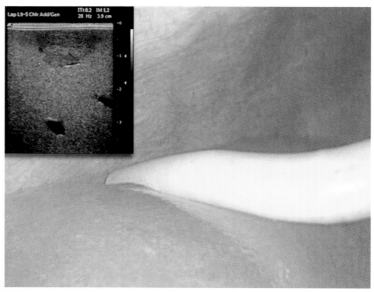

Fig. 16.5 Laparoscopic ultrasonography. A suspected liver metastasis is evaluated

phadenopathy. Subsequently, lesser sac endoscopy [86] is performed to visualize lymph node stations in the celiac trunk, left gastric artery, and splenic and common hepatic arteries.

The staging of the "T" parameter consists of evaluating the dimensions of the neoplasm, its fixation, and its relationship with close structures. With the operating table in the Trendelenburg position and moving the omentum toward the left superior quadrant, it is possible to identify the ligament of Treitz and to inspect the transverse mesocolon and middle colic vein, which is usually easily visible. In addition, vascular involvement can be carefully evaluated by LUS as well as color Doppler imaging. The probe can be introduced through one of the two lateral 10-mm trocars or through the periumbilical trocar, at the best angle possible, to scan and evaluate a specific vascular district. In particular, the course of the portal vein up to the confluence with the superior mesenteric vein is evaluated, introducing the probe through the left trocar and transversely for the hepatoduodenal ligament. During this phase, the hepatic artery, the extrahepatic biliary tree, and the back of the cava are also visualized. Subsequently, introducing the probe through the periumbilical trocar transversely with respect to the gastrocolic ligament, a sagittal scan of the superior mesenteric artery and vein can be obtained. The superior mesenteric artery, from the aorta origin and the mesenteric vein, are thus visualized up to the confluence with the portal vein.

Finally, the neoplasm and the pancreatic gland can be directly scanned in order to investigate multifocal lesions.

Laparotomic Exploration

Laparotomic exploration resolves any doubt regarding the resectability of pancreatic cancer. As the first step in any operation upon pancreatic tumors, surgical exploration aims to estimate whether it is technically possible to remove the tumor mass.

The surgical exploration is performed in a centripetal way, moving gradually towards the primary lesion. The liver and peritoneal surfaces are examined for unexpected extrapancreatic metastases. Intraoperative ultrasonography of the liver and regional lymph nodes may be used selectively when findings are suspicious, yet indeterminate by palpation. Routine biopsy of apparently normal lymph nodes is unnecessary, but suspect lesions and enlarged lymph nodes outside the planned field of dissection should be biopsied and examined by frozen section [87].

Surgical Technique

The steps of laparotomic exploration are as follows [87]:

- Palpation and visualization of the diaphragmatic domes, peritoneum, bowel, mesenteries, and pouch of Douglas, looking for peritoneal carcinomatosis implants.
- Exploration of the liver surface, searching for small subglissonian metastases, if necessary with the aid of intraoperative ultrasonography.
- Exploration of the celiac region through the gastrohepatic ligament. By holding the caudate lobe with a liver retractor, it is possible to search for enlarged interaortocaval and celiac axis lymph nodes. The hepatic pedicle is palpated by the thumb and the forefinger of the left hand, and the latter is then inserted in the foramen of Winslow. Thereafter, dissection of the first portion of the jejunum permits palpation of the superior mesenteric artery, allowing for further investigation of suspect lymph nodes.
- Finally, a closer exploration of the pancreatic gland and the primary lesion is performed in order to evaluate resectability. An important step is to lift the transverse colon in order to expose the mesenteric root, near the uncinate process. The presence of infiltration at the base of the mesocolon could indicate unresectability [87].

The following step allows dissection of the greater omentum with mobilization in particular of the right colic flexure, which permits excellent exposure of the anterior side of the entire pancreatic gland and evaluation of possible anterior extracapsular involvement. The access to the lesser sac allows exploration of the superior surface of the transverse mesocolon, mesenteric lymph nodes, and isthmus and body of the gland itself.

The next step is a wide dissection of the duodenum and head of the pancreas by the Kocher maneuver, up to the level of the right side of the aorta (Fig. 16.6a). In this phase, exposure of the aorta and vena cava allows the sampling of suspected lymph nodes that, if metastatic, compromise the possibility of radical resection. Once the head of the pancreas is mobilized and gently handled between the fingers of one hand, it is possible to evaluate the distance between the tumor and the isthmus. At this stage, it is possible to define the line of section of the pancreas, or to discover neoplastic infiltration of the retroportal tissue or the origin of the superior mesenteric artery, which would lead to a high risk of microscopic residue upon excision [87].

The last step of surgical exploration aims to evaluate the cleavage between the anterior wall of the mesenteric–portal axis and the posterior aspect of the pancreatic gland. This maneuver begins with exposure of the superior mesenteric vein, which is easily identifiable in the mesenteric root, just to the right of the superior mesenteric artery or following the middle colic vein. The portal vein is then identified above the pancreatic neck. The anterior surface of the vein is separated by blunt dissection from the pancreas, creating a tunnel behind the pancreatic neck, where a tape is passed (Fig. 16.6b) [87].

This exploration will reveal one of four different scenarios:

1. *The lesion is limited to the pancreas*, involving at least the near lymph nodes: curative resection is possible.
2. *Limited vascular (venous and or arterial) infiltration is present*, but curative resection is still possible through vascular reconstruction.
3. *Widespread vascular infiltration is present*: the neoplasm is unresectable.
4. *Distant metastasis is present* (peritoneal carcinosis, hepatic metastasis, metastatic lymph nodes of the celiac trunk, intercavoaortic lymph nodes): the tumor is unresectable.

For the above reasons, it may be stated that widespread neoplastic involvement of the mesenteric vessels and distant metastases contraindicate any attempt at resection. There is more debate as to the most appropriate choice of therapeu-

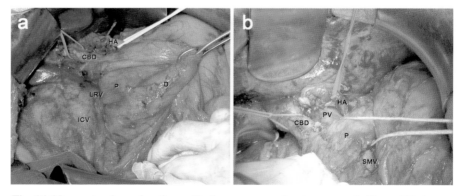

Fig. 16.6 Laparotomic exploration: **a** Kocher maneuver, **b** retropancreatic "tunnel" between the anterior surface of the portal–mesenteric vein and the pancreas (a surgical tape was passed). *ICV* inferior caval vein, *LRV* left renal vein, *CBD,* common bile duct; *HA,* hepatic artery; *P*, pancreas; *D*, duodenum; *PV,* portal vein; *SMV,* superior mesenteric vein

tic procedure when the tumor shows limited vascular infiltration, or when the tumor involves structures outside the field of the planned dissection [12, 13].

Conclusions

Pancreatic cancer is rarely diagnosed at an early stage; two-thirds of patients have locally advanced or metastatic disease at the time of diagnosis. At the present time, accurate staging represents, without a doubt, one of the primary objectives to be pursued in the treatment of this disease. The choice of the best therapeutic strategy is, in fact, strictly dependent upon accurate preoperative staging and evaluation of resectability.

An accurate and reliable preoperative evaluation is not provided by the imaging techniques that are currently available. In fact, no single radiological, endoscopic, or surgical method exists that is capable of precisely defining all three parameters ("T," "N," and "M"). In addition, there is no homogeneous and universally recognized definition of resectability criteria. Distant metastases and infiltration of the celiac–mesenteric arterial axis represent absolute contraindications for the removal of tumor masses, but involvement of the mesenteric–portal venous axis and lymphatic spread are not universally recognized as criteria for unresectability. Progress in surgical techniques and technological innovations have led some authors to perform en-bloc vascular resection for locally advanced tumors and extended lymph node dissection [12, 13]. Moreover, multidisciplinary treatments (adjuvant, neoadjuvant chemoradiotherapy) are now available for pancreatic cancer, and may offer more advantages in terms of survival when used appropriately [88]. The aim of current clinical research is to elucidate diagnostic–therapeutic algorithms that are able to avoid unnecessary treatments, and also to direct the patient towards so-called *stage-adapted* treatment [89–91].

MDCT, in association with EUS, appears to be the first step in investigations of clinical staging for pancreatic cancer. These two imaging techniques are at the present time considered the "gold standard" for conventional staging of pancreatic carcinomas, which aims to class tumors into one of four categories: resectable tumor, borderline resectable tumor, locally advanced tumor, and metastatic tumor [4]. ERCP has a therapeutic role in treating cases of obstructive jaundice complicated by sepsis. MRI, in conjunction with MRCP and PET/CT, is an optional procedure after initial staging [18].

Staging laparoscopy has a key role in the algorithm, as it relates to the treatment of patients affected by tumors clinically considered to be unresectable and nonmetastatic. These patients make up about 40% of all pancreatic cancer patients, and are the largest diagnostic group. Since surgical palliation (gastroenteroanastomosis and hepaticojejunostomy) has become obsolete in favor of more conservative endoscopic and radiological treatments, integrated radiochemotherapy is now the treatment of choice for these patients. Laparoscopy in these cases allows recognition of metastatic disease that is occult to imaging, thus avoiding unnecessary and harmful treatment. In well-selected patients, these treatments appear to improve survival and, if applied with a neoadjuvant purpose, may offer the chance for delayed curative resection when tumors are downstaged by treatment, with an outcome equal to that of patients with localized disease [77].

The routine use of laparoscopy for patients judged to have resectable tumors after conventional staging (resectable neoplasms and borderline resectable neoplasms) is more debatable. From the published literature, 10–36% of these patients are excluded from surgery after laparoscopic staging, although in these studies clinical staging did not involve MDCT and EUS. Furthermore, in these studies, LUS and peritoneal cytology were used during laparoscopy, which improve the accuracy of the procedure but also make it very expensive [77].

According to these considerations, an *evidence-based diagnostic–therapeutic algorithm* should be made, which would ideally be considered reliable and accurate for the preoperative study of pancreatic carcinomas (Fig. 16.7).

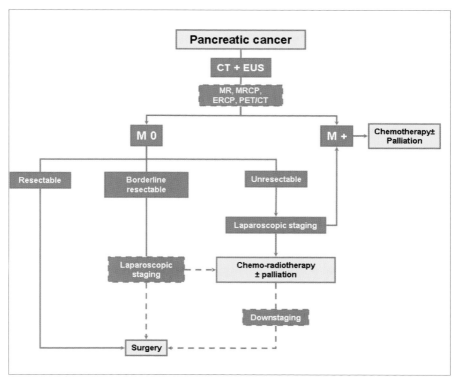

Fig. 16.7 Diagnostic–therapeutic algorithm. *Broken lines* show procedures not routinely used

References

1. Yeo CJ, Cameron JL (1999) Improving results of pancreaticoduodenectomy for pancreatic cancer. World J Surg 23:907–912
2. Parker SL, Tong T, Bolden S et al (1996) Cancer statistics, 1996. CA Cancer J Clin 46:5–27
3. Kalra MK, Maher MM, Mueller PR et al (2003) State-of-the-art imaging of pancreatic neoplasms. Br J Radiol 76:857–865
4. Soriano A, Castells A, Ayuso C et al (2004) Preoperative staging and tumor resectability assessment of pancreatic cancer: prospective study comparing endoscopic ultrasonography, helical computed tomography, magnetic resonance imaging, and angiography. Am J Gastroenterol 99:492–501
5. Liu RC, Traverso LW (2005) Diagnostic laparoscopy improves staging of pancreatic cancer deemed locally unresectable by computed tomography. Surg Endosc 19:638–642
6. Shoup M, Winston C, Brennan MF et al (2004) Is there a role for staging laparoscopy in patients with locally advanced, unresectable pancreatic adenocarcinoma? J Gastrointest Surg 8:1068–1071
7. Minnard EA, Conlon KC, Hoos A et al (1998) Laparoscopic ultrasound enhances standard laparoscopy in the staging of pancreatic cancer. Ann Surg 228:182–187
8. Merchant NB, Conlon KC (1998) Laparoscopic evaluation in pancreatic cancer. Semin Surg Oncol 15:155–165
9. Cuschieri A, Hall AW, Clark J (1978) Value of laparoscopy in the diagnosis and management of pancreatic carcinoma. Gut 19:672–677
10. Nieveen van Dijkum EJ, Romijn MG, Terwee CB et al (2003) Laparoscopic staging and subsequent palliation in patients with peripancreatic carcinoma. Ann Surg 237:66–73
11. Katz MH, Hwang R, Fleming JB et al (2008) Tumor-node-metastasis staging of pancreatic adenocarcinoma. CA Cancer J Clin 58:111–125
12. National Comprehensive Cancer Network (2008) NCCN practice guidelines for pancreatic cancer. Available at: http://www.nccn.org. Accessed May 2008
13. Varadhachary GR, Tamm EP, Abbruzzese JL et al (2006) Borderline resectable pancreatic cancer: definitions, management, and role of preoperative therapy. Ann Surg Oncol 13:1035–1046
14. Lawson TL (1978) Sensitivity of pancreatic ultrasonography in the detection of pancreatic disease. Radiology 128:733–736
15. Taylor KJW, Buchin PJ, Viscomi GN et al (1981) Ultrasonographic scanning of the pancreas. Radiology 138:211–213
16. Pasanen PA, Partanen KP, Pikkarainen PH et al (1993) A comparison of ultrasound, computed tomography and endoscopic retrograde cholangiopancreatography in the differential diagnosis of benign and malignant jaundice and cholestasis. Eur J Surg 159:23–29
17. Karlson BM, Ekbom A, Lindgren PG et al (1999) Abdominal US for diagnosis of pancreatic tumor: prospective cohort analysis. Radiology 213:107–111
18. Michl P, Pauls S, Gress TM (2006) Evidence-based diagnosis and staging of pancreatic cancer. Best Pract Res Clin Gastroenterol 20:227–251
19. Clarke DL, Thomson SR, Madiba TE et al (2003) Preoperative imaging of pancreatic cancer: a management-oriented approach. J Am Coll Surg 196:119–129
20. Tomiyama T, Ueno N, Tano S et al (1996) Assessment of arterial invasion in pancreatic cancer using color Doppler ultrasonography. Am J Gastroenterol 91:1410–1416
21. Morrin MM, Kruskal JB, Raptopoulos V et al (2001) State-of-the-art ultrasonography is as accurate as helical computed tomography and computed tomographic angiography for detecting unresectable periampullary cancer. J Ultrasound Med 20:481–490
22. Rosch T, Lightdale CJ, Botet JF et al (1992) Localization of pancreatic endocrine tumors by endoscopic ultrasonography. N Engl J Med 326:1721–1726
23. Yasuda K, Mukai H, Nakajima M (1995) Endoscopic ultrasonography diagnosis of pancreatic cancer. Gastrointest Endosc Clin N Am 5:699–712

24. Hunt GC, Faigel DO (2002) Assessment of EUS for diagnosing, staging, and determining resectability of pancreatic cancer: a review. Gastrointest Endosc 55:232–237
25. Kulig J, Popiela T, Zajac A et al (2005) The value of imaging techniques in the staging of pancreatic cancer. Surg Endosc 19:361–365
26. Buscail L, Pages P, Berthelemy P et al (1999) Role of EUS in the management of pancreatic and ampullary carcinoma: a prospective study assessing resectability and prognosis. Gastrointest Endosc 50:34–40
27. Ahmad NA, Lewis JD, Ginsberg GG et al (2000) EUS in preoperative staging of pancreatic cancer. Gastrointest Endosc 52:463–468
28. Akahoshi K, Chijiiwa Y, Nakano I et al (1998) Diagnosis and staging of pancreatic cancer by endoscopic ultrasound. Br J Radiol 71:492–496
29. Rosch T, Braig C, Gain T et al (1992) Staging of pancreatic and ampullary carcinoma by endoscopic ultrasonography. Comparison with conventional sonography, computed tomography, and angiography. Gastroenterology 102:188–199
30. Muller MF, Meyenberger C, Bertschinger P et al (1994) Pancreatic tumors: evaluation with endoscopic US, CT and MR imaging. Radiology 190:745–751
31. Midwinter MJ, Beveridge CJ, Wilsdon JB et al (1999) Correlation between spiral comuted tomography, endoscopic ultrasonography and findings at operation in pancreatic and ampullary tumours. Br J Surg 86:189–193
32. Brugge WR, Lee MJ, Kelsey PB et al (1996) The use of EUS to diagnose malignant portal venous system invasion by pancreatic cancer. Gastrointest Endosc 43:561–567
33. Aslanian H, Salem R, Lee J et al (2005) EUS diagnosis of vascular invasion in pancreatic cancer: surgical and histologic correlates. Am J Gastroenterol 100:1381–1385
34. Sahani DV, Shah ZK, Catalano OA et al (2008) Radiology of pancreatic adenocarcinoma: current status of imaging. J Gastroenterol Hepatol 23:23–33
35. Rösch T, Lorenz R, Braig C et al (1991) Endoscopic ultrasound in pancreatic tumor diagnosis. Gastrointest Endosc 37:347–352
36. Grimm H, Binmoeller KF, Soehendra N (1992) Endosonography-guided drainage of a pancreatic pseudocyst. Gastrointest Endosc 38:170–171
37. Erickson RA (2004) EUS-guided FNA. Gastrointest Endosc 60:267–279
38. Wiersema MJ, Vilmann P, Giovannini M et al (1997) Endosonography-guided fine-needle aspiration biopsy: diagnostic accuracy and complication assessment. Gastroenterology 112:1087–1095
39. Dupuy DE, Costello P, Ecker CP (1992) Spiral CT of the pancreas. Radiology 183:815–818
40. Taoka H, Hauptmann E, Traverso LW et al (1999) How accurate is helical computed tomography for clinical staging of pancreatic cancer? Am J Surg 177:428–432
41. Bluemke DA, Cameron JL, Hruban RH et al (1995) Potentially resectable pancreatic adenocarcinoma: spiral CT assessment with surgical and pathologic correlation. Radiology 197:381–385
42. Phoa SSKS, Reeders JWAJ, Rauws EAJ (1999) Spiral computed tomography for preoperative staging of potentially resectable carcinoma of the pancreatic head. Br J Surg 86:789–794
43. Vendenthan S, LU DSK, Reber HA et al (1998) Small peripancreatic veins; improved assessment in pancreatic cancer patients using thin section pancreatic phase helical CT. AJR Am J Roentgenol 170:377–383
44. Horton KM, Fishman EK (2000) 3D CT angiography of the celiac and superior mesenteric arteries with multidetector CT data sets: preliminary observations. Abdom Imaging 25:523–525
45. Fishman EK, Horton KM, Urban BA (2000) Multidetector CT angiography in the evaluation of pancreatic carcinoma: preliminary observations. J Comput Assist Tomogr 24:849–853
46. Bronstein YL, Loyer EM, Kaur H et al (2004) Detection of small pancreatic tumors with multiphasic helical CT. Am J Roentgenol 182:619–623
47. Li H, Zeng MS, Zhou KR et al (2005) Pancreatic adenocarcinoma: the different CT criteria

for peripancreatic major arterial and venous invasion. J Comput Assist Tomogr 29:170–175

48. Prokesch RW, Chow LC, Beaulieu CF et al (2002) Local staging of pancreatic carcinoma with multi-detector row CT: use of curved planar reformations – initial experience. Radiology 225:759–765

49. Furukawa H, Uesaka K, Boku N (2008) Treatment decision making in pancreatic adenocarcinoma: multidisciplinary team discussion with multidetector-row computed tomography. Arch Surg 143:275–280

50. Roche CJ, Hughes ML, Garvey CJ et al (2003) CT and pathologic assessment of prospective nodal staging in patients with ductal adenocarcinoma of the head of the pancreas. AJR Am J Roentgenol 180:475–480

51. Pisters PW, Lee JE, Vauthey JN et al (2001) Laparoscopy in the staging of pancreatic cancer. Br J Surg 88:325–337

52. Megibow AJ, Zhou XH, Rotterdam H et al (1995) Pancreatic adenocarcinoma: CT versus MR imaging in the evaluation of resectability: report of the radiology diagnostic oncology group. Radiology 195:327–332

53. Ichikawa T, Haradome H, Hachiya J et al (1997) Pancreatic ductal adenocarcinoma: preoperative assessment with helical CT versus dynamic MR imaging. Radiology 202:655–662

54. Semelka RC, Ascher SM (1993) MR imaging of the pancreas. Radiology 188:593–602

55. Saisho H, Yamaguchi T (2004) Diagnostic imaging for pancreatic cancer: computed tomography, magnetic resonance imaging, and positron emission tomography. Pancreas 28:273–278

56. Pamuklar E, Semelka RC (2005) MR imaging of the pancreas. Magn Reson Imaging Clin N Am 13:313–330

57. Semelka RC, Shouenut JP, Kroeker MA (1993) Chronic pancreatitis: MRI features before and after administration of gadopentate dimeglumine. J Magn Reson Imaging 3:79–82

58. Wallner BK, Schumaker KA, Weidenmaier W et al (1991) Dilated biliary tract: evaluation with MR cholangiography with a T2-weighted contrast-enhanced fast sequence. Radiology 181:805–808

59. Mehta SN, Reinhold C, Barkun AN (1997) Magnetic resonance cholangiopancreatography. Gastrointest Endosc Clin N Am 7:247–270

60. Adamek H, Albert J, Breer H et al (2000) Pancreatic cancer detection with MR cholangiopancreatography and endoscopic retrograde cholangiopancreatography: a prospective controlled study. Lancet 356:190–193

61. Lee MG, Lee HJ, Kim MH et al (1997) Extrahepatic biliary diseases: 3D MR cholangiopancreatography compared with endoscopic retrograde cholangiopancreatography. Radiology 202:663–669

62. Hirschowitz BI, Curtiss LE, Peters CW et al (1958) Demonstration of a new gastroscope, the "fiberscope". Gastroenterology 35:50

63. Siegel JH (1992) Endoscopic retrograde cholangiopancreatography. Technique, diagnosis and therapy. Raven, New York

64. Niederau C, Grendell JH (1992) Diagnosis of pancreatic carcinoma. Imaging techniques and tumor markers. Pancreas 7:66–86

65. Aly EA, Johnson CD (2001) Preoperative biliary drainage before resection in obstructive jaundice. Dig Surg 18:84–89

66. Flamm CR, Mark DH, Aronson N (2002) Evidence-based assessment of ERCP approaches to managing pancreaticobiliary malignancies. Gastrointest Endosc 56(6Suppl):S218–S225

67. Strasberg SM (2002) ERCP and surgical intervention in pancreatic and biliary malignancies. Gastrointest Endosc 56:S213–S217

68. Keogan MT, Tyler D, Clark L et al (1998) Diagnosis of pancreatic carcinoma: role of FDG PET. AJR Am J Roentgenol 171:1565–1570

69. Sendler A, Avril N, Helmberger H et al (2000) Preoperative evaluation of pancreatic masses with positron emission tomography using 18F-fluorodeoxyglucose: diagnostic limitations. World J Surg 24:1121–1129

70. Rose DM, Delbeke D, Beauchamp RD et al (1999) 18Fluorodeoxyglucose-positron emis-

sion tomography in the management of patients with suspected pancreatic cancer. Ann Surg 229:729–737

71. Friess H, Langhans J, Ebert M et al (1995) Diagnosis of pancreatic cancer by 2[18F]-fluoro-2-deoxy-d-glucose positron emission tomography. Gut 36:771–777

72. Annovazzi A, Peeters M, Maenhout A et al (2003) 18-Fluorodeoxyglucose positron emission tomography in nonendocrine neoplastic disorders of the gastrointestinal tract. Gastroenterology 125:1235–1245

73. Diederichs CG, Staib L, Vogel J et al (2000) Values and limitations of 18F-fluorodeoxyglucose-positron-emission tomography with preoperative evaluation of patients with pancreatic masses. Pancreas 20:109–116

74. Heinrich S, Goerres GW, Schafer M et al (2005) Positron emission tomography/computed tomography influences on the management of resectable pancreatic cancer and its cost-effectiveness. Ann Surg 242:235–243

75. Bernheim BM (1911) Organoscopy: cystoscopy of the abdominal cavity. Ann Surg 53:764–767

76. Cuschieri A, Hall AW, Clark J (1978) Value of laparoscopy in the diagnosis and management of pancreatic carcinoma. Gut 19:672–677

77. Stefanidis D, Grove KD, Schwesinger WH et al (2006) The current role of staging laparoscopy for adenocarcinoma of the pancreas: a review. Ann Oncol 17:189–199

78. White R, Winston C, Gonen M, D'Angelica et al (2008) Current utility of staging laparoscopy for pancreatic and peripancreatic neoplasms. J Am Coll Surg 206:445–450

79. Conlon KC, Dougherty E, Klimstra DS et al (1996) The value of minimal access surgery in the staging of patients with potentially resectable peripancreatic malignancy. Ann Surg 223:134–140

80. Leach SD, Rose JA, Lowy AM et al (1995) Significance of peritoneal cytology in patients with potentially resectable adenocarcinoma of the pancreatic head. Surgery 82:472–478

81. Merchant NB, Conlon KC, Saigo P et al (1999) Positive peritoneal cytology predicts unresectability of pancreatic adenocarcinoma. J Am Coll Surg 188:421–426

82. Nakao A, Oshima K, Takeda S et al (1999) Peritoneal washings cytology combined with immunocytochemical staging in pancreatic cancer. Hepatogastroenterology 46:2974–2977

83. Yachida S, Fukushima N, Sakamoto M et al (2002) Implications of peritoneal washing cytology in patients with potentially resectable pancreatic cancer. Br J Surg 89:573–578

84. Yamada S, Takeda S, Fujii T et al (2007) Clinical implications of peritoneal cytology in potentially resectable pancreatic cancer: positive peritoneal cytology may not confer an adverse prognosis. Ann Surg 246:254–258

85. Berber E, Garland AM, Engle KL et al (2004) Laparoscopic ultrasonography and biopsy of hepatic tumor in 310 patients. Am J Surg 187:213–218

86. Charukhchyan SA, Lucas GW (1998) Laparoscopy and lesser sac endoscopy in gastric carcinoma operability assessment. Am Surg 64:160–164

87. Jaeck D, Boudjema K, Bachellier P et al (1998) Exeresi pancreatiche cefaliche: duodeno-cefalo-pancreasectomie (DCP). In: Encyclopédie médico chirurgicale: Tecniche chirurgiche – Addominale. Elsevier, Paris, 40–880-B, 17 p

88. Brown KM, Siripurapu V, Davidson M et al (2008) Chemoradiation followed by chemotherapy before resection for borderline pancreatic adenocarcinoma. Am J Surg 195:318–321

89. Verslype C, Van Cutsem E, Dicato M et al (2007) The management of pancreatic cancer. Current expert opinion and recommendations derived from the 8th World Congress on Gastrointestinal Cancer, Barcelona, 2006. Ann Oncol 18(Suppl 7):vii1–vii10

90. Crane CH, Varadhachary G, Pisters PW et al (2007) Future chemoradiation strategies in pancreatic cancer. Semin Oncol 34:335–346

91. Russo S, Butler J, Ove R et al (2007) Locally advanced pancreatic cancer: a review. Semin Oncol 34:327–334

Chapter 17

Antibiotic and Antithrombotic Prophylaxis for Pancreatic Surgery

Domitilla Foghetti, Luciano Landa

Antibiotic Prophylaxis

Infection of the incised skin or soft tissue is a common but potentially avoidable complication of any surgical procedure. Some bacterial contamination of a surgical site is inevitable, either from the patient's own bacterial flora or from the environment [1]. The goals of prophylactic administration of antibiotics to surgical patients are:
- To reduce the incidence of surgical site infection
- To minimize adverse effects and antibiotic effects on the patient's normal bacterial flora
- To use antibiotics in a manner that is supported by evidence and effectiveness
  Surgical site infections (SSIs) are classified as being either incisional or organ/space infections. Incisional SSIs are further divided into "superficial incisional SSI," which involves only skin and subcutaneous tissue, and "deep incisional SSI," which involves deeper soft tissue of the incision. Organ/space SSIs involve any part of the anatomy, other than incised body wall layers, that was opened or manipulated during an operation [2].

Antibiotic prophylaxis consists of a brief course of antibiotics initiated preoperatively in order to decrease the risk of postoperative wound infection in the patient with a clean wound. The antibiotic should be started within 60 min before skin incision and continued for not more than 24 h. Prophylactic antibiotics are not a substitute for proper aseptic technique; rather, they are an additional measure used to decrease infection risk. Optimally, an antibiotic level exceeding the minimum inhibitory concentration of that antibiotic for the infecting organism should be maintained in the tissue from incision through to wound closure [3].

There are many reasons for postoperative wound infection, risk factors being related to the patient's clinical condition, categories of surgical operation, staff, theater design, equipment, and surgical procedure.

Operations can be classed into four categories with increasing incidence of bacterial contamination and subsequent postoperative infection: *clean, clean–contaminated, contaminated, dirty* [4] (Table 17.1). Contaminated and dirty operations require antibiotic therapy rather than prophylaxis.

W. Siquini (Ed.), *Surgical Treatment of Pancreatic Diseases*.
©Springer-Verlag Italia 2009

Table 17.1 Classification of operations

Class	Definition
Clean	Operation in which no inflammation is encountered and the respiratory, alimentary, or genitourinary tracts are not entered. There is no break in aseptic operating room technique
Clean-contaminated	The respiratory, alimentary, or genitourinary tracts are entered but without significant spillage
Contaminated	There is visible contamination of the wound (gross spillage from a hollow viscus or open injuries operated on within 4 h)
Dirty	Presence of pus, previously perforated hollow viscus, open injuries more than 4 h old

The insertion of any prosthetic implant, prolonged duration of surgery, and patient co-morbidities are associated with an increased risk of wound infection. The presence of the association of co-morbidity (indicated by an ASA physical status score above 2; Table 17.2) and prolonged operation (operations that lasted longer than 75th percentile for the procedure were classified as prolonged, based on data from the USA) can be used to calculate a "risk index": if neither risk factor is present, the risk index = 0; if either one of the risk factors is present, risk index = 1; if both risk factors are present, risk index = 2. Data from a large epidemiological study show that the risk of wound infection with a clean operation plus both risk factors is greater than the risk with a contaminated wound but no additional risk factor (5.4% vs. 3.4%; Table 17.3).

The value of surgical antibiotic prophylaxis is related to the severity of the consequence of SSI; it reduces postoperative mortality, decreases short-term morbidity, or reduces hospital stay in relation to the different kind of surgical operations. To rationalize surgical antibiotic prophylaxis, it is important to reduce the inappropriate use of antibiotics and to minimize the consequences of misuse.

Table 17.2 American Society of Anesthesiologists (ASA) classification of physical status

ASA score	Physical status
1	Normal healthy patient
2	Patient with a mild systemic disease
3	Patient with a severe systemic disease that limits his activity but is not incapacitating
4	Patient with an incapacitating systemic disease that is a constant threat to life
5	Moribund patient not expected to survive 24 h with or without operation

Table 17.3 Probability of wound infection by type of wound and risk index

Operation classification	Risk index		
	0	1	2
Clean	1.0%	2.3%	5.4%
Clean–contaminated	2.1%	4.0%	9.5%
Contaminated	3.4%	6.8%	13.2%

Thus, antibiotic prophylaxis depends on: the patient's risk of SSI, the potential severity of the consequences of SSI, the effectiveness of prophylaxis in that kind of operation, and the consequences of antibiotic use for that patient.

The following *evidence-based guidelines for the use of antibiotic prophylaxis* have been issued by the Scottish Intercollegiate Guideline Network [4]:

- *Highly recommended:* If prophylaxis unequivocally reduces mortality due to major morbidity, reduces hospital costs, and decreases overall consumption of antibiotics.
- *Recommended:* If it reduces short-term morbidity, and probably also reduces major morbidity, hospital costs, and overall consumption of antibiotics.
- *Recommended but local policy makers may identify exceptions:* If SSI incidence associated with specific operations is low, local policy makers may identify exceptions, as prophylaxis may not reduce hospital costs and could increase nonuseful consumption of antibiotics.
- *Not recommended:* Prophylaxis has not been proven to be clinically effective (for example, the consequences of infection are short-term morbidity); it is likely to increase hospital antibiotic consumption for a poor clinical benefit [4].

Antibiotic prophylaxis is recommended during these situations:

- Clean–contaminated surgical operations in which a hollow viscus is entered but without significant spillage.
- Clean surgery: when prosthetic implants are inserted, antibiotic prophylaxis reduces wound infection by 50%.
- When wound infection incidence is more than 10%.
- When the benefits of prophylaxis are greater than the adverse consequences (risk of anaphylaxis, allergy, resistance)
- When the consequences of SSI would be severe (clean surgery in patients with an ASA score of 3–4; operations lasting longer than 2 h; patient co-morbidity).

The antibiotics selected for prophylaxis must cover the common pathogens and can be the same used as those for active treatment of infection. For maximum effect, prophylaxis should ideally be started within 30–60 min of the induction of anesthesia. Intravenous administration is the most reliable method for ensuring effective serum antibiotic concentrations at the time of surgery. It may seem logical to give an additional dose of prophylaxis during operations that last for more than 2–4 h, because many of the drugs used have a relatively short half-life, although the data available show that surgical patients have slower clearance of drugs from their blood than do normal volunteers [4, 5]. An additional dose is, however, also indicated when there is a blood loss of up to 1,500 ml during surgery or hemodilution of up to 15 ml/kg.

The dose of antibiotic required for prophylaxis is the same as that used for therapy of infection. For all operations, the administration of additional doses after the end of surgery does not provide any additional prophylactic benefit.

In pancreatic surgery, the most common pathogens involved are enteric gram-negative bacilli, gram-positive cocci, and *Clostridium* spp. Cefazolin or cefoxitin are the recommended drugs (2 g i.v.) [6]. An additional dose should be administered if the operation is longer than 3 h. Clindamycin 600 mg plus gentamicin 120 mg or metronidazole plus gentamicin may be used in patients with documented penicillin or cephalosporin allergies.

When a preoperative biliary drainage (PBD) is done before pancreaticoduodenectomy, there is a significant increase in positive intraoperative bile cultures, postoperative infectious morbidity, and death. PBD has a notable influence on bile microbial contamination, including increasing the rate of antibiotic resistance. For this reason, specific antibiotic prophylaxis based on bile culture is required for preventing infectious complications during pancreatic surgery such as pancreaticoduodenectomy [7–15].

A Japanese group also investigated the use of perioperative probiotics to reduce the morbidity associated with pancreaticoduodenectomy. The probiotics seem to reduce postoperative infectious complications, making them a promising potential adjunct therapy for patients undergoing high-risk pancreatic surgery [16].

Antithrombotic Prophylaxis

Venous thromboembolism (VTE) in the lower venous system usually occurs as a complication of major surgery, especially if risk factors are present. Without antithrombotic prophylaxis, objective diagnostic measures have shown that 20–25% of patients develop venous thrombosis after major general surgery (29% of cancer patients). VTE manifests as pulmonary embolism in 1.6% of patients (the incidence of fatal pulmonary embolism is 0.9%).

Surgery is a predisposing condition to VTE because of the prolonged immobility of the patient during the postoperative period, to which may be added individual patient risk factors. Patients undergoing surgical procedures have VTE risks associated with the procedure, such as the site, surgical technique, duration, type of anesthesia, complications (infection, shock, etc.), and degree of immobilization [17]. More rapid mobilization, greater use of thromboprophylaxis, and other advances in perioperative care may tend toward reducing the thromboembolic risk. However, the performance of more extensive operative procedures in older and sicker patients, the use of preoperative chemotherapy, and the shorter lengths of stay in hospital (leading to shorter durations of prophylaxis) may heighten the risk of VTE.

Laparoscopic surgery of all types causes serum hypercoagulability of varying degrees, too: shorter (less than 1 h) and less complex laparoscopic procedures such as simple laparoscopic cholecystectomy have low risk of VTE, whereas longer and more complex laparoscopic procedures such as pancreatoduodenectomy are higher-risk.

As for the surgical patients themselves, it is possible to assign them to one of four VTE risk levels based on type of operation (e.g., minor or major), age (e.g., <40 years, 40–60 years, >60 years), and the presence of additional risk factors (e.g., cancer, medical illnesses, or previous VTE) [18] (Table 17.4). It is also possible to obtain a visualization of the risk level by combining the risk factors related to the patient's condition and to the surgical procedure (Fig. 17.1).

Table 17.4 Risk levels associated with surgery and patient's clinical condition [4]

Surgery	
Level 1	Nonmajor surgical procedure: appendicectomy, hernia repair, esophageal surgery, abdominal wall surgery, head and neck surgery, cholecystectomy
Level 2	Complicated appendicectomy, inflammatory small bowel disease
Level 3	Major cancer surgery: gallbladder, biliary tract, esophagus, pancreas, small bowel, colorectum, spleen, adrenal gland
Patient	
Level 1	Age
Level 2	Age >40 years, estrogen use in pharmacologic doses (oral contraception pills or hormone replacement therapy), major medical illnesses (acute myocardial infarction, ischemic stroke, congestive cardiac failure, acute respiratory failure), perioperative prolonged confinement to bed (>4 days), leg varicose veins, perioperative acute local or systemic acute infection, obesity, peripartum. *If two or more risk factors are present, patient is classified in the next level*
Level 3	Cancer, history of venous thromboembolism, myeloproliferative disorders, inherited hypercoagulable states (protein C or S deficiency, antithrombin deficiency)
Thromboembolism risk stratification for surgery patients	
Low risk	Age <40 years, no risk factors, minor uncomplicated surgery (minimal immobility postoperatively)
Moderate risk	Age <40 years, no risk factors, major surgery or cancer
	Age 40–60 years, no risk factors, any surgery
	Any age, minor surgery in patients with one or more risk factors
High risk	Age 40–60 years with one or more risk factors, major surgery or cancer
	Age >60 years, no risk factors, major surgery or cancer
Very high risk	Age >40 years, previous venous thromboembolism, major surgery or cancer
	Age >40 years, known hypercoagulable state, major surgery or cancer

Risk level related to surgery								
1			2			3		
Risk level due to patient condition								
1	2	3	1	2	3	1	2	3
Thromboembolic risk								
Low			Moderate			High		

Fig. 17.1 Visualization of patient's overall VTE risk level: the risk factors related to the patient's condition are combined with those relating to the surgical procedure

During the perioperative period, not only the VTE risk must be considered, but also the patient's risk of bleeding. The patient must be asked about any history of postoperative bleeding or bleeding after dental extraction, active hepatitis or hepatic insufficiency, acute peptic ulcer, and any pharmacologic therapy with anticoagulant agents.

Appropriate antithrombotic prophylaxis should be initiated for patient on the basis of risk levels. The choice is between mechanical or pharmacological measures, or a combination of both.

Mechanical Antithrombotic Prophylaxis

Nonpharmacologic methods act especially on the venous system: they increase venous outflow and/or reduce stasis within the veins of the legs [18]. These methods are considerations for patients at high risk of bleeding, because of their lack of potential for inducing bleeding, and they may be used alone or associated with pharmacologic measures. They include *graduated elastic compression stockings*, an *intermittent pneumatic compression device*, and *inferior vena cava filters*. These methods may be used alone in patients at low thrombotic risk; they should be combined with antithrombotic drugs in patients at high risk.

Graduated elastic compression stockings should be worn before the surgical operation and kept on for 1 or 2 weeks. They should be used as an alternative to pharmacologic agents in patients at moderate risk of VTE patients who are also at risk of bleeding, or in patients at high risk of VTE, combined with other measures. Contraindications are skin lesions, arterial insufficiency in the legs, and diabetic neuropathy.

Intermittent pneumatic compression (which provides rhythmic external compression at 35–40 mmHg for about 10 s every minute) may also be used in patients with skin lesions on the legs.

Inferior vena cava filters are retrievable filters that can be placed perioperatively and removed up to 1 year later or left in place. Their placement should be reserved for patients at very high risk of VTE in whom both anticoagulation and physical methods are contraindicated [19]. They should be used, for example, for an emergency operation in a patient with acute deep vein thrombosis. These filters tend to cause a long-term increase of recurrent deep vein thrombosis, although the immediate risk of postoperative pulmonary embolism is reduced.

Prophylactic Antithrombotic Drugs

Prophylactic drugs include low-dose unfractionated heparin (LDUH), low-molecular-weight heparin (LMWH), oral anticoagulant (such as coumarins), thrombin inhibitors (such as hirudin), and specific factor Xa inhibitors (such as fondaparinux).

The three issues that need to be addressed are choice of agent, dosage, and the duration of therapy. One meta-analysis [18] found that LMWH prophylaxis reduced the risk of asymptomatic deep vein thrombosis and symptomatic VTE in general surgery patients by more than 70% compared with no prophylaxis. LDUH and LMWH have similar efficacy and bleeding rates for general surgery patients. LDUH is cost-effective and effective in reducing the risk of postoperative VTE, while LMWH has the convenience of once-daily dosing but it is significantly more expensive.

As far as unfractionated heparin is concerned, the dose is 5,000 IU given subcutaneously started within 2 h of the operation and then every 8 or 12 h (every 8 h is probably more effective at preventing VTE and entails a similar risk of major bleeding). Continuous infusion of LDUH is as effective as the subcutaneous route but carries an increased risk of major bleeding and also requires hematologic monitoring.

The various brands of LMWH have different molecular weight distribution profiles, specific activities (anti-Xa to anti-IIa activities), and rates of plasma clearance, and each brand should therefore be considered as distinct and the doses set accordingly. Antithrombotic potencies and potential bleeding effects of different LMWHs cannot be extrapolated from one product to another on the basis of weights in milligrams [20]. The dosage and frequency for LMWH depends on the manufacturer. LMWHs cause less heparin-induced thrombocytopenia than LDUH, and they should be adjusted at prophylactic doses for patients with a creatinine clearance less than 30 ml/min; the dose must be increased in very obese patients (body mass index 35 or more) [17].

Intravenous dextran, a branched polysaccharide with a molecular weight of 40,000 or 70,000, has also been shown to be effective after major surgery; however, its use is expensive and associated with anaphylactic responses, and it is contraindicated in patients with renal insufficiency and limited cardiac reserve. Some studies showed that recombinant hirudin, started preoperatively, was more effective than unfractionated heparin, as was bivalirudin (hirulog) too, although these drugs are undergoing further clinical evaluation. Prophylaxis with the selective inhibitor of factor Xa fondaparinux, started postoperatively, was compared with prophylaxis with dalteparin started before surgery: the results showed no significant differences in the rates of VTE, major bleeding, or death between the two groups [18].

Risk of development of VTE continues beyond the hospital stay, so the need for postdischarge anticoagulation should be assessed especially in selected high-risk patients, including those who have undergone major cancer surgery [17, 18]. Prophylaxis with LMWH for 2–3 weeks after hospital discharge appears to reduce the incidence of asymptomatic deep vein thrombosis in cancer surgery patients [18].

Pharmacologic prophylaxis is not without risk. The patient's risk of thrombosis needs to be balanced against his or her risk of bleeding; however, for short-term prophylactic anticoagulation, there are relatively few conditions with excessive bleeding risk or other considerations that would contraindicate anticoagulation. Contraindications for pharmacologic prophylaxis are active major, significant bleeding; extreme thrombocytopenia (less than $50 \times 10^3/\mu l$); uncontrolled hypertension; bacterial endocarditis; active hepatitis; or hepatic insufficiency [17].

The following evidence-based guidelines for the use of *antithrombotic prophylaxis in general surgery patients* have been published [18]:

– *Low risk:* Early mobilization, early and persistent ambulation (grade 1C)
– *Moderate risk:* Low-dose unfractionated heparin (LDUH; 5,000 IU 12-hourly starting 2 ion elastic stockings or intermittent pneumatic compression
– *High risk:* LDUH 5,000 IU three times a day starting 2 h before surgery or LMWH >3,400 anti-Xa mpression stockings and/or intermittent pneumatic compression in patients with multiple risk factors (grade 1C)
– *Very high risk:* LMWH >3,400 anti-Xa IU daily plus compression elastic stockings, or prolonged LMWH therapy plus compression elastic stockings
– *High risk of bleeding:* Mechanical prophylaxis at least initially until the bleeding risk decreases (grade 1A)

VTE is an important health-care problem, resulting in significant mortality, morbidity, and resource expenditure. The prevalence of deep vein thrombosis may be expected to increase in future because the average age of the population and the number of cancer patients is increasing, advanced age is becoming a lesser contraindication for major surgery, and many surgical patients, young and old, are being discharged from hospital before they are fully ambulant [20].

The implementation of evidence-based and thoughtful prophylaxis strategies provides benefit to the patient, and should also protect the caregivers and the hospitals providing care from legal liability. So it may be useful for every hospital to develop a formal strategy to prevent thromboembolic complications, and that this should be in the form of a written thromboprophylaxis policy [18, 21– 24].

References

1. De Lalla F (2003) L'infezione postoperatoria. Clinica, terapia, profilassi. Edimes, Pavia
2. Mangram AJ, Horan TC, Pearson ML et al (1999) Guideline for prevention of surgical site infection. Infect Control Hosp Epidemiol 20:250–278
3. Holtom PD (2006) Antibiotic prophylaxis: current recommendations. J Am Acad Orthop Surg 14(10):98–100
4. Anonymous (2000) Antibiotic prophylaxis in surgery. Scottish Intercollegiate Guideline Network. Sign Publication 45. Available at: http://www.sign.ac.uk/pdf/sign45.pdf. Accessed 23 June 2008
5. Ohge H, Takesue Y, Yokoyama T et al (1999) An additional dose of cefazolin for intraoperative prophylaxis. Surg Today 29:1233–1236
6. Ueno T, Yamamoto K, Kawaoka T et al (2005) Current antibiotic prophylaxis in pancreatoduodenectomy in Japan. J Hepatobiliary Pancreat Surg 12:304–309
7. Sudo T, Murakami Y, Uemura K et al (2007) Specific antibiotic prophylaxis based on bile cultures is required to prevent prostoperative infectious complications in pancreatoduodenectomy patients who have undergone preoperative biliary drainage. World J Surg 31:2230–2235
8. Cortes A, Sauvanet A, Bert F et al (2006) Effect of bile contamination on immediate outcomes after pancreaticoduodenectomy for tumor. J Am Coll Surg 202:93–99
9. Lermite E, Pessaux P, Teyssedou C et al (2008) Effect of preoperative endoscopic biliary drainage on infectious morbidity after pancreatoduodenectomy: a case-control study. Am J Surg 195:442–446
10. Jethwa P, Breuning E, Bhati C et al (2007) The microbiological impact of pre-operative biliary drainage on patients undergoing hepato-biliary-pancreatic (HPB) surgery. Aliment Pharmacol Ther 25:1175–1180
11. Sohn TA, Yeo CJ, Cameron Jl et al (2000) Do preoperative biliary stents increase postpancreaticoduodenectomy complications? J Gastrointest Surg 4:258–267
12. Povosky SP, Karpeh MS Jr, Conlon KC et al (1999) Preoperative biliary drainage: impact on intraoperative bile cultures and infectious morbidity and mortality after pancreaticoduodenectomy. J Gastrointest Surg 3:496–505
13. Pisters PW, Hudec Wa, Hess KR et al (2001) Effect of preoperative biliary decompression on pancreaticoduodenectomy-associated morbidity in 300 consecutive patients. Ann Surg 234 :47–55
14. Grizas S, Stakyte M, Kincius M et al (2005) Etiology of bile infection and its association with postoperative complications following pancreatoduodenectomy. Medicina (Kaunas) 41:386–391
15. Jagannath P, Dhir V, Shrikhande S et al (2005) Effect of preoperative biliary stenting on immediate outcome after pancreaticoduodenectomy. Br J Surg 92:356–361
16. Nomura T, Tsuchiya Y, Nashimoto A et al (2007) Probiotics reduce infectious complications after pancreaticoduodenectomy. Hepatogastroenterology 54:661–663
17. Anonymous (2007) Venous thromboembolism prophylaxis.: Institute for Clinical System Improvement (ICSI), Bloomington, 52. Available at: http://www.guideline.gov/summary/summary.aspx?ss=15&doc_id=11286. Accessed 23 June 2008
18. Geerts WH, Pineo GF, Heit JA et al (2004) Prevention of venous thromboembolism. The Seventh ACCP Conference on Antithrombotic and Thrombolytic Therapy. Chest 124:338–400
19. Turpie AGG, Chin BSP, Lip GYH (2002) ABC of antithrombotic therapy. Venous thromboembolism: pathophysiology, clinical features, and prevention. BMJ 325:887–890
20. Verstraete M (1997) Fortnightly review: prophylaxis of venous thromboembolism. BMJ 314:123

21. De Franciscis S, Agus GB, Bisacci R et al (2008) Guidelines for venous thromboembolism and clinical practice in Italy: a nationwide survey. Ann Vasc Surg 22:319–327
22. Cohen AT, Tapson VF, Bergmann JF et al (2008) Venous thromboembolism risk and prophylaxis in the acute hospital care setting (ENDORSE study): a multinational cross-sectional study. Lancet 371:387–394
23. Michota FA (2007) Bridging the gap between evidence and practice in venous thromboembolism prophylaxis: the quality improvement process. J Gen Intern Med 2:1762–1770
24. Nutescu EA (2007) Assessing, preventing, and treating venous thromboembolism: evidence-based approaches. Am J Health Syst Pharm 64(11S7):5–13

Chapter 18

Operative Endoscopic Ultrasonography for Pancreatic Diseases

Silvia Carrara, Maria Chiara Petrone, Cinzia Boemo, Paolo Giorgio Arcidiacono

Introduction

Endoscopic ultrasonography (EUS) is a highly accurate method for staging gastrointestinal diseases, especially benign and malignant pancreatic lesions. As the probe can be placed so close to the pancreas (in the stomach and duodenum), EUS provides high-resolution images of the pancreas, with precise visualization of the biliary and pancreatic ducts and peripancreatic vessels.

The development of the linear array probe has extended the diagnostic potential of this technique for EUS-guided fine-needle aspiration biopsy (FNA) with cytological analysis (Fig. 18.1). From this operative diagnostic procedure, interventional EUS has moved on in both the diagnostic and therapeutic fields.

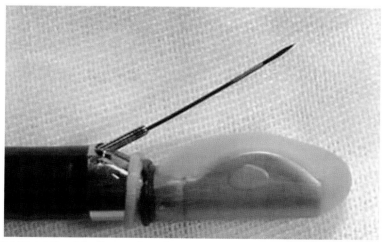

Fig. 18.1 Distal tip of the linear echoendoscope: the probe is covered with a balloon that is inflated with water and creates a tight interface between the transducer and the tissues. The needle is passed through the operative channel of the instrument and its track is followed under real-time endoscopic ultrasound (EUS). An elevator at the tip of the instrument guides the needle in the right direction

W. Siquini (Ed.), *Surgical Treatment of Pancreatic Diseases.*
©Springer-Verlag Italia 2009

Diagnostic Interventional EUS: EUS–FNA

EUS-FNA is a safe technique with a high accuracy [1, 2]. Pancreatic FNA is done under EUS guidance with the patient in left lateral decubitus. The lesion is carefully staged and vascular infiltration is evaluated. Lesions in the head and uncinate process are biopsied from the duodenum, and those in the body and tail from the stomach. Color Doppler equipment is used to avoid vascular structures along the path of the needle.

Once the target lesion has been visualized, with the transducer in a steady position, the up–down and left–right wheels are locked and the needle is inserted into the biopsy channel. It is easiest to insert the needle straight, because if the tip is too flexed or the echoendoscope looped, advancing the needle becomes difficult and may be dangerous for the instrument. In this case the instrument should be withdrawn and straightened until the needle passes easily, without resistance; then it can be repositioned close to the target lesion.

Many different needles have been developed, in different sizes from 19 to 25 gauge. The needle is equipped with a stylet covered by a protective sheath. The stylet prevents the needle clogging with tissue or blood while it is being advanced into the target lesion. Before the puncture, the stylet is withdrawn a few millimeters to expose the sharp tip of the needle, and the tip is advanced under real-time endoscopic ultrasound guidance until it can be seen as a hyperechoic line within the lesion (Fig. 18.2). If the needle cannot be seen fully, fine

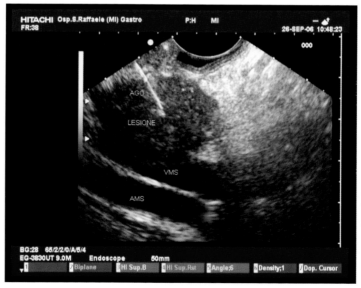

Fig. 18.2 EUS-guided fine-needle aspiration (FNA) of a solid lesion of the pancreatic head involving the superior mesenteric vein (*VMS*). The needle is visualized as a hyperechoic line in the mass *AMS*, Superior mesenteric artery

adjustments to the transducer position usually right the image. Once the needle has penetrated the lesion, the stylet is advanced back to the original position, then removed. Suction is applied through a 10-ml syringe and the needle is moved to and fro a few times inside the lesion. The suction is then released and the needle is retracted into the catheter and removed from the echoendoscope. The aspirated material is placed on glass slides for smears using Papanicolaou and Wright–Giemsa stains.

In cases of adenocarcinoma the desmoplastic reaction can sometimes make this kind of lesion difficult to puncture.

The sensitivity of the technique varies between 75 and 94%; the specificity is 100%, and the diagnostic adequacy 85–92% [3, 4]. With a cytopathologist in the endoscopy room during the procedure, the rate of inadequacy is less than 10% compared to 5–18% when the cytopathologist is not present [5, 6].

Molecular analysis of the specimen, for K-*ras* expression, for example, seems to improve the diagnostic adequacy of EUS-FNA for adenocarcinoma [7], while for cystic lesions (Fig. 18.3), cyst fluid analysis investigating tumor markers (CEA) increases the accuracy of diagnosis: less than 5 ng/ml normally indicates a benign lesion (serous cystoadenoma), while more than 192 ng/ml may be seen in mucinous tumors, which are more likely to progress to malignancy. The optimal cut-off of CEA varies according to different studies between 192 and 400 ng/ml, with 79–97% sensitivity [8, 9].

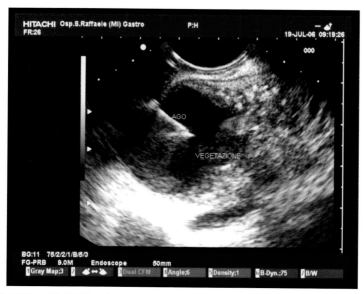

Fig. 18.3 EUS-guided FNA of an intraductal papillary mucinous neoplasm (IPMN) of the pancreatic head: a cystic lesion with vegetation. The material aspirated is sent for cytological analysis and investigation for tumoral markers (CEA)

Advances in needle technology have led to the 19-gauge Tru-cut needle, which can obtain enough material for histological examination. The main problem with these needles, however, is that they stiffen the distal part of the echoendoscope, especially when the needle is placed in the biopsy channel; this makes it hard to position the endoscope close enough to the lesion and keep it in place while taking the biopsy. The elevator function may lose 5–10° of movement [10].

On the whole, EUS-FNA is a safe procedure with a complication rate of about 1–2%, less for solid lesions than for cystic ones [11]. Bleeding is the most frequent complication, but it is usually self-limiting, with a frequency of 1% [12, 13]. The risk of infection is low, but cystic lesions, both tumors and pseudocysts, carry a greater risk of infection and the patient is usually given antibiotic prophylaxis, even though there is still no clinical evidence of its efficacy in randomized trials [11].

The risk of seeding of tumoral cells during the EUS-FNA is negligible since the peritoneum is not touched and the duodenum, through which lesions of the head are biopsied, is resected and removed with the mass.

Operative Therapeutic EUS

Pancreatic Pseudocyst Drainage

Endoscopic drainage is an effective treatment for pancreatic pseudocysts, but there is always a risk of bleeding or perforation of the vascular structures between the gastric wall and the cyst [14]. EUS-guided drainage is ideal for these lesions, thanks to its real-time imaging, its ability to identify vessels with the color-Doppler effect, and its precise localization of the cyst. EUS can guide the needle along the shortest and safest path (Figs. 18.4, 18.5): a distance of more than 1 cm between the gastric wall and the pseudocyst is a contraindication to endoscopic drainage.

There are three main techniques for EUS-guided pseudocyst drainage:
1. *EUS-assisted drainage*, in two steps: EUS is done before the operative procedure to identify and mark an optimal puncture site. In the second step the echoendoscope is withdrawn and a duodenoscope is used to puncture the site with a needle-knife and place a stent semi-blind, according to Cremer's standard procedure [15]. EUS can be done with a linear or a radial instrument – they are both adequate for topographic study of the region.
2. *EUS-guided drainage*, using a linear array echoendoscope, in one of two ways:
   – In *two steps:* EUS guides a plastic-sheathed needle-knife to puncture the pseudocyst, a guide wire is run down the plastic catheter, and the echoendoscope is withdrawn; a large-channel duodenoscope is used to place the stent over the wire.

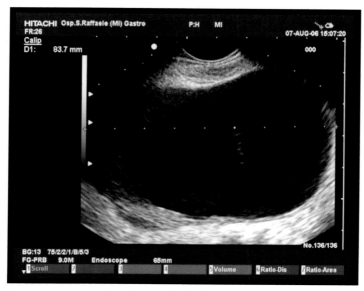

Fig. 18.4 Huge pseudocyst of the body and tail of the pancreas

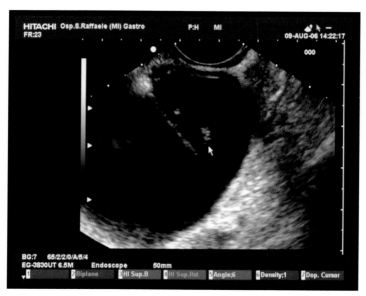

Fig. 18.5 One-step EUS-guided drainage of a pancreatic pseudocyst: the needle-knife is seen in the lesion

- In *one step:* the procedure is followed all the way under real-time EUS guidance using an echoendoscope with a large working channel (3.8 mm) and power Doppler to avoid vascular damage. A cystotome (Fig. 18.6) is passed through the operative channel and used to electrosurgically penetrate the gastric or duodenal wall and put a guide wire, then a stent, into a pancreatic pseudocyst [16, 17].

Celiac Plexus Neurolysis

Since EUS offers good accuracy for diagnosis in cases of suspected pancreatic cancer, it is used in early tumor staging, and is the best way to guide analgesic treatment for patient with painful advanced disease.

Pain in patients with pancreatic cancer is triggered by pancreatic neuropathy due to damage to intrapancreatic nerves, and perineural cancer cell invasion is one of the causes. So-called "neurogenic inflammation" can also contribute to causing pain in pancreatic cancer, just as in chronic pancreatitis.

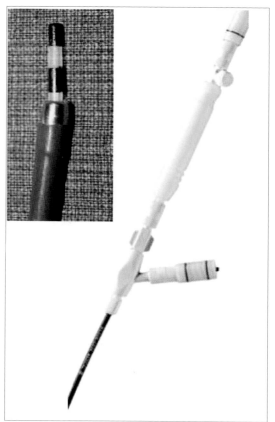

Fig. 18.6 Distal and proximal tip of the cystotome

The celiac plexus carries the neuropathic pain, which is acute and reduces the patient's quality of life. The plexus is composed of a network of nerve fibers and is situated retroperitoneally at the level of the T12 and L1 vertebrae, anterior to the crura of the diaphragm. It surrounds the abdominal aorta and the celiac artery. EUS is a safe way to place the needle inside the plexus or close to it without damaging vascular structures, thanks to the color Doppler technique.

The endosonographic marker for the celiac trunk is the point where the celiac artery emerges from the aorta. For EUS-guided cardiac plexus neurolysis (EUS-CPN), the needle punctures the gastric wall below the cardia and moves to the angle between the aorta and the celiac trunk. A 20-gauge needle is used for CPN. When the tip is in place, 3 ml of a local analgesic, usually bupivacaine 0.25–0.75%, is injected, followed by 10 ml of 98% alcohol (Fig. 18.7). After the injection, the alcohol is visualized as a periaortic echoic cloud. The whole procedure takes about 15–20 min [18].

EUS-CPN is simple to perform and avoids the serious complications such as paraplegia or pneumothorax that can be associated with the posterior approach. A tendency to improved survival of pancreatic cancer patients treated with EUS-CPN has been reported, but larger studies are needed to confirm this. Gunaratman showed a lasting benefit in 88% of treated patients, with 91% requiring fewer drugs [19].

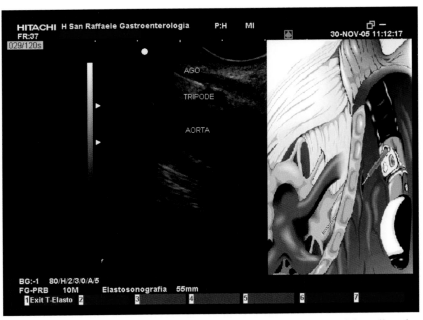

Fig. 18.7 EUS-guided celiac plexus neurolysis (CPN). *Right:* Anatomy of the celiac plexus which surrounds the aorta and the celiac trunk. *Left:* EUS image of the CPN

EUS-Cholangiopancreatography

Investigations of the common bile duct and the main pancreatic duct (duct of Wirsung) can be challenging after surgery or because of difficulty in cannulating the papilla. Detailed imaging of the biliopancreatic tract is possible with endosonography, and EUS-guided cholangiopancreatography offers an alternative method for achieving a diagnosis in patients in whom endoscopic retrograde cholangiopancreatography (ERCP) is unsuccessful. The pancreas is evaluated by following the path of the pancreatic duct, paying due attention to vascular structures. The tip of the echoendoscope is placed in the duodenum to puncture the distal portion of the ducts (in the pancreatic head).

A 22- or 23-gauge needle is followed under real-time imaging and guided to puncture the pancreatic or biliary duct (Fig. 18.8). Color Doppler imaging is helpful to avoid vessels such as the gastroduodenal artery, which runs very close to the duodenum and the biliary duct. A radiological contrast agent is injected under fluoroscopic guidance.

Wiersema reported the effectiveness of the EUS-guided procedure in 11 patients in whom ERCP was unsuccessful, with success in 73% of cases ($p < 0.001$) and only one case of pancreatitis [20].

EUS is a feasible technique for rendezvous drainage of obstructed biliary or pancreatic ducts. EUS-guided transgastric or transduodenal needle puncture is performed and a guide wire is placed through the obstructed pancreatic or bile

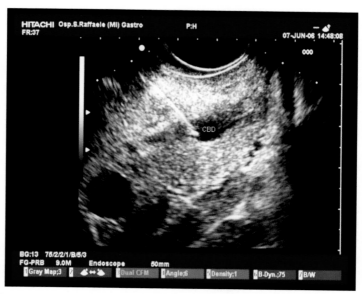

Fig. 18.8 EUS-guided puncture of the common bile duct (CBD) in a patient with a stricture of the distal biliary tract due to a scar of the ampullary region. The Endoscopic retrograde cholangiopancreatography was unsuccessful

duct. The guide wire is advanced antegrade across the papilla and, if passage is successful, rendezvous ERCP with stent placement is done using a duodeno-scope [21].

EUS-Guided Methylene Blue Injection into the Pancreatic Duct Before Ampullectomy

Endosonography-guided injection of methylene blue into the pancreatic duct has been described to identify the minor papilla after unsuccessful ERCP [22]. We used intraductal injection of methylene blue in patients with adenoma of the ampulla to help detect the pancreatic orifice and placed a stent after ampullecto-my [23].

Pancreatic duct stenting after endoscopic snare excision of the ampulla in patients with papillary tumors has been effective in preventing postprocedural pancreatitis [24]. However, pancreatic duct cannulation can be challenging, and edema and artifacts due to electrocautery during ampullectomy can make it even harder to identify and stent the pancreatic orifice.

In our tertiary referral center for pancreatobiliary diseases we follow two main steps in case of adenoma of the ampulla:

1. Linear EUS staging: if the lesion is superficial, without involvement of the ducts, the pancreatic duct is punctured with a 25 or 22-gauge needle and methylene blue (methylthionine 100 mg/10 Ml, dilution 1:20,000, 3 ml) is injected until leakage from the ampullary orifice is seen as a blue flow into the duodenum.

2. After EUS staging: during the same session, the echoendoscope is withdrawn and therapeutic resection is done with a duodenoscope. After ampullectomy, the methylene blue flow from the pancreatic orifice is a useful guide for plac-ing of a stent in the pancreatic duct (Fig. 18.9).

Future Applications of EUS for the Treatment of Tumors

EUS will be able to guide the application of biological or physical antitumoral agents to tumors. Recent phase I clinical trials have tested EUS-guided implan-tation of immunomodulating cells into pancreatic tumors in order to stimulate an immunological response from T-killer cells [25]. More studies are needed to assess the feasibility of these new techniques and their clinical impact.

A new field in the treatment of pancreatic tumors is EUS-guided ablation of tissues with radiofrequency (RF). Goldberg et al. investigated the feasibility and safety of RF ablation in the porcine pancreas under EUS guidance and the dis-crete zones of coagulation necrosis produced [26].

We used a new cryotherm probe (ERBE Elektromedizin GmbH, Tubingen, Germany) in the same animal model to create a larger coagulative lesion with less collateral damage. The new flexible bipolar probe created an ablation area

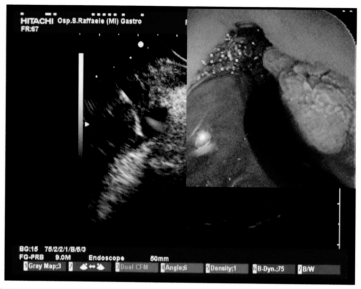

Fig. 18.9 EUS-guided injection of methylene blue into the main pancreatic duct. The blue flow from the ampullary orifice guides the placement of a stent into the pancreatic duct after ampullectomy

whose extent was related to the duration of application, and complications were fewer than with conventional RF ablation techniques [27].

References

1. Williams DB, Sahai AV, Aabakken L et al (1999) Endoscopic ultrasound-guided fine-needle aspiration biopsy: a large single-center experience. Gut 44:720–726
2. Gress F, Gottlieb K, Sherman S et al (2001) Endoscopic ultrasonography-guided fine-needle aspiration biopsy of suspected pancreatic cancer. Ann Intern Med 134:459–464
3. Chang KJ, Wiersema M, Giovannini M (1996) Multicenter collaborative study on endoscopic ultrasound-guided FNA of the pancreas. Gastrointest Endosc 43:A507
4. Eloubedi MA, Jhala D, Chhieng DC et al (2003) Yield of endoscopic ultrasound-guided fine-needle aspiration biopsy in patients with suspected pancreatic carcinoma. Cancer 99:285–292
5. Erickson RA, Sayage-Rabie L, Beisser RS et al (2000) Factors predicting the number of EUS-guided fine-needle passes for diagnosis of pancreatic malignancies. Gastrointest Endosc 51:184–190
6. Klapman JB, Logrono R, Dye CE et al (2003) Clinical impact of on-site cytopathology interpretation of endoscopic ultrasound-guided fine-needle aspiration. Am J Gastroenterol 98:1289–1294
7. Tada M, Komatsu Y, Kawabe T et al (2002) Quantitative analysis of K-ras gene mutation in pancreatic tissue obtained by endoscopic ultrasonography-guided fine-needle aspiration: clinical utility for diagnosis of pancreatic tumor. Am J Gastroenterol 97:2263–2270
8. Brugge WR, Lewandrowski K, Lee-Lewandrowski E et al (2004) Diagnosis of pancreatic

cystic neoplasms: a report of the cooperative pancreatic cyst study. Gastroenterology 126:1330–1336

9. Hernandez LV, Mishra G, Forsmark C et al (2002) Role of endoscopic ultrasound (EUS) and EUS-guided fine-needle aspiration in the diagnosis and treatment of cystic lesions of the pancreas. Pancreas 25:222–228

10. Wiersema MJ, Levy MJ, Harewood GC et al (2002) Initial experience with EUS-guided Tru-cut needle biopsies of perigastric organs. Gastrointest Endosc 56:275–278

11. Wiersema MJ, Vilmann P, Giovannini M et al (1997) Endosonography-guided fine-needle aspiration biopsy: diagnostic accuracy and complication assessment. Gastroenterology 112:1087–1095

12. Varadarajulu S, Eloubeidi MA (2004) Frequency and significance of acute intracystic hemorrhage during EUS-FNA of cystic lesions of the pancreas. Gastrointest Endosc 60:631–635

13. Affi A, Vasquez-Sequeiros E, Norton ID et al (2001) Acute extraluminal hemorrhage associated with EUS-guided fine-needle aspiration: frequency and clinical significance. Gastrointest Endosc 53:221–225

14. Barthet M, Bugallo M, Moreira LS et al (1993) Management of cysts and pseudocysts complicating chronic pancreatitis: a retrospective study of 143 patients. Gastroenterol Clin Biol 17:270–276

15. Cremer M, Deviare J, Engelholm L (1989) Endoscopic management of cysts and pseudocysts in chronic pancreatitis: long-term follow-up after 7 years of experience. Gastrointest Endosc 35:1–9

16. Seifert H, Dietrich C, Schmitt T et al (2000) Endoscopic ultrasound-guided one-step transmural drainage of cystic abdominal lesions with large-channel endoscope. Endoscopy 32:255–259

17. Giovannini M, Pesenti C, Rolland AL et al (2001) Endoscopic ultrasound-guided drainage of pancreatic pseudocysts or pancreatic abscesses using a therapeutic echo-endoscope. Endoscopy 33:472–477

18. Arcidiacono PG, Rossi M (2004) Celiac plexus neurolysis. JOP 5:315–321

19. Gunaratnam NT, Sarma AV, Noton ID et al (2001) A prospective study of EUS-guided celiac plexus neurolysis for pancreatic cancer pain. Gastrointest Endosc 54:316–324

20. Wiersema MJ, Sandusky D, Carr R et al (1996) Endosonography-guided cholangiopancreatography. Gastrointest Endosc 43:102–106

21. Mallery S, Matlock J, Freeman ML (2004) EUS-guided rendezvous drainage of obstructed biliary and pancreatic ducts: report of 6 cases. Gastrointest Endosc 59:100–107

22. DeWitt J, McHenry L, Fogel E et al (2004) EUS-guided methylene blue pancreatography for minor papilla localization after unsuccessful ERCP. Gastrointest Endosc 59:133–136

23. Carrara S, Arcidiacono PG, Diellou AM et al (2007) EUS-guided methylene blue injection into the pancreatic duct as a guide for pancreatic stenting after ampullectomy. Endoscopy 39(Suppl 1):E151–E152

24. Harewood GC, Pochron NL, Gostout CJ (2005) Prospective, randomized, controlled trial of prophylactic pancreatic stent placement for endoscopic snare excision of the duodenal ampulla. Gastrointest Endosc 62:367–373

25. Chang KJ, Nguyen PT, Thomson JA et al (1998) Phase I clinical trial of local immunotherapy (cyto-implant) delivered by endoscopic ultrasound (EUS)-guided fine-needle injection (FNI) in patients with advanced pancreatic carcinoma. Gastrointest Endosc 47:AB144

26. Goldberg SN, Mallery S, Gazelle GS, Brugge WR (1999) EUS-guided radiofrequency ablation in the pancreas: results in a porcine model. Gastrointest Endosc 50:392–401

27. Carrara S, Arcidiacono PG, Albarello L et al (2008) Endoscopic ultrasound-guided application of a new hybrid cryotherm probe in porcine pancreas: a preliminary study. Endoscopy 40:321–326

Chapter 19

Pancreaticoduodenectomy: Perioperative Management and Technical Notes

Stefano Cappato, Fiorenza Belli, Diego Dedola, Marco Filauro

Preparation of the Patient

Intestinal preparation is not routinely performed at our centre. Preoperative parenteral nutrition is only administered to debilitated patients. Antithrombotic prophylaxis with low-molecular-weight heparin (reviparin sodium, one ampoule, subcutaneously in the evening) and graduated compression stockings are the norm.

The day before surgery, the following are prepared:
- A *central venous catheter* (generally in the right subclavian vein) is useful during the procedure or in the postoperative period for infusion of hydroelectrolytic solutions, crystalloids and, if necessary, parenteral nutrition, both in debilitated patients and in case postoperative complications arise that delay the resumption of feeding by mouth.
- A *peridural catheter* is used both for combined anesthesia and, in the postoperative period, for analgesia.

Once the patient is asleep, a *vesical catheter* and a *nasogastric probe* are positioned. In addition, antibiotic prophylaxis with sulbactam-ampicillin is administered at the time of induction.

Position of the Patient on the Operating Table

The patient is supine with one of the two arms (preferably the left one), as requested by the anesthetist, exposed.

Good visualization of the operative field can be obtained by "dividing" the operating table at the level of the first thoracic vertebra. If a mobile operating table is not available, the same result can be obtained by positioning a support, such as a gel cushion, inflatable balloon, or folded blanket, under the patient's shoulders (Fig. 19.1). In order to obtain good exposure, an Olivier retractor is fixed to the appropriate supports on a small arch that must be positioned before the skin is disinfected.

W. Siquini (Ed.), *Surgical Treatment of Pancreatic Diseases.*
©Springer-Verlag Italia 2009

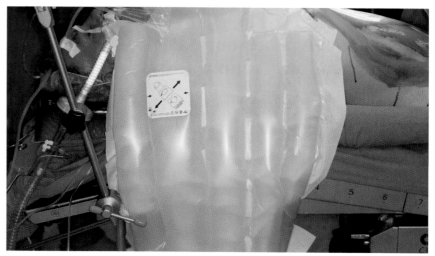

Fig. 19.1 Position of the patient

Position of the Operating Team

The first surgeon is positioned to the right of the patient, the first assistant opposite him/her, and the second assistant to the left of the first surgeon. The skin is then disinfected with iodinated solution. Surgical drapes (of cloth or disposable adhesive) are positioned. Usually, we place an adhesive film (such as Steri-drape) over the skin.

Start of the Procedure

Exploration of the Abdominal Cavity

1. *The incision:* A subcostal bilateral incision or, rarely, a median incision is made.
2. *Exploration of the abdominal cavity*: Extrapancreatic metastases are excluded by checking for the presence of peritoneal carcinosis and ascites fluid (if present, a sample is taken for cytological examination) as well as by assessing any duodenal or transverse mesocolon infiltration.
3. *Echography (IOUS)*: This technique enables the lesion to be accurately identified and permits the surgical team to ascertain the vascular relationships with respect to the superior mesenteric artery and the superior mesenteric vein. Scanning of the hepatic parenchyma identifies the presence of metastases that were not detected in the preoperative work-up.
   Exploration of the abdominal cavity and echography can also be conducted by laparoscopy with laparoscopic ultrasound. The indications for laparoscopy with echolaparoscopy are:

a)   Abdominal effusion detected at the preoperative diagnostic examination
b)   Preoperative imaging suspicion of hepatic and/or lymph node lesions
c)   High levels of tumor markers (CA 19-9) unjustified by cholestasis

A 10-mm umbilical trocar and a 10-mm trocar are used on the right side for the video camera and laparoscopic echographic probe, and a trocar in the left hypochondrium for the grasping forceps. This plays an important role in highlighting metastases that are "occult" to the various diagnostic imaging techniques employed in the preoperative work-up.

Echographic scans of the liver are conducted to search for signs of disease spread, with infiltrations staged in terms of their contiguity/continuity with surrounding structures. Laparoscopy provides useful information regarding the presence of lymphadenomegalies, some of which may simply be inflammatory but others already macroscopically metastatic. A biopsy sample can be obtained and an extemporary histological examination performed. The Mascagni lymph node and the periportal lymph nodes are particularly visible. It is possible to explore the retrocavity to search for peritoneal or lymph node tumor localizations.

4. *Lymph node biopsy*: The utility of extemporary histological examination of a lymph node biopsy is still a matter of debate, since in low-risk patients with localized resectable pancreatic cancer the presence of metastases in the locoregional lymph nodes is not necessarily an absolute contraindication to a pancreaticoduodenectomy (PD). A lymph node biopsy is performed in case the patient proves to be at high-risk with suspected adenopathies, and in whom the result of lymph node positivity could represent a contraindication to PD.

Pancreaticoduodenectomy: Traverso-Longmire Technique (with Preservation of the Pylorus)

As a mnemonic we use the clock-scheme of the M.D. Anderson Cancer Center of the University of Texas: colo-epiploic detachment; extended Kocher maneuver; portal dissection; section of the stomach; section of the jejunum; section of the pancreas.

Exploration of the Pancreas and of the Lesion To Evaluate the Resectability of the Head of the Pancreas

1. *Colo-epiploic detachment with liberation of the hepatic flexure:* This permits access to the retrocavity of the epiploon, evaluation of the upper side of the transverse mesocolon and the lymph nodes of the mesenteric pedicle, and exposure of the anterior face of the pancreas.

2. *Mobilisation of the duodenum and the head of the pancreas*: The so-called Kocher maneuver is the first operative stage in the surgical exploration of the pancreas head. It enables the duodenum to be mobilised as far as the superi-

or mesenteric vein in order to search, by means of palpation, for any vascular filtration. The Kocher maneuver must be supplemented by sectioning of the peritoneum from the right margin of the common bile duct up to the left margin of the superior mesenteric artery.

Demolitive Surgery

1. *Dissection of the hepatic pedicle with cholecystectomy and lymphectomy:* A bipolar forceps, scissors, and a suture passer are used to open the lesser omentum and isolate the elements of the hepatic pedicle, which are looped onto differently colored elastic vessel bands (yellow for the biliary duct, red for the hepatic artery, and blue for the portal vein).
First, the cystic artery is sectioned; the gallbladder is then separated from the hepatic bed. By means of traction towards the right of the bile duct and towards the left of the hepatic artery itself, the anterior face of the portal vein is exposed, which in turn is isolated with an elastic vessel band. This stage also enables the surgeon to check for any infiltration of the mesenteric-portal axis by the tumor. Lymphadenectomy of the hepatic pedicle is then performed. The main bile duct is sectioned proximally above the cystic duct. We use two Vicryl 4-0 sutures as anatomical reference points at the two margins of the section, fixed on mosquito-type forceps. The biliary stump should be clamped shut to avoid ischemia of the tissues; alternatively, a balloon catheter may be positioned to drain the bile away during subsequent stages of the procedure.

2. *Sectioning of the duodenum and of the first jejunal loop*: The duodenum is freed from its "anchor" with the hepatic pedicle and then sectioned. This is necessary to locate the posterosuperior pancreaticoduodenal vein on the right side of the portal vein.
The gastroduodenal artery is then located; it originates from the common hepatic artery. Of note, it should be ascertained that it is, in fact, the gastroduodenal artery and not the hepatic artery arising from the aorta or from the superior mesenteric artery, nor is it a vessel supplying the arterial vascularization of the liver, arising from the superior mesenteric artery. To do this, the gastroduodenal artery is temporarily clamped and the presence of a good pulsation of the arteries supplying the liver confirmed. The gastroduodenal artery is then sectioned. The duodenal section is performed 2–3 cm downstream from the pylorus, using a linear mechanical suture instrument, while respecting the gastroepiploic arch; the stomach is mobilized upwards and to the left.
The transverse colon is raised and displaced to the right of the mass of loops of small intestine, exposing the angle of Treitz and the fourth portion of the duodenum. The inferior mesenteric pedicle is displaced to the left, exposing the ligament of Treitz, which is sectioned. At approximately 10 cm from the duodenojejunal angle, the jejunum is sectioned using a linear mechanical suture instrument. The proximal segment is freed from the first jejunal vessels by sectioning between ligatures or by using Ligasure.

At this point the freed jejunal segment is replaced at the supramesocolic level by passing it from the left to the right and posteriorly to the superior mesenteric pedicle (retromesenteric skewing). During this maneuver, attention must be paid to several delicate veins that link the middle colic vein and the superior mesenteric vein to the inferior pancreaticoduodenal vein. Alternatively, it is possible to mobilize the Treitz and section the jejunum at the duodenal side after having applied gentle traction in a mediolateral direction.

3. *Pancreatic section*: By passing a swab mounted on a forceps or on the finger of the surgeon, retroisthmic detachment is performed and the isthmus is surrounded with tape. This maneuver must be carried out rigorously, keeping to the anterior wall of the portal vein without lateral or medial displacement in order to avoid laceration of the small venous collaterals, which can cause hemorrhages that are troublesome and difficult to control at this stage of the operation.

The pancreas is sectioned 2–3 cm to the left of the superior mesenteric vein, after it has been ensured that the splenic artery is accurately isolated. This artery sometimes appears as a lump in the anterolateral direction and it can prove dangerous if not identified. Dissection is performed with a cold scalpel. Hemostasis follows by ligation of the superior and inferior pancreatic arteries and of the small vessels of the pancreatic remnant, paying close attention to the duct of Wirsung, which must be identified and cannulated.

4. *Freeing of the pancreas from the superior mesenteric vein*: At this stage, the prepared block, including the duodenum, pancreas head, main biliary duct, and gallbladder, is mobilized, thereby providing access to the venous floor, which comprises the portal vein and the superior mesenteric vein. The head of the pancreas and the hooked process must be freed from the superior mesenteric vein. Gentle traction towards the right is applied to the head. This is the most delicate stage of the operation, involving sectioning of the superior and inferior pancreaticoduodenal vessels. Exposure of the retroportal laminar is then undertaken, selectively tying the small veins that arise in a perpendicular manner from it, close to the portal vein.

The superior mesenteric artery is meticulously examined. The exeresis thus performed exposes the mesentericoportal venous axis, which receives on the left the splenic vein and sometimes the inferior mesenteric vein.

5. *Lymphadenectomy:* Once the surgical specimen has been removed en bloc, skeletonization of the hepatic hilum is completed, both for oncological reasons and to prepare the biliary wall for construction of the anastomosis. At this point, the lymph nodes of the upper portion of the hepatoduodenal ligament are removed. (Station 12 lymph nodes: 12a1 $^1/_2$ superior to the hepatic artery itself, 12b1 $^1/_2$ superior to the bile duct, 12v1 $^1/_2$ superior to the portal vein, and superior and inferior pancreatic lymph nodes are station 13) according to the general rules proposed by the Japanese Pancreas Society classification. The decision as to the type of procedure must then be made, i.e., standard or radical?

The *standard* procedure consists of en bloc lymph node removal from the right side of the hepatoduodenal ligament (12b1, 12b2, and 12c), removal of the posterior pancreaticoduodenal lymph nodes (13a and 13b), nodes to the right of the superior mesenteric artery from its origin from the aorta up to the origin of the pancreaticoduodenal artery (14a and 14b) as well as the anterior pancreaticoduodenal lymph nodes (17a and 17b) and the removal of the lymph nodes from the anterosuperior portion of the common hepatic artery (8a).

The extent of the lymphadenectomy that we perform is recognized as falling exclusively within the "standard" lymphadenectomy procedure.

Reconstructive Surgery

The three stages of this scheme are described by the mnemonic clock-scheme of the M.D. Anderson Cancer Center of the University of Texas: proceeding in an anticlockwise direction, the pancreatic duct, biliary duct and alimentary tract are reconstructed.

1. *Pancreaticojejunal anastomosis (end-to-side Wirsung-jejunal anastomosis):* This is performed upstream of all the other anastomoses, approximately 2–3 cm downstream from the sinking of the jejunal loop. Our approach is a terminal anastomosis on the pancreas and a lateral anastomosis on the jejunum, at the level of the antimesenteric margin, in double layers. The procedure begins with a continuous suture using polypropylene 4-0, seromuscular on the jejunal side and capsuloparenchymal on the pancreatic side, subject to cannulation of the Wirsung duct in order to avoid accidental lesions or closures.

   In the second stage of suturing, interrupted stitches, 4-0 slow-absorbing parenchymal sutures are used on the pancreatic side and full-thickness sutures on the jejunal side. Suturing on the anterior floor is thus completed. If the dimensions of the Wirsung duct permit, a Wirsung-jejunostomy is then carried out (Fig. 19.2). This anastomosis entails two levels of sutures: pancreaticojejunal to fix the pancreatic remnant to the serosa of the loop and Wirsung-jejunal, in the literal sense, between the wall of the excretory duct and the jejunal mucosa. This is begun from the posterior plane. We usually position a Silastic drainage stent inside the Wirsung duct to drain the anastomosis. Then a continuous polypropylene 4-0 suture is applied with extramucosal stitches on the jejunal side and on the capsuloparenchymal pancreatic side.

   Once the posterior plane is completed, the more interior area is commenced; the stitches, using slow-absorbing suture of caliber 5-0 and in this case interrupted, are applied to the duct wall and the carefully opened jejunal mucosa. The anterior wall is completed in continuous sutures of polypropylene 4-0.

2. *End-to-side hepaticojejunal anastomosis:* In patients in whom the duct is dilated due to stasis, this is a technically straightforward procedure. Approximately 10 cm downstream of the pancreatic anastomosis, a jejunostomy is performed on the antimesenteric portion of the loop. The width of the jejunostomy should be suitable for the caliber of the bile duct. The jejunal incision should not be excessive, as it can easily widen during the course of the procedure and during stretching by the surgeon. The mucosa is then

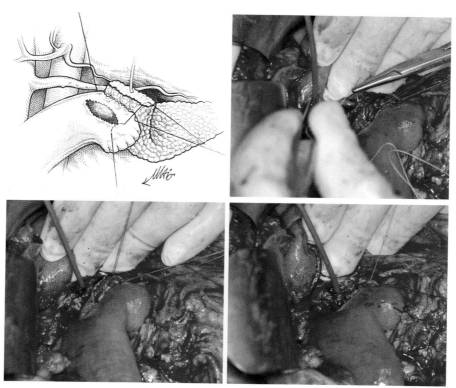

Fig. 19.2 Wirsung jejunal anastomosis

removed at the level of the jejunal breech, grasping the mucosa with anatomical forceps. It is lifted and removed with an electric scalpel (whose power should be reduced during this stage), creating a length of wall that is demucosated around the entire circumference of the jejunostomy (Fig. 19.3).

The common hepatic duct is fixed to the surface of the jejunum by means of two angled sutures; using a mounted swab, the assistant lowers the anterior part of the wall so as to better expose the posterior floor of the viscera. The anastomosis of the posterior wall is performed with full-thickness sutures using slow-absorption caliber 4-0 thread. Suturing is started at a central point and with interrupted stitches ("inside out/outside in") so as to obtain an extraluminal knot.

The anterior part is sutured beginning from the corners and moving towards the centre. The knot must be particularly delicate so as to avoid the possibility of any brusque movements that could cause longitudinal lacerations of the biliary duct wall, which may result in perianastomotic biliary filtration or dehiscence of the anastomosis. It is also possible to perform this anastomosis with two semi-continuous sutures, which must still be slow-absorbing and caliber 4-0.

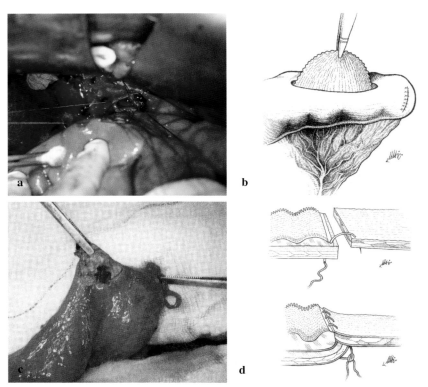

Fig. 19.3 a End-to-side hepaticojejunal anastomosis; **b** jejunal mucosectomy; **c** preparation
of the jejunal segment; **d** hepatico-jejunal anastomosis

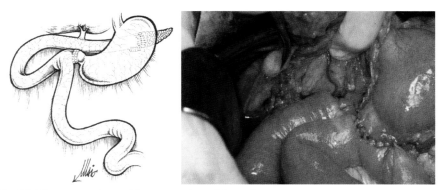

Fig. 19.4 Reconstruction, with preservation of the pylorus

3. *End-to-side duodenojejunal anastomosis*: This procedure is carried out at approximately 30 cm from the biliary anastomosis, with monolayered interrupted sutures using slow-absorbing caliber 4-0 thread (Fig. 19.4).

Surgical Removal Without Preservation of the Pylorus (Whipple Pancreaticoduodenectomy)

The second stage of radical surgery consists of removal of the distal third of the stomach.

1. *Section of the gastric antrum*: The terminal branches of the left gastric artery are ligated and sectioned along the lesser curvature. The stomach is dissected approximately 10 cm upstream of the pylorus with a mechanical suture instrument. The omentum is dissected at the level of the transection of the greater curvature. The line of mechanical suture is sunk for haemostatic reasons with an overcast stitch of reabsorbable monofilament suture. Reconstruction of the digestive continuity (*Child's reconstruction*) provides for the pancreas, bile duct, and stomach to be drained in succession by the proximal jejunum.
2. *End-to-side gastrojejunal anastomosis:* In this submesocolic approach, a breech in the left of the transverse mesocolon is fashioned and the gastric stump pulled downwards, in a double layer. The mechanical suture is removed, starting from the greater curvature, for 5–6 cm.
A posterior layer of seroserosal running suture is fashioned as a "support;" we then open the jejunum on the antimesocolic side and proceed with stitching of the posterior wall using interrupted slow-absorbing sutures and caliber 4-0 thread; occasionally, we use two semi-continuous sutures, still with the same type of thread, first for the posterior wall and then for the anterior wall. This anastomosis is carried out at least 40 cm downstream of the biliary anastomosis in order to avoid traction on it. Finally, two drainage collection devices are positioned: a Jackson-Pratt type near the pancreatic anastomosis, and a tubular drainage device near the biliary anastomosis.

Suggested Reading

Cameron JL (ed) (2001) American Cancer Society atlas of clinical oncology: Pancreatic cancer. BC Decker, Hamilton, Ontario, Canada
Evans DB, Lee JE, Pisters PWT (2004) Pancreaticoduodenectomy (Whipple operation) and total pancreatectomy for cancer. In: Baker RJ, Fischer JE (eds) Mastery of surgery, 4th edn. vol 2. Lippincott Williams & Wilkins, Philadelphia, pp 1322–1341
Gazzaniga GM, Filauro M, Bagarolo C et al (1997) Le neoplasie delle vie biliari extraepatiche: 99° Congresso della Società Italiana di Chirurgia : Padova, 19-22 ottobre 1997. Società Italiana di Chirurgia, Rome

Jaeck D, Boudjema K, Bachellier P et al (1998) Exeresi pancreatiche cefaliche: duodeno-cefalo-pancreasectomie (DCP). Encycl Méd Chir Elsevier, Paris Tecniche Chirurgiche Addominali, 40-880-B, p 17

Kremer K (ed) (1993) Atlas of operative surgery USES, vol 2. Gallbladder, bile ducts, pancreas. Tumours of the exocrine pancreas. Thieme, Stuttgart, New York, pp 199–234

Chapter 20

Surgical Treatment of the Pancreatic Stump: Technical Notes

Gianpaolo Balzano, Enrico Ortolano, Marco Braga

Introduction

The aim of this chapter is to give an overview of different ways of treating the pancreatic stump after pancreaticoduodenectomy, describing and illustrating the surgical techniques, but neither addressing results nor comparing these reconstructive techniques, because that will be the subject of the next chapter. Here we describe the techniques of pancreaticojejunostomy and pancreaticogastrostomy (and their main variations), and the technique of occlusion of the main pancreatic duct (with no anastomosis). First, we will briefly treat two further important aspects: the choice of sewing materials and the preparation of the pancreatic stump. And a final recommendation: whatever technique you choose, pancreatic anastomosis will require a long, plodding procedure. Pancreatic surgery is not suited to the hasty surgeon.

Suturing Materials

An in vitro study estimated the durability of different suturing materials: polydioxanone (PDS), Vicryl (polyglactin 910, coated Vicryl), polyglycolic acid (Dexon), plain catgut, chromic catgut, silk, polypropylene (Prolene). The materials were left in a solution of pancreatic secretion and bile. Those with the greatest tensile strength were PDS, silk, and polypropylene; Vicryl and Dexon lost almost all their tensile strength in 1 week [1]. A pancreatic fistula could therefore occur more often when an absorbable thread is used, or an initially low-output fistula could increase its output once the sutures have been digested. The advice is thus to use potentially tough threads, not absorbable ones such as silk or polypropylene or slowly absorbable ones as PDS. With regard to thread thickness, the use of a slightly thicker thread (3-0 or 4-0) for the external layer and a thinner one (4-0 or 5-0) for the internal layer is often reported. Authors rarely report which thread they use for the anastomosis; however, as an example the following are the suture materials used by some pancreatic surgeons: Büchler: PDS 5-0 [2]; Yeo: silk 3-0 for the external layer, an absorbable thread for the

W. Siquini (Ed.), *Surgical Treatment of Pancreatic Diseases*.
©Springer-Verlag Italia 2009

internal one [3]; Warshaw: a 3-0 nonresorbable thread for the external layer, a 4-0 absorbable thread for the internal one [4].

Preparation of the Pancreatic Stump

Once the existence of a cleavage between the posterior aspect of the pancreas and the mesenteric–portal vein has been verified, and after tumor invasion of mesenteric vessels (in the case of a tumor of the uncinate process) has been excluded, the indication for resection can be confirmed.

1. *Preparation of the neck.* The superior and inferior margins of the pancreatic neck are exposed (anterior to venous axis) in order to place four hemostatic 3–0 stitches passing through the whole thickness of the cranial and caudal margins of the pancreas, within 1 cm of the section line. The threads are pulled by a mosquito forceps to enable further mobilization of the stump.

2. *Section of the pancreas.* The section must be made anterior to the mesenteric–portal vein. To avoid vascular injuries, a large dissecting forceps (such as O'Shaughnessy) is positioned posterior to the pancreas. We advise using a cold scalpel with a large blade, taking great care to do a sharp-cut vertical section of the pancreatic parenchyma that will facilitate reconstruction. Otherwise the electric scalpel can be used, but only in the most superficial portion, to avoid injuring the duct of Wirsung (main pancreatic duct), which usually lies next to the posterior margin. After the section, the second operator exerts hemostatic pressure on the section margin of the pancreatic body, while the first operator obtains a new section of the margin towards the pancreatic head (always with the regular scalpel) for frozen section examination. The next step will be bleeding control: hemostasis on the head margin can be easily achieved by electrocautery, but manipulation of the pancreatic stump margin should be gentle and precise. First of all the duct of Wirsung must be identified, avoiding accidentally damaging it; then hemostasis is carried out. Most of the bleeding sources will be controlled by electrocauterization, but in the case of bleeding from vessels of larger diameter or next to the Wirsung duct, it will be safer to use a hemostatic suture (polypropylene 5-0).

3. *Preparation of the pancreatic stump.* The pancreatic remnant must be prepared for at least 2 cm; sutures on the external layer of the anastomosis will be made between this part of the mobilized pancreatic stump and the jejunal seromuscularis layer, as will be described below. The parenchyma must be properly exposed, separating it from the fat that usually enwraps it on the anterior surface, and from the lymphatic and adipose tissues that overlie the superior margin of the gland. Pulling gently on the two stitches on the superior and inferior margins of the pancreatic remnant facilitates its mobilization. It is always necessary to perform ligatures and sections of small collateral veins, tributaries of the splenic vein, to prepare the posterior layer.

Classical Pancreaticojejunostomy

This is the most common reconstruction after pancreaticoduodenectomy (Fig. 20.1). We use this technique for low-risk anastomoses (dilated duct, hard consistency of pancreatic parenchyma). Pancreatic, biliary, and jejunal (gastric) anastomoses are performed in sequence on the same jejunal segment, transposed through the transverse mesocolon. Recently we began to perform an antecolic duodenojejunostomy (or gastrojejunostomy) in order to distance it from the pancreaticojejunostomy, in the hope of reducing the incidence of delayed gastric emptying, which is usually due to complications relating to pancreaticojejunostomy.

Technique Used in the Case of a Dilated Pancreatic Duct

We set up the anastomosis leaving a jejunal remnant 2–3 cm in length (Fig. 20.2). The posterior wall of the pancreas (previously prepared) must be well exposed, pulling on the above-mentioned stitches or gently inserting an atraumatic instrument into the pancreatic duct to overturn the tip of the remnant. The posterior layer is started at the superior margin, stitching in a direction perpendicular to the pancreatic section, carefully leaving the pancreatic section margin free for at least 0.5 cm. This margin will be used to perform the internal layer. In this case (Fig. 20.3) a continuous external suture has been placed, but interrupted stitches can be used when utmost caution is required.

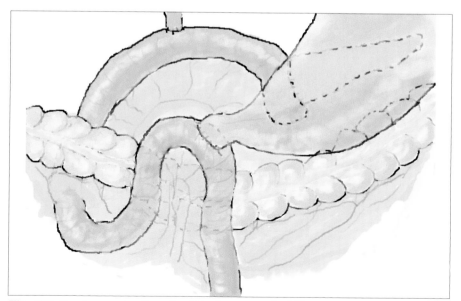

Fig. 20.1 Usual reconstruction after PD: the pancreatic, biliary and duodenal (or gastric) anastomoses are performed on the same jejunal limb

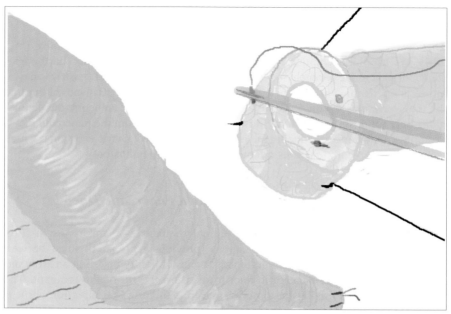

Fig. 20.2 Pancreaticojejunostomy in case of dilated Wirsung duct: the outer posterior suture is placed so that the cut margin remains free for the inner suture.

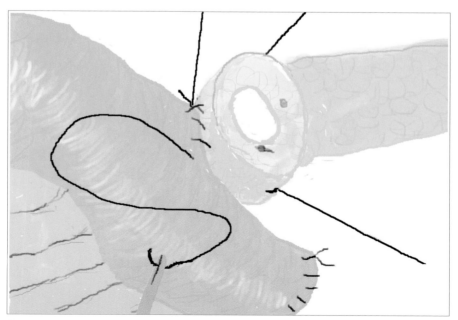

Fig. 20.3 Pancreaticojejunostomy in case of dilated Wirsung duct: the outer suture can be performed as a running suture (as in the figure), or with interrupted stitches

The external posterior layer is completed (Fig. 20.4); the jejunal limb is then opened 1 cm distal to the suture line, for a tract slightly longer than the pancreatic duct, but smaller than the diameter of the pancreatic remnant. Then the internal layer of suturing starts: the suture is placed piercing through the pancreas from the lumen of the Wirsung duct to the section margin left free in the previous phase (Fig. 20.5). If the duct is dilated and the parenchyma atrophic, the internal suturing could be continuous, but in any case we prefer interrupted sutures, as they are more precise (Fig. 20.6). All the sutures are placed before any are tied ("parachute" technique). In this way the knots will be inside the anastomosis, but using thin suture threads (5-0), especially if they are absorbable, prevents any long-term consequence.

The internal posterior layer is done and the internal anterior layer is started with the same interrupted parachute suture technique (Figs. 20.7, 20.8). A continuous suture on the external anterior layer completes the anastomosis (Fig. 20.9).

Technique in the Case of a Small Duct of Wirsung

The technique described here requires suturing the pancreatic duct as the first step. Other authors, when dealing with a small duct of Wirsung, prefer to pro-

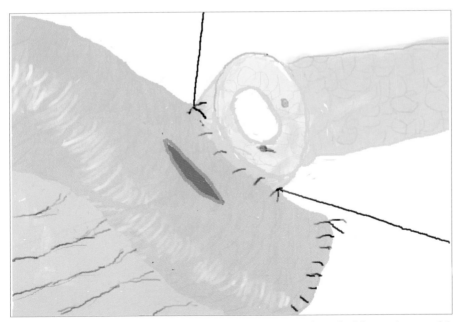

Fig. 20.4 Pancreaticojejunostomy in case of dilated Wirsung duct: the jejunum is opened 1 cm from the previous suture line; the incision is slightly longer than the duct.

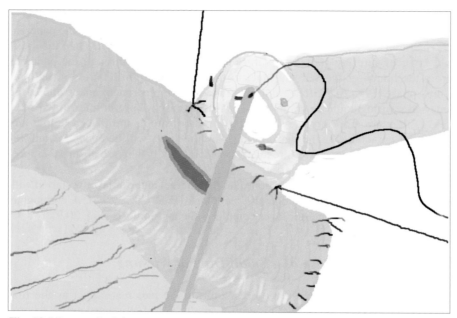

Fig. 20.5 Pancreaticojejunostomy in case of dilated Wirsung duct: the sutures of the inner posterior layer are placed from inside the duct and include the posterior cut end of the pancreas

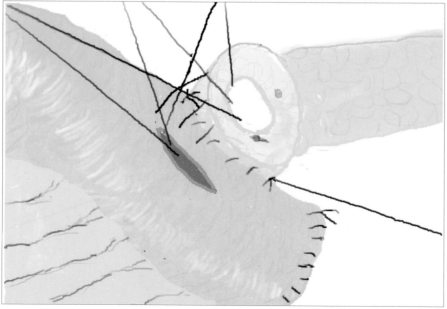

Fig. 20.6 Pancreaticojejunostomy in case of dilated Wirsung duct: the inner posterior layer is performed with interrupted sutures, tying the knots after placing all the stitches (parachute technique)

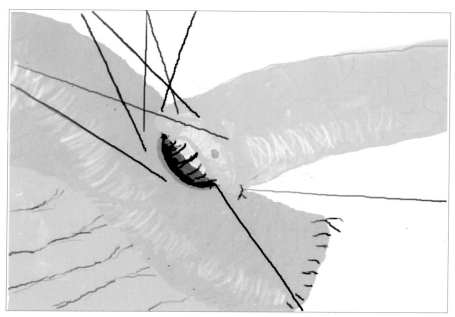

Fig. 20.7 Pancreaticojejunostomy in case of dilated Wirsung duct: also the inner anterior layer is performed with interrupted sutures (parachute technique)

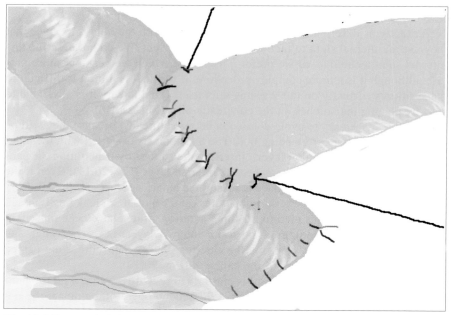

Fig. 20.8 Pancreaticojejunostomy in case of dilated Wirsung duct: the inner anterior layer has been completed

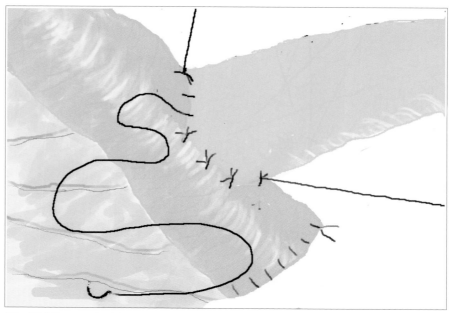

Fig. 20.9 Pancreaticojejunostomy in case of dilated Wirsung duct: the outer anterior layer can be performed with a running (or interrupted) suture

ceed exactly as described above for a dilated duct, with the only difference that they use an internal stent to facilitate suture of the duct. We do not describe this internal stent technique, as we prefer a technique which we consider more precise, although it is a more complex procedure. If the duct is thin, it is difficult to place sutures correctly on the Wirsung duct itself. That is why it is advisable to start by placing the stitches on the pancreatic duct (Fig. 20.10).

It will be necessary to avoid confusion between threads, because they will be there for a long time before being tied. The anastomosis is started with the anterior sutures (anterior internal layer), inserting the sutures by penetrating the pancreatic duct wall from the external to the internal layer (Fig. 20.11). Even if the duct is small, it is possible to place at least three anterior sutures (at the 10–12–2 o'clock positions) and three posterior sutures (at the 4–6–8 o'clock positions) in almost every case. In this picture the three anterior sutures have been placed.

Placing the posterior sutures (posterior internal layer) is the next step and will be facilitated by gently pulling the anterior sutures. The sutures are passed from the lumen to the cut end of the pancreas (Fig. 20.12).

The external posterior suturing is started (Fig. 20.13). Sutures on the pancreatic duct are pulled toward the side of the second operator, being careful not to tangle them, pulling the anterior and posterior sutures apart from the others. As described for the case of a dilated Wirsung duct, the posterior suture layer is started from the superior margin, suturing in a direction perpendicular to the

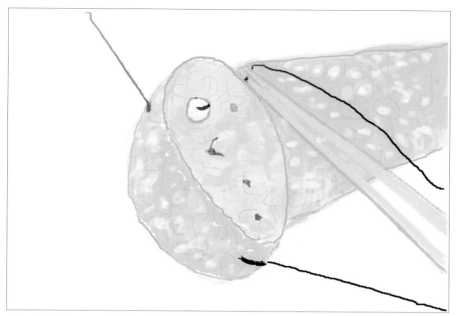

Fig. 20.10 Pancreaticojejunostomy in case of small Wirsung duct: ductal anterior stitches from outside the cut pancreatic margin are placed first

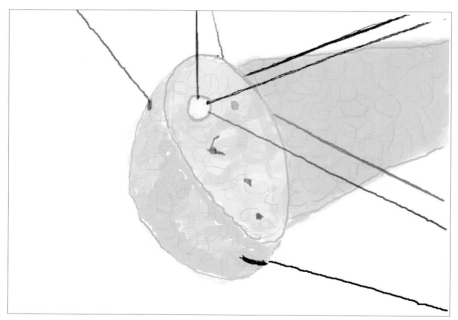

Fig. 20.11 Pancreaticojejunostomy in case of small Wirsung duct: at least 3 or 4 ductal stitches must be passed anterior

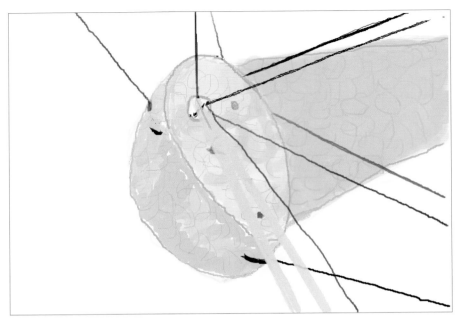

Fig. 20.12 Pancreaticojejunostomy in case of small Wirsung duct: after the placement of the anterior stitches, 3 or 4 posterior ductal stitches are passed from inside the duct to the posterior cut margin

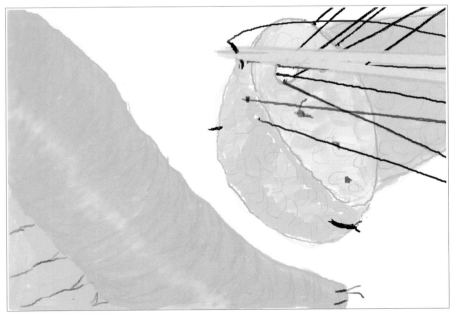

Fig. 20.13 Pancreaticojejunostomy in case of small Wirsung duct: the outer posterior suture is then started, paying attention to leave the cut margin free

cut end of the pancreas, leaving the pancreatic section margin free for at least 0.5 cm.

On the posterior external layer interrupted sutures are performed. All sutures are placed before any are tied ("parachute" technique) (Figs. 20.14; 20.15).

On the jejunal limb an incision is made not longer than 1 cm next to the transected end of the pancreatic duct, 1 cm distant from the previous suture line. The three posterior sutures previously passed through the pancreatic duct are inserted in the jejunal opening (Fig. 20.16).

The small opening on the jejunal limb does not include all the possible secondary ducts on the cut end of pancreas (which would anyway cause a "pure", and hence low-risk, pancreatic fistula. However, it has the advantage of limiting the jejunal fluid output should the anastomosis leak.

It is possible to fasten a duct-to-mucosa pancreaticojejunostomy with two sutures at the 3 o'clock (Fig. 20.17) and the 9 o'clock position. The posterior internal wall is completed with some interrupted sutures passed through the jejunal limb and pancreatic margin (Fig. 20.18). Then sutures on the anterior wall of the Wirsung duct are passed (Fig. 20.19) and the anterior internal layer is completed with sutures passed through the pancreatic margin and jejunal limb (Fig. 20.19). The anastomosis is completed by oversewing the anterior external wall with interrupted sutures (parachute technique) (Fig. 20.20).

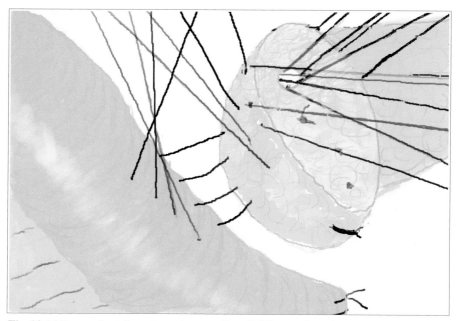

Fig. 20.14 Pancreaticojejunostomy in case of small Wirsung duct: the outer posterior suture is performed by interrupted sutures tying the knots after the placement of all the stitches

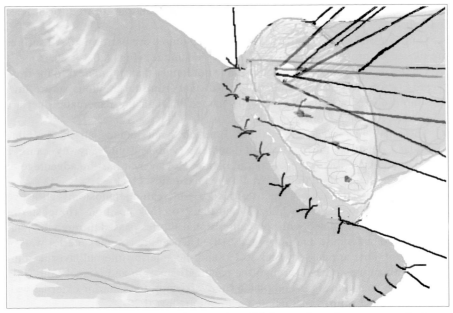

Fig. 20.15 Pancreaticojejunostomy in case of small Wirsung duct: the outer posterior layer has been completed

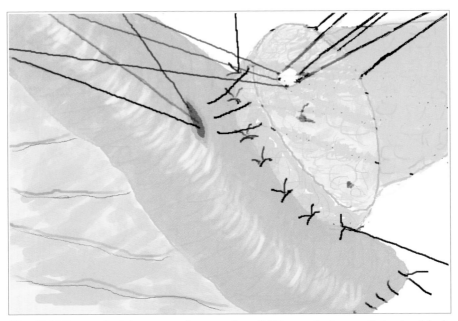

Fig. 20.16 Pancreaticojejunostomy in case of small Wirsung duct: a small duodenal incision has been made (1 cm from the previous suture line) and the previously placed ductal posterior sutures have been passed through the jejunal opening

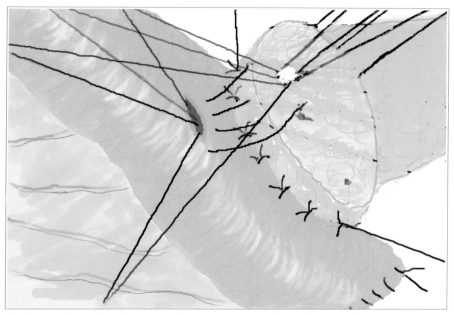

Fig. 20.17 Pancreaticojejunostomy in case of small Wirsung duct: two further sutures can be passed at 3 and 9 o'clock

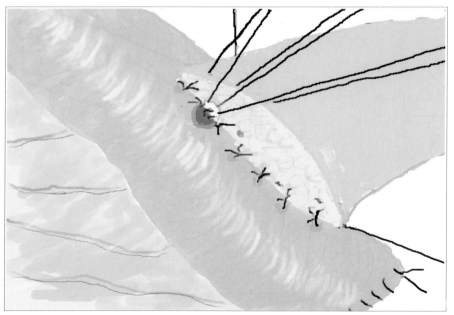

Fig. 20.18 Pancreaticojejunostomy in case of small Wirsung duct: the inner posterior layer is completed by some stitches passed from the pancreatic margin to the jejunal wall

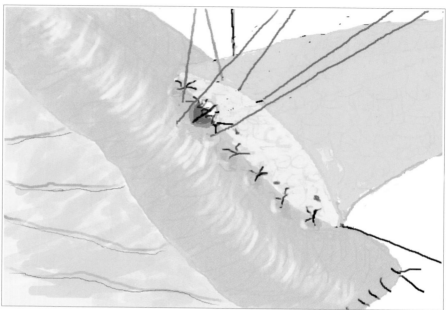

Fig. 20.19 Pancreaticojejunostomy in case of small Wirsung duct: the inner anterior layer is performed by passing the previously placed ductal sutures through the jejunal incision

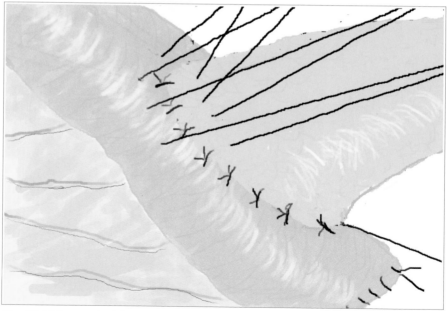

Fig. 20.20 Pancreaticojejunostomy in case of small Wirsung duct: after the completion of the inner layer, the last interrupted suture row (outer anterior layer) is placed with the parachute technique.

Isolated Roux-en-Y Loop Pancreaticojejunostomy

In a case of pancreatic fistula, Roux-en-Y pancreaticojejunostomy should prevent activation of pancreatic enzymes, as pancreatic juice is not activated by bile. The proximal jejunal limb is passed through a transmesocolic opening different (more medial) from the one for the jejunal limb for biliary and duodenal or (gastric) anastomoses. Isolated Roux-en-Y for pancreatic anastomosis has to be 40 cm long at least, to prevent biliary and alimentary reflux on the pancreatic anastomosis itself (Fig. 20.21).

Pancreaticojejunostomy with External Diversion of Pancreatic Juice

This technique can be used to further reduce the risk in cases of a high-risk pancreatic stump (small duct of Wirsung, soft pancreas). A catheter is passed through the jejunal limb; the upper extremity is inserted into the pancreatic duct, the latter is brought externally, using the Volker or Witzel technique. In Fig. 20.22 this anastomosis is performed with an isolated Roux-en-Y limb as this is

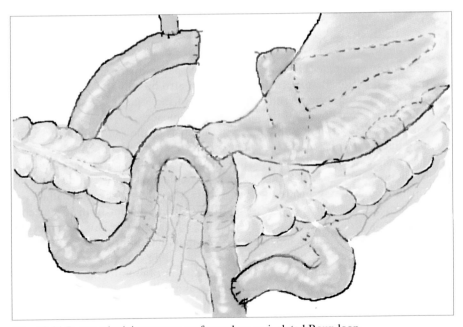

Fig. 20.21 Pancreaticojejunostomy performed on an isolated Roux loop

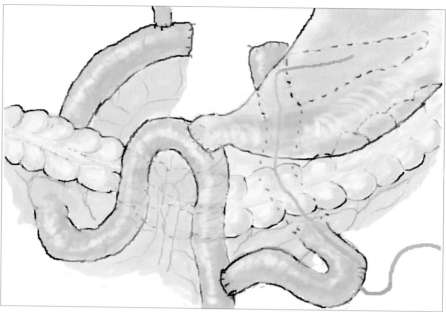

Fig. 20.22 Isolated Roux loop pancreaticojejunostomy with external stenting of the pancreatic duct

our preferred technique in cases of high-risk pancreatic remnant. However, external diversion of the pancreatic juice could also be combined with a "standard" reconstruction, bringing the catheter out of the jejunal segment wall between the biliary and duodenal (or gastric) anastomoses.

A blunt catheter (to prevent damage to the duct) of the same diameter as the Wirsung duct is usually used; it must also have multiple side openings to drain as much pancreatic secretion as possible. It is important to check that there are no obstructions to its insertion into the pancreatic duct (stenoses, angles); all the side openings must stay inside the duct itself. After this check, the catheter is passed through an opening of the jejunal limb 30 cm distant from its cut end; then it is brought out 3–4 cm distant from the jejunal stump. This step must be performed before the anastomosis starts: the manipulation of the jejunal limb necessary for the passage of the catheter is impossible once the posterior layer of the anastomosis is done. To take the catheter out of the limb, we advise pushing it against the wall (as in Fig. 20.23) and making an incision in this point by electrocauterization.

The ductal stitches are passed, as described above, in the case of a small duct. The posterior external layer is then started, as already described (Fig. 20.24) and the posterior external and internal walls completed (Fig. 20.25).

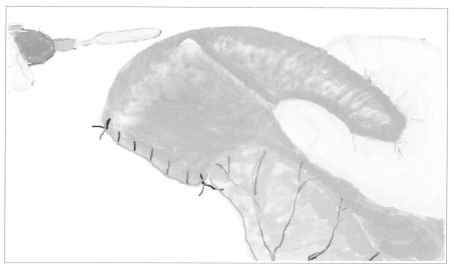

Fig. 20.23 External stenting of the pancreatic duct: after passing the stent inside the jejunal limb, the stent tip is pushed against the jejunal wall to facilitate its extraction

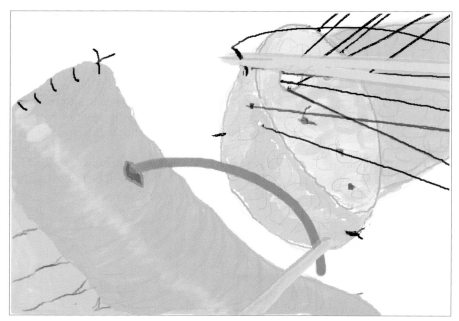

Fig. 20.24 External stenting of the pancreatic duct: ductal stitches have been passed as previously described; the outer posterior layer is beginning

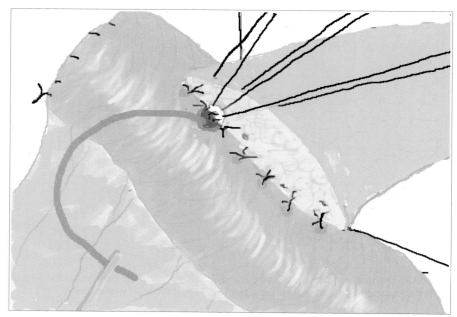

Fig. 20.25 External stenting of the pancreatic duct: the inner posterior layer is performed with the same modalities of the technique in case of small Wirsung duct

The catheter is fastened to the jejunal limb, so as to prevent its displacing, a 5-0 absorbable (e.g. Monocryl or Vicryl) suture. A suture is placed 1 cm distant from the jejunal opening (Fig. 20.26); the catheter is pierced 1–2 cm distant from the last opening, leaving all the side openings inside the duct; suture is passed again through the jejunal limb, bringing it out next to the point of entry, so that the knot remains outside the jejunal opening. The catheter insertion is then complete.

The anastomosis is completed with the same technique already described for the case of a small Wirsung duct (Fig. 20.27). The catheter will be removed after reabsorption of the fastening suture (mean: 30–40 days).

Pancreaticogastrostomy

Classical Pancreaticogastrostomy

Several authors consider anastomosis between the pancreatic stump and posterior gastric wall a good alternative to pancreaticojejunostomy. Technical details concerning sutures or the differences when dealing with a dilated or a small pancreatic duct are similar to what we described for pancreaticojejunostomy (Fig. 20.28).

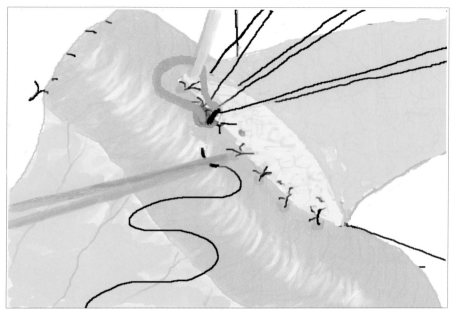

Fig. 20.26 External stenting of the pancreatic duct: a stitch is passed to fasten the stent; the stitch enters the jeunum 1 cm distant from the opening margin. The catheter is pierced so that all its holes remain inside the pancreatic duct. The stitch is then passed again into the jejunal opening and brought outside next to its insertion point, so that the knot remains outside the jejunum

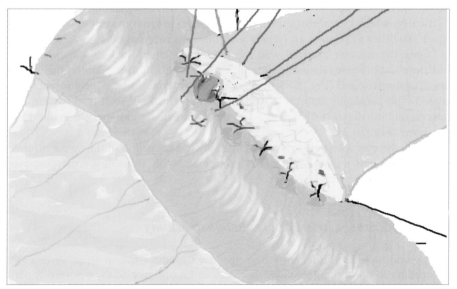

Fig. 20.27 External stenting of the pancreatic duct: the catheter has been inserted in the duct; anterior ductal stitches have been passed through the jejunal opening. The completion of the anastomosis will be accomplished as previously described.

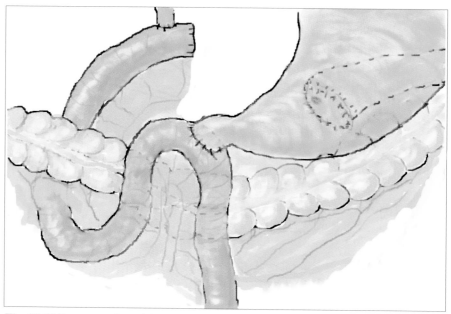

Fig. 20.28 Reconstruction with pancreaticogastrostomy

The pancreatic stump must be adequately mobilized (at least 2–3 cm). The second operator exposes the posterior gastric wall. The anastomosis will be set vertically at least 5 cm distant from the pylorus (or from the cut end of the stomach) in order to prevent an ischemia of the visceral margin (Fig. 20.29).

Once the anterior external wall has been completed, then, at a distance of 1 cm from the previous suture, a gastric wall incision, shorter than the pancreatic stump, is performed (Fig. 20.30). The anterior internal layer is performed completed with parachute interrupted sutures as described above It is always necessary to include the duct of Wirsung and the pancreatic stump margin in the internal layer (Fig. 20.31).

The posterior internal layer is sutured (always parachute interrupted sutures) (Fig. 20.32) and the anastomosis is completed with suturing of the posterior external layer (Fig. 20.33).

Anterior Transgastric Pancreaticogastrostomy

This variation has been recently described by Claudio Bassi et al. of Verona [5]. According to them this technique is easier and more precise than posterior pancreaticogastrostomy (for illustrations see [5]). The pancreatic stump must be widely mobilized (for almost 5 cm) and an extended incision performed on the anterior gastric wall. The posterior wall is vertically opened at a level correspon-

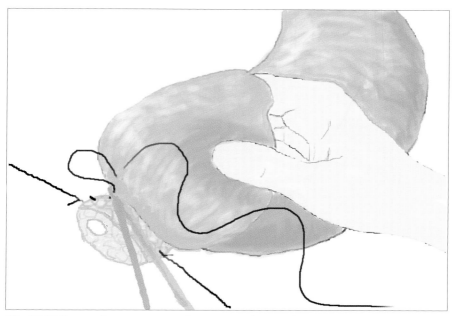

Fig. 20.29 Pancreaticogastrostomy: the anastomosis must be set at least at 5 cm from the pyloric (or gastric) margin. The first layer to be performed is the outer anterior one

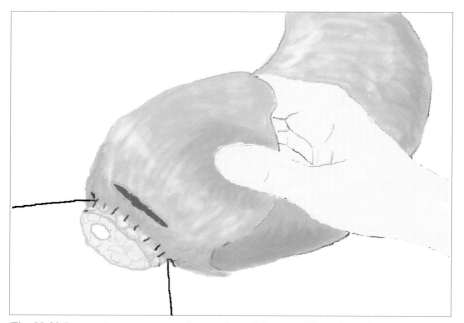

Fig. 20.30 Pancreaticogastrostomy: the gastric wall is opened 1 cm from the suture line

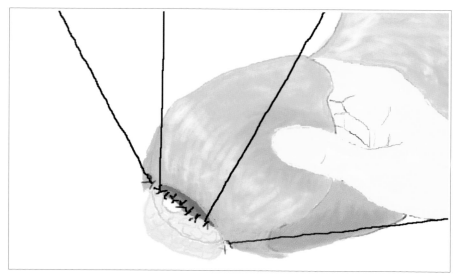

Fig. 20.31 Pancreaticogastrostomy: the inner anterior layer is performed by interrupted sutures

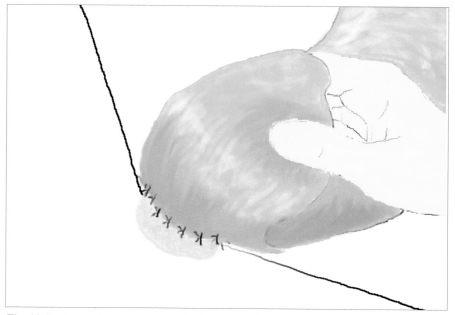

Fig. 20.32 Pancreaticogastrostomy: the inner posterior layer has been completed

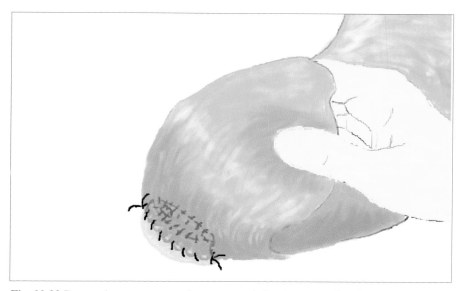

Fig. 20.33 Pancreaticogastrostomy: the anastomosis has been completed

ding to the anterior opening. The pancreatic stump is brought into the gastric lumen through the posterior opening for at least 3–4 cm, using pulling sutures placed on the stump. The external layer is sewn as the first step, placing interrupted sutures between seromuscular margin of the gastric wall and the pancreatic parenchyma; a further internal layer is then sutured, oversewing the gastric mucosa and the pancreatic wall. Additional blanket stitches passed through the pancreas and seromuscular gastric wall can be placed externally.

Occlusion of the Duct of Wirsung

This technique has been proposed as an alternative to pancreatic anastomosis and implies the abolition of exocrine pancreatic secretion. The pancreatic stump is prepared as usual (for 2–3 cm). A 4-0 purse-string suture is performed on the Wirsung duct; it is better to pass sutures through the duct, as in Fig. 20.34, rather than only through the pancreatic parenchyma, lest they could rip through the pancreas when the purse-string suture is being closed. The pancreatic stump is then closed by "fish-mouth" interrupted sutures, or by multiple U-shaped sutures (Fig. 20.35). This technique aims to prevent secretion leaks from secondary ducts onto the pancreatic cut end.

The next step consists of injection of an occluding substance into the pancreatic duct: this could help in reducing exocrine secretion. The only approved substance for this use is prolamine, although others have been used in the past, such as Neoprene, fibrin glue, and cyanoacrylate. The duct is cannulated with a catheter (Fig. 20.36) and the substance slowly injected, gradually retracting the catheter itself; the

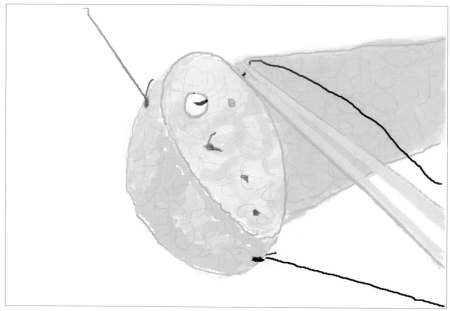

Fig. 20.34 Occlusion of the pancreatic duct: a purse-string suture is passed through the Wirsung duct

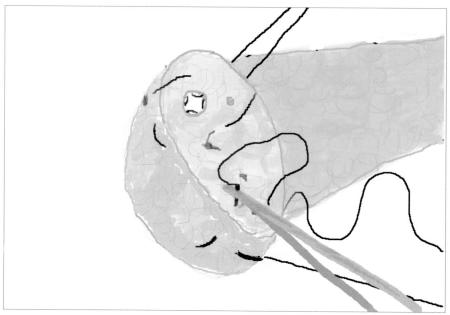

Fig. 20.35 Occlusion of the pancreatic duct: closure of the pancreatic margin by interrupted sutures

second operator is ready to tie the purse-string suture when catheter is completely retracted. The procedure is now complete (Fig. 20.37).

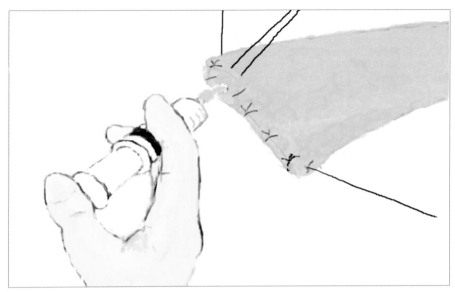

Fig. 20.36 Occlusion of the pancreatic duct: the occluding substance is gently injected through a catheter inserted in the duct, gradually withdrawing the catheter. The second operator must be ready to tie the purse-string when the catheter is completely retracted

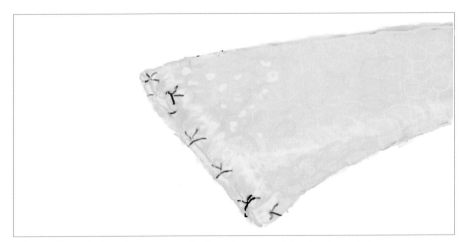

Fig. 20.37 Occlusion of the pancreatic duct: the purse-string has been tied

References

1. Muftuoglu MA, Ozkan E, Saglam A (2004) Effect of human pancreatic juice and bile on the tensile strength of suture materials. Am J Surg 188:200–203
2. Z'graggen K, Uhl W, Friess H, Büchler MW (2002) How to do a safe pancreatic anastomosis. J Hepatobiliary Pancreat Surg 9:733–737
3. Winter JM, Cameron JL, Campbell KA et al (2006) Does pancreatic duct stenting decrease the rate of pancreatic fistula following pancreaticoduodenectomy? Results of a prospective randomized trial. J Gastrointest Surg 10:1280–1290
4. Warshaw AL, Thayer SP (2004) Pancreaticoduodenectomy. J Gastrointest Surg 8:733–741
5. Bassi C, Butturini G, Salvia R et al (2006) Open pancreaticogastrostomy after pancreaticoduodenectomy: a pilot study. J Gastrointest Surg 10:1072–1080

Chapter 21

Surgical Treatment of the Pancreatic Stump: Comparing Different Techniques

Gianpaolo Balzano, Alessandro Zerbi, Valerio Di Carlo

Introduction

The pancreatic stump is the major source of morbidity and mortality of pancreatoduodenectomy (PD). Any surgeon experienced in pancreatic surgery is often dealing with the dramatic consequences of the failure of the technique he or she adopted; thus we ask ourselves what technical errors we have committed, or whether it would have been better to perform a different reconstruction, maybe an anastomosis with the stomach, or an interrupted suture instead of a continuous one, or to use a Roux-en-Y limb, or to close the stump without anastomosis. In these circumstances the questions are many and legitimate, because pancreatic surgery requires an extremely accurate technique and we need to choose the proper solution based on the pancreas' characteristics and on our own experience. However, it is important, first of all, to realize that the main actor in the dramatic consequences of pancreatic surgery is the pancreas itself, with the destructive potential of its digestive secretions. There is no evidence that any given technique is able to solve the problems of the pancreatic remnant, and no comparative study has proved one specific technique to be clearly better than another. Nevertheless, if our aim is to expose our patient who is a candidate for a PD to the smallest possible risk of death (for that is what is at issue), there is one vital element that is frequently ignored.

The "V" Factor

The international literature agrees upon one only factor that can reduce the mortality rate of PD: the "V" factor, the hospital's patient volume – that is, the number of PDs performed every year in a given hospital. It is well known that, the more complex a procedure is, the more a better outcome will depend upon the frequency with which the procedure is performed. This has been confirmed for complex surgical procedures in the fields of cardiac, vascular, thoracic, and esophageal surgery, but the procedure that by far most proved the existence of this relation is PD. Since the mid 1990s, many American and European studies

W. Siquini (Ed.), *Surgical Treatment of Pancreatic Diseases.*
©Springer-Verlag Italia 2009

have demonstrated a high mortality risk after PD in centers where it is rarely performed [1, 2]. This risk reduces significantly and progressively as the frequency of performance of the procedure rises.

The situation in Italy is analogous, and has been described in a recently published article [3]: in Italy the surgical mortality after PD is 12.4% in low-volume centers (those performing 1–5 PDs per year), while the risk decreases by a factor of 5 (adjusted OR 0.208) in hospitals with greater experience (very-high-volume centers performing 80–100 PDs per year), with a mortality rate of 2.6%. This difference is not only due to the experience of the operating surgeon, but also to the ability to recognize and manage the complications occurring in a consistent number of patients. Therefore, before embarking upon a PD, surgeons must ask questions not only about their own experience, but also about the hospital's resources. An appropriate intensive care unit is mandatory; the operating room must be available 24 h a day; at least two surgeons with appropriate training in pancreatic surgery are needed (one of them always available for an emergency procedure). The hospital must be equipped with interventional radiology and endoscopy available 24 h a day.

The guidelines on pancreatic surgery published in the UK [4] and Ontario [5] follow these directions and aim to reduce the mortality rate following PD below 5% (on a national basis). In Italy, 75% of hospitals performing PD are low-volume centers (1–5 PDs per year). It is desirable that this percentage should drastically fall in the next few years, but until the health authorities regulate this issue, it is up to the individual surgeon to recognize whether his or her experience and the hospital conditions are adequate to control the risk of mortality after PD.

Comparing Techniques

Comparing different studies is difficult, since their primary aims may vary, and moreover because the definition of pancreatic fistula frequently differs. For these reasons the results of meta-analyses and the conclusions of collective reviews should always be interpreted with particular caution.

Pancreaticojejunostomy or Pancreaticogastrostomy?

A number of retrospective studies and three prospective randomized trials [6–8] have addressed this question. Generally, retrospective studies suggest an advantage of the pancreaticogastrostomy, but the randomized trials have not confirmed it. A meta-analysis regarding this topic was also recently published (though it does not include two of the three randomized trials!) [9]. It shows a superiority of pancreaticogastrostomy in terms of mortality (factor of 2.5), global morbidity (factor of 1.4), and pancreatic fistula (factor of 2.6); however, the same study remarks on the impossibility of reaching a formal conclusion due to the variations in methodology of nonrandomized trials.

Considering the cases of the three randomized studies, which included a total of 450 patients, no difference was observed between the two techniques in relation to overall morbidity and mortality rates: morbidity rate was 43.8% (95/222 patients) following pancreaticojejunostomy compared to 41.7% (93/223) after pancreaticogastrostomy. The incidence of pancreatic fistula is harder to calculate, due to differences in its definition; nevertheless, none of the three trials showed a significant difference in the pancreatic fistula rate (Table 21.1), and considering the overall data, no significant difference has been observed (15.8% after pancreaticojejunostomy and 13.9% after pancreaticogastrostomy).

If we consider the long-term outcomes for pancreatic exocrine function associated with the two techniques, few data are available, but one study reports a greater rate of pancreatic exocrine failure after pancreaticogastrostomy compared to pancreaticojejunostomy [10].

In conclusion, it is not possible to recommend either of the two techniques on the basis of the published data: the advice is to use the reconstruction with which one is most familiar.

Table 21.1 The incidence of pancreatic fistula after pancreaticojejunostomy and pancreaticogastrostomy in the three prospective randomized studies

Author	Year	Incidence of pancreatic fistula	
		Pancreaticojejunostomy (%)	Pancreaticogastrostomy (%)
Yeo et al. [6]	1995	11	12
Duffas et al. [7]	2005	21	16
Bassi et al. [8]	2005	16	13
Total		15.8	13.9

Perform All Anastomoses on the Same Limb or Use a Roux-en-Y Limb for the Pancreaticojejunostomy?

The use of a Roux-en-Y limb for the pancreatic anastomosis may reduce the danger of a pancreatic fistula in two ways: (1) the pancreatic secretions do not come in contact with the bile, so enzyme activation is lower (although contact with the jejunal secretions may be enough to activate the enzymes); (2) the volume of the fistula will be lower since the bile component is missing. The disadvantages of this technique are: (1) a slightly longer operative time (an additional anastomosis has to be performed); (2) a jejunal tract of 40–50 cm (the defunctionalized bowel) will not take part in the digestive process. The literature does not help us in regard to the results of this technique: only a few retrospective studies on this topic are available [11].

Internal Stent or No Stent?

Some authors suggest the use of a stent inside the pancreatic anastomosis, regardless of the type of anastomosis. This technique should allow a safer anastomosis for two reasons: the stent could facilitate the suture between the pancreatic duct and the jejunum; moreover, it would also protect the anastomosis, conveying the pancreatic secretions directly into the jejunal lumen. However, when in regard to the last item, it is hard to believe that a reflux of pancreatic juice does not occur at the anastomotic site.

A prospective randomized study on this topic, including 234 patients, has been recently published [12]. The use of pancreatic duct stenting brought no advantage in terms of total morbidity (58% vs. 57.4%) and pancreatic leakage: using the definition of pancreatic fistula suggested by the International Study Group on Pancreatic Fistula (ISGPF) [13], the incidence was 27% in the stent group versus 21.9% in the group without stent. Even in the group of patients whose pancreas was soft, the internal stent had no protective effect: the fistula rate was 40.7% (stent) versus 47.4% (no stent).

External Stent? (External Diversion of Pancreatic Secretions)

Theoretically, the use of a catheter to convey the pancreatic secretions externally in the first postoperative weeks has the advantage of avoiding contact between the pancreatic secretions and the anastomosis. Moreover, if a fistula occurs, it should be pure biliary or jejunal; it should not carry the digestive potential of the pancreatic component, and it should have a lower output. Unfortunately, the authors' experience does not support these expectations. This does not mean that this technique could not be useful; however, results are poorer than we would have expected from the theoretical assumptions.

This has two possible explanations:

1. This technique cannot achieve complete external diversion of the secretions and a variable amount of pancreatic juice is not drained externally, but remains at the anastomotic level. This fact is proved by the variability of the amount of secretion (in some patients 20–50 ml/day, in others >500 ml/day), and by the finding of a high amylase concentration in the peripancreatic drain fluid in cases of fistula.

2. A progressive reduction of the output, secondary to possible displacement or obstruction of the external stent, can be observed. Therefore, this technique does not exclude all pancreatic secretions from the anastomotic site, but it just reduces their amount to a greater or lesser extent and for a variable period (the external drainage of secretions may dry up within a few days or it may persist until removal of the stent).

At the beginning of 2003 we started using this technique (together with the use of a Roux-en-Y limb) in cases of "difficult" pancreas (small pancreatic duct, soft texture). Comparing this to other techniques (standard anastomosis, duct occlusion), we observed a benefit in patients with a difficult stump. The advantage was not due to a reduction in the overall fistula rate, but to a reduction of the dramatic consequences that may occur in cases of fistula, measured in terms of mortality rate and number of relaparotomies (Table 21.2). After this first evaluation, in patients with a "difficult" pancreatic stump we decided to adopt the following technique: the pancreaticojejunostomy on a Roux-en-Y limb, with external diversion of the pancreatic secretions. From 2003 we have used this technique in 125 "difficult" patients in a total of 410 PDs (Table 21.3). In this highly selected group, we recorded a mortality rate of 4%, a reoperation rate of 5.6%, and an incidence of pancreatic fistula (ISGPF definition [13]) of 42.4%. The mortality associated with the fistula and the relaparotomy rate were very low (5.7% for both of them). The incidence of fistulas may seem extremely high to those not used to performing pancreatic surgery, but it must be remembered that we are

Table 21.2 Severity of pancreatic fistula related to the reconstruction performed. The group is composed of 68 patients with "difficult" pancreas (soft texture, nondilated duct), who underwent a pancreaticoduodenectomy (PD) between the years 2000 and 2004

	Standard anastomosis (N = 22)		Occlusion with Ethibloc[b] (N = 16)		Two limbs with external stent (N = 30)	
	n	%	n	%	n	%
Pancreatic fistula[a]	9	41	9	56	14	46
Mortality in patients with fistula	2	22	1	11	0	
Reoperation in patients with fistula	3	33	3	33	1	7

[a] As defined by the International Study Group on Pancreatic Fistula [13]. *N*, number of patients
[b] Ethicon, Norderstedt, Germany

Table 21.3 Results of pancreaticojejunostomy on defunctionalized Roux-en-Y limb with external diversion of the pancreatic secretions in 125 patients with "difficult" pancreas (soft texture, nondilated duct), who underwent PD between the years 2003 and 2007

	No. of patients	%
Mortality	5	4
Reoperations	7	5.6
Pancreatic fistula[a]	53	42.4
Mortality in patients with fistula	3	5.7
Reoperation in patients with fistula	3	5.7

[a] As defined by the International Study Group on Pancreatic Fistula [13]

considering cases of "difficult" pancreas here, and that the pancreatic fistula rate is strictly linked to its definition; it is worth mentioning as a reminder that, in the event of a soft pancreas, the incidence of pancreatic fistula (ISGPF definition) recorded at the Johns Hopkins Hospital was greater than 40% [12].

In the published literature there is just one randomized trial comparing the external diversion of pancreatic secretions with the standard technique: it reports a significant reduction of the pancreatic fistula rate when external diversion is used [14].

Anastomosis or Occlusion of the Pancreatic Duct?

The occlusion technique was proposed during the 1980s and 1990s to avoid pancreatic anastomosis and the potentially dramatic consequences of its failure. With this technique, the postoperative rate of pancreatic fistula was generally greater, but it was a "benign" pancreatic fistula: inactive, and so less dangerous. The authors adopted this technique until the pros and cons of duct occlusion were made clear by a prospective randomized study conducted by our institute in cooperation with a Dutch group [15]. In this trial, duct occlusion was compared with standard pancreaticojejunostomy. No significant difference was recorded between the two groups in terms of surgical complications (mortality, morbidity, and pancreatic leakage), but patients who underwent duct occlusion had a higher rate of postoperative diabetes than did patients treated with anastomosis (34% vs. 14%, p <0.001). In accordance with these results, we ceased using this technique in elective PD.

Nevertheless, the duct occlusion technique can still sometimes be indicated. We previously said that in Italy mortality after PD in low-volume hospitals is greater than 12%, and the majority of these deaths are probably due to anastomotic failure. In the patients' interest, low-volume hospitals should not perform PD; but until this attitude changes, the duct occlusion method could perhaps be useful to reduce mortality in these circumstances, because of the safer pancreatic fistula when the enzymes are not activated. In this case the higher postoperative diabetes rate would be easier to accept, as diabetes is less harmful than anastomotic failure

A second possible indication for duct occlusion is that of reoperation after PD for serious adverse events such as sepsis or hemorrhage due to pancreatic anastomosis leakage. In these cases, duct occlusion could be an alternative to the completion of pancreatectomy (total pancreatectomy): duct occlusion could "simplify" the procedure, avoiding the consequences of a total pancreatectomy.

Conclusions

There is no evidence that any given technique is able to solve the problems of the pancreatic stump, and no comparative study has proved any specific technique to be clearly better than another. The only element that drastically reduces the risk of operative mortality is the hospital's patient volume.

In regard to the choice of operative technique, pancreaticojejunostomy and pancreaticogastrostomy are equivalent in terms of results, and the use of a stent inside the anastomosis does not seem to be useful in reducing complications.

In the authors' experience, the use of a Roux-en-Y limb for the pancreatic anastomosis and external diversion of the pancreatic secretions can be useful in anastomosis in patients with a higher risk (small duct, soft pancreas). Occlusion of the residual pancreatic stump is associated with a greater risk of developing postoperative diabetes, but maybe, in low-volume hospitals, it could be useful in reducing the high operative mortality.

References

1. Birkmeyer JD, Siewers AE, Finlayson EV et al (2002) Hospital volume and surgical mortality in the United States. N Engl J Med 346:1128–1137
2. van Heek NT, Kuhlmann KF, Scholten RJ et al (2005) Hospital volume and mortality after pancreatic resection: a systematic review and an evaluation of intervention in the Netherlands. Ann Surg 242:781–788
3. Balzano G, Zerbi A, Capretti G et al (2008) Effect of hospital volume on outcome of pancreaticoduodenectomy in Italy. Br J Surg 95:357–362
4. Anonymous (2002) Guidance on Commissioning Cancer Services. Improving outcomes in upper gastro-intestinal cancers. Available at: www.dh.gov.uk/assetRoot/04/08/02/78/04080278.pdf. Accessed 23 June 2008
5. Marcaccio M, Langer B, Rumble B, Hunter A; Expert Panel on HPB Surgical Oncology (2006) Hepatic, pancreatic, and biliary tract (HPB) surgical oncology standards. Available at: www.cancercare.on.ca/pdf/pebchpbf.pdf. Accessed 23 June 2008
6. Yeo CJ, Cameron JL, Maher MM et al (1995) A prospective randomized trial of pancreaticogastrostomy versus pancreaticojejunostomy after pancreaticoduodenectomy. Ann Surg 222:580–592
7. Duffas JP, Suc B, Msika S et al; French Associations for Research in Surgery (2005) A controlled randomized multicenter trial of pancreatogastrostomy or pancreatojejunostomy after pancreatoduodenectomy. Am J Surg 189:720–729
8. Bassi C, Falconi M, Molinari E et al (2005) Reconstruction by pancreaticojejunostomy versus pancreaticogastrostomy following pancreatectomy: results of a comparative study. Ann Surg 242:767–771
9. Mc Kay A, Mackenzi S, Sutherland Fr et al (2006) Meta-analysis of pancreaticojejunostomy versus pancreaticogastrostomy reconstruction after pancreaticoduodenectomy. Br J Surg 93: 929–936
10. Rault A, SaCunha A, Klopfenstein D et al (2005) Pancreaticojejunal anastomosis is preferable to pancreaticogastrostomy after pancreaticoduodenectomy for longterm outcomes of pancreatic exocrine function. J Am Coll Surg 201:239–244
11. Sutton CD, Garcea G, White SA et al (2004) Isolated Roux-loop pancreaticojejunostomy: a series of 61 patients with zero postoperative pancreaticoenteric leaks. J Gastrointest Surg 8:701–705
12. Winter JM, Cameron JL, Campbell KA et al (2006) Does pancreatic duct stenting decrease the rate of pancreatic fistula following pancreaticoduodenectomy? Results of a prospective randomized trial. J Gastrointest Surg 10:1280–1290
13. Bassi C, Dervenis C, Butturini G et al; International Study Group on Pancreatic Fistula Definition (2005) Postoperative pancreatic fistula: an International Study Group (ISGPF) definition. Surgery 138:8–13
14. Poon RT, Fan ST, Lo CM et al (2007) External drainage of pancreatic duct with a stent to

reduce leakage rate of pancreaticojejunostomy after pancreaticoduodenectomy: a prospective randomised trial. Ann Surg 246:425–433

15. Tran K, Van Eijck C, Di Carlo V et al (2002) Occlusion of the pancreatic duct versus pancreaticojejunostomy: a prospective randomized trial. Ann Surg 236:422–428

Chapter 22

Resection Criteria in Pancreatic Surgery: Lymphadenectomy and Vascular Resections

Marco Del Chiaro, Ugo Boggi, Franco Mosca

Introduction

Pancreatic carcinoma is generally considered a systemic disease; at diagnosis the disease is often metastatic [1], and its early spread via the lymphatic and blood circulation is well documented by the identification of tumor cells at the level of the cardiovascular system in around 28% of cases and of the marrow in around 24% of cases [2]. However, the poor resectability of pancreatic cancer is also due to local progression, which is also often detected at diagnosis. Approximately 30% of patients diagnosed as having pancreatic carcinoma are excluded from resective surgery owing to suspected involvement of the large vessels of the retropancreatic region (portal mesenteric venous axis, superior mesenteric artery, celiac trunk) [3]. In the early 1970s, Fortner [4] introduced the concept of regional pancreatectomy as a way to achieve higher surgical resection for improved local control of the disease and better lymphatic clearance. Fortner's experience has been reproduced by various authors with different results and sometimes controversial conclusions.

Lymphadenectomy in Pancreatic Surgery

Results of Pancreatectomy with Extended Lymphadenectomy

At the end of the 1980s the interest of the scientific world in the role of lymphadenectomy in pancreatic cancer increased massively following the results reported by Ishikawa et al. [5] and Manabe et al. [6], who had shown significant survival advantages in patients subjected to pancreatectomy with extended lymphadenectomy compared to those subjected to standard lymphadenectomy. Since then, many studies have been carried out to check the data reported by these authors, but the results have proved discrepant and no clear survival has been shown in patients undergoing extended lymphadenectomy. Firstly, a comparison between the data for extended and those for standard lymphadenectomy shows that only four prospective randomized studies exist on this subject [7–10]

W. Siquini (Ed.), *Surgical Treatment of Pancreatic Diseases.*
©Springer-Verlag Italia 2009

(Table 22.1). The results were unable to demonstrate a survival advantage in patients who underwent extended lymphadenectomy compared to those who underwent standard lymphadenectomy. Only the study by Pedrazzoli et al. [9] showed survival advantage in the subgroup of patients with metastatic lymph nodes who underwent the extended procedure. Even the meta-analysis by Michalski et al. [11], who examined the results of 484 published studies, showed no significant differences in survival between extended and standard lymphadenectomy in pancreatic cancer, but did show increased morbidity associated with more extended clearances. In particular, in some studies extended lymphadenectomy with circumferential clearance of the superior mesenteric artery (SMA) seems to be associated with severe diarrhea in up to 48% of cases [10].

So far, we have been unable to define the exact role of lymphadenectomy in pancreatic cancer because, as shown by Pisters et al. [12], the patients who could benefit from extended lymphadenectomy are only those with negative margins (80%), second-level metastases in lymph nodes (10%), and absence of distant metastases (5%). According to the conclusions of Pisters et al., expressed by the mathematical formula [R0(80%) x N2(10%) x M0(5%) = 0.4%], we would need a total of 238,000 patients per arm in order to construct a randomized prospective study able to demonstrate an advantage between the two study groups. Thus the question of lymphadenectomy remains open, and will need to be reassessed once an adjuvant therapy able to affect lymph node involvement and metastases becomes available for pancreatic cancer.

Another problem in the assessment of the studies on lymphadenectomy regards the definitions of extended and standard lymphadenectomy. The surgical techniques reported in the literature are very inhomogeneous, and the definition of extended lymphadenectomy in one group is not very different from the standard lymphadenectomy of another group. For this reason there has been an

Table 22.1 Randomized prospective studies of pancreatectomy with extended lymphadenectomy (ELC) versus standard lymphadenectomy (SLC)

Study	Year	No. of patients	Survival (%)		
			1-Year	3-Year	5-Year
Farnell et al. [7]	2005	SLC 40	71	25	17
		ELC 39	82	41	16
Yeo et al. [8]	2002	SLC 81	77	36	14
		ELC 82	74	38	33
Pedrazzoli et al. [9]	1998	SLC 40	–	–	–
		ELC 41	5	22	–
Nimura et al. [10]	2004	SLC 51	78	32	–
		ELC 50	51	16	–

attempt to standardize the concept of extended lymphadenectomy during a consensus conference which took place at Castelfranco Veneto in 1999. What follows are the definitions of extended lymphadenectomy developed by this study group.

Surgical Technique of Lymphadenectomy (Castelfranco Veneto Consensus Conference)

The Castelfranco Consensus Conference of 1999 brought together the representatives of the most important European pancreatic cancer research centers with a high patient volume in order to define the European technical standards for pancreaticoduodenectomy (PD). Three types of PD were defined: standard, radical, and extended.

Standard Pancreaticoduodenectomy

The standard PD procedure included the following steps:
- En-bloc cholecystectomy with the surgical specimen and section of the bile duct above the cystic outlet
- Section of the neck of the pancreas above the mesenteric–portal vein at a distance of at least 1 gin at extemporaneous histological examination
- Preservation of the pylorus, considered equivalent to the traditional Whipple procedure, with the exception of lesions derived from the dorsal part of the pancreas
- Resection of the portal mesenteric venous trunk and/or accessory organs (stomach, colon, spleen, small bowel, kidney) justifying R0 resection
- En-bloc lymphadenectomy, implying resection of the lymph nodes to the right of the hepatoduodenal ligament, posterior pancreaticoduodenal lymph nodes, lymph nodes on the right margin of the SMA from its origin to the inferior pancreaticoduodenal artery, anterior pancreaticoduodenal arteries, and lymph nodes of the superoanterior region of the common hepatic artery.

Radical Pancreaticoduodenectomy

In addition to what has been described for the standard procedure, radical PD includes the following steps:
- Section of the pancreas on the left margin of the mesenteric–portal axis
- Removal of Gerota's fascia during Kocher's maneuver, carried out en bloc with the surgical specimen
- Compared with the standard procedure, extension of the lymphatic clearance with the addition of: skeletonization of the common and proper hepatic artery, removing the lymph nodes at the Haller's tripod and lymph nodes dis-

posed along the right-hand and left-hand sides of the hepatoduodenal ligament; circumferential skeletonization of the SMA from its origin to the inferior pancreaticoduodenal artery, removing the preaortic and precaval lymph
nodes en-bloc with Gerota's fascia from its origin on the tripod to the origin
of the inferior mesenteric artery in adjunct to the standard procedure.

Extended Pancreaticoduodenectomy

In addition to the "radical" procedure, extended PD includes the following step:
– Removal of the lymphatic–connective fascia starting 3 diaphragm to the iliac
bifurcation (Fig. 22.1).

Indications For the Type of Lymphadenectomy

Although there is no evidence about the type of lymphadenectomy to be used,
clinical practice has provided some useful suggestions. Although standard lymphadenectomy showed no significant negative impact on prognosis, in many

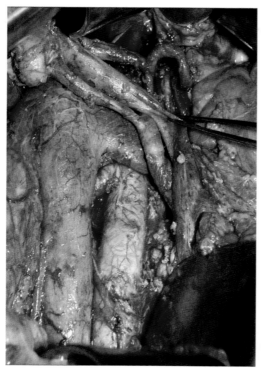

Fig. 22.1 Pancreaticoduodenectomy
with extended lymphadenectomy

studies it was associated with a shorter survival period and with a high rate of local disease recurrence. Extended lymphadenectomy shows a small although insignificant survival advantage; however, it is associated with higher morbidity and in particular with worse quality of life due to diarrhea caused by circumferential clearance of the SMA and intestinal denervation. The use of radical lymphadenectomy, with clearance of the right side of the SMA, may suggest improved local control of the disease without affecting the morbidity, as is traditionally associated with more extended clearance. Therefore, in our opinion, radical lymphadenectomy aimed at saving the tissue on the left side of SMA in order to prevent diarrhea could be considered a standard technique for pancreatic cancer. However, the present authors also believe that extended lymphadenectomy can play a role in young patients with early tumors (T1) and in those who are responding to neoadjuvant chemotherapy.

Vascular Resection in Pancreatic Surgery

Results of Pancreatectomy Combined with Vascular Resection

The reasons traditionally adduced to discourage resection surgery in patients with pancreatic carcinoma are high operative risk on the one hand and long-term prognosis on the other. However, although early pancreatectomy experiences with vascular resections were expected to increase operative risk [13], an examination of the recent literature suggests that the results surpass those of "conventional" pancreatectomy (Table 22.2) [14].

Table 22.2 Morbidity and mortality associated with pancreatectomy combined with vascular resection

Study	Year	No. of patients	Mortality (%)	Morbidity (%)
Harrison	1996	58	5	ND
Leach	1998	31	0	30
Bachellier	2001	21	4.7	38.1
Shibata	2001	28	4	32
Van Greenen	2001	34	0	41
Hartel	2002	68	4	27
Sasson et al. [21]	2002	37	2.7	35
Nakagohri	2003	33	6.1	ND
Capussotti	2003	22	0	33.3
Howard et al. [20]	2003	13	ND	54
Total		345	3.7	34

As regards the prognostic significance of this surgery, a clarification is necessary. The sometimes unsatisfactory results relate principally to cases for which surgery was forced in an unplanned way (i.e., in cases in which vascular infiltration was diagnosed intraoperatively and following irreversible actions, or cases in which vascular resection became necessary due to intraoperative accidents) [15]. By contrast, in the case of planned vascular resections the results were far more encouraging. However, although venous resections are associated with long-term survival times better than those following standard resections (Table 22.3), the problem is more complex with regard to arterial resections and even more with regard to arteriovenous combined resections. In particular, tumors involving multiple vascular segments would appear to reflect locally advanced disease with lymphangitic involvement of the peripancreatic tissues, and would therefore be associated with short survival times even after surgery aiming at radical resection [23, 24]. Nonetheless, owing to the steady improvement of oncological treatment available nowadays, the number of patients defined as "responders" is increasing [25]. These patients are suitable candidates for surgical resection following neoadjuvant chemotherapy, also combined with multiple vascular resection [26]. In the case of small tumors originating close to the artery trunks, pancreatectomy associated with artery resection seems to obtain results superior to those of conventional pancreatectomy [27].

Table 22.3 Long-term survival of pancreatectomy with resection of the portal mesenteric vein performed for pancreatic carcinoma

Study	Year	No. of patients	Survival (%)		
			3-Year	5-Year	Median (months)
Mosca et al. [14]	2008	102	15	10.5	15
Al-Haddad et al. [22]	2007	22	20	20	–
Carrere et al. [16]	2006	45	22	–	15
Zhou et al. [17]	2005	32	16	–	–
Poon et al. [18]	2004	12	–	–	19.5
Tseng et al. [19]	2004	110	–	–	23
Howard et al. [20]	2003	13	–	–	13
Sasson et al. [21]	2002	37	–	16	26

Preoperative Work-Up

Preoperative assessment of all patients should include clinical examination, blood tests, chest X-ray examination, and CT. Like angiography, explorative laparoscopy can be used in selected cases [28]. There seems to be no indication nowadays for routine angiography in the preoperative assessment if careful vascular examination is carried out by CT [29].

Surgical Techniques

Venous Resection

In the authors' experience, when preparing for a possible pancreatectomy with vascular resection, as well as the abdomen, it is advisable to include a laterocervical region and the groins with the thighs in the operative field, so that these regions are available to allow withdrawal of autologous vascular grafts if needed (Fig. 22.2). Following surgical incision (which in the case of the authors generally consists of an extended left subcostal incision) the abdominal cavity is explored to exclude the presence of distant metastatic spread (hepatic metastases or carcinosis). The state of local advancement of the disease or the presence of small occult hepatic lesions can be assessed with the aid of intraoperative contact ultrasonography. When the portal–mesenteric venous axis is involved or when the tumor is not clearly cleavable with respect to one of the large peripancreatic vessels, the surgical intervention is continued by programming a planned vascular resection with no direct attempt at resection of the tumor from the vessel (no-touch technique) [30]. In these cases the portal vein is immediately surrounded within the context of the hepatoduodenal ligament and the superior mesenteric vein (SMV) in the context of the mesenteric root. The right colon and the small bowel can be completely mobilized in order to allow better exposure of the field and to facilitate the reconstructive phase [31–33].

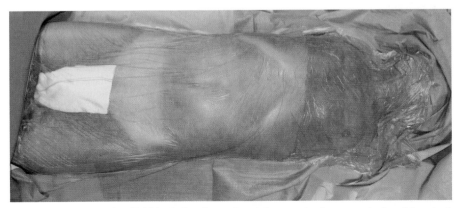

Fig. 22.2 The operative field includes the entire abdomen, the laterocervical and inguinal regions, and the proximal part of the thighs

The retroperitoneal margin is approached on the left-hand side of the SMV upwards, skeletonizing the right lateral margin of the SMA without reaching the peritumoral floor. At the end of this stage the head of the pancreas will remain connected only with the portal–mesenteric venous trunk (Fig. 22.3) [30]. Therefore, clamping the vessel at both ends, the surgical specimen is removed en bloc with the vascular segment. In the case of resections of the portal–mesenteric venous axis some technical variants are possible. If only the SMV is involved, it is often possible to clamp it in the root of the mesentery and then immediately proximal to the confluence of the portal vein, retaining a small amount of portal flow through the splenic vein (Fig. 22.4) [30]. Reconstruction may occur by end-to-end anastomosis, which in most cases is more rapid and feasible (Fig. 22.5) [30]. Whenever it is necessary to resect the splenic portal junction as well, the authors prefer to reimplant the splenic vein. In this case it is often better to interpose an autologous venous graft replacing the resected vascular segment (Fig. 22.6) [30].

For tumors adhering to the right lateral wall of the portal–mesenteric vein, tangential resection of the venous wall is also possible, but it requires a broad venous resection, in keeping with the concept of no-touch resection in healthy tissue. In these cases the size of the vascular breach is such that it is necessary to perform a venous patch [30]. The left internal jugular vein is the most suitable segment for the cases in which it is necessary to use a venous graft, but for total pancreatectomy it is sometimes possible to use a segment of splenic vein rotated clockwise and downwards, when the resected segment is SMV. In those rare cases in which a tangential venous resection is sufficient, it is possible to use the right gonadal vein, the saphenous vein, or even the internal jugular vein to obtain

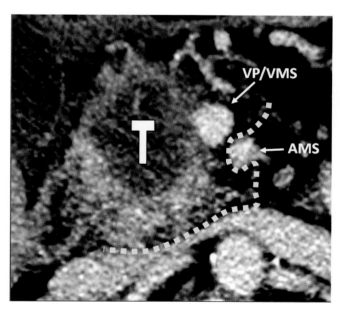

Fig. 22.3 Carcinoma of the head of the pancreas (*T*) in which the cleavage plane with the wall of the portal-mesenteric venous axis is not visible (*VP/VMS*). The *dotted line* shows the approach to the retroperitoneal margin using the no-touch technique, passing to the left of the venous axis and skeletonizing the right margin of the superior mesenteric artery (*AMS*)

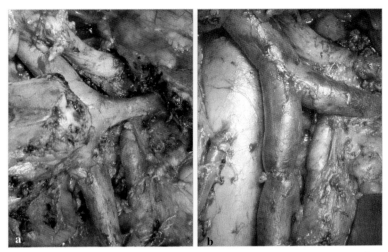

Fig. 22.4 a Head of the pancreas with the tumor adhering to the right lateral surface of the superior mesenteric artery (SMV) after section of the retroperitoneal margin. **b** Reconstruction after resection of the SMV and interposition of autologous graft in the internal jugular vein

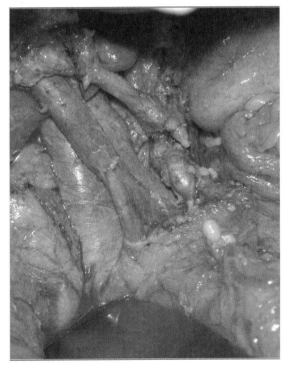

Fig. 22.5 Total pancreatectomy for pancreatic carcinoma with en-bloc resection of the portal–mesenteric junction and reconstruction by end-to-end anastomosis between the SMV and the portal vein.

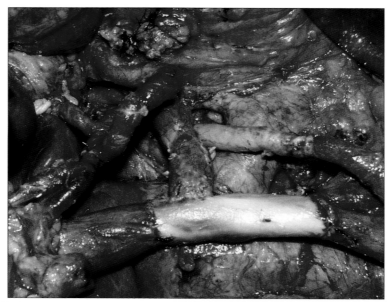

Fig. 22.6 Pancreaticoduodenectomy with en-bloc resection of the portal–mesenteric junction and reconstruction by interposition of heterologous venous graft (from a cadaveric donor) and reimplantation of the splenic vein

a vascular patch. In the absence of an autologous graft one can use a venous graft from a cadaveric donor (generally the iliac vein), stored at a temperature between 0 and 4 °C in a Terasaki solution (ICN Biomedicals, Illkirch, France) for the shortest possible time and in any case for no longer than 7 days. The use of prosthetic material is not advisable owing to the risk of abdominal infections associated with pancreatectomy interventions [30].

If collateral venous circles are present, as in the case of partial occlusion of the portal–mesenteric venous axis, their preventive ligature is associated with acute venous hypertension and increased blood loss as well as onset of intestinal edema. In these cases the SMA can be clamped during the surgical maneuvering of resection and venous reconstruction [30]. Furthermore, reconstruction of the venous axis may be worth considering, using a bridge graft, before completing the resection is completed. Proximal involvement of the SMV in the mesenteric root can represent an important technical problem in the planning of venous resection. In these cases resection can take place not at the level of the principal trunk, but of the jejunal branches. Before passing the "point of nonreversibility," it is advisable to check the technical feasibility of the intervention carefully. The venous branches must be isolated and clamped individually to enable the decision as to which ones need to be reconstructed and which ones can be tied on the basis of the existing collateral circles. Before starting the resection, it is first necessary to have at one's disposal a vascular segment suitable for reconstruction. In these cases, and whenever prolonged reconstruction times are envisioned (more than 15 min), it is advisable to clamp the SMA to reduce intestinal edema [34].

The patient undergoing venous resection does not generally need heparin treatment.

Arterial Resection

Pancreatic carcinomas originating from the isthmus or from the medial part of the pancreatic body may occasionally cause "isolated" involvement of adjacent arterial structures (hepatic artery, celiac trunk) in the same way as lesions of the pancreatic head can involve, for example, an individual superior mesenteric or hepatic artery. When the tumor of the body allows preservation of the head, vascularization of the liver following resection of the celiac trunk or of the common hepatic artery can be guaranteed by the gastroduodenal artery (Fig. 22.7) [35]. Alternately, reconstruction of these vascular segments can take place by direct anastomosis of the stumps or by interposition of autologous graft (generally the saphenous vein).

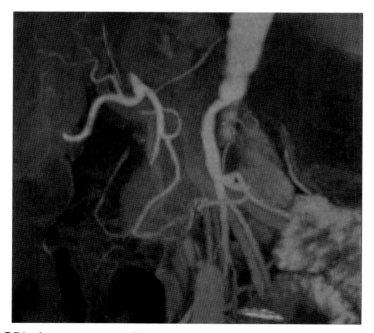

Fig. 22.7 Distal pancreatectomy with en-bloc resection of the celiac trunk (Haller's tripod). Vascularization of the liver, as evidenced in this postoperative CT scan, is preserved by the gastroduodenal artery

Arteriovenous Resections

This type of resection, reserved for selected cases, presents technical problems which are definitely more complex than the ones listed above. A priority problem is to reduce liver and bowel ischemic times as much as possible. Total enbloc pancreatectomy with total gastrectomy can facilitate resection and guarantee better oncological resection. The resection stage generally begins with a duodenal Kocher maneuver and complete mobilization of the right colon and small bowel. In the case of tumors involving the SMV proximally, it is advisable to perform right hemicolectomy followed by precaval and preaortic lymphadenectomy, from the iliac bifurcation to the origin of the SMA and of the celiac trunk at the aortic level. The splenopancreatic bloc is mobilized up to the aortic plane, followed by identification, from left to right, of the origin of the SMA and of the celiac trunk. We proceed to isolation in the context of the mesenteric root of the SMV and SMA, leaving the small bowel connected only through these two vessels. We then isolate the portal vein and the proper hepatic artery in the hepatoduodenal ligament.

Starting from the top we resect the stomach at the level of the cardia and move downwards in the direction of the celiac trunk along the pillars of the diaphragm. The small bowel is sectioned at the level of the first jejunal loop. The gastrosplenopancreatic bloc is completely mobilized, connected exclusively through its major vascular peduncles. When a "trivascular" resection is necessary, the first step consists in resection of the common hepatic artery–celiac trunk, retaining vascularization of the liver through the portal vein. The next step consists in reconstruction through interposition of an autologous graft from the large saphenous vein or the internal iliac artery. SMA clamping is performed at the start of the aorta and in the context of the mesenteric root, and clamping of the portal vein in the hepatoduodenal ligament and of the SMV in the mesenteric root are performed. At this point the gastropancreaticosplenic bloc can be resected. After complete mobilization of the bowel, reconstruction of the mesenteric vascular segments can be done by direct endto-end anastomosis or interposition of (preferably autologous) grafts. During this stage the bowel is ischemic and the liver is partially supplied by the hepatic artery (Fig. 22.8) [30].

Indications for Vascular Resection

Nowadays, extended venous infiltration involving less than 180° of the vessel circumference, in the absence of thrombosis, presents no surgical contraindication, allowing survival comparable to that of standard pancreatectomy. In particular, tumors contiguous to the wall of the mesenteric–portal axis, in the absence of clear signs of infiltration, appear to be suitable for R0 resection, independent of vessel infiltration. The same oncological principles appear to be valid for the rare small tumors growing close to the artery trunk.

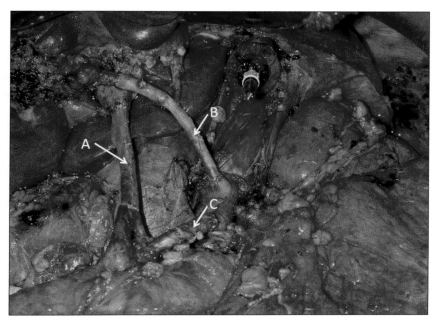

Fig. 22.8 Total pancreatectomy, total gastrectomy, right hemicolectomy with en-bloc resection of the portal–mesenteric vein (reconstructed with autologous graft from the internal jugular vein [A]), celiac trunk and hepatic artery (reconstructed by interposition of autologous graft from the saphenous vein [B]) and SMA (reconstructed by interposition of autologous graft from the internal iliac artery [C]), in patients responding to neoadjuvant therapy

The benefits of surgery are less evident for the locally more advanced tumors involving a number of vessels simultaneously, at least when the histotype is pancreatic ductal carcinoma. However, recent data suggest that surgery can prolong survival of these patients when they respond to neoadjuvant treatment protocols (Table 22.4).

Table 22.4 Indications for vascular resection in pancreatic cancer

Resection type	Indications
Venous resection	Vessel involvement <180° in the absence of thrombosis
	Vessel involvement >180° in responders to neoadjuvant therapy?
Arterial resection	Vessel involvement <180° in the absence of thrombosis
	Vessel involvement >180° in responders to neoadjuvant therapy?
Arteriovenous resection	Responders to neoadjuvant therapy

References

1. Pawlik TM, Abdalla EK, Barnett CC et al (2005) Feasibility of a randomized trial of extended lymphadenectomy for pancreatic cancer. Arch Surg 140:584–589; discussion 589–591
2. Picozzi VJ, Kozarek RA, Traverso LW (2003) Interferon-based adjuvant chemoradiation therapy after pancreaticoduodenectomy for pancreatic adenocarcinoma. Am J Surg 185:476–480
3. Tseng JF, Raut CP, Lee JE et al (2004) Pancreaticoduodenectomy with vascular resection: margin status and survival duration. J Gastrointest Surgery 8:935-949
4. Fortner JG (1973) Regional resection and pancreatic carcinoma. Surgery 73:799–800
5. IshikawaO, OhhigashiH, Sasaki Y et al (1988) Practical usefulness of lymphatic and connective tissue clearance for the carcinoma of the pancreas head. Ann Surg 208:215–220
6. Manabe T, Ohshio G, Baba N et al (1989) Radical pancreatectomy for ductal cell carcinoma of the head of the pancreas. Cancer 64:1132–1137
7. Farnell MB, Pearson RK, Sarr MG et al (2005) A prospective randomized trial comparing standard pancreatoduodenectomy with pancreatoduodenectomy with extended lymphadenectomy in resectable pancreatic head adenocarcinoma. Surgery 138:618–628; discussion 628–630
8. Yeo CJ, Cameron JL, Lillemoe KD et al (2002) Pancreaticoduodenectomy with or without distal gastrectomy and extended retroperitoneal lymphadenectomy for periampullary adenocarcinoma, part 2: randomized controlled trial evaluating survival, morbidity, and mortality. Ann Surg; 236:355–366; discussion 366–368
9. Pedrazzoli S, DiCarlo V, Dionigi R et al (1998) Standard versus extended lymphadenectomy associated with pancreatoduodenectomy in the surgical treatment of adenocarcinoma of the head of the pancreas: a multicenter, prospective, randomized study. Lymphadenectomy Study Group. Ann Surg; 228:508–517
10. Nimura Y, Nagino M, Kato H et al (2004) Regional versus extended lymph node dissection in radical pancreaticoduodenectomy for pancreatic cancer: a multicenter, randomized controlled trial. HPB 6(Suppl 1):2 (abstract)
11. Michalski CW, Kleeff J, Wente MN et al (2007) Systematic review and meta-analysis of standard and extended lymphadenectomy in pancreaticoduodenectomy for pancreatic cancer. Br J Surg 94:265–273
12. Pisters PWT, Evans DB, Leung DHY et al (2001) Re: Surgery for ductal adenocarcinoma of the pancreatic head. World J Surg 25:533–534
13. Fortner JG (1973) Regional resection and pancreatic carcinoma. Surgery 73:799–800
14. Mosca F, Boggi U, Del Chiaro M (2008) Management of tumor invasion/adhesion to the superior mesenteric-portal vein during pancreatectomy. In: Disease of the pancreas. Springer, Berlin Heidelberg, pp 593–610
15. Cusack JC, Fuhrman GM, Lee JE et al (1994) Managing unsuspected tumor invasion of the superior mesenteric–portal venous confluence during pancreaticoduodenectomy. Am J Surg 168:352–354
16. Carrere N, Sauvanet A, Goere D et al (2006) Pancreaticoduodenectomy with mesentericoportal vein resection for adenocarcinoma of the pancreatic head. World J Surg 30:1–10
17. Zhou GW, Wu WD, Xiao WD et al (2005) Pancreatectomy combined with superior mesenteric-portal vein resection: report of 32 cases. Hepatobiliary Pancreat Dis Int 4:130–134
18. Poon RT, Fan ST, Lo CM et al (2004) Pancreaticoduodenectomy with en bloc portal vein resection for pancreatic carcinoma with suspected portal vein involvement. World J Surg 28:602–608
19. Tseng JF, Raut CP, Lee JE et al (2004) Pancreaticoduodenectomy with vascular resection: margin status and survival duration. J Gastrointest Surg 8:935–950
20. Howard TJ, Villanustre N, Moore SA et al (2003) Efficacy of venous reconstruction in patients with adenocarcinoma of the pancreatic head. J Gastrointest Surg 7:1089–1095
21. Sasson AR, Hoffman JP, Ross EA et al (2002) En bloc resection for locally advanced cancer of the pancreas: is it worthwhile? J Gastrointest Surg 6:147–158

22. Al-Haddad M, Martin JK, Nguyen J et al (2007) Vascular resection and reconstruction for pancreatic malignancy: a single center survival study. J Gastrointest Surg 11:1168–1174

23. Ishikawa O, Ohigashi H, Imaoka S et al (1992) Preoperative indications for extended pancreatectomy for locally advanced pancreas cancer involving the portal vein. Ann Surg 215:231–236

24. Nakao A, Harada A, Nonami T et al (1995) Clinical significance of portal invasion by pancreatic head carcinoma. Surgery 117:50–55

25. Mehta VK, Fisher G, Ford JA et al (2001) Preoperative chemoradiation for marginally respectable adenocarcinoma of the pancreas. J Gastrointest Surg 5:27–35

26. Boggi U, Del Chiaro M, Mosca I et al (2007) En-bloc resection of superior mesenteric vessels and mesenteric root followed by intestinal auto-transplantation for locally advanced pancreatic cancer: a pilot study. HPB 9(Suppl 2):60

27. Hirano S, Kondo S, Hara T et al (2007) Distal pancreatectomy with en bloc celiac axis resection for locally advanced pancreatic body cancer: long-term results. Ann Surg 246:46–51

28. Pietrabissa A, Caramella D, Di Candio G et al (1999) Laparoscopy and laparoscopic ultrasonography for staging pancreatic cancer: critical appraisal. World J Surg 23:998–1002; discussion 1003

29. Mazzeo S, Cappelli C, Caramella D et al (2007) Evaluation of vascular infiltration in resected patients for pancreatic cancer: comparison among multidetector CT, intraoperative findings and histopathology. Abdom Imaging Mar 27 [Epub ahead of print]

30. Boggi U, Del Chiaro M et al (2006) Le resezioni vascolari in chirurgia pancreatica. In: Trattato di tecnica chirurgica. Volume pancreas, surrene, milza, peritoneo, retroperitoneo. UTET, Turin, pp 111–122

31. Varty PP, Yamamoto H, Farges O et al (2005) Early retropancreatic dissection during pancreatectomy. Am J Surg 189:488–491

32. Machado MC, Penteado S, Cunha JE et al (2001) Pancreatic head tumors with portal vein involvement: an alternative surgical approach. Hepatogastroenterology 48:1486–1487

33. Leach SD, Davidson BS, Ames FC et al (1996) Alternative method for exposure of retropancreatic mesenteric vasculature during total pancreatectomy. J Surg Oncol 61:163–165

34. Tseng JF, Tamm EP, Lee JE et al (2006) Venous resection in pancreatic cancer surgery. Best Pract Res Clin Gastroenterol 20:349–364

35. Makary MA, Fishman EK, Cameron JL (2005) Resection of the celiac axis for invasive pancreatic cancer. J Gastrointest Surg 9:503–507

Chapter 23

Distal Splenopancreatectomy: Indications for Surgery and Technical Notes

Carmine Napolitano, Luca Valvano, Maurizio Grillo

Embryological Notes

The pancreas is a large gland located across the back of the abdomen. The organ develops from two buds that first appear as evaginations of the primitive anterior foregut at around the 5th week of gestation. The first, called the dorsal pancreas, develops rapidly into the mesoduodenum and crosses in front of the portal vein. Due to selective expansion of the duodenum, by about the 7th week the second bud, called the ventral pancreas, rotates with the gut, passing behind the duodenum from right to left and eventually fusing with the dorsal pancreas. The ventral pancreas forms the inferior part of the head of the pancreas and the uncinate process whereas the dorsal pancreas becomes the tail and the body. After the fusion of the two buds, the right mesoduodenal layer is reabsorbed and the pancreas, covered only by the left mesoduodenal layer, becomes retroperitoneal [1].

Anatomical Notes

The pancreas is fixed to the abdominal cavity through the posterior parietal peritoneum, the vessels passing through it and in close connection with the duodenum. It is interesting to note that the pancreas is surrounded by two connective layers, one anterior and the other posterior (Treitz's fascia). The vessels run through the gland and these layers. The body and the tail of the pancreas have the following relations: in front, through the omental bursa, with the stomach and lesser omentum; at the back, through the Gerota layer, with the left kidney and adrenal gland, left renal vein, aorta, and celiac plexus. The inferior side of the pancreas, on the left of the head and through the root of the mesocolon, has relation with the duodenojejunal flexure and mesenteric intestinal mesenteric loops. The pancreatic tail, inserted in the splenopancreatic ligament, becomes an intraperitoneal organ and therefore it becomes movable. The pancreas has posterior connections with the major vessels, so the lumbar approach is dangerous, whereas the anterior approach is possible because of the presence of Treitz's fascia.

W. Siquini (Ed.), *Surgical Treatment of Pancreatic Diseases.*
©Springer-Verlag Italia 2009

The pancreatic body and tail are mainly supplied by branches of the splenic artery. The main pancreatic arteries, which are small and fragile, branch to the organ surface before penetrating.

The splenic artery on the superior pancreatic margin gives off many small-caliber branches and commonly three of significant caliber:

1. The *dorsal pancreatic artery* arises from the initial portion of the splenic artery. It runs downwards and is divided in two branches. The right branch anastomoses with the anterior pancreatic trunk, while the left branch contributes to making the transverse or inferior pancreatic artery, that is, the left terminal branch of the dorsal pancreatic artery; it runs on the dorsal surface of the inferior margin of the body and tail.

2. The *great pancreatic artery* arises further left than the dorsal artery and reaches the pancreatic parenchyma at the junction of the middle and distal thirds of the gland and the caudal arteries, originating mainly from the left gastroepiploic artery and from the main trunk of the splenic artery. It comes down and anastomoses with the dorsal pancreatic artery.

3. The *artery for the pancreatic tail* arises from branches of the splenic artery and anastomoses with branches of the transverse pancreatic artery.

The pancreatic veins are generally satellite to the arteries, but are much more variable and are located more superficially. They drain into the portal vein, the superior mesenteric vein, the splenic vein at different sites and, rarely, into the inferior mesenteric vein. The splenic vein runs behind the pancreas, below the artery, and contrary to the artery. It results from the confluence of the gastric veins, the right gastroepiploic vein, the pancreaticoduodenal veins, and the inferior mesenteric vein [2].

Distal Splenopancreatectomy

Introduction

In a distal pancreatectomy the pancreas is commonly divided on the left of the superior mesenteric–portal venous trunk. The line of section depends on the exact site of the lesion. At present, the indications for distal pancreatectomy are benign and malignant tumors, chronic pancreatitis, and trauma. There are two kinds of surgical procedure: distal splenopancreatectomy, and spleen-preserving distal pancreatectomy.

Technical Notes

A support of 20 cm below the spine allows the most comfortable exposure of the pancreas. The choice of laparotomy is limited to two incisions: a median incision for a long-limbed person, and a left subcostal incision, extended to the right, for the brachymorphic type.

Once the abdominal cavity has been opened and the autostatic retractors placed, the procedure starts with seeking for contraindications such as hepatic metastases, peritoneal carcinosis, and infiltration of the mesenteric root (relative contraindications in surgery of neuroendocrine tumors) [3]. The epiploic retrocavity is fully opened below the gastroepiploic arterial arch; on the left it is necessary to proceed upward to the short gastric vessels. The stomach is mobilized and pulled upwards; therefore the inferior border of the body–tail region is separated from the upper leaflet of the transverse mesocolon. The common hepatic artery is identified on the superior border of the pancreatic neck and is encircled on a vessel loop. Its dissection toward the celiac trunk allows identification of the origin of the splenic artery, which is also loaded on a vessel loop.

Operative Technique

Anterograde

The operative steps are: ligature and division of the splenic artery, creation of the retropancreatic tunnel at the neck level, pancreatic division, and ligature and division of the splenic vein. In this procedure the mobilization and subsequent division of the splenopancreatic complex are performed from right to left. This technique derives from the *no-touch technique* and is important in cases of distal localization with contiguous organ invasion, requiring en-bloc division [4]. The organs often involved are the colon, stomach, adrenal gland, and kidney.

The main identification of the vessels is an essential element of safety and oncologic radicality [5]. In addition, it allows resection and local control of tumor staged as inoperable.

Hirano et al. [6], starting from the observation that tumors of the body of the pancreas often involve the celiac trunk and common hepatic artery, have proposed, for locally advanced tumors, en-bloc resection of the celiac trunk without arterial reconstruction. The operation produces en-bloc resection of the celiac trunk, common hepatic artery, left gastric artery, superior celiac–mesenteric complex and its lymph nodes, a portion of the pillar muscles of the diaphragm with Gerota's fascia, artery of the left adrenal gland, lymph nodes of the left kidney hilum, the layer of transverse mesocolon that covers the pancreatic body, and the inferior mesenteric vein (Fig. 23.1). Preoperative embolization of the common hepatic artery induces the development of collateral arterial pancreaticoduodenal circulation. In the experience of Hirano et al., this operation carries a mortality of 0%, morbidity of 48%, and median survival of 21 months, but particularly it allows a local control of the disease in 91% of cases, with clear advantages for pain control.

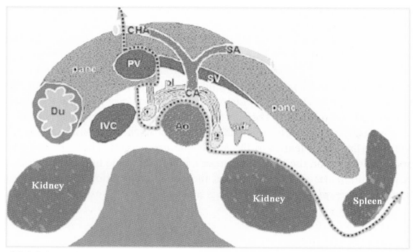

Fig. 23.1 Schematic representation of distal splenopancreatectomy with en-bloc resection of the celiac trun. The *dotted line* shows the dissection plane. *PV*, Portal vein; *IVC*, inferior vena cava; *Ao*, aorta; *adr*, adrenal gland; *g*, celiac nodes; *CHA*, common hepatic artery; *SA*, splenic artery; *SV*, splenic vein; *CA*, celiac trunk; *pl*, celiac plexus; *Du*, duodenum

Retrograde

The operation continues with division among the ligature of the gastrosplenic ligament with the short gastric vessels. After release of the lower pole of the spleen through the division of the splenocolic ligament, the surgeon's left hand is passed behind the spleen and draws it towards the medial line This maneuver stretches the splenorenal ligament, facilitating its division.

Subsequently the spleen and the pancreatic tail, connected by the pedicle, are brought out through the laparotomy. The maneuver is easy so long as care is taken not to open the kidney area and not to damage the left adrenal gland. The splenic vessels are covered and protected by Treitz's fascia.

One or more laparotomy gauzes are placed on the splenic area hemostasis. At the level of the splenomesenteric confluence the splenic vein and artery are isolated and ligated. The inferior mesenteric vein may be divided because the venous circulation depends on Riolan's arch. The pancreas is then divided.

Lymphadenectomy

Extended lymphadenectomy, if performed with low morbidity and mortality, plays a role in determining the extent of lymph node involvement and thus in the staging of disease. In this procedure the retroperitoneal structures, included Gerota's fascia and the left adrenal gland artery, are removed.

The Japanese Pancreas Society has identified regional (N1), peripancreatic (N2), and para-aortic (N3) lymphadenectomy [7]. The *regional lymph nodes* (N1) are the nodes of the common hepatic artery, the splenic artery, the inferior pancreatic border, and the splenic hilum. The *peripancreatic lymph nodes* (N2) are the nodes of the left gastric artery, the celiac trunk, the SMA and middle colic artery. The para-aortic lymph node dissection area reaches from the celiac trunk to the origin of the IMA and from the right margin of the inferior vena cava to the left margin of the left gonadal vein.

In the paper by Shimada et al. [8], according to the paper by Nakao et al. [9], involvement of peripancreatic (N2) and para-aortic (N3) nodes is observed respectively in 6 and 14% of cases, and this is the most important prognostic variable influencing long-term survival.

In fact, N2 or N3 patients do not survive for more than 2 years. Consequently, the effectiveness of this aggressive approach needs more evaluation in randomized, controlled studies. Nevertheless, this surgical procedure may be performed without mortality and seems to offer accurate nodal staging and free margins for resection.

Vascular Resection

Infiltration of the splenic artery or vein is not a problem in distal splenopancreatectomy. However, infiltration of the splenopancreatic trunk requires a different approach, which, as in duodenopancreatectomy, though without the need for splenic artery reimplantation, may require resection and anastomosis with or without vascular graft.

Venous resections of few centimeters with an adequate Cattel maneuver allow direct reconstruction of the mesenteric portal trunk without the need for grafting. However, over the simple technical data, histologic infiltration of the portal vein is associated with worse survival; moreover, according to Nakagohri et al. [10], infiltration of the portal intima layer is related to infiltration of the extrapancreatic plexus, involvement of para-aortic nodes, and positive resection margins.

Another negative association is the presence of hepatic metastases, which is the most significant aspect of disease recurrence after curative operation [11].

Infiltration of the common hepatic artery or the celiac trunk is covered in our description of anterograde technique.

Spleen-Preserving Distal Pancreatectomy

The spleen-preserving distal pancreatectomy is an interesting operation for preventing postoperative infections and decreasing the thrombotic risk that follows from severe thrombocytosis after splenectomy [12]. The indications for this operation are neuroendocrine tumors [13], benign lesions, and trauma. The main contraindication is the presence of adenocarcinoma [14].

Preservation of the spleen is obtained by one of two procedures.

Spleen-Preserving Pancreatectomy by Saving the Splenic Artery and Vein

After detachment of the root of the transverse mesocolon and opening of the inferior margin of the pancreas up to the splenic hilum, the dissection is continued by clearing the posterior pancreatic surface from the retroperitoneum.

The splenic artery and vein are loaded on a vessel loop. Thus the progressive and meticulous dissection runs from left to right [15] and from right to left [16]: this last method is the one most used.

After the pancreatic dissection, the distal stump is raised and gently moved to the left: the numerous small arterial and venous branches are ligated between clips and divided.

The dissection continues distally until the pancreatic tail cannot be separated from the splenic hilum. This direction is best because at the splenic hilum the vein is already divided into small vessels that may be damaged. By contrast, the arterial clearing is easier in the opposite direction, besides less tedious, because of the smaller number of branches in the proximal tract of the hilum.

Spleen-Preserving Pancreatectomy by Saving the Short Gastric Vessels and Gastroepiploic Artery

This is the operation planned by Warshaw [17]. The omental bursa is opened and the origin of the splenic artery and splenic vein identified on the posterior pancreatic surface. After detachment of the mesocolic root, the splenic vessels may be dissected between ligatures [18]: this must be done near the point of the pancreatic section. By contrast, distally the splenic vessels have to be ligated closer to the pancreas, to save the collateral circulation through the short vessels and gastroepiploic arch. In this mode, too, the mobilization may be anterograde or retrograde; the former allows better identification of anatomic planes.

Complications of this intervention are splenic necrosis and abscesses, owing to insufficiency of splenic perfusion by means of the collateral circulation described.

Treatment of the Pancreatic Stump

In high-volume centers, the mortality associated with distal pancreatectomy is nowadays under 5%, while the morbidity varies between 30 and 40% [19, 20].

Morbidity in distal pancreatectomy relates to pancreatic fistulas. The method of dividing the pancreas and how to treat the pancreatic duct are still the subject of debate. In practice two techniques are used most: the linear stapler technique, and section of the pancreas with elective ligature of the pancreatic duct. For the sake of completeness, we also mention the following possibilities:

- Pancreaticojejunal anastomosis, in cases of hypertension of the duct of Wirsung (i.e., chronic pancreatitis)
- Gastric or jejunal seromuscular patch on the line of pancreatic section [21, 22]
- Obliteration of the duct of Wirsung using fibrin glue [23]

Use of the Linear Stapler

Deployment of the linear stapler is preceded by blunt dissection of the retroperitoneal tissue of the pancreatic region on which the stapler will be used. The vein, unlike the artery, which is usually isolated and dissected separately, does not need isolation and therefore may be dissected with the pancreatic parenchyma in the stapler stroke: this makes the procedure quicker and bloodless. This maneuver is made easier by the new stapler with larger and longer jaws.

This technique is easy because it is unnecessary to ligate the main pancreatic duct and to add further stitches in order to approach the margins of resection, and safe because it limits the loss of blood [24]. However, it is subject to a rate of pancreatic fistulas of about the 15% in the literature. Some authors reinforce the metal suture with thread sutures, particularly near the pancreatic duct; others add onto the stump a patch of collagen covered with fibrinogen and thrombin; another authors again use resorbable prostheses that are inserted on the stapler. The large number of surgical approaches is indicative of the fact that no technique has been proven to lead to a notable reduction in the incidence of pancreatic fistulas.

Elective Ligature of the Pancreatic Duct

The pancreatic section may be carried out with a blade scalpel, an electric scalpel, or with an ultrasound dissector [25]. The hemostasis of the pancreatic stump needs a lot of fine sutures (i.e., 4/0).

Ligature of the pancreatic duct with nonresorbable sutures must be elective. This is a more difficult technique with more bleeding, but with a fistula rate around 0% [26].

References

1. Netter FH (1985) Atlante di anatomia fisiopatologica e clinica, vol 6. Collezione CIBA
2. Testut L, Latarjet A (1977) Trattato di anatomia umana, vol 5. UTET, Torino

3. Jaeck D, Boudjema K (1986) Pancréatectomie gauche ou distales. Enycl Méd Chir. Technique chirurgicales- Appareil digestif. Elsevier, Paris, 40–880-D, 6p
4. Brennan MF, Moccia RD, Klimstra D (1996) Management of adenocarcinoma of the body and tail of the pancreas. Ann Surg 223:506–512
5. Nikfarjam M, Warshaw AL, Axelrod L et al (2008) Improved contemporary surgical management of insulinomas: a 25-year experience at the Massachusetts General Hospital. Ann Surg 247:165–172
6. Hirano S, Kondo S, Hara T et al (2007) Distal pancreatectomy with en bloc celiac axis resection for locally advanced pancreatic body cancer. Long term results. Ann Surg 246:46–51
7. Japan Pancreas Society (2003) Classification of pancreatic carcinoma, 2nd edn. Kanehara, Tokyo
8. Shimada K, Sakamoto Y, Sano T et al (2006) Prognostic factors after distal pancreatectomy with extended lymphadenectomy for invasive pancreatic adenocarcinoma of the body and tail. Surgery 139:288–295
9. Nakao A, Harada T, Nonami T et al (1997) Lymph node metastasis in carcinoma of the body and tail of the pancreas. Br J Surg 84:1090–1092
10. Nakagohri T, Konoshita T, Konishi M et al (2003) Survival benefits of portal vein resection for pancreatic cancer. Am J Surg 186:149–153
11. Ishikawa O, Ohigashi H, Imaoka S et al (1992) Preoperative indications for extended pancreatectomy for locally advanced pancreas cancer involving the portal vein. Ann Surg 215:231–236
12. Rodríguez JR, Germes SS, Pandharipande PV (2006) Implications and cost of pancreatic leak following distal pancreatic resection. Arch Surg 141:361–365
13. Fernández-Cruz L, Blanco L, Cosa R, Rendón H (2008) Is laparoscopic resection adequate in patients with neuroendocrine pancreatic tumors? World J Surg 32:904–917
14. Bruzoni M, Sasson AR (2008) Open and laparoscopic spleen-preserving, splenic vessel-preserving distal pancreatectomy: indications and outcomes. J Gastrointest Surg Apr 24 (epub ahead of print)
15. Warren DW (1986) Splenopancreatic disconnection. Ann Surg 204:346
16. Blumgart LH (2007) Surgery of the liver, biliary tract and pancreas, vol 1, 4th edn. Saunders Elsevier, Philadelphia, p 893
17. Warshaw AL (1988) Conservation of the spleen with distal pancreatectomy. Arch Surg 123:550–553
18. Rodríguez JR, Madanat MG, Healy BC (2007) Distal pancreatectomy with splenic preservation revisited. Surgery 141:619–625
19. Kleeff J, Diener MK, Z'Graggen K et al (2007) Distal pancreatectomy: risk factors for surgical failure in 302 consecutive cases. Ann Surg 245:573–582
20. Lillemoe KD, Kausha S, Cameron JL (1999) Distal pancreatectomy: indications and outcomes in 235 patients. Scientific Papers of the Southern Surgical Association. Ann Surg 229:693
21. Moriura S, Kimura A, Ikeda S et al (1995) Closure of the distal pancreatic stump with a seromuscular flap. Surg Today 25:992–994
22. Kluger Y, Alfici R, Abbley B et al (1997) Gastric serosal patch in distal pancreatectomy for injury: a neglected technique. Injury 28:127–129
23. Ohwada S, Ogawa T, Tanahashi Y et al (1998) Fibrin glue sandwich prevents pancreatic fistula following distal pancreatectomy. World J Surg 22:494–498
24. Kajiyama Y, Tsurumaru M, Udagawa H et al (1996) Quick and simple distal pancreatectomy using the GIA stapler: report of 35 cases. Br J Surg 83:1711
25. Sugo H, Mikami Y, Matsumoto F (2001) Comparison of ultrasonically activated scalpel versus conventional division for the pancreas in distal pancreatectomy. J Hepat Pancreat Surg 8:349–352
26. Bilimoria MM, Cormier JN, Mun Y et al (2003) Pancreatic leak after left pancreatectomy is reduced following main pancreatic duct ligation. Br J Surg 90:190–196

Chapter 24

Indications and Technique of Central Pancreatectomy

Riccardo Casadei, Claudio Ricci, Nicola Antonacci, Francesco Minni

Definition

Central pancreatectomy, also referred to as medial pancreatectomy, is a segmental, conservative resection of the pancreas of about 5 cm length with sparing of the surrounding structures (spleen, duodenum, biliary tree, and gallbladder). Some authors [1–3] have defined the extent of this surgical resection: the central segment is limited on the right by the gastroduodenal artery, and on the left by the need to leave at least 5 cm of pancreatic tissue in order to perform the reconstruction on the distal pancreatic stump.

Indications

Central pancreatectomy, described for the first time by Guillemin and Bessot [4] in 1957, was indicated at the beginning mainly for benign lesions of the pancreatic neck or proximal body, such as chronic pancreatitis or traumatic lesions. Proponents of central pancreatectomy focus on the maintenance of endocrine and exocrine function; additionally, spleen preservation, especially in younger patients, may also be a benefit.

In 1988 Fagniez et al. [5] for the first time extended the indication to perform this operation in patients with benign tumors of the neck and body of the pancreas. Subsequently the method has been proposed for borderline tumors too, but never for malignant ones. There is anyway the evidence that central pancreatectomy is performed only rarely and only on very selected cases: in 2000, in fact, a literature review reported only 78 published cases [6]. The tumors were mainly well differentiated, benign, or borderline (according to the WHO classification [7]) neuroendocrine tumors, and cystic neoplasms, in particular mucinous, serous, and papillary solid forms.

Regarding intraductal papillary mucinous neoplasm (IPMN), the multicenter French study [8], which has collected the highest number of central pancreatectomies (n = 53), suggests performing this surgery only in patients with a diagnosis of benign IPMN, strictly located in the branch duct of the midpancreas

W. Siquini (Ed.), *Surgical Treatment of Pancreatic Diseases.*
©Springer-Verlag Italia 2009

(branch duct type or type II), because the risk of in situ or invasive carcinoma is low in this setting.

The main purpose of this surgical technique is to reduce both exocrine and endocrine pancreatic insufficiency, sparing normal pancreatic parenchyma. At the same time it must maintain the same oncologic radicality and the same complication rate as are associated with more extended resections such as pancreaticoduodenectomy and distal pancreatectomy.

Surgical Technique

Central pancreatectomy is technically closer to left pancreatectomy than to pancreaticoduodenectomy because central pancreatectomy preserves gastroenteric and bilioenteric continuities and only changes pancreaticoenteric drainage of the body and tail.

Central pancreatectomy is usually performed with open technique, because the laparoscopic approach for pancreatic resection that requires pancreaticoenteric reconstruction remains undetermined. Only a few laparoscopic central pancreatectomies have been reported in the literature [9–11].

The open technique requires a midline incision, from over the xiphoid to below the umbilicus, or a subcostal incision a righ, enlarged to the left, or bilateral subcostal incision. It can be subdivided into three main surgical stages [12]:
1. Surgical exploration and pancreatic mobilization
2. Resection of the neoplastic pancreatic tissue
3. Restoration of gastrointestinal continuity

The *surgical exploration* is performed by carefully checking the whole abdominal cavity. The liver is examined by manual palpation in order to detect metastatic lesions in patients with neoplasms, as are the common bile duct, gallbladder, hepatoduodenal ligament, stomach, duodenum, and spleen. The whole peritoneal surface is investigated for the presence of carcinosis. The mesenteric root is uncovered by lifting the transverse colon to identify the presence of any infiltrating neoplastic leak or metastatic lymph nodes. Finally, venous dilatations are looked for, inside the gastrocolic and hepatoduodenal ligaments, in order to identify venous hypertension in the mesenteric region that could be due to portal infiltration, which would be a contraindication to resective surgery. At this time the anterior surface of the pancreatic head can already be palpated between the left thumb and forefinger through the foramen of Winslow or through the stomach or duodenum.

At this point it is necessary to expose the pancreas through some maneuvers:
1. Transection of the gastrocolic ligament
2. Cattell maneuver
3. Kocher maneuver
4. Opening of lesser omentum
5. Identification of the portal–mesenteric trunk

Transection of the gastrocolic ligament is the first maneuver to perform and allows access to the anterior surface of the pancreas. The stomach is retracted upward and the pancreatic gland is exposed.

The opening of gastrocolic ligament is continued, outside the gastroepiploic vessels, to the right up to the angle located between the middle colic artery and the right gastroepiploic vessels and to the left up to the gastrosplenic ligament, which can be dissected to allow exploration of the splenic hilum. Section of the splenocolic ligament can also be important, giving a complete view of the inferior border of the pancreas, after moving the colic flexure downward.

The stomach is lifted upward, allowing exposure of the anterior surface of the pancreas. This will be even better viewed, in the head area, by sectioning the connective tissue in which are the right gastroepiploic vessels, which together with the middle colic vein and the anterior inferior pancreaticoduodenal vein form the gastrocolopancreatic trunk or venous trunk of Henle, which drains directly in the superior mesenteric vein. Clearly much attention is needed while tractioning the stomach upward and the colon downward, because if not accurately executed it could cause ruptures of the venous trunk of Henle. These can be particularly dangerous because the junction can be located close to the superior mesenteric vein, with consequently much significant blood loss.

The *Cattel maneuver* begins with the incision of the lateral avascular peritoneal layer next to the proximal portion of the ascending colon and continues up to the right colic flexure. The peritoneum which separates this from the descending portion of the duodenum is cut, allowing detachment of the peritoneal layers between the colon and the duodenum itself, making possible the separation of the right colonic flexure from the anterior wall of the second and third portions of the duodenum and from the anterior surface of the head of the pancreas. The colon can then be pulled downward and medially in order to completely expose the duodenal curve, allowing access to the pre-duodenopancreatic submesocolic Fredet fascia. This maneuver is usually performed for pancreatic lesions located at the level of the head of the organ; its use is more limited for body–tail lesions.

The *Kocher maneuver* allows appropriate exposure of the duodenum and of the posterior surface of the pancreatic head; it is very useful for pathologies of the head of the pancreas but is also performed for those of the body and tail, although less extensively.

The maneuver starts with incision of the avascular posterior peritoneal layer (known as Toldt's fascia) at 2–3 cm distance from the duodenal margin, next to the descending portion of the duodenal margin, and continues up to the foramen of Winslow and to the bottom of the mesenteric root. Posterior dissection continues as far as Gerota's fascia and gives access to the retroduodenopancreatic region of Treitz, where the anterolateral surface of the inferior vena cava becomes evident together with the aortic tract between the root of the inferior mesenteric artery and the upper border of the left renal vein. Exactly below the right renal vein, the right spermatic/ovarian vein can be identified.

Opening the lesser omentum allows us to explore better the lymphatic and vascular structures of the right portion of the pancreas. The liver is retracted and the stomach pulled down: in this way the gastrohepatic ligament is extended, and the surgeon can divide it, close to the "pars flaccida", which is avascular, using an electric scalpel or scissors. In this way, the anterior surface of the upper part of the pancreatic head can be visualized and the celiac axis, common hepatic artery, and gastroduodenal artery identified.

Identification of the portal–mesenteric trunk begins with the search for the superior mesenteric vein. This can be identified directly at the lower border of the pancreas, by incision of the parietal peritoneum which covers the vein itself, or following either the right gastroepiploic vein or the middle colic vein, which end, through the venous trunk of Henle, on its right margin or anterior surface. After identification of the portal–mesenteric trunk, the avascular anterior surface is detached from the posterior surface of the pancreatic neck, going from the bottom to the top as far as the superior border of the pancreas.

This maneuver must be extremely delicate and must be performed with extreme caution even though the anterior surface of the portal–mesenteric trunk is avascular, as there is a risk of lacerating some small collateral vessels draining the lateral borders.

In order to complete the mobilization of the body and tail of the pancreas, the peritoneum is incised close to the inferior and superior margins of the pancreas, beginning from the body, on the left of the superior mesenteric vein, all the way to the tail as far as the splenic hilum (Fig. 24.1a). Pancreas and splenic vessels are then lifted to expose completely the posterior surface of the pancreas (Fig. 24.1b). At this point the splenic vessels are separated from the pancreatic parenchyma so that the central pancreatic resection can be performed.

In order to perform a central pancreatectomy some rules must be followed:

– The tumor or the pancreatic lesion must be located to the left of the gastroduodenal artery, which therefore is always maintained.

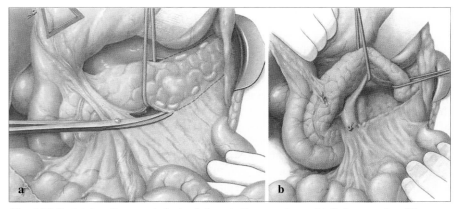

Fig. 24.1 Parietal peritoneum is incised close to the superior and inferior margin of the pancreas (**a**). This maneuver allows complete mobilization of the body and tail of the pancreas (**b**)

- Proximal and distal resection borders must be at least 1 cm away from the tumor.
- The extent of the resection to the left must allow at least 5 cm length of pancreatic parenchyma to be saved.

Thus, a central pancreatectomy is limited on the right by the gastroduodenal artery, while on the left at least 5 cm of pancreatic tissue should be kept. Regarding the portal–mesenteric trunk, the proximal resection margin can be on either the left or the right of it (Fig. 24.2).

The *pancreatic resection* is performed: first the proximal portion, then the distal one is resected. A knife or cautery is used to divide the pancreas.

The intermediate resection of the organ is now complete. Before starting the reconstructive stage, it is mandatory to proceed with the histologic examination of both resection margins, proximal and distal, in order, in the case of a neoplasm, to verify its complete resection.

The *reconstructive stage* concerns the management of the proximal and distal pancreatic stumps. The proximal one is usually closed by a mechanical stapler (GIA or TA, depending on the surgeon's preference), but can also be managed with a manual suture, by identifying and ligating the main pancreatic duct, separately. The distal pancreatic stump can very rarely be closed with a stapler or manually; usually it can be anastomosed with a jejunal loop (pancreaticojejunostomy) or with the posterior surface of the stomach (pancreaticogastrostomy).

The pancreaticojejunostomy, usually in a Roux-en-Y jejunal loop, can be performed with two different techniques: end-to-end or end-to-side. The end-to-end pancreaticojejunostomy (Fig. 24.3) has to be performed by opening the jeju-

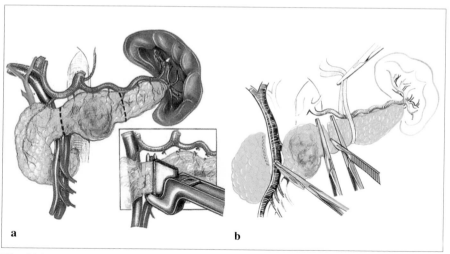

a   b

Fig. 24.2 Extent of central pancreatectomy: proximal resection to the left (**a**) or the right (**b**) of the portal–mesenteric trunk. Moreover, the gastroduodenal artery is always preserved and, to the left, at least 5 cm length of pancreatic parenchyma must be spared

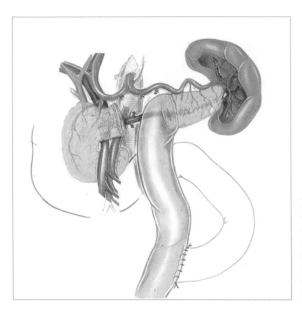

Fig. 24.3 Treatment of the pancreatic stumps: the proximal one is closed by a mechanical stapler (GIA or TA), while the distal one is anastomosed with a jejunal loop (end-to-end pancreaticojejunostomy in a Roux-en-Y jejunal loop)

nal loop completely. Subsequently this loop is anastomosed to the pancreatic stump with a double layer of 3/0 absorbable interrupted sutures, posterior and anterior. The end-to-side anastomosis is performed by suturing first the jejunal serosa and the posterior surface of the pancreas; then a small incision of 1 cm length is made on the jejunum and this is connected with the main pancreatic duct by a double layer of 5/0 absorbable interrupted sutures; finally the jejunal serosa is sutured with the anterior surface of the pancreas.

Some authors prefer to leave a free-floating silicon tutor between the jejunum and the main pancreatic duct to ensure patency of the anastomosis.

As previously mentioned, pancreaticogastrostomy is performed between the pancreatic parenchyma and the posterior wall of the gastric body, in a double layer of 3/0 absorbable interrupted sutures. No statistically significant differences in outcomes have been shown between these different reconstructive methods (pancreaticojejunostomy versus pancreaticogastrostomy). For this reason both the techniques are nowadays used, depending on the surgeon's experience.

If central pancreatectomy is performed with a laparoscopic approach, the patient is placed supine in the lithotomy position. The surgeon stands between the legs of the patient, the first assistant on the right, the second on the left of the operator. The scrub nurse stays on the right side of the first operator. The laparoscopic approach requires four trocars (2 of 10 mm, 2 of 5 mm). The first trocar (10 mm) is placed just above the umbilicus and is used to insufflate the pneumoperitoneum and to insert the 30° optical camera. The other three trocars are placed respectively: (1) on the right hemiclavear line (Conradi's line) (5 mm trocar), about 3 cm above the transverse line passing through the umbilicus, where a grabber forceps is usually inserted; (2) on the left hemiclavear line (10 mm trocar), about 2 cm above the transverse line passing through the umbilicus, where a specific cutting and coagulating instrument is used (electrical ultrasound or radiofrequency tools); (3) (5 mm trocar) immediately below the xiphoid process, where a grabber is placed (Fig. 24.4).

The surgical stages for the laparoscopic technique are the same as for the open technique. In the laparoscopic surgery the proximal pancreatic stump is usually sutured with a linear endoGIA stapler of 60 mm. The distal stump is sectioned using a bipolar electrocoagulation instrument and is subsequently anastomosed to the posterior wall of the stomach. Laparoscopic pancreaticogastrostomy is technically easier than pancreaticojejunostomy because of the anatomic proximity of the stomach and the pancreas and because laparoscopic pancreaticogastrostomy reduces the number of anastomoses. The specimen is extracted after widening one of the holes used to introduce a 10-mm trocar.

The *disadvantages of central pancreatectomy* are related to the necessity of treating two different pancreatic stumps, so the incidence of postoperative complications, especially pancreatic fistulas, can be high. A recent international literature review [13] reported an overall morbidity rate of 33% (range 0–60%), with an incidence of pancreatic fistulas of 22% (0–36%). Postoperative mortality is usually very low and ranges between 0 and 2%.

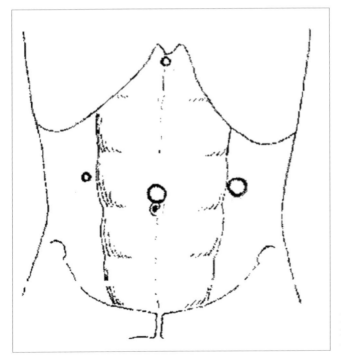

Fig. 24.4 Trocar placement for laparoscopic central pancreatectomy

The *advantages* of this operation relate to the more conservative resection of the pancreatic parenchyma, with sparing of the exocrine and endocrine function of the pancreas. Long-term results show well-preserved exo- and endocrine function of the organ with a 3% incidence of exocrine insufficiency (range 0–8%) and a 3.6% incidence of endocrine insufficiency (range 0–10%) [13].

In conclusion, central pancreatectomy is a safe and technically feasible surgical approach for removing tumors of the pancreatic neck in well-selected patients, with no mortality but high morbidity, and allowing preservation of the spleen, pancreatic parenchyma, and exocrine–endocrine function.

References

1. Sperti C, Pasquali C, Ferronato A et al (2000) Median pancreatectomy for tumors of the neck and body of the pancreas. J Am Coll Surg 190:711–716
2. Efron DT, Lillemoe KD, Cameron JL et al (2004) Central pancreatectomy with pancreatico-gastrostomy for benign pancreatic pathology. J Gastrointestinal Surg 8:532–538
3. Iacono C, Bortolasi L, Serio G (2005) Indications and technique of central pancreatectomy – early and late results. Langenbecks Arch Surg 390:266–271
4. Guillemin P, Bessot M (1957) Pancréatite chronique calcifiante chez un tuberculeux rénal: pancréato-jéjunostomie selon une technique originale. Mem Acad Chirurg 83:869–871
5. Fagniez PL, Kracht M, Rotman N (1988) Limited conservative pancreatectomy for benign tumours: a new technical approach. Br J Surg 75:719
6. Johnson MA, Rajendran S, Balachandar TG et al (2006) Central pancreatectomy for benign pancreatic pathology/trauma: is it a reasonable pancreas-preserving conservative surgical strategy alternative to standard major pancreatic resection? ANZ J Surg 76:987–995
7. Solcia E, Kloppel G, Sobin LH (2000) Histological typing of endocrine tumours. Springer, New York Berlin Heidelberg
8. Sauvanet A, Partensky C, Sastre B et al (2002) Medial pancreatectomy: a multi-institutional retrospective study of 53 patients by the French Pancreas Club. Surgery 132:836–843
9. Ayav A, Bresler L, Brunaud L et al (2005) Laparoscopic approach for solitary insulinoma: a multicentre study. Langenbecks Arch Surg 390:134–140
10. Orsenigo E, Baccari P, Bissolotti G et al (2006) Laparoscopic central pancreatectomy. Am J Surg 191:549–552
11. Sa Cunha A, Rault A, Beau C et al (2007) Laparoscopic central pancreatectomy: single institution experience of 6 patients. Surgery 142:405–409
12. Minni F, Casadei R, Marrano N, Marrano D (2006) Chirurgia del pancreas. UTET, Torino
13. Roggin KK, Rudloff U, Blumgart LH et al (2006) Central pancreatectomy revisited. J Gastrointest Surg 10:804–812

Chapter 25

Total Pancreatectomy: Indications, Technique, and Postoperative Problems

Roberto Santoro

Definition

Total pancreatectomy (TP) consists in removing the entire pancreas, together with part of stomach, duodenum, common bile duct, gallbladder, spleen, and nearby lymph nodes.

Alternative procedures may be pylorus-preserving, spleen-preserving, and duodenum-preserving surgery, with the latter technique envisaging preserving a portion of pancreas a few millimeters thick, thus being called duodenum-preserving near-total pancreatectomy.

Indications

In the 1960s, TP was considered the surgery of choice for ductal carcinoma of the pancreas. It entailed a twofold advantage, eliminating any risk of pancreatic leak and reducing recurrence rates, which were higher when a portion of the pancreas was preserved. In the 1980s, TP was abandoned as it did not show any advantage in terms of survival rates, and, most importantly, intraoperative morbidity and mortality rates were high. Moreover, it resulted in poor postoperative quality of life, due to the serious metabolic consequences of endocrine and exocrine pancreatic insufficiency. This is why, although over the last 20 years intraoperative mortality rates have been decreasing significantly, indications for TP are now limited to a few specific situations, and this surgical procedure only accounts for 5% of all pancreatic resections performed in specialized departments of major referral centers.

Technically speaking, the presence of an *extremely soft pancreatic stump* or an *excessively thin main pancreatic duct* (duct of Wirsung), which make a sturdy anastomosis impossible, are *not considered indications for TP*. Numerous techniques have been suggested to treat the pancreatic stump, and diagnosis and treatment methods for pancreatic fistula are now consolidated. This has allowed specialized centers to reduce pancreaticoduodenectomy-related mortality rates

W. Siquini (Ed.), *Surgical Treatment of Pancreatic Diseases.*
©Springer-Verlag Italia 2009

to less than 5%, meanwhile maintaining the endocrine function of the remaining portion of pancreas, which is the cause of the most serious metabolic problems of TP.

Hence, TP is necessary on the basis of the pancreatic pathology when the latter is widespread and affects the whole gland, and/or when resection margins are infiltrated by a malignancy proceeding towards the pancreatic tail. Currently, TP is a therapeutic option for pancreatic duct carcinoma, as well as other malignancies including intraductal papillary mucinous neoplasms of the pancreas, and benign conditions such as chronic pancreatitis and pancreatic trauma.

Total Pancreatectomy for Cancer

The overall prognosis for pancreatic cancer is severe. Survival for 5years is reported in only 3–5% of all cases, and more than 80% of patients die within 12months after they are diagnosed with the disease. No adjuvant treatment has proved to be effective in reducing the remarkable biological aggressiveness of this cancer and improving the prognosis.

Today, surgery is the only treatment option available, but, unfortunately, the resectability rate is low and only major referral centers report rates of 15–30%. In a literature review covering the years up to 1987, Gudjonsson [1] reported an 11% resectability rate in a total of 37,000 patients suffering from this cancer. Survival at 5years was reported for only 156 patients, who accounted for 0.4% of all patients, thus showing 3.8% survival after resection. More recently, 20–25% 5-year actuarial survival rates have been reported for patients who underwent curative resection, but, overall, the national and international literature shows substantially similar results to the past. In patients suffering from localized and resectable disease, primary prognostic factors for local and/or distal recurrence include tumor size, lymph node metastases, perineural spreading, and residual disease (R1/R2). With the lack of adjuvant treatments, improved outcome seems to be due to more timely and thorough surgical treatment. In this framework, extending the resection seems to be the only way to obtain R0 curative resections.

Extended resection is usually applied when performing *pancreaticoduodenectomy (PD)*, which is the most frequent surgical procedure. The extension includes lymphadenectomy, vascular resections, splenectomy, and regional TP.

TP is recommended as the treatment of choice for pancreatic carcinoma in patients with multicentric neoplasms; to eliminate the risk of infiltration of the pancreatic resection margin; when lymphadenectomy is extended to the whole pancreatic region; and to eliminate any potential risk of sepsis following a complicated pancreatic leak. However, nowadays, TP is no longer popular as a first-choice procedure (Table 25.1). Not only is there no evidence of significant advantages in terms of survival, but this surgical procedure is also associated with higher intraoperative mortality, the onset of unstable diabetes, and malabsorption syndrome due to the ablation of the pancreas. Andren-Sandberg [2] and

Table 25.1 Results of total pancreatectomy (TP) for ductal adenocarcinoma of the pancreas

Author	Period	Surgery performed	No. of patients	Node-positive (%)	Mortality (%)	Morbidity (%)	Survival 1-year (%)	3-year (%)	5-year (%)	Median duration
Van Heerden et al. [4]	1951–85	TP	89	47	10		54	11	7	12 months
	1951–85	PD	101		4			9	4	16.5 months
Brooks et al. [5]	1970–86	TP	41	65	10	27	52	38	14	
Launois et al. [6]	1968–86	TP	47		15	53	42	12	8	8 months
Ishe et al. [3]	1959–84	TP	89	49	27	52			4.5	7 months
	1985–92	PD	36	61	3	28			7.4	11 months
Karpoff et al. [7]	1983–98	TP	35	29	3	55			11	7.9 months

PD, Pancreaticoduodenectomy

Ishe [3] were strong supporters of TP for many years, and they performed it from 1959 to 1982. High mortality (27%) was combined with 5-year survival as low as 5% (median survival: 7 months), with two out of four surviving patients dying during the 6thyear after surgery. In addition, two patients died from hypo-glycemic coma. After this, these authors abandoned TP to adopt the standard Whipple procedure, and observed a significant decrease in intraoperative mor-tality (3%) and a long-term survival rate of 7.4% (median survival: 11 months), which was similar to that of TP. The authors themselves confirmed the therapeu-tic failure of TP as a first-choice procedure, and advised against its routine per-formance, preferring PD. Other authors [4–6, 8] confirmed that 30% of patients who underwent TP had multicentric neoplasms and, despite this, although they supported TP, its results were discouraging as they showed that TP entailed no significant advantage compared to the PDs they had performed in the same peri-od, in same-stage disease. Hence, indications for TP were restricted to those cases where it was difficult to perform sturdy pancreatic anastomosis, and for those where intraoperative frozen section showed neoplastic infiltration of the resection margin extending towards the pancreatic tail. In conclusion, TP has been abandoned as a procedure of choice and is performed only in cases where there is no other alternative, i.e., in the presence of neoplastic infiltration of the pancreatic resection margin.

At present, TP is associated with higher mortality than standard procedures; it also causes major metabolic problems in most patients and, most importantly, does not show any significant long-term prognostic advantage. In addition, a 1983–1998 review carried out by the Sloan-Kettering Cancer Center [9] on TP performed as a last resort showed a markedly more severe prognosis in patients who had undergone TP compared to those who had had subtotal curative resec-tion, and went so far as to challenge its therapeutic value. In fact, 27 out of 28 patients died from neoplasm recurrence.

TP is also a mainstay for so-called *regional pancreatectomy (RP)*, which is an extension of the standard Whipple resection in all directions, based on a "regional" approach. This "regional" approach, proposed by Fortner in 1973 [10] as the new radical treatment for pancreatic cancer, consisted in en-bloc resection of pancreas, spleen, and duodenum, as well as lymph node removal from the diaphragm to the inferior mesenteric artery, with vascular skeletoniza-tion and ablation of the nervous connective tissue (Fortner type 0). This proce-dure could be combined with *resection–anastomosis of the retropancreatic por-tion of the portal vein* (Fortner type 1) and *resection–anastomosis of the initial portion of the superior mesenteric artery* and/or the *celiac trunk* (Fortner type 2). The advantages of RP in controlling the disease have never been clearly proven (Table 25.2), and this procedure undoubtedly entails excessively high intraoperative morbidity and mortality rates, even when performed by experts and, most importantly, causes serious and crippling metabolic problems in patients who survive surgery. RP has never been included with full rights in the list of therapeutic options for pancreatic cancer treatment, as Whipple's proce-dure showed similar results to RP, but very much lower intraoperative mortality

Table 25.2 Results of regional pancreatectomy (RP) for ductal adenocarcinoma of the pancreas

Author	Period	Surgery performed	No. of patients	Node-positive (%)	Mortality (%)	Morbidity (%)	Survival			Median
							1-year (%)	3-year (%)	5-year (%)	
Fortner [11]	1972–82	56	64	26	26	67	40	3		12.5 months
Sassol et al. [12]	1973–84	41	34	22	15	70	65	20	10	12 months
Nagakawa et al. [13]	1973–86	49	70	10	15	37		20[a]	15[a]	
Sindelar [14]	<1989	20	75	8	20	50	50	10		12 months
Fortner et al. [15]	1979–91	56	58	4	9	85			14	17 months

[a] Including intraoperative mortality

rates (5–10%) and no metabolic change, unlike RP. RP has therefore been abandoned, and is today performed only on rare occasions.

TP in Intraductal Papillary Mucinous Tumor of the Pancreas

Intraductal papillary mucinous neoplasms (IPMNs) of the pancreas are considered preneoplastic lesions with potentially neoplastic foci at diagnosis affecting the canal of Wirsung (main pancreatic duct), but also secondary ducts. The involvement of pancreatic ducts varies depending on the disease localization and spread. It may be extremely localized and confined to some sections of the main duct or individual secondary ducts, or it may involve the whole canalicular system of the pancreas.

The most appropriate treatment for IPMN has not been identified yet, as no final data are available about the natural history of the disease and long-term follow-up of patients who have undergone surgery. This being said, there are grounds for saying that untreated IPMNs will become malignancies, following the dysplasia–carcinoma–metastasis process. Surgery aims at ablating preneoplastic lesions, easing symptoms of duct obstruction, and providing curative treatment to already developed carcinomas. The diagnosis of IPMN is made on the basis of computed tomography (CT) and magnetic resonance (MR) cholangiopancreatography, as well as ultrasonography and endoscopic retrograde cholangiopancreatography (ERCP), showing dilatation of ducts filled with solid content. In most cases, only histological examination of the ablated pancreas allows the presence of carcinoma to be ascertained. The presence of a neoplasm has been proven in 35–45% of patients who underwent cephalic pancreatectomy or distal pancreatectomy due to IPMN.

The decision about the extent of the exeresis is based on preoperative imaging together with intraoperative frozen section of the pancreatic resection margin. Isolated dilatation of a secondary duct is more often observed in the head and in the uncinate process of the pancreas, and a distinction has to be made between the latter and any benign cystic lesion of a different nature (pseudocysts, simple cysts, serous cystadenoma). Lesions of the head of the pancreas can be treated by a head pancreatectomy, just as main duct segmental dilatation, which is mainly observed in the body–tail region, can be treated by subtotal distal pancreatectomy. Should dilatation affect the whole of the canal of Wirsung and reach the secondary ducts, TP must be performed. These are the forms where malignant degeneration is most often observed. Malignant recurrences are frequent (60–70% of cases) in invasive IPMNs, regardless of the resection extent.

Today, IPMNs are the second most frequent indication for pancreatic resection after ductal adenocarcinoma. The surgical procedure of choice is partial pancreatectomy, which is planned depending on the extent of the disease. TP does not entail any survival advantage compared to partial resection when it comes to invasive forms which turn into malignancies, and should only be performed if there is no suitable alternative.

Total Pancreatectomy for Neuroendocrine Tumors

Neuroendocrine tumors (NET) include a wide family of rare neoplasms showing variable clinic behavior, ranging from benign and differentiated forms to undifferentiated metastasized malignancies. More than 50% of NETs are functioning tumors, less than 50% of them being malignant. Distal subtotal pancreatectomy and, more rarely, total pancreatectomy, are therapeutic options for clinically unidentifiable insulinomas or forms relating to benign multicentric pancreatic diseases, including adenomatosis, nesidioblastosis, or hyperplasia of the pancreatic islets. In the very few cases in which insulinomas are not preoperatively or intraoperatively localized (<5%), the left half of the pancreas must be resected, with a frozen section being performed by the pathologist; if necessary, the resection must be extended rightwards, thus including up to 80–90% of the gland. Total pancreatectomy is rarely necessary. In fact, subtotal distal pancreatectomy allows insulin levels to be reduced significantly, facilitating medical treatment of the disease, and thus also easing symptoms, even in multicentric benign pathologies.

Total Pancreatectomy for Chronic Pancreatitis

Chronic pancreatitis is a progressive disease that destroys the pancreatic exocrine tissue and entails pain, making the patient's quality of life remarkably worse. Almost 50% of patients suffering from chronic pancreatitis need to resort to surgery to eliminate pain or other complications relating to the disease, and 30–50% of them have additional subsequent problems due to their pancreatic pathology. Primary TP is rarely performed in the treatment of chronic pancreatitis. It can be considered as the treatment of choice in selected patients reporting untreatable chronic pain that does not respond to medical treatment, caused by chronic pancreatitis with minor dilatation of the canal of Wirsung. In most cases, TP is performed as a second step after a previous resection (including pancreaticoduodenectomy or distal pancreatectomy), or after drainage procedure (Puestow) that proved to be ineffective after long-term follow-up, with crippling pain recurrence or new complications arising. Unfortunately, eliminating pain means triggering near-uncontrollable "unstable" insulin-dependent diabetes mellitus.

Total Pancreatectomy for Acute Pancreatitis and Pancreatic Trauma

TP is not a standard procedure in the treatment of acute pancreatitis, as it is a particularly difficult procedure to be performed in cases of multicentric hemorrhagic necrosis, with a high risk of vascular lesions, as well as peripancreatic, biliary, and digestive lesions. It has been replaced by necrosectomy or sequestrectomy, which cannot even be considered as pancreatectomies.

Both closed and open abdominal injury can entail a wide variety of pancreatic lesions, in terms of types and severity. They can include simple hematoma as well as more serious injuries such as partial or total rupture of the isthmus on the vertebral body and the destruction of the pancreatic head, with rupture of the duodenum, the common bile duct, or even major regional vascular axes and pedicles. Such injuries are rarely isolated and can seldom be the targets for elective treatment. In fact, they are often combined with other major injuries affecting other organs and systems, in the framework of a polytrauma causing rapid death, with no possibility for surgery. Should emergency surgery be required, it would be necessary to explore the pancreatic region carefully with a view to identifying possible lesions before edema and the foci of steatonecrosis may hide them. In cases of partial or total rupture of the isthmus, the simplest solution consists in performing body and tail pancreatectomy, avoiding the temptation to try conservative procedures. Pancreatic head lesions are often complex and difficult to define. It is necessary to ascertain the integrity of the duodenum and common bile duct as well as the surrounding vascular axes. When injuries are widespread, extended resection is, again, necessary. If major injuries are not treated radically, they may entail serious complications, including hemorrhage, sepsis, and pancreatitis.

Technique

TP can be performed in two different situations, namely:
1. *TP as a second step after pancreaticoduodenectomy.* This is the most frequent situation, which takes place after PD due to neoplastic infiltration of the pancreatic resection margin found at frozen section. In such cases, left pancreatectomy is performed after PD, as described in previous chapters concerning left pancreatectomy.
2. *TP as an "at once" procedure.* In this case, an en-bloc resection is performed of the entire pancreas, part of the stomach, duodenum, jejunum, common bile duct, gallbladder, and spleen.

The preferred approach is via a bilateral subcostal laparotomy. The abdominal region must be carefully explored, with a view to identifying any small liver metastases, retroperitoneal lymph node metastases, and any metastatic or neoplastic infiltration of the celiac trunk and its main branches (hepatic artery and splenic artery). Opening the lesser omentum and retracting downward the lesser gastric curvature allow good exposure of the celiac region. Total coloepiploic detachment with mobilization of the right and left colic flexures and section of the short vessels allows the retrocavity to be thoroughly explored, and verification of whether the disease has also affected the mesocolon and mesenteric vessels. Kocher's maneuver, extended up to the right wall of the aorta, allows retroperitoneal neoplastic infiltration to be excluded and mobilization of the duodenopancreatic complex to be started. Next, the elements of the hepatic peduncle are prepared, cholecystectomy is performed, and the pancreatic isthmus is mobilized from the retropancreatic vascular axis, as in pancreaticoduodenectomy.

Once operability has been ascertained, irreversible actions can be taken. The body and tail of the pancreas are mobilized from left to right, in order to dissect and isolate the complex on the pancreatic isthmus and reflect it to the right. This procedure is easier if started with the ligation and section of the splenic artery at its origin, thus reducing bleeding and decongesting the spleen. The spleen and pancreatic tail are held with the left hand, lifted, and moved to the right. The right hand performs the detachment from the posterior retroperitoneum, dissecting the ligaments with the diaphragm, and detaching the lower margin of the pancreas from the root of the mesocolon. The mesenteric–portal venous trunk is freed by sectioning the splenic vein, located on the posterior side of the pancreatic body, upstream of its connection to the superior and inferior mesenteric vein.

Once the distal splenopancreatic complex has been entirely mobilized and the retropancreatic vessels have been freed, the procedure envisages the detachment of the cephalic duodenopancreatic complex, as in standard pancreaticoduodenectomy. Section between the ligatures of the gastroduodenal artery at its origin, section of the biliary duct upstream of its intersection with the cystic duct, and section of the gastric antrum between the body and the antrum allow fully mobilization of the upper part of the duodenopancreatic complex. Inferiorly, the mobilization of the angle of Treitz and the first jejunal loop allow the mesenteric complex to be detached. At this point, the duodenosplenopancreatic complex is medially dissected and isolated on the uncinate process. Reflecting the gastric antrum, splenopancreatic complex, and first jejunal loop to the right allows full exposure of the uncinate process and retropancreatic sheat, which is resected; the afferent pancreaticoduodenal vessels of the superior mesenteric artery undergo selective ligature.

Various reconstruction techniques exist. The simplest consists in using a single jejunal loop to perform transmesocolic biliodigestive anastomosis and, subsequently, transmesocolic gastrojejunal anastomosis, in order to restore digestive continuity.

Postoperative Metabolic Problems

TP entails complete endocrine and exocrine pancreatic failure. Post-TP diabetes is characterized by barely controllable major instability, due to the absence of endogenous insulin and glucagon, which entail alternating hyperglycemia – with related symptoms – and hypoglycemia. The instability of the glycemic values is mainly due to the lack of glucagon, a hormone responsible for controlling long-term glycemia after meals, as well as hepatic glucidic metabolism; this leads to *severe postprandial hyperglycemia*, and *serious nocturnal hypoglycemia*. This condition, which appears immediately after surgery, may last a long time and can lead to renewed hospitalization with the aim of stabilizing glycemia. Specific deaths due to severe hypoglycemia have also been reported. Total exocrine insufficiency contributes to increase glycemic instability.

Malabsorption caused by TP is particularly significant in the initial period. This condition typically entails fat malabsorption steatorrhea and fatty stools, where the fat concentration in the stool is more than doubled. *Malabsorption syndrome* may entail diarrhea and weight loss, and is caused by multiple factors. The absence of pancreatic enzymes is combined with the metabolic and digestive consequences of gastrectomy; extended lymphectomy may result in diarrhea; some patients also show difficulties in adjusting to the new diet. In some cases, it is necessary to continue total parenteral feeding at home for quite a long time. Long-term sequelae of malabsorption include osteoporosis and liver steatosis, which can result in terminal cirrhosis. Osteoporosis is probably due to the reduction in calcium absorption after gastrectomy, while fatty stools seem to be linked to changes in liver lipogenesis due to alterations of glucidic metabolism.

Correct postoperative management allows most patients to reach a balanced condition, with diarrhea disappearing and weight loss ceasing. Calorie and supplemental pancreatic enzyme needs have to be accurately calculated for each patient, as well as their need of vitamin D and antidiarrheal drugs, also envisaging a high-calorie diet and the administration of fat-soluble vitamins. This being said, the *post-pancreatectomy glycemic balance is closely related to good nutritional balance*. Post-TP patients must follow a diet that will allow their glycemic values to stabilize within a safe range, below a safety threshold of 200mg/dl. Controlling glycemia is difficult, as continuous monitoring is necessary, which influences patients' quality of life. Unfortunately, despite great effort, some patients do not succeed in reaching stable equilibrium, and glycemic decompensation episodes can keep on occurring over time.

Regional pancreatectomy (RP) entails severe and crippling metabolic consequences. In addition to TP-related problems, it also entails problems related to extended lymphectomy, with the ablation of regional sympathetic plexuses, which entail more severe diarrhea. Dresler and Fortner reported that all patients who underwent RP showed severe and crippling postoperative diarrhea, which improved after 1year but continued in 10% of patients.

Autotransplantation of pancreatic islets and *cadaveric islet or pancreas transplantation* are options for the treatment of diabetes in candidates for TP due to benign pathologies. The 1980s saw the introduction of autotransplantation of autologous pancreatic islets taken and prepared when the pancreas was ablated, and immediately engrafted through the portal circulation in order to favor their implantation in the hepatic parenchyma. Over the last few years, this procedure has been remarkably improved in terms of the isolation, preservation, and infusion of a higher number of islets, and excellent results have been obtained in terms of independence from insulin and the disappearance of hypoglycemic crises. For this reason, TP with autotransplantation of pancreatic islets could become the future surgery of choice in the treatment of complicated chronic pancreatitis that does not respond to medical treatment. Furthermore, over the last few years, transplantation of cadaveric pancreas and pancreatic islets has also been performed, with encouraging results.

References

1. Gudjonsson B (1987) Cancer of the pancreas. 50 years of surgery. Cancer 60:2284–2303
2. Andren-Sandberg A, Ishe I (1983) Factors influencing survival after total pancreatectomy in patients with pancreatic cancer. Ann Surg 198:605–610
3. Ishe I, Anderson H, Andren-Sandberg A (1996) Total pancreatectomy for cancer of the pancreas: is it appropriate? World J Surg 20:288–294
4. Van Heerden JA, McIlrath DC, Ilstrup DM, Weiland LH (1988) Total pancreatectomy for ductal adenocarcinoma of the pancreas: an update. World J Surg 12:658–662
5. Brooks JR, Brooks DC, Levine JD (1989) Total pancreatectomy for ductal cell carcinoma of the pancreas. An update. Ann Surg 209:405–410
6. Launois B, Franci J, Bardaxoglou E et al (1993) Total pancreatectomy for ductal adenocarcinoma of the pancreas with special reference to resection of the portal vein and multicentric cancer. World J Surg 17:122–127
7. Karpoff HM, Klimstra DS, Brennan MF, Conlon KC (2001) Results of total pancreatectomy for adenocarcinoma of the pancreas. Arch Surg 136:44–47
8. Sperti C, Pasquali C, Piccoli A, Pedrazzoli S (1996) Survival after resection for ductal adenocarcinoma of the pancreas. Br J Surg 83:625–631
9. Karpoff HM, Klimstra DS, Brennan MF, Conlon KC (2001) Results of total pancreatectomy for adenocarcinoma of the pancreas. Arch Surg 136(1):44–7; discussion 48
10. Fortner J (1973) Regional resection of cancer of the pancreas. A new surgical approach. Surgery 73:307–320
11. Fortner JG (1984) Regional pancreatectomy for cancer of the pancreas, ampulla, and other related sites. Ann Surg 199:418–425
12. Sassol C, Joyeux H, Yakoun M et al (1984) La pancreatectomie régionale dans le traitement de l'adénocarcinome du pancréas. Gastroenterol Clin Biol 8:17–21
13. Nagakawa T, Konishi I, Ueno K et al (1991) Surgical treatment of pancreatic cancer. The Japanese experience. Int J Pancreatol 9:135–143
14. Sindelar WF (1989) Clinical experience with regional pancreatectomy for adenocarcinoma of the pancreas. Arch Surg 124:127–132
15. Fortner JG, Klimstra DS, Senie RT, Maclean B (1996) Tumor size is the primary prognosticator for pancreatic cancer after regional pancreatectomy. Ann Surg 223:147–153

Suggested Reading

Balcom JH, Rattner DW, Warshaw AL et al (2001) Ten years experience with 733 pancreatic resections. Arch Surg 136:391–398

Baumel H, Huguier M, Manderscheid JC et al (1994) Results of resection for cancer of the exocrine pancreas: a study from the French Association of Surgery. Br J Surg 81:102–107

Besselink MG, Verwer TJ, Schoenmaeckers EJ et al (2007) Timing of surgical intervention in necrotizing pancreatitis. Arch Surg 142:1194–1201

Billing BJ, Christein JD, Harmsen WS et al (2005) Quality-of-life after total pancreatectomy: is it really that bad on long-term follow-up? J Gastrointest Surg 9:1059–1066

Conlon KC, Klimstra DS, Brennan MF (1996) Long term survival after curative resection for pancreatic ductal adenocarcinoma. Ann Surg 223:273–279

Doi R, Fujimoto K, Wada M, Imamura M (2002) Surgical management of intraductal papillary mucinous tumour of the pancreas. Surgery 132:80–85

Dresler CM, Fortner JG, McDermott K, Bajorunas D (1991) Metabolic consequences of (regional) total pancreatectomy. Ann Surg 214:131–140

Falconi M, Salvia R, Bassi C et al (2001) Clinicopathological features and treatment of intraductal papillary mucinous tumour of the pancreas. Br J Surg 88:376–381

Fortner JG, Kim DK, Cubilla A et al (1977) Regional pancreatectomy: en bloc pancreatic, portal vein and lymph node resection. Ann Surg 186:42–50

Gruessner RW, Sutherland DE, Dunn DL et al (2004) Transplant options for patients undergoing total pancreatectomy for chronic pancreatitis. J Am Coll Surg 198:559–567

Gruessner RW, Sutherland DE, Drangstveit MB et al (2008) Pancreas allotransplant in patients with previous total pancreatectomy for chronic pancreatitis. J Am Coll Surg 206:458–465

Heidt DJ, Burant C, Simeone DM (2007) Total pancreatectomy: indications, operative technique, and postoperative sequelae. J Gastrointest Surg 11:209–216

Hirata K, Sato T, Mukaiya M et al (1997) Results of 1001 pancreatic resections for invasive ductal adenocarcinoma of the pancreas. Arch Surg 132:771–777

Kim SC, Park KT, Lee YJ et al (2008) Intraductal papillary mucinous neoplasms of the pancreas: clinical characteristic and treatment outcomes of 118 consecutive patients from a single center. J Hepatobiliary Pancreat Surg 15:183–188

Maire F, Hammel P, Terris B et al (2002) Prognosis of malignant intraductal papillary mucinous tumour of the pancreas after surgical resection. Comparison with pancreatic ductal adenocarcinoma. Gut 51:717–722

Ministero della Sanità (1997) Relazione sullo stato sanitario del Paese 1992/96. Ministero della Sanità, Rome

Muller MW, Friess H, Kleff J, Dahmen R et al (2007) Is there still a role for total pancreatectomy? Ann Surg 246:966–974

Rodriguez Rilo HL, Ahmad SA, D'Alessio D et al (2003) Total pancreatectomy and autologous islet cell transplantation as a means to treat severe chronic pancreatitis. J Gastrointest Surg 7:978–989

Rosso S, Casella C, Crocetti E et al (2001) Sopravvivenza dei casi di tumore in Italia negli anni novanta: i dati dei Registri Tumori. Epidemiol Prev 25:1–375

Schmidt CM, Glant J, Winter JM et al (2007) Total pancreatectomy (R0 resection) improves survival over subtotal pancreatectomy in isolated neck margin positive pancreatic adenocarcinoma. Surgery 142:572–578

Stitzemberg KB, Watson JC, Roberts A et al (2008) Survival after pancreatectomy with major arterial resection and reconstruction. Ann Surg Oncol 15:1399–1406

Sugiyama M, Atomi Y (1998) Intraductal papillary mucinous tumour of the pancreas. Ann Surg 228:685–691

Trede M, Schwall G, Saeger H (1990) Survival after pancreaticoduodenectomy. Ann Surg 211:447–458

Yamaguchi K, Konomi H, Kabayashi K et al (2005) Total pancreatectomy for intraductal papillary-mucinous tumor of the pancreas: reappraisal of total pancreatectomy. Hepatogastroenterology 52:1585–1590

Yang AD, Melstrom LG, Bentrem DJ et al (2007) Outcome after pancreatectomy for intraductal mucinous neoplasms of the pancreas: an institutional experience. Surgery 142:534–537

Yeo CJ, Cameron JL, Lillemoe KD et al (1995) Pancreaticoduodenectomy for cancer of the head of the pancreas. Ann Surg 221:721–733

Chapter 26

Laparoscopic Pancreatic Surgery: What Have We Learnt in 10 Years?

Micaela Piccoli, Barbara Mullineris, Domenico Marchi, Gianluigi Melotti

The first great lesson we learned is that to achieve the best results you need skills and enthusiasm. Ten years ago two great Schools joined efforts to start a wonderful adventure: the Verona University school of pancreatic surgery, directed by Professor Paolo Pederzoli, and the Modena Hospital school of laparoscopic surgery, directed by Professor Gianluigi Melotti. This made it possible to standardize technique, to achieve very good results, and to specify indications and contraindications. Once again, Italy had climbed to the top of the international literature.

Indications

The first dilemma we addressed concerned the indications for laparoscopic pancreatic surgery. Under this heading we can consider two main aspects: the site and the type of the pathology.

Site

The laparoscopic approach to the **head of the pancreas** is still the subject of numerous discussions. Diagnostic laparoscopy, before excision of the duodenum and head of the pancreas for tumor, is a simple and accurate way to avoid a laparotomy that will be useless if there are micrometastases in the liver and peritoneum. In the absence of peritoneal carcinosis and liver micrometastases, a laparoscopic evaluation carried out by an experienced surgeon with suitable equipment can be even more accurate in assessing the resectability of a pancreatic neoplasm: the characteristics of the lesion can be inspected with laparoscopic ultrasound probes to reveal possible vascular (portal vein, mesenteric vein and artery) and biliary infiltration and lymph node involvement and to perform biopsies. In some cases, a regular Kocher's maneuver allows evaluation of any duodenal and vena caval infiltrations. In inoperable cases, *biliary and digestive tract reconstructive procedures* are also feasible with the laparoscopic approach (Fig. 26.1).

W. Siquini (Ed.), *Surgical Treatment of Pancreatic Diseases.*
©Springer-Verlag Italia 2009

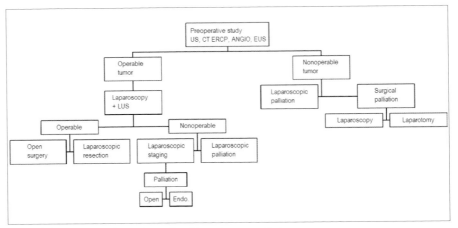

Fig. 26.1 Laparoscopic staging of malignant pancreatic tumors

As to *laparoscopic pancreaticoduodenectomy,* however, the procedure has been proven to be feasible, but its reproducibility was not equally clearly demonstrated. It is a difficult and often lengthy technique requiring a phase of demolition followed by a reconstruction time (with three anastomoses). To overcome all this, a number of artifices and hybrid techniques have been attempted, to the detriment of the advantages of the technique: laparoscopic demolition and laparotomic or hand-assisted reconstruction. The results are not optimal in terms of operating time and intraoperative and postoperative complications, and the technique does not seem to lend itself to standardization. The robotic technique perhaps yields better results, but the problems related to reproducibility are left unsolved. The laparoscopic approach, on the other hand, is feasible for enucleation of benign lesions of the head, provided, however, that very good preoperative imaging is performed (Fig. 26.2) and a laparoscopic ultrasound probe is used during the procedure to locate the lesion and ascertain its relation to the pancreatic ducts and the blood vessels.

Laparoscopic enucleation of benign or low-malignancy lesions on the anterior surface of the **body of the pancreas** is a simple technique. *Central pancreatectomy*, by contrast, should only be used when a pancreatic body lesion is located either too deeply to allow enucleation or too far proximally to perform distal pancreatectomy, which would entail too great a sacrifice of pancreatic parenchyma. This technique, tested in the open surgery approach and proven reliable for benign or low-malignancy lesions, has already been used in laparoscopy but only in sporadic cases. If the anastomosis is fashioned between the pancreatic stump and the posterior wall of the stomach, reconstruction can be easier than with a jejunopancreatic anastomosis with Roux-en-Y loop, as it does not produce discontinuity of the jejunum and it requires one anastomosis fewer.

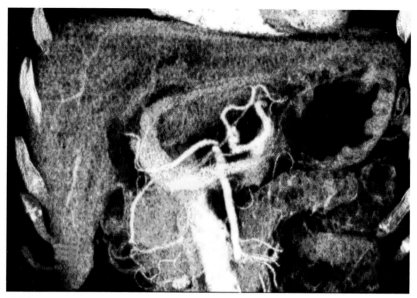

Fig. 26.2 Neuroendocrine tumor of uncinate process of the pancreas

The laparoscopic treatment options for lesions involving the **tail of the pancreas** include enucleation, distal pancreatectomy, and distal splenopancreatectomy. Enucleation seems to produce a higher incidence of postoperative fistula than distal pancreatectomy: therefore, if the lesion is distal and the loss of parenchyma not too great, a major resection should be chosen even in the case of superficial lesions.

Pathology

Considering only the standardized pancreatic lesions – that is, body and tail lesions – it may be safely stated that:

- There is general consensus that the laparoscopic approach is almost a "gold standard" for all benign lesions or low-grade malignancies (pancreatitis, neuroendocrine tumors, cystic tumors, etc.)
- Malignancies (again in the area of the body and tail of the pancreas) show resectability rates of 8–12% in various centers of excellence

What is required in terms of oncological radicality is splenopancreatectomy and the resection of splenic vessels at their site of origin, without performing a broad retroperineal lymphadenectomy (as a substantial number of lymph nodes is excised when the vessel are resected at their origin and with the splenectomy). All this is feasible with the laparoscopic approach, but the literature data cannot be assessed clearly as yet: most papers on laparoscopic distal pancreatectomy include both benign and malignant pathology; in most patients with malignant lesions, other lesions are also present besides adenocarcinomas; there are no randomized trials, no long-term follow up is reported. Therefore, distal pancreatectomy for malignant tumors is still an option open to discussion.

Position of the Patient

Usually the patient lies supine with legs apart, and is tilted to a slight (35°) anti-Trendelenburg position. The operating surgeon stands between the patient's legs, with the first and second assistant placed at his or her left and right, respectively. The scrub nurse stands at the right of the operating surgeon. The monitor is at the patient's left shoulder (Fig. 26.3). Some authors use the supine position, with a pillow supporting the patient's left side so that a semilateral right decubitus is obtained (Fig. 26.4), as for a splenectomy. Others prefer the right lateral decubitus proper (Fig. 26.5), as for a left adrenalectomy. In a 2005 European multicenter trial, the positions used for 122 patients undergoing laparoscopic resection of pancreatic body–tail lesions were: 61 (50%) supine decubitus, 51 (42%) right semilateral decubitus, and 10 (8%) right lateral decubitus. In our

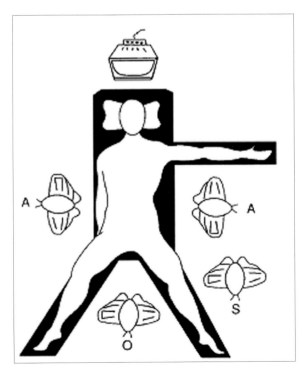

Fig. 26.3 Supine decubitus. *A*, Assistant surgeons; *O*, operating surgeon; *S*, scrub nurse

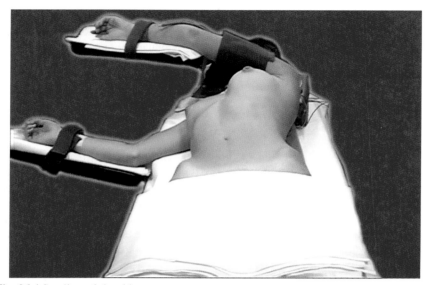

Fig. 26.4 Semilateral decubitus

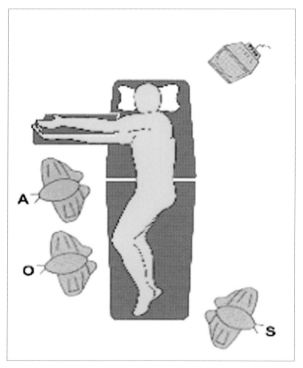

Fig. 26.5 Right lateral decubitus. *A*, Assistant surgeon; *O*, operating surgeon; *S*, scrub nurse

experience, the surgical isolation and dissection of splenic vessels is not made any easier by the right lateral position and previous mobilization of the spleen, which may even complicate these surgical maneuvers. The semilateral right position, on the other hand, favors a partial elevation of the spleen and can therefore be useful in the carrying out of distal splenopancreatectomy.

Position of the Trocars

A pneumoperitoneum is created by inserting a Veress needle, then the first trocar bearing the scope is inserted in the umbilicus. The other operative trocars are placed as follows: one (5 mm) left paraxiphoid, one (5–12 mm) in the right upper quadrant of the abdomen, one (5–12 mm) in the left side (Fig. 26.6). It is useful to add a further trocar, placed more laterally in the left side, which facilitates dissection and at the end of the procedure can be used to place a drain that slopes downward enough to allow the thorough draining of any potential pancreatic postoperative fistulas.

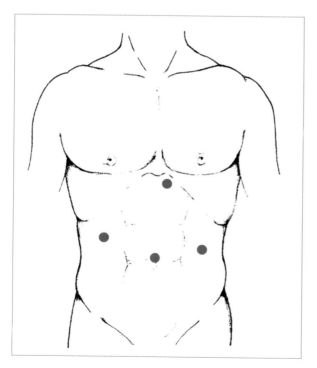

Fig. 26.6 Trocars placement

Access to the Pancreatic Recess and Exploration of the Pancreas

The pancreas can be explored through a supragastric or infragastric access. The supragastric route through the lesser omentum, however, does not allow full exploration of the pancreas. It can be used for fine-needle aspiration or biopsy of cystic or solid lesions mainly of the head but also of the pancreatic tail and body, if they protrude from the superior pancreatic margin. The infragastric route, on the other hand, allows a full view of the whole anterior surface, not only of the body and tail, but also of the head (Fig. 26.7). With an atraumatic grasper introduced through the left paraxiphoid trocar, the first assistant lifts the stomach, grasping it at the greater curvature and then at its posterior surface. The operating surgeon opens a window in the gastrocolic ligament, under the gastroepiploic arch; the window is then enlarged so as to expose the pancreas. *To the left, the enlargement should stop at the first short gastric vessel, especially if the initial intent is to spare the spleen: an injury to the splenic vessels and their ligature, after ensuring blood supply through the short gastric vessels, could spare the need for splenectomy (Warshaw's technique).*

Enucleation

Once the lesion has been identified through the scopes or using the ultrasound probe, and the enucleation judged feasible without the risk of traumatizing the duct of Wirsung and the vessels, dissection can be initiated. The utmost care

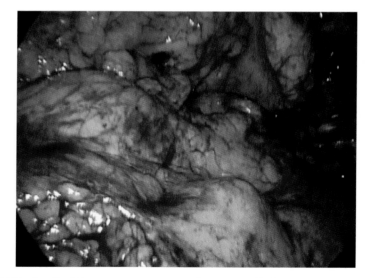

Fig. 26.7 Body-tail of the pancreas: exposure after gastrocolic legament opening

should be taken to ablate the lesion together with the whole capsule, but without going too deep into the parenchyma, so as not to damage the pancreatic duct and create postoperative pancreatic fistulae. The ultrasound dissector will make the procedure much easier, but often the unipolar hook will make it possible to perform fine dissections not feasible otherwise. It can be useful to introduce into the operating field a gauze soaked in adrenaline solution, to check modest parenchymal bleeding. The residual pancreatic recess can be coated with fibrin glue. The excised neoplasm is put in a bag and exteriorized through the umbilicus. A Penrose or Jackson-Pratt drain is always placed adjacent to the residual recess and left in situ. To prevent it from dislodging, it can be attached to the pancreatic fat with a thin resorbable stitch.

"Spleen-Preserving" Distal Pancreatectomy

In distal pancreatectomy, the pancreas can be dissected from the vessels via the antegrade route (from the right to the left) or the retrograde route (from the left to the right). The multicenter European trial cited above reports that out of 96 distal pancreatectomies, 82% were carried out using the antegrade route, and in only 18% was the retrograde route used.

The advantage of the *retrograde technique* is that the surgeon can decide the exact position of the pancreatic section, depending on where the neoplasm is located, thus sparing as much parenchyma as possible. With the antegrade technique, the pancreas is always resected at the isthmus and all too often this means sacrificing too much pancreatic parenchyma. The surgeon should be familiar with both techniques – which we will now expound briefly – in order to make the right decision on the basis of the patient's anatomy and the site of the lesion.

Retrograde Technique

The dissection begins at the inferior margin of the body of the pancreas, at the site of insertion of the root of the transverse mesocolon (which, if opened accidentally, should be carefully sutured), and proceeds towards the tail, looking for the splenic vein which, once identified, is gently dissected from the pancreas (Fig. 26.8).

The small branches originating from the splenic vein and going to the pancreas are easily coagulated and only rarely are clips or ligatures necessary. Then the tail of the pancreas is mobilized and verticalized medially (Fig. 26.9). The pancreatic parenchyma should be grasped very gently, to avoid damage and bothersome bleeding which would dim the light during the laparoscopic procedure and fog the vision of the operating field. Following dissection of the posterior surface of the pancreas, the splenic vessels become fully visible (Fig. 26.10). The splenic artery is usually dissected in the opposite direction to the vein, i.e., from left to right. This maneuver is generally easier than it is on the

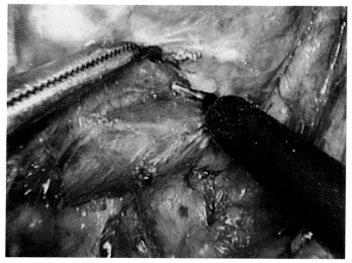

Fig. 26.8 Splenic vein dissection at the inferior edge of the pancreas

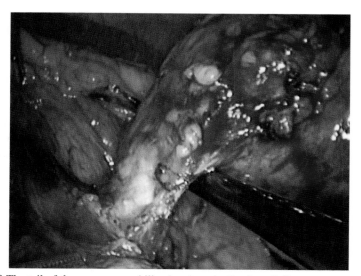

Fig. 26.9 The tail of the pancreas mobilized and verticalized medially

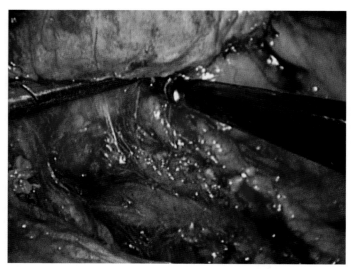

Fig. 26.10 Retrograde technique. Splenic vessels dissected from the posterior surface of the pancreas

vein, as the arterial walls are firmer, the collateral vessels are less numerous, and the artery is more loosely connected to the pancreatic parenchyma. Hemostatic stitches can be used to repair any small arterial tear, without converting the procedure to laparotomy. The vascular dissection can be extended medially beyond the splenomesenteric–portal confluence (Fig. 26.11). Lesions – especially cystic ones – should be handled very cautiously, taking care to avoid rupture and seeding, which in the case of malignancy would invalidate the oncological radicality of the procedure. The rupture of a cystic lesion, however, does not require, per se, conversion to laparotomy: the fluid should be immediately and completely aspirated and the lesion closed by a ligature, clips, or suture stitches.

Antegrade Technique

The dissection begins at the inferior margin of the pancreatic isthmus, thus creating a true subpancreatic tunnel (Fig. 26.12). The pancreas is detached from the splenic vessels, at the splenomesenteric venous confluence. The dissection plane is avascular, as it runs between the posterior mesogastric fascia, behind the pancreas, and Gerota's fascia. The pancreatic isthmus is lifted to introduce a rubber band which will facilitate dissection (Fig. 26.13). The pancreas is dissected proceeding towards the hilum, from right to left, to detach the body–tail from the remaining splenic vessels.

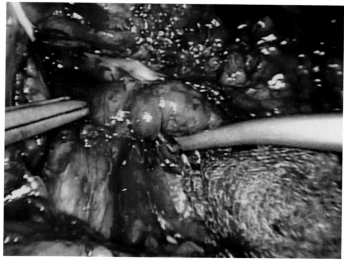

Fig. 26.11 The splenic vein isolated at the splenomesenteric-portal confluence

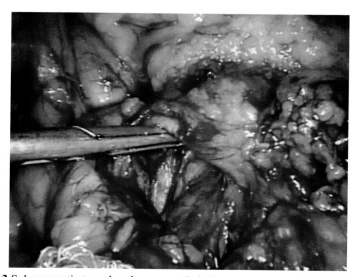

Fig. 26.12 Subpancreatic tunnel at the pancreatic isthmus

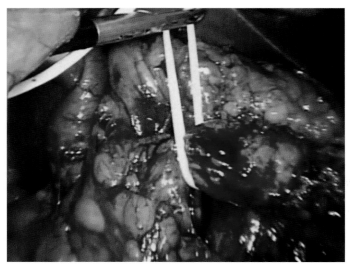

Fig. 26.13 The pancreatic isthmus is lifted with a rubber band

Warshaw's Technique

Some authors describe the distal pancreatectomy technique as entailing ligature and dissection of the splenic vessels on both sides of the resected pancreas, without spleen ablation. Thus the spleen would continue to be vascularized by the short gastric vessels and through the splenocolic ligament. We believe that the surgeon should always endeavor to spare the splenic vessels, to prevent spleen necrosis and abscesses. If, however, the splenic artery or vein are accidentally injured during the procedure, Warshaw's technique is a useful option.

Sectioning the Pancreas

One of the most challenging problems in pancreatic surgery – including open surgery – is safe section of the pancreas, which should prevent, or at least minimize, postoperative pancreatic fistulae.

The use of a mechanical stapler is the most common technique in laparoscopy; the same European multicenter trial reports that mechanical staplers are used in 90% of cases, ultrasound dissectors in 9%. A reinforcing manual suture is used respectively in 4% and 20% of cases. Fibrin glue is used only in 16% of cases (Fig. 26.14).

A mechanical stapler with large staples (Fig. 26.15), indicated for thick tissues, will only minimally crush the pancreatic parenchyma, allow a good seal of the duct of Wirsung and safe hemostasis. A 60-mm cartridge is also useful, and

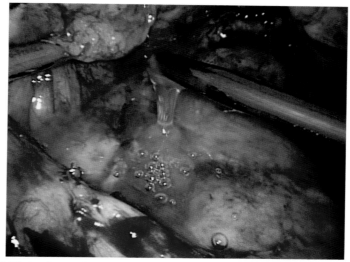

Fig. 26.14 Fibrin glue on the pancreatic staple line

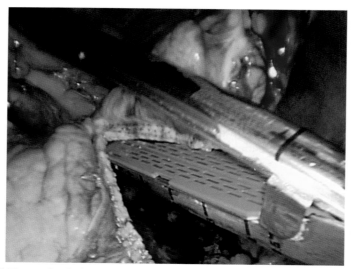

Fig. 26.15 The mechanical stapler with large staples

possibly a roticulator to cut the pancreas in one surgical session (Fig. 26.16). It is also possible to equip the mechanical stapler's jaws with a slow-absorption reinforcement made of preformed porous bioabsorbable sheets held into the form of sleeves through the use of a nonabsorbable polyester braided suture

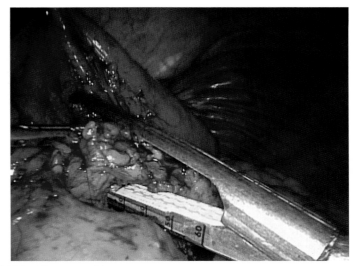

Fig. 26.16 The 60 mm cartridge

(Gore Seamguard bioabsorbable staple line reinforcement; Gore Medical, Flagstaff, Arizona, USA). If no satisfactory results are obtained with the mechanical stapler, clips can be applied or a continuous suture can be executed on the segment of the pancreatic section. A laminar drain such as a Penrose drain is always left in situ adjacent to the pancreatic section. To prevent it from dislodging, the drain can be secured to the peripancreatic fat by a thin resorbable wire. It is important that the drain be positioned to slope downward as much as possible: if the left side position does not ensure an adequate angle of slope, a counterincision can be made to place the drain in a more suitable site.

Distal Splenopancreatectomy

The technique entails the en-bloc resection of the distal pancreas and the spleen. The procedure is initiated with the antegrade technique, creating a subpancreatic tunnel at the isthmus. After dissecting the splenic vein from the pancreatic parenchyma, however, the surgeon proceeds to section it between clips or with a mechanical vascular stapler (white cartridge with smaller staples – 2.5 mm). Similarly, the artery is detected on the superior margin of the pancreatic body and then sectioned between clips or with a mechanical vascular stapler (Fig. 26.17). If the resection of the pancreatic parenchyma is carried out very far medially, great care should be taken to identify the splenic artery, which might be confused with the other arteries of the celiac tripod (hepatic artery and left gastric artery) (Fig. 26.18). It is advisable to look for the splenic artery always

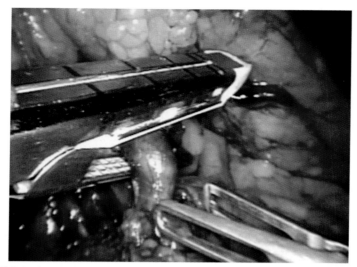

Fig. 26.17 Splenic artery section at the superior edge of the pancreas

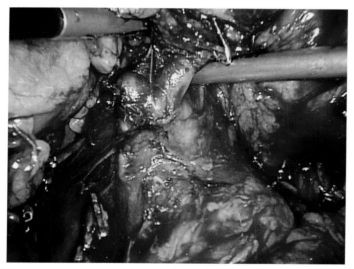

Fig. 26.18 Hepatic artery sectioned instead of splenic artery

on the upper margin of the pancreas, quite far distally. Following pancreas resection, if the arterial stump is too long, it can be further shortened. If it is impossible to dissect the vessels from the pancreatic parenchyma, a transparenchymal section of both the vein and the artery can be carried out with a mechanical stapler (large staple cartridge). Once the pancreatic portion is sectioned, the spleen can be mobilized.

Extraction of the Specimen

The excised specimen is introduced into a sterile bag and exteriorized through an umbilical minilaparotomy on the left side or in the suprapubic area, depending on cosmetic needs.

Conclusions

So what questions are still open, to be answered, perhaps, in the next 10 years?
- How can we cut down on the long learning curve, given the relatively small number of cases to be treated?
- Will a safe method be found to section and seal the pancreas?
- Will technology assist us in the management of the reconstruction of pancreas head resections?
- Will pancreatic malignancies be amenable to laparoscopy, safely and on the basis of suitable randomized trials and long-term follow up?
- Will robotic surgery have real prospects in this field?
- Will it be possible to treat the pancreas with endocavitary surgery?

Suggested Reading

Assalia A, Gagner M (2004) Laparoscopic pancreatic surgery for islet cell tumours of the pancreas. World J Surg 28:1239–1247

Ayav A, Bresler L, Brunaud L et al (2005) Laparoscopic approach for solitary insulinoma: a multicentre study. Langenbecks Arch Surg 390:134–140

Butturini G, Crippa S, Bassi C et al (2007) The role of laparoscopy in advanced pancreatic cancer diagnosis. Dig Surg 24:33–37

Corcione F, Marzano E, Cuccurullo D et al (2006) Distal pancreas surgery: outcome for 19 cases managed with laparoscopic approach. Surg Endosc 20:1729–1732

Dulucq Jl, Wintringer P, Mahajn A (2006) Laparoscopic pancreaticoduodenectomy for benign and malignant diseases. Surg Endosc 20:1045–1050

Fernandez Cruz L, Cosa R, Blanco L et al (2007) Curative laparoscopic resection for pancreatic neoplasm: a critical analysis from a single institution. J Gastrointest Surg 11:1607–1621

Lebedyev A, Zmora O, Kurinasky J et al (2004) Laparoscopic distal pancreatectomy. Surg Endosc 18:1427–1430

Mabrut Jy, Fernandez-Cruz L, Azagra JS et al (2005) Laparoscopic pancreatic resection: result of a multicenter European study of 127 patients. Surgery 137:597–605

Melotti G, Butturini G, Piccoli M et al (2007) Laparoscopic distal pancreatectomy: results on a consecutive series of 58 patients. Ann Surg 246:77–82

Melotti G, Cavallini A, Butturini G et al (2007) Laparoscopic distal pancreatectomy in children: case report and review of the literature. Ann Surg Oncol 14:1065–1069

Melotti G, Piccoli M, Bassi C et al (2000) L'approccio laparoscopico ai tumori cistici del corpo-coda del pancreas: indicazioni e tecnica. Osp Ital Chir 6:441–445

Melotti G, Piccoli M (2005) La laparoscopia nella stadiazione dei tumori. In: Pezzangora V (ed) Manuale di day surgery. Piccin, Padua, pp 443–445

Sa Cunha A, Rault A, Beau C et al (2007) Laparoscopic central pancreatectomy: single institution experience of 6 patients. Surgery 142:405–409

Siech M, Tripp K, Schmidt-Rohlfing B et al (1998) Cystic tumours of the pancreas: diagnostic accuracy, pathologic observations and surgical consequences. Langenbecks Arch Surg 383:56–61

Staudacher C, Orsenigo E, Baccari P et al (2005) Laparoscopic assisted duodenopancreatectomy. Surg Endosc 19:352–356

Takaori K, Tanigawa N (2007) Laparoscopic pancreatic resection: the past, the present and the future. Surg Today 37:535–545

Toshiyuki M, Nobutsugu A, Masanori S et al (2005) Laparoscopic pancreatic surgery. J Hepatobiliary Pancreat Surg 12:451–455

Willingham FF, Brugge WR (2007) Taking NOTES: translumenal flexible endoscopy and endoscopic surgery. Curr Opin Gastroenterol 23:550–555

Chapter 27

Laparoscopic Pancreatectomy: Indications and Description of the Technique

Carlo Staudacher, Elena Orsenigo, Saverio Di Palo,
Shigeki Kusamura

Introduction

The advent, continuous development, and systematization of the laparoscopic method has represented a revolution in surgery. Since the first successful laparoscopic cholecystectomy in 1989 [1], several other types of procedures have been performed by means of the minimally invasive technique. Despite several factors that argue against this approach, such as the long learning curve, high cost, and concerns relating to oncological radicality, the laparoscopic method continues to gain increasing popularity among the scientific community.

Several recent studies have demonstrated the efficacy of laparoscopic surgery in the treatment of neoplastic disease. On the other hand, the problem of the learning curve still remains unsolved. It is universally accepted that the major challenge to the routine execution of minimally invasive surgical procedures is the inherent ability of the operator to accomplish the procedure without conversion to laparotomy. Advanced laparoscopic surgery requires a long and specific program of training.

The laparoscopic technique has been applied in increasing numbers of clinical situations and recently also in diseases of the pancreas. The pancreas is located in a not easily accessible retroperitoneal region and consequently can be reached only after several mobilization maneuvers. In spite of this natural difficulty, several techniques have been described in the literature aiming to treat specific diseases of the pancreas such as endocrine lesions or pseudocyst [2, 3]. On the other hand, only anecdotal accounts of laparoscopic treatment of lesions affecting the head of the organ have been reported [4, 5]. Since the pancreaticoduodenectomy described by Whipple [6, 7] and its pylorus-preserving variation [8] are complex procedures, most authors are of the opinion that they should not be performed using the minimally invasive method. The first pancreaticoduodenectomy was described by Gagner [5]. The successive results thus far have been invariably favorable to the traditional open approach. Recently the laparoscopic approach has regained interest with the introduction of a hand-assisted technique as it allows easy manipulation of the structures, with preservation of the tactile sensitivity of the surgeon and rapid control of any bleeding [4, 9]. In theory, every pancreatic surgical operation could potentially be performed laparoscopically.

There is no consensus in the literature about the application of the laparoscopic method in the field of oncology. To accept it as a valid surgical option [10, 11] in the treatment of pancreatic diseases one should expect at least the same low rates of morbidity and mortality as are associated with conventional open pancreaticoduodenectomy in referral centers. Moreover, the minimally invasive approach must assure oncological radicality equivalent to that obtained with the open technique.

The advantages of the laparoscopic surgery are evident (cosmetic, reduction of in-hospital stay, better control of postoperative pain), making minimally invasive surgery increasingly frequently requested. While proximal pancreaticoduodenectomies reported in the literature are few, more cases of distal resections of the organ have been reported by referral centers specializing in laparoscopic surgery.

Technique of Laparoscopic Pancreaticoduodenectomy

The patient is under general anesthesia and is positioned in the supine lithotomy position (Fig. 27.1). The pneumoperitoneum is induced after introduction of a Hasson trocar through a supraumbilical minilaparotomy. The abdominal cavity is systematically inspected using a 30° laparoscope. Under direct vision three operative ports are placed: one in the epigastric and two in the paraumbilical regions (Fig. 27.2).

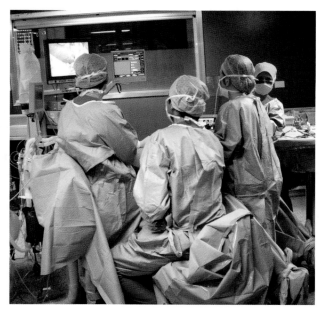

Fig. 27.1 The patient is placed in the supine position with legs abducted

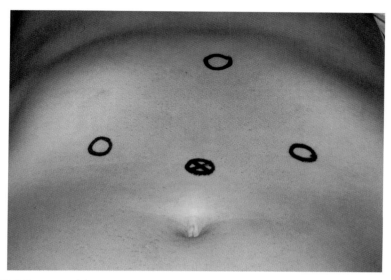

Fig. 27.2 Trocar positions

The first surgical step consists of laparoscopic cholecystectomy. The common bile duct is sectioned with an endoscopic linear stapler 2–3 cm cephalad to the pancreatic margin. The gastrocolic ligament is sectioned in order to expose the pancreas. The procedure is performed with wide use of the ultrasonic scalpel and continues with the Kocher maneuver.

At the level of the inferior margin of the pancreas the inferior mesenteric artery is identified and prepared. The gastroduodenal artery is sectioned and ligated with metallic clips. Once full access has been obtained to the anterior plane of the superior mesenteric artery with the harmonic scalpel, the pancreatic parenchyma is transected and the duct of Wirsung identified. The duodenum is resected 2–3 cm distal to the pylorus. If the surgical aim is to perform the procedure according to Whipple, the stomach is resected. After resection of distal jejunum with a linear endoscopic stapler 10–20 cm from the Treitz ligament, en-bloc mobilization of the duodenum, pancreas, and distal biliary duct is done. The attachment between the uncinate process and the superior mesenteric vein is gently divided and any branches of the latter ligated with metallic clips; the superior mesenteric artery is identified and the retroportal lamina sectioned with a linear endoscopic stapler or through a minilaparotomy. The hepatic and splenic arteries are dissected along the superior margin of the pancreas. The lymphadenectomy takes in the following regions: celiac, perihepatic, pyloric, superior and inferior margins of the pancreas, liver hilum, and intercavo-aortic. After inserting a plastic ring sleeve for wound protection, the surgical specimen is extracted through a minilaparotomy that is performed in the subcostal region or in the supraumbilical region and should measure 7 cm.

The reconstructive step is performed through the minilaparotomy and encompasses the performance of a pancreaticojejunostomy, hepaticojejunostomy, duodenojejunostomy, or gastrojejunostomy.

Technique of Middle Laparoscopic Pancreatectomy

The patient is under general anesthesia and is positioned in the supine lithotomy position. Pneumoperitoneum is induced after introduction of a Hasson trocar through a supraumbilical minilaparotomy. The abdominal cavity is systematically inspected using a 30° laparoscope. Under direct vision three operative ports are placed: one in the epigastric and two in the paraumbilical regions.

The gastrocolic ligament and gastroepiploic vessels are sectioned to expose the body and tail of the pancreas. The inferior margin of the pancreas is isolated from the attachment of the transverse mesocolon and from the retroperitoneal fatty tissue using the ultrasonic scalpel. The superior mesenteric vein is gently isolated from the anterior fascia of the pancreas. With the ultrasonic scalpel the middle portion of the pancreatic parenchyma is resected. The Wirsung duct is identified, and a small portion of it, a few millimeters in size, is dissected and cannulated with a pediatric 5F nasogastric tube. The proximal pancreatic stump is approached using a Endoloop ligation and sutured with separate stitches (Fig. 27.3). Then the jejunum is sectioned with a linear endoscopic stapler 20 cm

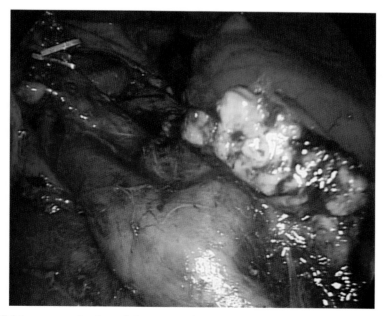

Fig. 27.3 Laparoscopic view of the pancreatic stump

from the ligament of Treitz and transposed transmesocolically. This segment is used to perform the end-to-side Wirsung-jejunostomy through laparoscopy. The reconstructive phase is concluded with the performance of a laparoscopic side-to-side entero-enteroanastomosis using an Endo-GIA stapler. The surgical specimen is extracted through a supraumbilical incision used for the Hasson trocar positioning.

Technique of Distal Splenopancreatectomy Technique

The patient is under general anesthesia and is positioned in the supine lithotomy position. Pneumoperitoneum is induced after introduction of a Hasson trocar through a supraumbilical minilaparotomy. The abdominal cavity is systematically inspected using a 30° laparoscope. Under direct vision three operative ports are placed: one in the epigastric and two in the paraumbilical regions.

The gastrocolic ligament is sectioned to expose the body and tail of the pancreas. The inferior margin of the pancreas is isolated from the attachment of the transverse mesocolon using the ultrasonic scalpel. The splenic arteries are dissected along the superior margin of the pancreas and successively sectioned and ligated with metallic clips. The pancreatic tail is sectioned with a linear stapler and the next step is to mobilize the splenopancreatic specimen. In the supraumbilical region a 5-cm minilaparotomy is performed and the surgical specimen is extracted using a specimen extraction bag.

Spleen-Preserving Distal Pancreatectomy

Not all pancreatic neoplasms require the performance of splenectomy to assure oncological radicality. Small benign endocrine neoplasms may be treated conservatively with a spleen-preserving approach. The technique is similar to distal splenopancreatectomy with the difference of an additional phase in which the posterior surface of the pancreas is dissected from the splenic vessels. These structures should be respected absolutely. There is a variation of the technique described by Warshaw in which splenic vessels are ligated both at the level of transection of the pancreas and again at the splenic hilum and the spleen preserved, leaving the spleen to survive on blood flow through the short gastric vessels [12]. This type of procedure, which is indicated in cases of pancreas transplantation from a living donor, unfortunately is associated with a 10–20% rate of ischemia. This, in turn, implies reoperation, during which splenectomy could become mandatory.

Discussion

The treatment of choice for neuroendocrine and ductal tumors of the pancreas is surgery. In particular, surgical resection is the only treatment for ductal adeno-carcinoma, which shows very aggressive biological behavior. Lesions of the pancreatic head may be treated with the classic Whipple procedure [6] or with the pylorus-preserving technique [7]. The mortality associated with these proce-dures has been minimized to less than 5%, but the mortality remains considera-ble, reaching rates higher than 40–60% [13]. Thus, every pancreatic resection, regardless of the technique being employed (open or minimally invasive), requi-res not only high surgical expertise but also an acquaintance with this complex anatomic region. The pancreas is located deep in the retroperitoneal space and is close to fundamental structures such as the mesenteric vessels [14]. Moreover, it is well known that referral centers present better results in terms of morbidity and mortality. The 5-year overall survival after resection of ductal adenocarcino-ma is less than 15% [15]. The modest increment in survival and treatment-rela-ted mortality rate of up to 10% outweighs the potential benefit associated with pancreatic surgery in the treatment of malignant ductal neoplasia [15]. This fact, together with the technical difficulty, warrants extremely judicious indication for the procedure, in particular in the treatment of lesions located in the head of the organ [2, 3, 7, 10–12]. In addition, several authors argue against the procedure when there is any doubt concerning the feasibility of a radical resection [16] and when the potential benefit to the patient seem to be questionable.

Laparoscopic techniques are complex, and only surgeons with expertise who are familiar with advanced minimally invasive surgery are suitable to approach pancreatic disorders in this way. On the other hand, distal laparoscopic resec-tions have been increasingly indicated and some authors consider it the gold standard, in particular in the treatment of endocrine neoplasia. In contrast with previous experiences [2–5, 9, 17], recent clinical results suggest that in the field of pancreatic disease, laparoscopic surgery offers advantages to patients in terms of shorter hospital stay, postoperative course, and the possibility of adequate oncological clearance.

An important step is an accurate instrumental preoperative work-up, which should provide the basis for planning the surgical strategy and minimizing the risk of laparotomic conversion. The objections against the procedure reported in the literature concerning the possibility of oncological radicality [16] have not been confirmed in most recent experiences, although the median follow-ups of the published series are still too short to allow more consistent conclusions to be drawn.

The preliminary data reported in the literature suggest that surgical laparosco-pic resection of the pancreas could potentially benefit the patient mainly in the case of distal resections. The higher cost related to the laparoscopic approach is due to the longer duration of surgery and the requirement for a larger number of technological devices such as staplers. With the progress of the experiences in the various centers, one would intuitively expect operative times to come down.

On the basis of the promising preliminary results, we are of the opinion that laparoscopic distal resection of the pancreas is safe and technically feasible. However, this presupposes the involvement of a surgical team highly skilled not only in advanced laparoscopic surgery but also in traditional open pancreatic surgery. Laparoscopic pancreaticoduodenectomy, although feasible, does not seem to present superior outcomes with respect to its open counterpart.

References

1. Dubois F, Berthelot G, Levard H (1989) Cholecystectomy by coelioscopy. Presse Med 18:980–982
2. Cuschieri A (1994) Laparoscopic surgery of the pancreas. J R Coll Surg Edinb 39:178–184
3. Gagner M, Pomp A (1997) Laparoscopic pancreatic resection: is it worthwhile? J Gastrointest Surg 1:20–26
4. Gagner M, Gentileschi P (2001) Hand-assisted laparoscopic pancreatic resection. Semin Laparosc Surg 8:14–125
5. Gagner M, Pomp A (1992) Laparoscopic pylorus-preserving pancreaticoduodenectomy. 2nd Annual Congress, Canadian Society for Endoscopic and Laparoscopic Surgery, 10–11 September 1992, Ottawa, ON, Canada, pp 26–29
6. Whipple AO, Parsons WB, Mullins CR (1935) Treatment of carcinoma of the ampulla of Vater. Ann Surg 102:763–769
7. Whipple AO (1941) The rationale of radical surgery for cancer of the pancreas and ampullary region. Ann Surg 114:612–615
8. Traverso LW, Longmire WP Jr (1978) Preservation of the pylorus in pancreaticoduodenectomy. Surg Gynecol Obstet 146:959–962
9. Ammori BJ (2003) Pancreatic surgery in the laparoscopic era. JOP 4:187–192
10. Balcom JH 4th, Rattner DW, Warshaw AL et al (2001) Ten-year experience with 733 pancreatic resections: changing indications, older patients, and decreasing length of hospitalisation. Arch Surg 136:391–398
11. Bramhall SR, Allum WH, Jones AG et al (1995) Treatment and survival in 13,560 patients with pancreatic cancer, and incidence of the disease, in the West Midlands: an epidemiological study. Br J Surg 82:111–115
12. Warshaw AL (1988) Conservation of the spleen with distal pancreatectomy. Arch Surg 123:550–553
13. Buchler MW, Friess H, Wagner M et al (2000) Pancreatic fistula after pancreatic head resection. Br J Surg 87:883–889
14. Ho V, Heslin MJ (2003) Effect of hospital volume and experience on in-hospital mortality for pancreaticoduodenectomy. Ann Surg 237:509–514
15. Kotwall CA, Maxwell JG, Brinker CC et al (2002) National estimates of mortality rates for radical pancreaticoduodenectomy in 25,000 patients. Ann Surg Oncol 9:847–854
16. Park A, Schwartz R, Tandan V, Anvari M (1999) Laparoscopic pancreatic surgery. Am J Surg 177:158–163
17. Tagaya N, Kasama K, Suzuki N et al (2003) Laparoscopic resection of the pancreas and review of the literature. Surg Endosc 17:201–206

Chapter 28

The Role of Robotics in Pancreatic Surgery

Graziano Pernazza, Pier Cristoforo Giulianotti

Introduction

The role of minimally invasive surgery in the diagnosis and treatment of pancreatic pathologies, although fully evolved, remains controversial and the subject of lively scientific discussions. Despite a growing number of documented studies clearly showing the safety and feasibility of minimally invasive procedures, their advantages and tremendous value to patients, with respect to staging, palliation and therapy of pancreatic pathologies, are still far from obvious. Traditional open surgery is considered the standard procedure both for treatment and palliation, while the laparoscopic approach is reserved for a small number of patients and performed only by a selected group of highly skilled surgeons. Robotic surgery, a genuine improvement to current conventional laparoscopic interventions, may broaden the applications of minimally invasive surgery and thereby extend its indications.

The "Da Vinci" Robotic System

Since the early 1980s, following the initial positive experiences, the applications of laparoscopic surgery have grown progressively. Accordingly, the indications have increased accompanied by strong technological support and development. The advantages of this minimally invasive approach quickly became apparent, i.e. reduced trauma to the abdominal wall, less scarring and improved cosmetics, less postoperative pain and discomfort, shorter hospital stay, and reduced postoperative ileus. The decreased risk of infection and the negligible blood losses not only supported the hypothesis of reduced stress to the immune system but also resulted in enhanced patient recovery in postoperative rehabilitation programs.

Nevertheless, some drawbacks to carrying out the surgical procedure itself became evident: the dissociated hand-eye alignment of laparoscopy generates unnatural positions and poor ergonomics for the surgeon; the reduced degrees of freedom in using the instruments made it difficult for the surgeon to perform

W. Siquini (Ed.), *Surgical Treatment of Pancreatic Diseases.*
©Springer-Verlag Italia 2009

precise and delicate dissections, and the 2-dimensional visualization resulted in limited depth perception.

The initiative in the second half of the 1990s to supplement minimally invasive surgery with robotic technology coincided with two developments. First, there was the military's development of automatic systems that could partially or absolutely replace human intervention in war or disaster situations. Second, there was the scientific application of robotic technology to laparoscopy in an attempt to overcome its limitations. The first prototypes were designed to be used outside the medical field, but later a medical device was developed, manufactured and put on the market. This device was capable of reproducing the motion of a surgeon's hand positioned away from the operating table.

In 1997, Intuitive Surgical (Menlo Park, CA, USA) delivered the only available and fully functional robotic surgical system. Their "da Vinci Surgical System" has been recently updated to the improved "da Vinci S Surgical System."

The system consists of three fundamental elements: a surgeon's console, a patient-side cart with four interactive robotic arms, and the vision system. The surgeon operates while seated at the surgical console, viewing a 3-dimensional image of the surgical field and grasping the master controls with his or her hands such that the wrists are naturally positioned relative to the eyes. The surgeon's hand, wrist, and finger movements are translated by the system into matching movements of the surgical instruments inside the patient.

One of the system's distinctive features is its high-resolution stereoscopic endoscope, which allows real 3-dimensional sight (Insite vision system), giving the surgeon the feeling of practically being immersed in the operating field. The field's natural depth, the high-quality contrast, and the image magnification provide a spatial perception much higher than that available with a 2-dimensional system. Furthermore, by activating the robotic arm, the surgeon can position the endoscope unassisted and without the physiologically induced movements and shaking that even a highly trained and capable assistant would make in an open or laparoscopic surgery environment.

Activating the two "masters," the surgeon sets in motion the robotic surgical tools that due to the special mechanical articulations (EndoWrist) are able to reproduce all of the motions of the surgeon's wrists, but allowing the use two or three small hands inside the operating field. The EndoWrist system allows the robotic structure to reach a degree of surgical precision superior to the human capacity, electronically scaling the motions of the surgeon and those of the tools and suppressing the psychological human tremor.

The robotic cart consists of a central support onto which three or four robotic arms are connected. The fourth robotic arm is optional and extends the ability of the surgeon operating at the console, who can activate it alternately with one of the two main robotic arms in order to perform complementary maneuvers. This fourth arm was designed to potentially eliminate the need of an assistant at the operating table.

The relative simplicity of the control systems and the very straightforward use of the system are elements that promote applications of this technology. Moreover, these features may indeed reduce the learning curves even for complex minimally invasive procedures. The ability of the surgeon to operate while seated and with good hand-eye alignment is in contrast to the situation characteristic of most traditional laparoscopic procedures. The operating position possible with the da Vinci system is not only more natural and comfortable, but it also decreases the fatigability that normally occurs during long procedures.

Diagnosis and Staging

Diagnostic laparoscopy, especially when associated with intraoperative ultrasonography, is indicated in cases that require further investigations at the end of the study phase, even though, due to the high reliability of the last generation of radiological diagnostic, the percentage of such patients is extremely small. Nevertheless, careful evaluation of vascular involvement in locally advanced disease remains challenging in any patient. Moreover, macroscopic vascular adherence does not always imply histological changes; in this case, the feasibility of the intervention depends more on the technical skill of the surgeon and on the surgical approach rather than on the diagnostic imaging findings.

Laparoscopy is characterized by its high sensibility and specificity in identifying small peritoneal implants and superficial metastases of the liver, as demonstrated in a minority of the patients radiologically diagnosed as candidates for pancreatic resection.

Palliation

The importance of the minimally invasive approach is obviously greater when, after the diagnostic step, palliative or curative treatment is possible as well. There is no question about the safety and feasibility of laparoscopic biliary and gastrointestinal diversions, in addition to the clear benefits for such patients. However the most complex and challenging maneuver in laparoscopy is high-precision microsuturing, in which robotically performed anastomoses are one of the most interesting and promising procedures in the evolution of the minimally invasive surgery.

The fixed, deep and very small operative field has determined the features of this technology, for example, in gastrojejunostomy, which is a recommended option in biliodigestive bypass in order to prevent the development of gastric outlet syndrome.

Our behavioral algorithm in diagnosis and treatment requires patients to be divided into three groups based on clinical presentation and CT scan findings.
1. Patients with metastatic disease, not resectable
   a. Minimally invasive approach for palliation
2. Patients with potentially resectable disease

    a. Diagnostic laparoscopy (useful in 50–60% of cases)
       i. Palliation with minimally invasive techniques
      ii. Conversion to traditional open surgery for resection
3. Patients with highly resectable disease
    a. Diagnostic laparoscopy (useful in some cases)
    b. Resection performed using traditional techniques
    c. Resection performed using minimally invasive technique (in selected cases)

Surgical Technique

Minimally Invasive Palliative Hepaticogastrojejunostomy

Hybrid laparorobotic procedures are some of the most interesting developments in minimally invasive surgical techniques. To make the procedure as short as possible, some steps are completed using traditional laparoscopic technique, as these are more versatile for some maneuvers, while the robotic system is employed in selected steps during the intervention, i.e. when there is a need for greater accuracy in high-precision suturing, such as in the construction of delicate anastomoses.

The gastrojejunal anastomosis and the preparation of the Roux-en-Y jejunal loop are performed by conventional laparoscopy. The patient is placed on the operating table in supine position with a 30° reverse-Trendelenburg. A five-ports approach is used. The preliminary laparoscopic exploration should be meticulous since it is essential in determining the feasibility of the procedure.

The presence of massive carcinosis or excessive bulging of the neoplastic mass can hamper access to the hepatoduodenal ligament. The gallbladder is emptied, if necessary, with a suction device, and the right colic flexure is widely mobilized and lowered. To identify the first jejunal loop, it is necessary to retract the transverse mesocolon upwards. The transverse mesocolon is then opened in the middle of its avascular portion, obtaining a breach such that a portion of the gastric posterior wall is pulled down and fixed with one stitch to the first jejunal loop. The jejunal and gastric walls are incised and a side-to-side stapled anastomosis is performed. The anterior wall is then closed with interrupted stitches. Next, a jejunal loop is prepared 30–40 cm distal to the gastrojejunal anastomosis, isolated, stapled, and transected. A 60-cm loop is prepared to perform a Roux-en-Y reconstruction, with a side-to-side stapled anastomosis at the base of the loop. The jejunal loop is then pulled up through the transverse mesocolon and temporarily anchored with a stitch in the subhepatic region.

It is now that the robotic phase begins. It includes dissection of the hepatoduodenal ligament and hepaticojejunal anastomosis. The robotic cart is brought close to the operating table and placed alongside the patients between his or her head and right shoulder. The robotic arms are then connected to the ports.

The cystic duct and the artery are identified, ligated, and sectioned. The gallbladder is not completely detached from the liver, as it will be used as a grasping site to obtain optimal liver retraction until the very end of the procedure. The fourth robotic arm is very helpful in this task and the maneuver gives a fixed, stable operative field and accurate access to the subhepatic region.

The common bile duct is prepared and sectioned. The distal stump can be tied or sutured with a 2-0 stitch. The hepaticojejunal anastomosis is performed using 5-0 absorbable stitches, with two half-running sutures or frontal interrupted stitches depending on the caliber of the bile duct. The robotic handling of the needle is delicate enough and the 3-dimensional view so clearly defined that the anastomosis can be perfectly constructed, achieving extramucosal passage of the needle without leakage or stenosis. The procedure is concluded with completion of the retrograde cholecystectomy. A subhepatic drainage is preferably inserted.

Resection

The first minimally invasive pancreatic resections were carried out by Ganger and Pomp, in 1992. Other experiences were subsequently described, with opinions varying from enthusiasm to severe skepticism. The current consensus is that distal pancreatectomy (with or without preservation of the spleen) is a relatively simple procedure in selected cases, with low morbidity and clear benefits for the patient, while pancreatoduodenectomy requires an excessively long intervention for minimally invasive surgery, with a high complication rate and without apparent clinical advantages for the patient. Some investigators have strongly recommended that it be abandoned.

Scientific discussion of distal resections has focused on two fundamentally critical matters: (a) the "oncologic radicalism" and appropriateness of the procedure for the treatment of pancreatic malignancies and (b) the possibility to preserve the spleen in patients with benign pathologies.

On the one hand, the lack of evidence-based data in the medical literature about the long-term results of minimally invasive pancreatic resection and, on the other, the lack of definitive proof regarding the curative potential of extended lymphadenectomies makes it advisable to reserve minimally invasive treatment for benign lesions, small tumors, and less-aggressive or less-advanced malignancies. Spleen preservation, recommendable in distal pancreatic resection in patients with more favorable pathologies, is feasible in traditional surgery as well as in laparoscopy, even if technically challenging and may result in increased blood losses.

The medical literature reports variable results for spleen preservation during distal pancreatic resections. The robotic technique, due to the high-quality 3D view it provides together with the stability of the operating field, suppression of tremor, and articulation of the tools allows a more precise and bloodless dissection and thus can secure a more radical lymphadenectomy and increased rate of spleen preservation. This assertion is supported by the experience acquired in the Department of Surgery of "Misericordia" Hospital in Grosetto, Italy, where very careful and precise dissection of the splenic vessels has made it possible to achieve spleen preservation in every distal pancreatic resection performed in which the declared objective was preserving the spleen (Table 28.1).

Table 28.1. Minimally invasive robot-ic assisted pancreatic surgery: procedures performed since October 2000

Surgical procedure	N
Duodenopancreatectomy	
Hybrid technique[a]	
–Whipple	11
–Longmire	4
Full robotic technique[b]	
–Whipple	25
–Longmire	6
Distal splenopancreatectomy	21
Spleen-preserving total pancreatectomy	1
Spleen-preserving distal pancreatectomy	16
Spleen-preserving distal pancreatectomy + islet-cell transplant	1
Middle-segment pancreatectomy (pancreatogastric anastomosis)	4
Enucleation (insulinoma)	2
Total	91

[a]In the hybrid technique, exploration and preliminary dissection are performed in conventional laparoscopy, as described in the text
[b]In full robotic technique, the entire procedure is performed with robotic assistance
N, Number of patients

Robotic 'Spleen-Preserving' Distal Pancreatectomy

The patient is supine and tilted 30° on the right side, in a light reverse-Trendelenburg (10°) position. Five ports are placed: the first is periumbilical for the endoscope, two ports are subcostal (one on the left flank and one paramedian right) and the two accessory ports are in the epigastric area and paramedian left (Fig. 28.1). The robotic cart is placed in the vicinity of the patient's left shoulder. Preliminary exploration of the abdominal cavity should be completed by ultrasonographic scanning and using a laparoscopic probe.

After assessing the feasibility of the procedure, the left colic flexure is mobilized and the lesser sac opened. The splenic artery is prepared and surrounded by tape, in case clamping is required. The stomach is lifted up with the grasp installed on the fourth arm in order to open the operating field. It may be neces-

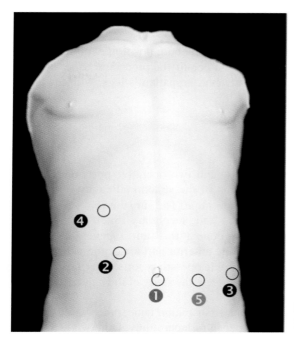

Fig. 28.1 Distal pancreatectomy
port placement

sary to transect some of the short gastric vessels to obtain effective control of the splenic hilum. The tail of the pancreas is detached and lifted, starting at the inferior border and moving toward the splenic hilum. Each small branch of splenic vein and artery from and to the pancreas is dissected, tied and sectioned using absorbable 5-0 sutures and several 5-0/6-0 transfixed stitches. The tasks of the assistant are to lift up the pancreatic tail, keep the operative field clean, control suctioning, supply suture and sponges and remove residual threads. Meticulous dissection continues along the gland until the planned sections are reached. The gland can be divided with the ultrasonic scalpel and the proximal stump is sutured with a few interrupted stitches. The specimen can be placed in a bag and removed through a light broadening of one of the port sites.

The robotic phase is essentially the same as in laparoscopy, with the difference that the use of the robot significantly improves manipulation of the small and delicate branches of the splenic vessels. Unexpected bleeding is rare but possible. The surgeon at the console should keep in mind that, if bleeding occurs, it may be quick and difficult to control, because he or she does not have the possibility to manage the suction tool. Thus, preventive preparation of the splenic artery is of fundamental importance in order to decrease blood flow and to repair the lesion with a few stitches at the bleeding point. The fourth arm can prove to be extremely useful in achieving a steady and delicate retraction of the pancreas. The stability of the surgical field increases the precision of the dissection and facilitates surgical maneuvering.

Robotic Pancreatoduodenectomy

The patient is in a supine, light reverse-Trendelenburg position, with legs parted and both arms along the body. The surgeon begins the procedure using conventional laparoscopy and is positioned between the patient's legs, with the assistants to the sides of the patient.

Exploration and Exhibition

One optical port is placed subumbilically and two operative ports on the right and left sides (Fig. 28.2). Full exploration of the abdominal cavity is easier in conventional laparoscopy using a 30° endoscope. The surgeon looks for regional carcinomatosis, lymphadenopathies, and secondary liver localizations. Peritoneal cytology and biopsies may be done at this time. Opening of the gastrocolic ligament allows exploration of the anterior surface of the pancreas. An accessory port, between the optical and left operative ports, may be placed to introduce the ultrasound probe and to complete the study of the pancreatic gland, the mesentericoportal axis, and the liver.

If, at this point, there is any element of suspicion concerning vascular invasion, it is advisable to immediately proceed to laparotomy. Otherwise, the right subcostal port is placed. A slight rotation of the table to the right makes it easi-

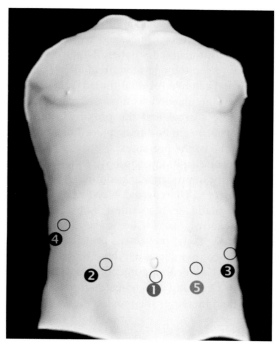

Fig. 28.2 Pancreatoduodenectomy port placement

er to explore the duodenojejunal flexure and detach the Treitz ligament. This is important to evaluate the uncinate process and the superior mesenteric vessels from the left side. Any infiltration at this level implies the presence of unresectable disease and the operation should be converted to a minimally invasive palliative procedure (gastrojejunostomy and hepaticojejunostomy).

The robotic cart, located near the head of the patient, is moved close to the table and restored to its original position. The operative arms should be arranged to avoid external collisions, offering the outside element the greater possible range of motion and allowing the assistant to easily provide complementary interactions. While the fourth arm, or the assistant, is retracting the stomach upwards, the surgeon at the console cuts the insertion of the mesocolon on the inferior margin of the pancreas. Following the middle colic vein, he or she exposes the confluence in the superior mesenteric vein and gently frees the neck of the pancreas from the anterior aspect of the portal axis.

Kocher Maneuver

The right colonic flexure is mobilized to expose the second duodenal portion and the anterior capsule of the pancreatic head. Since no major vessels have been transected until this point, the dissection can only be performed using the monopolar cautery hook. At the end of the dissection, the vena cava is cleaned and exposed, and the cavoaortic lymph nodes removed.

As the assistant retracts the liver and lifts the duodenum, the surgeon can advance the dissection along the pre-cavoaortic plane, using, alternately, the ultrasonic scalpel and the monopolar cautery hook. Once the duodenojejunal junction is reached, joining the previously dissected plane from the left, the origin of the superior mesenteric artery is exposed from the anterior aortic wall by removing the right celiac ganglia. The right aspect of the superior mesenteric vein is clearly evident at this stage.

Hepatoduodenal Ligament Dissection

The hepatic hilum is easily exposed by retracting the gallbladder upward using the fourth arm. Meanwhile the assistant helps by pushing down the antropyloric region and keeping the surgical field clean by suction and irrigation. The lymphadenectomy may be carried out by proceeding from top to bottom, opening the hepatoduodenal ligament. Sometimes it may be necessary to empty the gallbladder. Cholecystectomy is performed at the end of the maneuver, because the gallbladder is an optimal grasping site for the safe and effective retraction of the liver. The hepatoduodenal ligament is meticulously inspected, looking for aberrant or accessories hepatic arteries. The gastric artery is sectioned between bindings. The proper and common hepatic arteries are surrounded with tape. The common bile duct is sectioned at the confluence with the cystic duct, ligating the distal stump with a stitch and temporarily closing the proximal one with a delicate micro-clamp. This section of the bile duct allows access to the portal vein and easier preparation of the origin of the gastroduodenal artery, which is double-ligated and transected (Fig. 28.3).

Gastric Transection

Depending on the selected procedure (Whipple operation or pancreatoduodenectomy), the distal portion of the stomach or the proximal portion of the duodenum is sectioned using an endoscopic linear stapler and ensuring hemostasis with several interrupted stitches along the stapled line. The gastroepiploic arcade and the left gastric vessels on the lesser curve can be controlled using ultrasound shears. Sectioning of the stomach provides a complete view of the region of the pancreatic isthmus. The surgical field is now fully exposed by retracting the antrum and the duodenum laterally on the right and temporarily leaving the gastric stump in the left hypochondrium.

Pancreatic Neck Transection

Formation of the tunnel under the pancreatic neck has to be carried out with extreme gentleness. For this step as well, the safety of the maneuver is assured

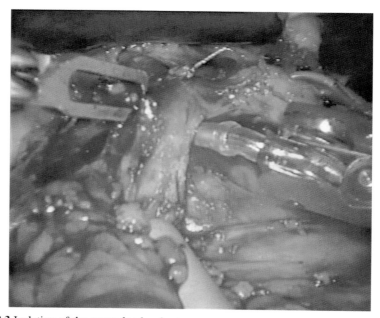

Fig. 28.3 Isolation of the gastroduodenal artery

by the steadiness of the robotic instruments, the three-dimensional view, and the EndoWrist capabilities which allow the surgeon to perform tangential motions in relation to the vascular axes (Fig. 28.4).

Once the tunnel is completed, a tape is passed through that provides traction on the pancreas, which can be divided with the ultrasound shears. Any unexpected bleeding from the line of sectioning can be controlled by precise 4-0/5-0 stitches or by bipolar coagulation. A pancreatic sample of the proximal section margin may be taken at this time and sent for examination.

Retroportal Lamina Dissection and Uncinate Process Detachment

Dissection of the retroportal lamina and detachment of the uncinate process are the very last and most difficult steps of the pancreatoduodenectomy. They are reported to be the primary cause of intraoperative complications and the most frequent cause of conversion, such that some authors invoke the use of a mini-laparotomy for hand assistance.

Robotic technology has completely changed and improved these crucial surgical steps, Some of the technical landmarks of the procedure deserve particular note. First of all, the dissection is different from open surgery in that it proceeds as a bottom-up pathway, along the mesentericoportal axis. In addition, the duo-denojejunal flexure (preventively prepared from the left side) is preliminarly sta-

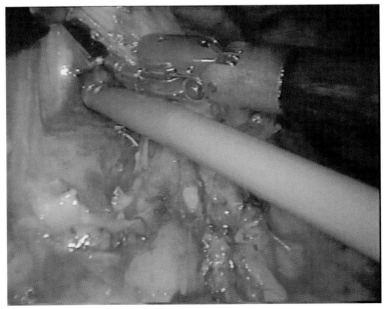

Fig. 28.4 Dissection behind the pancreatic neck. Exposure of the anterior aspect of the mesenteric vein

pled and transected from the right side. It is advisable to expose and preliminarily prepare the right side of the superior mesenteric artery. The inferior pancreaticoduodenal artery is preferably dissected, tied, and sectioned individually. The specimen is retracted sideways by the surgical assistant, using a few traction stitches if necessary (Fig. 28.5).

A cautery hook and ultrasound shears are used for the dissection. It is always necessary to pick up the tissue in small pieces. The surgical field should be kept clean and dry at all times. Any bleeding, no matter how small, should be controlled immediately with 5-0 stitches.

The main role of the assistant at this stage is to provide accurate suctioning and to carry out the delicate left retraction of the portal vein. The superior pancreaticoduodenal vein is transected as a last step, to avoid venous congestion and back-bleeding from the specimen.

The optimal place for a laparotomy should be carefully selected in advance, in case of emergency conversion, keeping the instruments for open surgery available from the beginning of the intervention. If such a situation should arise, the robotic cart can be removed from the surgical site in seconds.

The specimen, at the end of the procedure, is enclosed in a bag and retrieved through a small laparotomy in which one of the port sites is enlarged or a Pfannenstiel incision is made (Figs. 28.6 and 28.7).

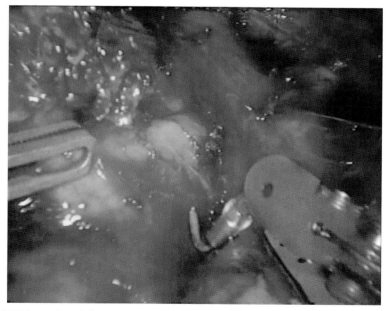

Fig. 28.5 Dissection of the retroportal lamina

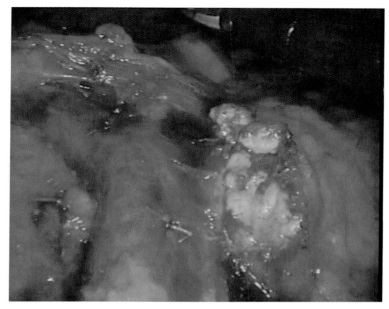

Fig. 28.6 The operative field at the end of the demolition. The pancreatic stump, the hepatic artery and the mesenterico-portal trunk are visible

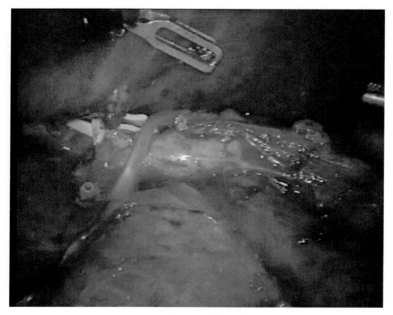

Fig. 28.7 The operative field at the end of the dissection: vena cava, mesenterico-portal trunk, common hepatic artery, proximal stump of the common bile duct

Reconstruction

The pancreatic stump is preferably sclerosed with glue and the Wirsung duct sealed with a purse-string prepared with a 3-0 Prolene. Nevertheless, the option of an anastomosis is not excluded. The decision should be based on the glandular thickness and on the caliber of the Wirsung duct, as in open surgery. With robotic assistance, it is possible to perform a safe Wirsung-jejunal anastomosis using 6-0 Prolene (Fig. 28.8).

Hepaticojejunostomy is performed, as previously described, on the first jejunal loop, which is passed behind the superior mesenteric vessels. A mechanical or robotic gastrojejunostomy is constructed about 40–50 cm distal to the anastomosis. In case of sclerosis, two drains are left close to the pancreatic stump; a benign pancreatic fistula occurs in about 20% of patients.

Conclusions

Robotic technology is exponentially spreading in the field of minimally invasive general surgery, offering the surgeon the ability to overcome the limitations of conventional laparoscopy while preserving its well recognized advantages. The optimal three-dimensional view and the precise articulation of the tools allow

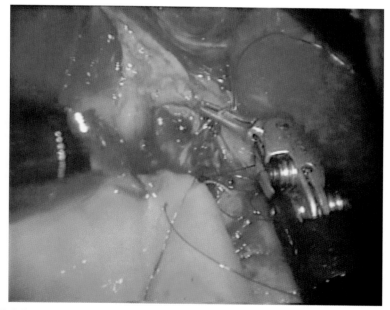

Fig. 28.8 Operative field at the end of the dissection

the execution of complex surgical maneuvers, and thus an extremely exact and accurate dissection, by improving tissue manipulation and simplifying microsuturing. These advantages will no doubt broaden the spread and extent of the indications for minimally invasive techniques.

Since October 2000, we and our colleagues at the Department of Surgery in Grosseto have performed more than 750 interventions using minimally invasive robotic techniques, directed by Prof. P.C. Giulianotti [Note: Prof. P.C. Giulianotti is now Distinguished Lloyd M. Nyhus Chair in Surgery, Professor and Chief of the Division of General, Minimally Invasive, and Robotic Surgery, University of Illinois-Chicago] (Table 1). Based on this experience, we have divided the operations in three classes with respect to conventional laparoscopy: those in which robotic assistance does not provide substantial advantages, those in which robotic assistance substantially improves the procedure, and those in which without robotic assistance minimally invasive surgery does not otherwise appear to be feasible.

In the field of pancreatic surgery, the advantages conferred by robotic technology are clearly apparent. In diagnostic exploration, traditional laparoscopy, supported by intraoperative ultrasonography, appears to suffice; however, the features that enable micro-suturing and anastomosis emphasize the role of robotic assistance in the execution of minimally invasive palliative procedures that include construction of gastrojejunal and hepaticojejunal anastomoses.

In distal pancreatic resections, robotic assistance improves the performance of laparoscopic surgery, which, according to the literature, is already considered a good surgical option at it better guarantees preservation of the spleen. By contrast, proximal pancreatic resections should still be considered as highly complex procedures with respect to minimally invasive surgery. Nevertheless, it may be possible to overcome many of the limitations and difficulties posed by traditional laparoscopic approaches, which have strongly limited its spread. Operating times, conversion rates and blood losses will likely continue to decrease as experience is gained.

Suggested Reading

Croce E, Olmi S, Azzola M et al (1999) Surgical palliation in pancreatic head carcinoma and gastric cancer: the role of laparoscopy. Hepatogastroenterology 46:2606–2011

Cuschieri A (2006) Laparoscopic surgery in Europe. Where are we going? Cir Esp 79(1):10–21

Dulucq JL, Wintringer P, Mahajna A (2006) Laparoscopic pancreaticoduodenectomy for benign and malignant diseases. Surg Endosc 20(7):1045–1050

Dulucq JL, Wintringer P, Stabilini C et al (2005) Are major laparoscopic pancreatic resections worthwhile? A prospective study of 32 patients in a single institution. Surg Endosc 19(8):1028–1034

Fernández-Cruz L, Martínez I, Gilabert R et al (2004) Laparoscopic distal pancreatectomy combined with preservation of the spleen for cystic neoplasms of the pancreas. J Gastrointest Surg 8(4):493–501

Freeny PC, Traverso LW, Ryan JA (1993) Diagnosis and staging of pancreatic adenocarcinoma with dynamic computed tomography. Ann J Surg 165:600–606

Friess H, Kleef J, Silva JC et al (1998) The role of diagnostic laparoscopy in pancreatic peri-ampullary malignancies. J Am Coll Surg 186:675–682

Gagner M, Pomp A (1994) Laparoscopic pylorus preserving pancreatoduodenectomy. Surg Endosc 8:408–410

Giulianotti PC (2004) Minimally invasive and robotic-assisted pancreatic surgery in primer of robotic and telerobotic surgery. In: Ballantyne GH, Marescaux J, Giulianotti PC (eds) Primer of robotic and telerobotic surgery. Lippincott Williams & Wilkins, Philadelphia, p 155

Giulianotti PC, Coratti A, Angelini M et al (2003) Robotics in general surgery: personal experience in a large community hospital. Arch Surg 138(7):777

Himpens J, Leman G, Cadiere GB (1998) Telesurgical laparoscopic cholecistectomy. Surg Endosc 12:1091

Intuitive Surgical – daVinci Surgical System. Available at: www.intuitivesurgical.com

Kavoussi LR, Moor RG, Adams JB et al (1995) Comparison of robotic versus human laparoscopic camera control. J Urol 154:2134–2136

Melotti G, Butturini G, Piccoli M et al (2007) Laparoscopic distal pancreatectomy: results on a consecutive series of 58 patients. Ann Surg 246(1):77–82

Milone L, Turner P, Gagner M (2004) Laparoscopic surgery for pancreatic tumors, an uptake. Minerva Chir 59(2):165–173

Nieveen Van Dijkum EJ (2003) et al Laparoscopic staging and subsequent palliation in patients with peripancreatic carcinoma. Ann Surg 237:66–73

Palanivelu C, Jani K, Senthilnathan P et al (2007) Laparoscopic pancreaticoduodenectomy: technique and outcomes. J Am Coll Sur 205(2):222–230

Park AE, Henriford T (2002) Therapeutic laparoscopy of the pancreas. Ann Surg 236:149–158

Pisters PW, Vauthey JN, Charnsangavej C et al (2001) Laparoscopy in the staging of pancreatic cancer. Br J Surg 88:325–337

Ruurda JP, van Dongen KW, Broeders IA et al (2003) Robot-assisted laparoscopic choledocho-jejunostomy. Surg Endosc 17(12):1937–1942

Sackier JM, Wang Y (1994) Robotically assisted laparoscopic surgery. From concept to development. Surg Endosc 8:63–66

Sanchez BR, Mohr CJ, Morton JM et al (2005) Comparison of totally robotic laparoscopic Roux-en-Y gastric bypass and traditional laparoscopic Roux-en-Y gastric bypass. Surg Obes Relat Dis 1(6):549–554

Schachter PP, Auni Y, Shimonov M et al (2000) The impact of laparoscopy and laparoscopic ultrasonography on the management of pancreatic cancer. Arch Surg 135:1303–1307

Shimizu S, Tanaka M, Konomi H et al (2004) Laparoscopic pancreatic surgery: current indications and surgical results. Surg Endosc 18(3):402–406

Stojadinovic A, Brooks A, Hoos A et al (2003) An evidence-based approach to the surgical management of resectable pancreatic adenocarcinoma. J Am Coll Surg 196:954–964

Tang CN, Siu WT, Ha JP et al (2007) Laparoscopic biliary bypass – a single centre experience. Hepatogastroenterology 54(74):503–507

Warshaw AL, Gu Z, Wittemberg J et al (1990) Preoperative assessment of resectability of pancreatic cancer. Arch Surg 125:230–237

Yu SC, Clapp BL, Lee MJ et al (2006) Robotic assistance provides excellent outcomes during the learning curve for laparoscopic Roux-en-Y gastric bypass: results from 100 robotic-assisted gastric bypasses. Am J Surg 192(6):746–749

Zheng MH, Feng B, Lu AG et al (2006) Laparoscopic pancreaticoduodenectomy for ductal adenocarcinoma of common bile duct: a case report and literature review. Med Sci Monit 12(6):CS57-CS60

Chapter 29

Nutritional Support in Acute Pancreatitis and Pancreatic Cancer

Simona Irma Rocchetti, Aldo Alberto Beneduce, Marco Braga

Introduction and Definition of Malnutrition

All pancreatic diseases, whether inflammatory or neoplastic, cause a change in the function of the organ that translates into a digestive impairment. Furthermore, pancreatic cancer is frequently responsible for cachexia, due to its late diagnosis and the peculiar characteristics of this type of tumor. It is also known that food consumption by pancreatic patients can frequently trigger or exacerbate pain – a typical and recurrent symptom of these diseases – forcing the patient to reduce food intake. Thus it is clear why moderate to severe malnutrition can be found in patients suffering from pancreatic disease, resulting in increased morbidity, mortality, hospital stay, and management expenses for these patients. This being so, it is obvious that, for malnourished patients, the correct approach and nutritional care can optimize their management, improving outcome and reducing costs.

The first step required for correct nutritional support is an assessment of the patient's nutritional status. This procedure aims at identifying the metabolic consequences of a nonphysiological state such as fasting or poor nutrient intake that leads to malnutrition. A combination of clinical and biochemical parameters should be used to determine the nutritional status and identify the metabolic consequences of malnutrition. A comprehensive history and physical examination are essential for a proper nutritional assessment. The main indicator used to determine the degree of malnutrition is body weight loss. The degree of weight loss that will cause a worsening of clinical conditions is variable in the literature; however, in several studies an unintentional weight loss greater than 10% compared to the previous usual weight, or greater than 5% in 1 month, is considered significant. If the usual body weight is unknown, less than 20% of ideal weight can be used as a measure of malnutrition [1]. Despite being simple and inexpensive, this tool often remains surprisingly unused in daily clinical practice.

In addition to the loss of body weight, malnutrition induces a number of changes in various clinical and biochemical parameters that can be measured to assess the nutritional status of the patient. In particular, some serum proteins

W. Siquini (Ed.), *Surgical Treatment of Pancreatic Diseases.*
©Springer-Verlag Italia 2009

correlate well with the nutritional status and severity of the main disease:
- Albumin is the chemical marker that has the strongest link with postoperative morbidity and mortality. Albumin levels lower than 3.5 g/l are strongly related to a worse prognosis [1].
- Transferrin, with its short half-life (8 days) and its relatively low level of body storage, gives a true reflection of the loss and recovery of protein mass [1, 2].
- Prealbumin, with a half-life of 2–3 days, can help monitor the effectiveness of nutritional support [3–5].

A classification of malnutrition status based on anthropometric, immunological, and biochemical indicators is given in Table 29.1.

It is important to note that most serum parameters are not specific markers of nutritional status because they can also be modified in paraphysiological conditions (e.g., hypoalbuminemia could result from simple hemodilution, or from maldistribution between intravascular and extravascular compartments, or reduced liver synthesis, or it could be due to a reallocation in the priority of the liver's synthetic pathways in sepsis). Consequently, although these parameters are often markers of the presence or severity of the disease, they do not necessarily represent the need for nutritional support, nor is their modification an indication of treatment efficacy.

Table 29.1 Parameters for the evaluation of nutritional status

Anthropometric parameters
Nutritional history
- Quantity/quality of nutrition
- Anorexia
- Nausea
- Vomiting
- Diarrhea
- Weight loss

Physical examination
- Weight
- Mid-arm circumference
- Triceps skinfold thickness

Biochemical parameters
- Serum albumin (g/dl)
- Serum transferrin (mg/dl)
- Prealbumin (mg/dl)
- Retinol binding protein (mg/dl)

Immunological parameters
- Skin tests
- Lymphocytes/mm^3

In the past years the body mass index (BMI) (body weight in kilograms divided by the square of the height in meters) has been commonly adopted as an indicator of nutrition status. A BMI of less than 18.5 is considered an indicator of malnutrition, a BMI of less than 15 is associated with a significant increase in mortality, a BMI of 25.0–29.9 indicates overweight, while a BMI above 30 indicates obesity. This last condition can also be considered as a state of malnutrition, implying an increase in morbidity and mortality similar to the one in malnourished patients. However, the use of BMI as a measure of nutritional assessment is useless particularly for patients usually in the lower range or obese patients who can experience weight loss of several kilos but still remain overweight. Thus it is clear that weight loss is, as previously stated, the most accurate and reliable marker by which to assess effective nutritional status.

In clinical practice several assessment protocols can be adopted. Nutritional screening should be performed within 48 h after hospitalization to identify malnourished patients or at risk of malnutrition, in order to implement artificial nutritional support if indicated. The following are the most sensitive, accurate, reproducible, cost-effective, easy, quick and most frequently used markers for nutritional assessment [6]:
− The disease itself
− Weight change
− Food intake
− Possible nutrient loss
− Physical activity level
− Clinical assessment, relying on physical examination and focusing on loss of skeletal muscle mass (in particular of temporal, deltoid, triceps, quadriceps muscles and interosseous muscles of the hand), and subcutaneous fat, the possible presence of cachexia, edema, glossitis, stomatitis, altered wound healing, and the level of albuminemia and total lymphocyte count

Furthermore, since artificial nutrition represents a preventive rather than a therapeutic tool, it is also indicated for patients presenting a tangible risk of malnutrition (e.g., patients with a planned period of inadequate nutritional intake greater than 10 days). For the same purpose, a variety of standardized groups of markers has been created to allow the formulation of an evaluation score, e.g., the SGA (Subjective Global Assessment) [7] or the MNA (Mini Nutritional Assessment) in elderly patients [8]. The SGA includes the taking of a history (weight loss, food intake, gastrointestinal symptoms, diagnosis of disease, functional capacity) and physical examination of the muscular masses, fat mass, and presence of edema. Despite its limitations, in the event of limited resources and lack of objective markers for the nutritional status, the SGA represents a valid tool that can assess the need for nutritional support in hospitalized patients [1, 9].

The evaluation of nutritional status also includes a metabolic assessment including investigation of organ and apparatus functions and changes in metabolism that can influence the loss of lean mass and the metabolic response to nutritional treatment. There is a very close link between nutritional status and severity of disease, so nutritional support can improve the efficacy of the disease-specific therapy prevent the development of malnutrition, and promote healing [10]. A recent study of 1410 patients undergoing surgery for gastrointestinal malignancies clearly demonstrated that malnutrition is closely related to increased postoperative morbidity and mortality, mostly caused by infective complications. Nutritional support, either enteral or parenteral, can noticeably reduce this trend [11].

Because of the close link between malnutrition and disease, nutritional assessment is not a static evaluation; in addition to identifying the patient who is malnourished or at risk of malnutrition, it must also be employed to monitor the nutritional changes and possible deficiencies that can arise during the course of the disease.

Malnutrition and Nutritional Support in Pancreatic Cancer

Cachexia represents, without doubt, one of the most debilitating complications of malignant disease, and in particular one of the most frequent symptoms of pancreatic cancer. The pathogenesis of cachexia in pancreatic cancer is typically multifactorial, because of multiple concomitant causes such as abdominal pain, depression, constipation, intestinal obstruction, malabsorption, side effects of radio- and chemotherapeutic treatments, changes in the sense of taste, and sharp alterations in energy balance. Several studies have demonstrated how metabolic alterations are mediated by a complicated network of proinflammatory cytokines, neuroendocrine hormones, neurotransmitters, and various factors produced by the tumor itself or by our body in response to the tumor, even if the complex interactions between these mediators in determining the clinical syndrome still remain partly unknown. In cancer-related cachexia, tumor-derived substances, or those originating from the hypothalamus, are released into the blood stream. The presence of neoplasia produces a systemic inflammatory response with proinflammatory cytokines, mainly interleukin 1 and 6 (IL-1, IL-6), TNF-α, IFN-γ, and leukemia inhibitory factor (LIF). Chronic administration of these cytokines, alone or combined, can lead to a reduction in food intake and reproduce the characteristics of the cancer anorexia–cachexia syndrome [10]. Results from therapeutic trials with eicosapentaenoic acid (EPA) and thalidomide were recently published. Fish oil fatty acids have been shown to decrease production of proinflammatory cytokines and hepatic acute-phase proteins in in-vitro models. Oral supplementation with EPA (variable dose from 2 to 12 g/day) in cachectic patients affected by pancreatic cancer led to a significant reduction in serum levels of C-reactive protein and IL-6, and on the clinical side showed a maintenance of body weight in the short term, as seen in several clinical studies [12, 13]. Thus it is clear that pancreatic cancer patients, and cancer patients in general, are a heterogeneous category of patients who in terms of nutritional support indications should be divided into the following groups:

1. Those with present oncologic disease, eligible for surgical, chemotherapeutic, and radiotherapeutic treatment.

2. Those with advanced oncologic disease, not suitable for conventional onco-logic treatment.

In patients with present oncologic disease need to be distinguished further into two subgroups: those who are well-nourished, for whom nutritional support is indicated, either enterally or parenterally, only if a starvation period greater than 10 days is planned; and those who are malnourished, who require major surgery, in whom perioperative nutritional support should begin 5 days before surgery if there is no contraindication to delay the operation, and continue for at least 1 week after surgery or until oral food intake is resumed, with the achieve-ment of, at least, 60% of energy and protein requirements [14–17].

When the tumor location and the type of surgery allow, the enteral route of nutritional support is preferable to parenteral nutrition since it is just as good in terms of nutritional and immune function in well-nourished patients. Moreover, enteral nutrition gives rise to lower sanitary costs and a lower incidence of seri-ous complications [18]. Parenteral nutrition requires a central venous access, usu-ally by the subclavian or jugular vein, while enteral nutrition is performed through a nasojejunal or nasogastric probe, endoscopically or radiologically posi-tioned; otherwise a nutritional jejunostomy or gastrostomy can be performed dur-ing surgery (Figs. 29.1, 29.2). These devices are connected to a continuous peri-staltic pump that can finely regulate the daily product intake (Fig. 29.3).

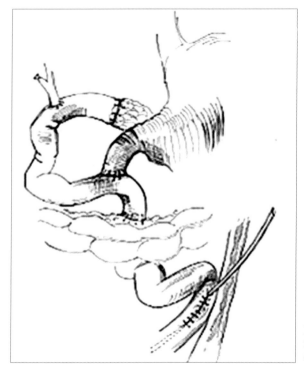

Fig. 29.1 Jejunostomy per-formed during pancreatoduo-denectomy

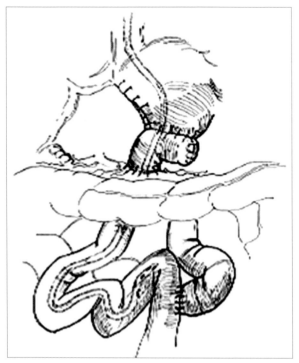

Fig. 29.2 Nasojejunal tube

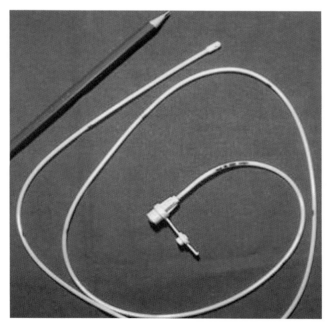

Fig. 29.3 Peristaltic pump

On this subject, at the moment there is no unanimous agreement on the desirable calorie and protein intake. However, a daily supply of 20–35 kcal/kg body weight and of 0.2–0.35 g nitrogen/kg body weight is recommended for both enteral and parenteral nutrition, with a balanced contribution of glucose and lipids, and supplementation of electrolytes, trace elements, and vitamins [19]. Oral or enteral administration of immune-stimulating substrates such as arginine, Ω-3 fatty acids, RNA, and glutamine has been shown to lead to a significant reduction in postoperative complications and length of hospital stay [20]. As a matter of fact, several clinical trials demonstrated the key role of these substrates in modulating systemic immune response, postsurgical stress response, and acute-phase protein synthesis regulation. They also improve gut oxygenation, thus preventing bacterial translocation capacity, resulting in a reduction of postoperative infectious complications and postoperative mortality [21–24]. Consequently, immunonutrient-enriched diets have been used as pharmacological and nutritional support in clinical practice to modulate proinflammatory response and to prevent immunometabolic alterations occurring after surgery which alone result in an increase in postoperative complications.

It is the same with the use of immunonutrition in well-nourished patients undergoing surgical procedures. For example, Gianotti et al. recorded a 15% reduction in postoperative infectious complications with subsequent reduction in hospital stay in well-nourished patients treated with immunonutrition compared to patients treated with standard nutritional support. However, preoperative treatment is crucial in achieving biochemical and immunologic modifications in order to prepare the patient for surgical stress [25]. Nevertheless, the real cost and benefit balance in the use of these substrates is still under debate, and for this reason immunonutrition still has not been introduced as a standard treatment in daily clinical practice.

In advanced pancreatic cancer patients who are eligible for radio- and chemotherapy, there is unanimous agreement, despite the absence of randomized clinical trials, that nutritional treatment is indicated for those who are malnourished or hypophagic. Enteral nutrition, even in these circumstances, seems to give benefit in terms of reducing post-treatment diarrhea [26].

In terminally ill patients the use of nutritional support is controversial [27] for ethical and economic reasons, mostly because of the lack of randomized clinical studies. Nutritional support in these patients is indicated in situations in which the nutritional problem is a priority, such as the risk of death due to malnutrition and not to the malignant disease, so that nutritional care can be continued at home. Artificial nutrition must aim at improving quality of life and survival. Therefore, in individuals with a life expectancy of less than 2–3 months and a Karnofsky performance status of less than 50%, artificial nutrition is not indicated [28, 29].

Nutritional Support in Acute Pancreatitis

Only in the last few years have the indications and modality of nutritional support in acute pancreatitis been better outlined. This topic represents a very interesting issue, but still little is known [30].

First of all, artificial nutrition is indicated only in cases of severe acute pancreatitis [31], which results in a hypercatabolic stress response due to the active acute pancreatic disease leading the patients to prolonged fasting, usually for more than 10 days, with a high risk of malnutrition and subsequent increase in infection rate, morbidity, and mortality. No scientific rationale exists for treating patients with mild pancreatitis, despite what frequently happens in usual clinical practice.

What the correct route of administration is for artificial nutrition is another matter of debate. Enteral nutrition should be the first choice in severe acute pancreatitis, starting as soon as the diagnosis is made [32–35]. Thus it is very important to quickly assess the severity of acute pancreatitis using the APACHE II score or, after the first 48 h, the Ranson or Imrie (Glasgow) scores, in order to start adequate nutritional support. Almost 80% of cases of acute pancreatitis are clinically mild, and here there is no indication for artificial nutrition since patients are able to start oral eating within 4–7 days, before damage due to malnutrition and prolonged fasting may appear [31, 32, 36, 37]. Adequate fluid-electrolyte support should be administered during the fasting period.

The remaining 20% of patients experience severe acute pancreatitis, with pancreatic necrosis. A minority of these patients requires intensive care support or surgical intervention, with a considerable mortality rate ranging from 30 to 50% according to various case studies.

Placement of a nutritional nasojejunal tube is recommended in the first phase of severe acute pancreatitis, coupled with a nasogastric tube for gastric aspiration to palliate nausea and vomiting. Currently double-lumen nasogastrojejunal tubes are also available. Usually during this period the BMI is inside the normal range, or not different from the usual value. Severe acute pancreatitis in obese individuals (BMI >30) is associated with a worse prognosis, just as major surgery is [38]. Patients must be readily treated, and first efforts must be taken to preserve and restore blood volume and adequate circulation [37–39], with careful and strong fluid resuscitation. This should be performed even before a definite prognosis has been made, which requires the use of the APACHE II score at diagnosis and/or the Ranson or Imrie score 48 h after the onset of symptoms, and specific imaging (contrast-enhanced CT at least 48 h after onset of symptoms). In severe acute pancreatitis large amounts of fluids can be retained in retro- and intraperitoneal cavities, leading to hypoperfusion of the splanchnic circulation, an important factor in developing organ dysfunction and intestinal impairment [40]. Fluid sequestration and a prolonged period of fasting, which lead to mucosal atrophy, represent the basis for bacterial translocation into the blood stream. Bacterial translocation, furthermore, seems to be responsible for pancreatic necrosis infection, carrying a worse prognosis. There is much scientific evidence supporting the use of enteral nutrition versus total parenteral nutrition (TPN) in severe acute pancreatitis [41]; among other elements are its role in preventing bacterial translocation, in conserving adequate intestinal blood perfusion, which avoids mucosal atrophy, and in preserving the function of the gut immune system [42].

At the present time no agreement exists on the correct time to start enteral nutrition, but data from the literature suggest that fluids and nutrients should be provided initially through parenteral nutrition in combination with an increasing amount of nutrients supplied with enteral nutrition via the jejunal route, in order to attain calorie and nitrogen requirements within 3–4 days. The combined approach is necessary since enteral nutrition alone is not enough to readily reach nutritional goals and satisfy the patient's energy requirements [30, 36, 38, 39]. It is advisable to start out with a minimum amount of enteral nutrition to test the patient's tolerance (10–20 ml/h), progressively increasing the infusion rate in the following days. When side effects occur, such as diarrhea, abdominal distension, nausea, intolerance, it is usually enough to reduce the infusion rate and if necessary administer symptomatic drugs. Sometimes, however, intolerance to enteral nutrition can only be solved after complete suspension of enteral feeding, which should be replaced with TPN to reduce the adverse effects of nutrient deprivation.

The jejunal route for enteral nutrition is usually preferred in order to minimize the pancreatic secretory response [43, 44] and reduce the risk of aspiration, even though recent reports found no difference between nasojejunal or nasogastric feeding in terms of clinical benefit and adverse events [45, 46].

The combination of enteral and total parenteral nutrition also allows the target of artificial nutrition, in terms of calorie and nitrogen level, to be achieved promptly and at lower risk. Calorie and nitrogen requirements are the following: 25–35 kcal/kg body weight per day (up to a maximum of 35 kcal/kg per day in the event of septic complications) and 1.2–1.5 g of protein/kg per day. This intake can change depending on the patient's clinical course, nitrogen balance, need for a surgical procedure, or mechanical ventilation [30, 34, 38, 43].

Different opinions exist on the appropriate enteral nutrition formula to administer; polymeric diets are usually preferred to elemental or semi-elemental diets, but in the end none of the employed formulas has proved better in the treatment of these patients. When TPN is indicated the glucose/lipids ratio should be 60/40 or 70/30. The only contraindications in the use of lipid emulsions is hyperlipidemia (serum triglycerides >400 mg/dl). Artificial nutrition in severe acute pancreatitis can continue for weeks, and perhaps months. The quality and quantity of nutrients should be adjusted according to the patient's general condition, onset of complications (e.g., organ failure, sepsis), clinical course, or in the event of surgery. During surgery it is always convenient to perform a nutritional jejunostomy [47].

When the patient's condition allows it, artificial nutrition should be gradually diminished while oral refeeding proceeds [48].

References

1. Charnery P (1995) Nutrition assessment in the 1990's, where are we now? Nutr Clin Pract 10:131–139
2. Heymsfield SB, Tighe A, Wang Z-M (1994) Nutritional assessment by anthropometric and biochemical methods. In: Shils ME, Olson JA, Shike M (eds) Modern nutrition in health and disease. Lea & Febiger, Philadelphia, pp 812–841
3. Ireton-Jones C, Hasse J (1992) Comprehensive nutritional assesment: the dietitian's contribution to the team effort. Nutrition 8:75–81
4. Barnsein L, Bachman TE, Meguid M et al. (1995) Measurement of visceral protein status in assessing protein and energy malnutrition: standard of care. Prealbumin in Nutritional Care Consensus Group. Nutrition 11:163–171
5. Mears E (1996) Outcomes of continuous process improvement of a nutritional care program incorporating serum prealbumin measurements. Nutrition 12:479–484
6. Barrocas A Belcher D, Champagne C et al (1995) Nutrition assessment practical approaches. Clin Geriatr Med 11:675–713
7. Edington J, Kon P, Martyn CN (1996) Prevalence of malnutrition in patients in general practice. Clin Nutr 15:60–63
8. Detsky AS, Mclaughlin JR Baker LP et al (1987) What is subjective global assessment of nutritional status? JPEN J Parenter Enteral Nutr 11:8–13
9. Giugoz Y, Vellas B, Gary PJ (1996) Assessing the nutritional status of the elderly: the mini nutritional assessment as part of the geriatric evaluation. Nutr Rev 54:S59–S65
10. Barton BE (2005) Interleukin-6 and new strategies for the treatment of cancer, hyperproliferative diseases and paraneoplastic syndromes. Expert Opin Ther Targets 9:737–752
11. Bozzetti F, Gianotti L, Braga M et al (2007) Postoperative complications in gastrointestinal cancer patients: the joint role of the nutritional status and the nutritional support. Clin Nutr 26:698–709
12. Brown TT, Zelnik DL, Dobs AS (2003) Fish oil supplementation in the treatment of cachexia in pancreatic cancer patients. Int J Gastrointest Cancer 34:143–150
13. Gordon JN, Trebble TM, Ellis RD, et al (2005) Thalidomide in the treatment of cancer cachexia: a randomised placebo controlled trial. Gut 54:540–545
14. Trujillo EB, Chertow GM, Jacobs DO (2001) Metabolic assessment. In: Rombeau JL, Rolandelli RH (eds) Parenteral nutrition. Saunders, Philadelphia, pp 80–108
15. Klein S, Kinney J, Jeejeebhoy K et al (1997) Nutrition support in clinical practice: review of published data and recommendations for future research directions Am J Clin Nutr 66:683–706
16. Meguid MM, Curtas MS, Meguid V et al (1998) Effects of pre-operative TPN on surgical risk – preliminary status report. Br J Clin Pract 42(Suppl 63):53–58
17. Bozzetti F, Gavazzi C, Miceli R, et al (2000) Perioperative total parenteral nutrition in malnourished, gastrointestinal cancer patients: a randomized clinical trial. JPEN J Parenter Enteral Nutr 24:7–14
18. Mercadante S (1998) Parenteral versus enteral nutrition in cancer patients: indications and practice. Support Care Cancer 6:85–93
19. Nitenberg G, Raynard B (2000) Nutritional support of the cancer patient: issues and dilemmas. Crit Rev Oncol Hematol 34:137–168
20. Braga M, Gianotti L, Nespoli L et al (2002) Nutritional approach in malnourished surgical patients: a prospective randomized study. Arch Surg 137:174–180
21. Daly JM, Lieberman MD, Goldfine J et al (1992) Enteral nutrition with supplemental arginine, RNA, and omega-3 fatty acids in patients after operation. Immunologic, metabolic and clinical outcome. Surgery 112:56–67
22. Senkal M, Kemen M, Homann HH et al (1995) Modulation of postoperative immune response by enteral nutrition with a diet enriched with arginine, RNA, and omega-3 fatty acids in patients with upper gastrointestinal cancer. Eur J Surg 161:115–122

23. Gianotti L, Alexander JW, Pyles T et al (1993) Arginine supplemented diets improve survival in gut-derived sepsis and peritonitis by modulating bacterial clearance: the role of nitric oxide. Ann Surg 217:644–654

24. Braga M, Gianotti L, Costantini E et al (1994) Impact of enteral nutrition on intestinal bacterial translocation and mortality in burned mice. Clin Nutr 13:256–261

25. Gianotti L, Braga M, Nespoli L et al (2002) A randomized controlled trial of preoperative oral supplementation with a specialized diet in patients with gastrointestinal cancer. Gastroenterology 122:1763–1770

26. Craighead PS, Young S (1998) Phase II study assessing the feasibility of using elemental supplements to reduce acute enteritis in patients receiving radical pelvic radiotherapy. Am J Clin Oncol 21:573–578

27. Barber MD, Fearon KCH, Delmore G et al (1998) Current controversies in cancer: should cancer patients with incurable disease receive parenteral or enteral nutrition support? Eur J Cancer 34:279–285

28. Bachmann P, Marti-Massaud C, Blanc-Vincent MP et al (2001) Standards, options and recommendations: nutritional support in palliative or terminal care of adult patients with progressive cancer [in French]. Bull Cancer 88:985–100

29. Scolapio JS, Fleming R, Kelly D, et al (1994) Survival in parenteral nutrition treated patients: 20 years of experience at the Mayo Clinic. Mayo Clin Proc 74:217–222

30. ASPEN Board of Directors and the Clinical Guidelines Task Force (2002) Guidelines for the use of parenteral and enteral nutrition in adult and pediatric patients. JPEN J Parenter Enteral Nutr 26(1 Suppl):1SA-138SA

31. SINPE (1995) Pancreatite acuta (Linee Guida). RINPE 13 S-2:22–24

32. Kalfarentzos F, Kehagias J, Mead N et al (1997) Enteral nutrition is superior to parenteral nutrition in severe acute pancreatitis: results of a randomized prospective trial. Br J Surg 84:1665–1669

33. Windsor ACJ, Kanwar S, Li AGK et al (1998) Compared with parenteral nutrition, enteral feeding attenuates the acute phase response and improves disease severity in acute pancreatitis. Gut 42:431–435

34. Olah A, Pardavi G, Belagyi T, et al (2002) Early nasojejunal feeding in acute pancreatitis is associated with a lower complication rate. Nutrition 18:259–262

35. Eckerwall G, Anderson R (2001) Early enteral nutrition in severe acute pancreatitis: a way of providing nutrients, gut barrier protection, immunomodulation, or all of them? Scand J Gastroenterol 36:449–458

36. Meier R, Beglinger C, Layer P et al (2002) ESPEN Consensus Group: ESPEN guidelines on nutrition in acute pancreatitis. Clin Nutr 21:173–183

37. Banks PA (1997) Practice guidelines in acute pancreatitis. Am J Gastroenterol 92:377–86

38. Toouli J, Brooke-Smith M, Bassi C et al (2002) Guidelines for the management of acute pancreatitis. J Gastroenterol Hepatol 17(Suppl):S15–S39

39. Glazer G, Mann DV (1998) United Kingdom guidelines for the management of acute pancreatitis. British Society of Gastroentrology. Gut 42(Suppl 2):S1–S13

40. Kingsnorth A, O'Reilly D (2006) Acute pancreatitis. BMJ 332:1072–1076

41. Mora J, Casas M, Cardona D, Farrè A (2007) Effect of enteral versus parenteral nutrition on inflammatory markers in severe acute pancreatitis. Pancreas 35:292

42. Nathens AB, Curtis JR, Beale RJ, et al (2004) Management of the critically ill patient with severe acute pancreatitis. Crit Care Med 32:2524–2536

43. Zaloga GP, Roberts PR (1998) Bedside placement of enteral feeding tubes in the intensive care unit. Crit Care Med 26:987–988

44. Zaloga GP, Roberts PR, Marik P (2003) Feeding the hemodynamically unstable patient: a critical evaluation of the evidence. Nutr Clin Pract 18:285–293

45. Eckerwall GE, Axelsson JB, Andersson RG (2006) Early nasogastric feeding in predicted acute pancreatitis: a clinical, randomized trial. Ann Surg 244:959–965; discussion 965–967

46. Ho KM, Dobb GJ, Webb SAR (2006) A comparison of early gastric and post-pyloric feeding in critically ill patients: a meta analysis. Intensive Care Med 32:639–649

47. UK Working Party on Acute Pancreatitis (2005) UK Guidelines for the management of acute pancreatitis. Gut 54(Suppl 3):iii 1–9
48. McClave SA, Chang WK, Dhaliwal R, Heyland DK (2006) Nutrition support in acute pancreatitis: a systematic review of the literature. JPEN J Parenter Enteral Nutr 30:143–156

Chapter 30

Pancreatic Fistulas after Pancreaticoduodenectomy or Distal Pancreatectomy

Giovanni Butturini, Despoina Daskalaki, Claudio Bassi, Paolo Pederzoli

Definition

Pancreatic fistula is defined as an abnormal communication between the pancreatic ductal system and any other space, internal or external to the peritoneal cavity, caused by an interruption to the integrity of the ductal epithelium itself [1]. Pancreatic fistulas are thus divided into *internal* and *external*, the former being by far the most frequent and almost the only ones that occur after pancreatic resection. In fact, whenever a postoperative fistula develops, in the absence of adequate drainage the result will be an abdominal collection that evolves into an abscess or a pseudocyst rather than an internal fistula.

However, the anatomic definition of pancreatic fistula is of little use in clinical practice. As a consequence, pancreatic surgeons have tried over the years to produce their own definition of fistula based on parameters such as drainage output, presence of amylase in the drained fluid, and radiological demonstration of communication with the pancreatic ductal system. Analyzing the various parameters in more detail, it is clear that in order to talk about fistula, the presence of drainage is necessary, and in fact this is how resective pancreatic surgery most commonly terminates, although recent evidence tends to call this practice into question [2].

There is still no agreement among various authors about the use of suction or nonsuction drains. The output of each drain should be checked daily, and its macroscopic appearance should be assessed as well as determining the presence or absence of amylase in the drained fluid. The cut-off value of amylase considered significant for the development of pancreatic fistula is still debatable and is the parameter on which there is most divergence amongst the various studies. Time is also a parameter of great importance, since it has been demonstrated that the amylase content in the drained fluid is physiologically high in the first days after operation, being significantly reduced after approximately 1 week [3]. However, the parameters mentioned above are not used by all authors, and so comparison of the different definitions and consequently of the different experiences is even more difficult. This particular aspect was further complicated at

W. Siquini (Ed.), *Surgical Treatment of Pancreatic Diseases.*
©Springer-Verlag Italia 2009

the beginning of the 1990s, when extremely accurate and strict definitions of fistula prevailed. These definitions were closely tied to clinical trials that were attempting to understand the influence of inhibitors of pancreatic secretion on the production of pancreatic juice by the gland itself, irrespective of the clinical relevance of the leakage that was defined as fistula [4, 5]. Since the year 2000, the same authors have modified their definition of fistula, extending the concept and trying to include also cases with some clinical impact [6]. The result of this effort made by the individual authors to define their own complication (which today is still the most common and difficult complication of all, leading to others such as late hemorrhage) is that dozens of such definitions, sometimes very different one from another, are to be found in the literature, such that, even if we applied these definitions to the same group of patients, operated by the same surgical team, we would have a significantly different incidence of pancreatic fistula [7].

From this realization, a group of expert pancreatic surgeons from all over the world, coordinated by Professor Claudio Bassi, developed a definition of pancreatic fistula that aimed to synthesize the various experiences and different definitions [1]. It was agreed that the clinical impact of a fistula on the postoperative course of the patient should be the predominant element by which to distinguish and classify pancreatic fistulas (Table 30.1). This definition represents the first attempt at an international agreement and is in use by the major groups in pancreatic surgery [8–10].

Pancreatic Fistula after Pancreaticoduodenectomy

Pancreatic fistula still represents the main postoperative complication after pancreaticoduodenectomy. It influences the outcome of the operation and explains nearly half of the postoperative mortality of this procedure. The risk factors for the development of pancreatic fistula are the following: soft pancreatic remnant; Wirsung duct diameter less than 3 mm [8, 11, 13]; presence of coronary disease and absence of arterial hypertension [8, 12]; high-tension anastomosis (increased risk of anastomotic leakage); re-operation; emergency surgery; jaundice; renal failure; cirrhosis; cardiovascular disease; and malnutrition [8, 12, 14, 15].

As for the texture of the pancreatic stump, the incidence of fistula will be greater in diseases that do not create an obstruction of the duct of Wirsung with subsequent chronic pancreatitis, as for example neoplasms of the distal common bile duct or benign neoplasms of the pancreatic head with expansive growth. On this point there has been an effort to avoid the development of fistula using inhibitors of pancreatic secretion, like somatostatin analogues that are still now widely used, even though there is great controversy on the subject. Use of the antiprotease gabexate mesilate has not been demonstrated to have any efficacy in preventing pancreatic fistula [18, 19] and is not in routine use today.

The correlation between the fistula and the diameter of the main pancreatic duct (<3 mm) has induced surgeons to place a stent in the Wirsung duct so as to

Table 31.1 Grading for the evaluation of the clinical impact of postoperative pancreatic fistulas (*POPF*), developed by the International Study Group of Pancreatic Fistula (ISGPF)

	Grade A	Grade B	Grade C
Clinical impact	None ("transitory" fistula)	Clinically significant fistula	Potentially life-threatening fistula
Patient's clinical condition	Well	Abdominal pain, fever, leukocytosis	Severe, possible signs of sepsis and/or organ failure
Ultrasound or CT	No peripancreatic collections	Potential intra-abdominal collections	Problematic peripancreatic collections
Treatment	Slow removal of the drains placed intraoperatively. No need for antibiotics, TPN, EN, or somatostatin analogues. The patient can be discharged from hospital and will be monitored as an outpatient	No oral feeding. TPN or EN, antibiotics, and somatostatin analogues are usually employed. Repositioning of the drains under radiological guidance, in the presence of peripancreatic collections	Aggressive. No oral feeding. TPN or EN, intravenous antibiotics and somatostatin analogues are required. Possible ICU. Re-operation
Prolonged hospital stay	No	Yes	Yes
Higher cost	No	Yes	Yes
In situ drain after 3 weeks	No	Frequently	Yes
Postoperative death	No	No	Possible

CT, Computed tomography; *TPN*, total parenteral nutrition; *EN*, enteral nutrition; *ICU*, intensive care unit

perform the pancreatic anastomosis safely. However, there are no prospective studies that support the utility of this technique [8, 12, 14]. The reconstruction of the pancreatic stump can be achieved with either a pancreaticojejunal or a pancreaticogastric anastomosis, but once again there are no statistically significant data that support the superiority of one technique over the other in reducing the development of fistula – although there is a certain trend in favor of the pancreaticogastric anastomosis, which seems to reduce the incidence of complex fistulas and thus the subsequent postoperative intra-abdominal collections [20]. If the pancreatic stump is particularly friable and the main pancreatic duct presents a diameter of 1–2 mm, a pancreaticogastric anastomosis might be indicated. In this case, wide mobilization of the residual pancreas should be obtained so that the stump can be introduced in the gastric cavity for at least 3–4 cm. This result can be easily achieved by performing an anterior gastrotomy [21]. If a pancreaticojejunal anastomosis is to be made, we suggest the use of single-layer absorbable sutures and the placement of a probe in the main pancreatic duct while the anastomosis is being performed, in order to avoid enclosing the duct, especially during the posterior wall step. Despite the already mentioned controversy that exists, we suggest the placement of two drains, one to the right and one to the left, at the end of the operation so as to protect the anastomosis.

During the postoperative course the drainage output should be monitored as to both quality and quantity. The amylase content of the drained fluid is of particular importance, because the data available allow us to establish a safe cut-off value that determines the risk of development of a pancreatic fistula. This value is 5000 U/l of amylase measured in the drained fluid on the 1st postoperative day [3]. If the amylase content is less than 5000 U/l, early removal of the drains should be considered, whereas if it is more than 5000 U/l, the risk of pancreatic fistula is high and further decisions should be postponed until the 5th postoperative day. The importance of the early removal of the drains is emphasized by the high risk of infection, which becomes notable after the 7th postoperative day [22].

When a fistula develops it is necessary to establish whether this event will lead to important changes in the clinical condition of the patient. Body temperature, common signs of inflammation, and bowel function should be monitored, and a first ultrasound scan should be done to rule out the presence of intra-abdominal collections. If the fistula is well-drained, it may have a simple, indolent postoperative course without severe consequences, and the patient may even start oral feeding. If the output of the fistula though is remains significantly high for some days, or if it assumes suspicious characteristics, fistulography will be necessary. This is performed by injecting hydrosoluble contrast medium through the drainage placed during the operation and can show opacification of any intra-abdominal collections, even small ones, in the path of the fistula and the anastomosed jejunal loop. It is also possible to optimize the position of the drain, which in many cases will have direct communication with the anastomosed loop keeping the fistula active [3]. This simple radiological method allows us to resolve a considerable number of fistulas after pancreaticoduodenectomy, just by targeted mobilization of the drainage.

When the fistula is sustained by pancreatitis of the pancreatic stump, a change in the postoperative management will be necessary. This event appears when serum amylase is elevated in the immediate postoperative course and is confirmed by contrast-enhanced abdominal CT. Treatment should include antibiotic therapy and total parenteral or enteral nutrition. The hospital stay will be prolonged. If intra-abdominal collections are present, drainage is mandatory. This can be achieved by percutaneous insertion of a pigtail drain tube under ultrasound or CT guidance with local anesthesia. During this procedure a sample of the liquid should be taken for microbiological and biochemical study. In the days that follow it will be possible to wash the pigtail drain tube with physiological solution, in order to keep it open and also favor the outflow of any intra-abdominal collection through the intraoperatively placed drain. If the drainage output does not rapidly reduce, the pigtail can also be used for fistulography. With these methods even grade B and C fistulas can be managed without the necessity for re-operation. This procedure should be considered only when all noninvasive methods have failed, since it is associated with significant morbidity and mortality [1, 9, 11, 23, 24].

Re-operation will in fact be necessary in the following cases:

- Sepsis sustained by significant intra-abdominal collections not sufficiently drained by percutaneous methods. During the procedure the area of the anastomosis should be exposed and the collections causing the sepsis should be drained. The drains placed during the operation can be used in the postoperative course to perform lavages with physiological solution.
- Complete anastomotic dehiscence with evidence of air bubbles near the anastomosis on CT scan, septic status, malfunction of the drains placed percutaneously. The procedure is more complex in this case, because a major anastomotic dehiscence might even require total pancreatectomy, with increased risk of morbidity and mortality.
- Late hemorrhage caused by the fistula. This is a frightful event with a high mortality rate, generally caused by the formation of an arterial pseudoaneurysm. The procedure should be anticipated by selective arteriography, so as to identify the exact source of the bleeding and embolize the vessel involved. Re-laparotomy should be performed afterwards in order to drain the hematoma, which otherwise will cause an intraperitoneal infection.

Pancreatic Fistula after Distal Pancreatectomy

Benign neoplastic diseases such as cystic and endocrine tumors, which are the most frequent indications for distal pancreatectomy.

Regarding the incidence of this complication, the same reasoning on various definitions as for fistulas after pancreaticoduodenectomy is still valid. Particular care is needed with regard to the congruency of reported rates and complications. For example, whenever a low incidence of pancreatic fistula is associated with a high rate of re-operation for abdominal abscess, the possibility must be considered that such infected intra-abdominal collections are just improperly drained fistulas [25–27]. Various techniques have been studied over the years in order to reduce the incidence of pancreatic fistula [19, 25, 28–36], but without any evidence of superiority of one technique over the other. A recent meta-analysis of the literature has identified a certain trend toward using the mechanic stapler for dissecting the pancreatic stump, although it is not yet statistically significant [30]. Moreover, since there is evidence that octreotide provokes spasm of the sphincter of Oddi [37], its use is not advisable after distal pancreatic resection.

During the operation a soft, nonsuction drain should be placed near the pancreatic stump. In the period that follows the operation the presence of amylase in the drained fluid should be determined, applying the cut-off value of 5000 U/l in order to regulate the postoperative management of the patient. It is highly recommended to carry out an ultrasound scan before removing the drains, so that any intra-abdominal collections will be demonstrated.

If a fistula develops, conservative management is effective in most cases. The patient's clinical course should be monitored, and in absence of intra-abdominal collections it will be brief and indolent, with rapid restoration of the digestive functions. The patient can be discharged from hospital and monitored in an outpatient setting until the fistula output stops and the drain can be safely removed.

To underline the limited clinical relevance of this type of fistula, it has been suggested to grade the definition of fistula itself, and grade A fistula in fact is the most common type after distal pancreatic resection. Nonetheless, if the drain is not well positioned, or is for any other reason displaced, an intra-abdominal collection might develop near the pancreatic stump with possible development into an abscess. This situation might even be characterized by a drop in the amylase in the drained fluid to within normal levels, but it will be accompanied by a deterioration in the patients' clinical status. An abdominal CT scan is indicated to evaluate the morphology of the collection and drain it if necessary. If with the percutaneously placed drainage the patient's clinical condition does not improve within 1 week, the surgeon is obliged to proceed with re-operation and therefore to drain the collection surgically.

The collections that might form after distal pancreatectomy, because of their particular position, can also be successfully drained endoscopically [38, 39]. Major indications for this approach include well-limited, capsulated collections with a thick pseudowall, that have a compressive effect on the stomach. When an area of necrosis is individuated within the collection [40] – event which is frequent in the case of fistula causing pancreatitis of the pancreatic stump – the endoscopic approach is more likely to be unsuccessful. In order to perform an endoscopic drainage more safely, it is opportune to use ultrasound endoscopy, which permits visualization of the vascular structures that are in contact with the wall of the collection [41, 42]. The positioning of a double stent between the gastric wall and the collection is advisable to reduce the risk of early closure of the path created endoscopically and consequent relapse of the pseudocyst.

References

1. Bassi C, Dervenis C, Butturini G et al (2005) Postoperative pancreatic fistula: an international study group (ISGPF) definition. Surgery 138:8–13
2. Conlon KC, Labow D, Leung D et al (2001) Prospective randomized clinical trial of the value of intraperitoneal drainage after pancreatic resection. Ann Surg 234:487–493; discussion 493–494
3. Molinari E, Bassi C, Salvia R et al (2007) Amylase value in drains after pancreatic resection as predictive factor of postoperative pancreatic fistula. Results of a prospective study in 137patients. Ann Surg 246:281–287
4. Pederzoli P, Bassi C, Falconi M et al (1994) Efficacy of octreotide in the prevention of complications of elective pancreatic surgery. Br J Surg 81:265–269
5. Buchler M, Frieb H, Klempa I et al (1992) The role of somatostatin analogue octreotide in the prevention of postoperative complications following pancreatic resection. The results of a multicentre controlled trial. Am J Surg 163:125–131
6. Buchler MW, Friess H, Wagner M et al (2000) Pancreatic fistula after pancreatic head resection. Br J Surg 87:883–889
7. Bassi C, Butturini G, Molinari E et al (2004) Pancreatic fistula rate after pancreatic resection. The importance of definitions. Dig Surg 21:54–59
8. Lermite E, Pessaux P, Brehant O et al (2007) Risk factors of pancreatic fistula and delayed gastric emptying after pancreaticoduodenectomy with pancreaticogastrostomy. J Am Coll Surg 204:588–596
9. Pratt W, Maithel SK, Vanounou T et al (2006) Postoperative pancreatic fistulas are not equivalent after proximal, distal, and central pancreatectomy. J Gastrointest Surg 10:1264–1278; discussion 1278–1279
10. Iannitti DA, Coburn NG, Somberg J et al (2006) Use of the round ligament of the liver to decrease pancreatic fistulas: a novel technique. J Am Coll Surg 203:857–864
11. Aranha GV, Aaron JM, Shoup M et al (2006) Current management of pancreatic fistula after pancreaticoduodenectomy. Surgery 140:561–568; discussion 568–569
12. Lin JW, Cameron JL, Yeo CJ et al (2004) Risk factors and outcomes in postpancreaticoduodenectomy pancreaticocutaneous fistula. J Gastrointest Surg 8:951–959
13. Muscari F, Suc B, Kirzin S et al (2006) Risk factors for mortality and intra-abdominal complications after pancreatoduodenectomy: multivariate analysis in 300 patients. Surgery 139:591–598
14. DeOliveira ML, Winter JM, Schafer M et al (2006) Assessment of complications after pancreatic surgery: A novel grading system applied to 633 patients undergoing pancreaticoduodenectomy. Ann Surg 244:931–937; discussion 937–939
15. Sierzega M, Niekowal B, Kulig J et al (2007) Nutritional status affects the rate of pancreatic fistula after distal pancreatectomy: a multivariate analysis of 132 patients. J Am Coll Surg 205:52–59
16. Moon HJ, Heo JS, Choi SH et al (2005) The efficacy of the prophylactic use of octreotide after a pancreaticoduodenectomy. Yonsei Med J 46:788–793
17. Connor S, Alexakis N, Garden OJ et al (2005) Meta-analysis of the value of somatostatin and its analogues in reducing complications associated with pancreatic surgery. Br J Surg 92:1059–1067
18. Büchler MW, Binder M, Friess H (1994) Role of somatostatin and its analogues in the treatment of acute and chronic pancreatitis. Gut 35(3 Suppl):S15–S19
19. Takeuchi K, Tsuzuki Y, Ando T et al (2003) Distal pancreatectomy: is staple closure beneficial? ANZ J Surg 73:922–925
20. Bassi C, Falconi M, Molinari E et al (2005) Reconstruction by pancreaticojejunostomy versus pancreaticogastrostomy following pancreatectomy: results of a comparative study. Ann Surg 242:767–771, discussion 771–773
21. Bassi C, Butturini G, Salvia R et al (2006) Open pancreaticogastrostomy after pancreaticoduodenectomy: a pilot study. J Gastrointest Surg 10:1072–1080

22. Kawai M, Tani M, Terasawa H et al (2006) Early removal of prophylactic drains reduces the risk of intra-abdominal infections in patients with pancreatic head resection: prospective study for 104 consecutive patients. Ann Surg 244:1–7

23. Payne RF, Pain JA (2006) Duct-to-mucosa pancreaticogastrostomy is a safe anastomosis following pancreaticoduodenectomy. Br J Surg 93:73–77

24. Munoz-Bongrand N, Sauvanet A, Denys A et al (2004) Conservative management of pancreatic fistula after pancreaticoduodenectomy with pancreaticogastrostomy. J Am Coll Surg 199:198–203

25. Bassi C, Butturini G, Falconi M et al (1999) Prospective randomised pilot study of management of the pancreatic stump following distal resection. HPB 1:203–207

26. Brennan M, Moccia RD, Klimstra D (1996) Management of adenocarcinoma of the body and tail of the pancreas. Ann Surg 223:506–512

27. Fabre JM, Houre S, Manderscheid JC et al (1996) Surgery for the left-sided pancreatic cancer. Br J Surg 83:1065–1070

28. Kuroki T, Tajima Y, Kanematsu T (2005) Surgical management for the prevention of pancreatic fistula following distal pancreatectomy. J Hepatobiliary Pancreat Surg 12:283–285

29. Pannegeon V, Pessaux P, Sauvanet A et al (2006) Pancreatic fistula after distal pancreatectomy: predictive risk factors and value of conservative treatment. Arch Surg 141:1071–1076; discussion 1076

30. Knaebel HP, Diener MK, Wente MN et al (2005) Systematic review and meta-analysis of technique for closure of the pancreatic remnant after distal pancreatectomy. Br J Surg 92:539–546

31. Fahy BN, Frey CF, Ho HS et al (2002) Morbidity, mortality, and technical factors of distal pancreatectomy. Am J Surg 183:237–241

32. Sheehan MK, Beck K, Creech S et al (2002) Distal pancreatectomy: does the method of closure influence fistula formation? Am Surg 68:264–267

33. Bilimoria MM, Cormier JN, Mun Y et al (2003) Pancreatic leak after left pancreatectomy is reduced following main pancreatic duct ligation. Br J Surg 90:190–196

34. Adam U, Makowiec F, Riediger H et al (2001) Distal pancreatic resection –indications, techniques and complications. Zentralbl Chir 126:908–912

35. Suzuki Y, Fujino Y, Tanioka Y et al (1999) Randomised clinical trial of ultrasonic dissector or conventional division in distal pancreatectomy for non-fibrotic pancreas. Br J Surg 86:608–611

36. Ohwada S, Ogawa T, Tanahashi Y et al (1998) Fibrin glue sandwich prevents pancreatic fistula following distal pancreatectomy. World J Surg 22:494–498

37. Di Francesco V, Angelini G, Bovo P et al (1996) Effect of octreotide on sphincter of Oddi motility in patients with acute recurrent pancreatitis: a manometric study. Dig Dis Sci 41:2392–2396

38. Buscail L, Faure P, Bournet B et al (2006) Interventional endoscopic ultrasound in pancreatic diseases. Pancreatology 6(1–2):7–16

39. Baron TH (2003) Endoscopic drainage of pancreatic fluid collections and pancreatic necrosis. Gastrointest Endosc Clin N Am 13:743–764

40. Papachristou GI, Takahashi N, Chahal P et al (2007) Peroral endoscopic drainage/debridement of walled-off pancreatic necrosis. Ann Surg 245:943–951

41. Kahaleh M, Shami VM, Conaway MR et al (2006) Endoscopic ultrasound drainage of pancreatic pseudocyst: a prospective comparison with conventional endoscopic drainage. Endoscopy 38:355–359

42. Giovannini M, Pesenti C, Rolland AL et al (2001) Endoscopic ultrasound-guided drainage of pancreatic pseudocysts or pancreatic abscesses using a therapeutic echo endoscope. Endoscopy 33:473–477

Chapter 31

Inhibitors of Pancreatic Secretion and Antiproteases in Acute Pancreatitis and Pancreatic Surgery

Ezio Caratozzolo, Marco Massani, Nicolò Bassi

Acute pancreatitis is a common and potentially life-threatening condition that requires a multidisciplinary team for diagnosis and correct treatment [1]. Although it is one of the most studied conditions in the history of medicine, acute pancreatitis still remains a demanding and dreadful disease. It may be considered as self-digestion of the pancreas, and progress in recent years in our understanding of the pathophysiology has led to some improvement in the diagnosis and outcome for patients suffering from the severe form of the disease [2–4]. Usually the pancreatic enzymes, in the form of proenzymes, are transported from pancreatic ducts in the duodenum, where they are activated. In acute pancreatitis there is early activation of intracellular zymogens with a complex phenomenon that leads to inflammation and tissue damage [4]. The severe course of the disease is characterized by a systemic inflammatory response that can induce multiorgan failure. Comprehension of this early activation of proenzymes represents the basis from which to understand the disease and develop its treatment [5, 6]. In the assessment of therapy we believe it is essential to distinguish between the acute phase, treatment of the causal factor, and the prevention of pancreatic fistula after surgical resection. This last aspect will form the final part of this chapter.

Adequate treatment should be started as soon as possible. Although the mild forms of acute pancreatitis rarely develop into severe disease, all attacks of acute pancreatitis should be regarded as life-threatening until proven otherwise. Treatment of the mild forms consists of brief fasting and fluid-electrolyte replacement, combined with analgesic therapy to be continued until the healing [7, 8]. However, in any case, the severity of the pancreatitis should be settled in order to diagnose deterioration that will require more specific treatment.

Treatment of the severe forms of pancreatitis, on the other hand, can be very complicated, and for the best results it is necessary to involve an expert team. Looking at the treatment of severe acute pancreatitis from 1950 to the present day, several phases have been gone through, and we have seen the alternation of very aggressive surgical treatments with other treatments based on complete abstention. Many drugs have been tested, all united in their attempt to reduce pancreatic activity. Medical therapy is in any case the treatment of choice for

W. Siquini (Ed.), *Surgical Treatment of Pancreatic Diseases.*
©Springer-Verlag Italia 2009

severe forms; the role of surgery is to treat early complications such as abscesses, septic necrosis, hemorrhage, peritonitis, and multiple organ failure, and late complications (mostly represented by pseudocysts). The role of therapy is to control the pain, maintain homeostasis, monitor multiorgan dysfunction, and prevent complications and infections [9].

The literature reports various experiences of different specific drugs used to control the process of self-digestion that characterizes acute pancreatitis, for example, antisecretion and antiprotease drugs. Regarding antisecretion agents such as somatostatin or octreotide, many studies have not demonstrated their effectiveness in the treatment of acute pancreatitis, whereas positive expectations worthy of consideration are reported in the prevention of fistulas after pancreatic surgery (see the end of this chapter). Looking at the results of some published controlled trials, the only drug that has shown real activity in the treatment of severe pancreatitis is gabexate mesilate [10]. This is an antiprotease drug that because of its low molecular weight is able to get inside the parenchyma, reducing the activation of pancreatic enzymes. It was well demonstrated that it is particularly active against the activation of trypsin, phospholipase A, plasmin, thrombin, and kallikrein, interfering with pancreatic elevation of proteases, the system of fibrinolysis, coagulation, and kinins. Gabexate mesilate is active against platelet binding. Studies on rats and rabbits have demonstrated a protective effect in experimentally induced pancreatitis, a direct effect to inhibit the disseminated intravascular coagulation as well as protective action in various types of shock [10]. In addition, in a dog model a clear relaxing action on the sphincter of Oddi was shown. The active principle was introduced many years ago and is administered by continuous intravenous infusion at a dose which can vary between 900 mg and 3000 mg per day.

To maximize the results of therapy, administration should be started as early as possible (within 24 h after onset of symptoms). In our experience, although the indication to use this drug is linked to the severity of the pancreatitis, administration of gabexate to all patients with a proven diagnosis of acute pancreatitis gave good results. Our policy is to stop the use of gabexate for the mild form within 48–72 h if the clinical course is favorable. Severe forms, on the other hand, require prolonged antiprotease therapy. The dosage and duration of treatment is closely related to the course of the disease. The standard duration of treatment is 7 days that could be suspended unless it is proved benefit. Considering the pharmacological action of this drug, its use for more than 7 days, after consolidation of the damage to the gland, should be unnecessary. Our experience, like that reported by many others groups, showed a clear benefit of using gabexate mesilate in severe pancreatitis, with a significant reduction of the number of complications requiring a surgical approach.

The particular mechanism of action of gabexate mesilate suggested a possible role in preventing pancreatitis induced by endoscopic retrograde cholangiopancreatography (ERCP), especially operative ERCP (for example for the removal of gallstones, or stent positioning). Although not all published articles prove that it is effective in preventing ERCP pancreatitis, our experience, in agreement with that of many other centers, clearly gave encouraging results. The dosage for preventing post-ERCP pancreatitis is 300 mg administered in continuous infusion in 12 h, starting at least 30 minutes before the procedure.The administration of gabexate mesilate should be continued in the presence of symptoms of acute pancreatitis or abnormalities documented with blood tests or instrumental studies.

Other antiproteases with molecular weight lower than that of gabexate mesilate and therefore greater penetration into pancreatic parenchyma have been introduced onto the market, and there are some positive experiences of their administration directly into the gastroduodenal artery. These experiences are reported by Japanese authors and require invasive and sometime difficult maneuvers performed by interventional radiologists [11]. Other data will be needed to see whether some drugs such as lexipafant may have an important role in the treatment of severe forms of acute pancreatitis. Lexipafant is one of a category of cytokine inhibitors that as we know play an important role in the pathogenesis of severe forms of acute pancreatitis (tumor necrosis factor, interleukin 1, and platelet-activating factor).

In any case, every patient who suffers from a severe form of pancreatitis should be carefully monitored in order to recognize as early as possible signs of clinical worsening that could require monitoring in intensive care. It is worth remembering that for each critical patient, the need for an appropriate caloric intake is very high, and a malnourished patient is a patient with an immune deficiency, with all the implications that this entails [12]. The incredible rapidity of depletion of fat and protein in severe forms of acute pancreatitis is well known, and in such patients it will be necessary to establish total parenteral nutrition as soon as possible. Many experiences in this regard have shown equal effectiveness of an enteral nutrition through a nasojejunal tube or through enterostomy in the case of patients who have undergone surgical treatment. Generally it is better to not overdo administration of lipids, although their total abolition does not seem to represent an advantage.

Finally, it is best to remember that, thanks to improved radiological knowledge, we have increasing evidence of autoimmune pancreatitis. These forms of the disease, in addition to the aforementioned organ therapy, benefit from early administration of high-dose steroids, to be maintained for at least 30 days.

As has been often pointed out, if the antiproteases have found a role in the treatment of acute pancreatitis, inhibitors of pancreatic secretions can rationally be used in the prevention of postoperative pancreatic fistula. Since 1912, the year which the first pancreatectomy was described by Kausch and subsequently improved by Whipple, resection has remained the best option for the cure of cancer and certain forms of chronic pancreatitis [13, 14]. The operation, despite all the improvements of technology and pathophysiological knowledge, still remains burdened by the fearsome complication of anastomotic fistula which, even in high-volume centers, is responsible for 30–60% of postoperative complications [15]. As has already happened for acute pancreatitis, efforts have therefore been concentrated on finding a drug that could help to reduce the incidence of fistulas based on the pathophysiological mechanism. Fistula is an event that has a strong influence on the outcome for the patient, resulting in abdominal infections, functional disorders of the digestive tract, and worsening of renal and respiratory functionality, leading to the death of the patient in 5–10% of cases of duodenocephalopancreatectomies. The use of inhibitors of pancreatic secretion minimizes the production of enzymes, allowing proper healing of the anastomosis, which is more at risk of developing fistula after pancreatic resection for cancer than in the case of chronic pancreatitis, where the fibrous pancreatic tissue is exposed to already reduced secretion of enzymes [16].

Over the years various drugs have been used; the most tested is somatostatin [17, 18]. This is a cyclic peptide compound of 14 amino acids that, in addition to its role as regulator of growth hormone production and modulator of the central nervous system, inhibits the exocrine and endocrine pancreatic secretions as well as reducing total secretions from all over the digestive tract (suffice it to recall its use in intractable diarrhea). The first descriptions of its use in pancreatic surgery date back to 1979, when it was administered in a continuous intravenous infusion at a dose of 250 µg/h [19]. A later introduction was octreotide, a synthetic analogue of somatostatin that can be administered subcutaneously because of its different absorption characteristics and far longer half-life [20]. In the treatment or prevention of pancreatic fistulas, the recommended dosage is of 0.1 mg three times daily; it can be increased up to 0.25 mg three times daily. The drug must be given at least one 1 h before operation and should be continued for a maximum of 5–7 days after. In most departments octreotide has supplanted somatostatin both because of its more limited cost and because of the possibility of subcutaneous administration. We must, however, stress that in the literature there is no agreement as to the current role of inhibitors of pancreatic secretions in the prevention or treatment of fistulas after pancreatic surgery, but it is well to remember that some authors have demonstrated a rationale for their use [21]. In our opinion, the use of octreotide as prophylaxis is always recommended, especially in low-volume centers.

This brief overview of a disease that has attracted much interest over the years is of necessity limited to certain fundamental principles for the best management of this disease that still today carries a high mortality. Figures 31.1 and 31.2 show flow-charts used in the management of acute pancreatitis in our department which are the result of data relating to over 1,000 patients observed over the course of 13 years.

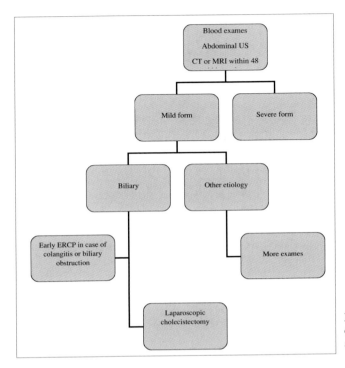

Fig. 31.1 Management of mild acute pancreatitis

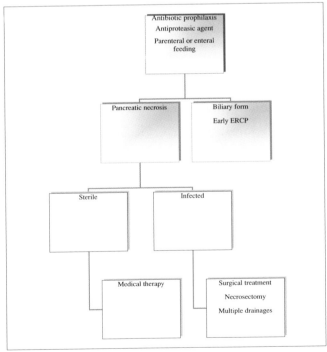

Fig. 31.2 Management of the severe acute pancreatitis

References

1. Cirenei A, Hollender LF (1997) Le pancreatiti acute oggi. Piccin Nuova Libraria, Padua, pp 15–64
2. Nagar AB, Gorlick FS (2004) Acute pancreatitis. Curr Opinion Gastr 20:439–443
3. Balthazar EJ (2002) Acute pancreatitis: assessment of severity with clinical and CT evaluation. Radiology 223:602–613
4. Wang ZE, Pan CE, Lu Y et al (2003) The role of inflammatory mediators in severe acute pancreatitis and regulation of glucocorticoids. Hepatobiliary Pancreat Dis Int 2:458–462
5. Hentic, Levy P, Hammel P et al (2003) Are the causes similar for benign and severe forms of acute pancreatitis? Gastroenterol Clin Biol 27:403–406
6. Ghen X, Wu H, Hang X et al (2002) The alteration of inflammatory cytokine during acute pancreatitis. Hua Xi Yi Ke Da Xue Xue Bao 33:238–240
7. Gruppo Italiano AISP (2001) La pancreatite acuta in Italia: studio osservazionale su 1005 pazienti. Press Service
8. Gruppo Italiano AISP (2004) La pancreatite acuta: storia naturale e terapia medica ragionata In: AISP (ed) Attualità in pancreatologia. AISP, pp 3–12
9. Haraldsen P, Sun SW, Börjesson A et al (2003) Multimodal management: of value in fulminant acute pancreatitis? Pancreatology 3:14–25
10. Kitagawa M, Hayakawa T (2007) Antiproteases in the treatment of acute pancreatitis. JOP 8(Suppl):518–525
11. Takeda K (2007) Antiproteases in the treatment of acute necrotizing pancreatitis: continuous regional arterial infusion. JOP 8(Suppl):526–532
12. Pezzilli R, Fantini L, Morsilli-Labate AM (2006) New approaches for the treatment of acute pancreatitis. JOP 7:79–91
13. Kausch W (1912) Das Carcinoma der Papilla duodeni und seine radikale Entfernung. Beitr Klin Chir 78:439–451
14. Whipple AO (1942) Present-day surgery of the pancreas. N Engl J Med 226:515–518
15. Stojadinovic A, Brooks A, Hoos A et al (2003) An evidence-based approach to the surgical management of resectable pancreatic adenocarcinoma. J Am Coll Surg 196:954–964
16. Li-Ling J, Irving M (2001) Somatostatin and octreotide in the prevention of postoperative pancreatic complications and the treatment of enterocutaneous pancreatic fistulas: a systematic review of randomized controlled trials. Br J Surg 88:190–199
17. Büchler M, Friess H, Klempa I et al (1992) Role of octreotide in the prevention of postoperative complications following pancreatic resection. Am J Surg 163:125–130
18. Büchler M, Friess H (1993) Prevention of postoperative complications following pancreatic surgery. Digestion 54(Suppl):41–46
19. Klempa L, Schwedes U, Usadel KH (1979) Verhütung von postoperativen pankreatischen Komplikationen nach Duodenopankreatekomie durch Somatostatin. Chirurgie 50:427–431
20. Lambert SWJ, Van Der Lely AJ, De Herder WW et al (1996) Octreotide. N Engl J Med 334:246–254
21. Yeo CJ, Cameron JL, Maher MM et al (1995) A prospective randomized trial of pancreaticogastrostomy versus pancreaticojejunostomy after pancreaticoduodenectomy. Ann Surg 222:580–588

Chapter 32

Complications After Pancreatic Surgery

F. Francesco di Mola, Giuseppe Mascetta, Antonio De Bonis,
Pierluigi di Sebastiano

Introduction

Pancreatic cancer is the fourth-leading cause of death from malignant disease; each year about 33,000 individuals in the United States are diagnosed with this condition and more than 60,000 in Europe [1]. It is a devastating disease with a very poor prognosis and has a death rate roughly equal to its incidence rate. Contributing to the high death rate is the often late diagnosis at a stage when the tumor has already metastasized, the possibility of a curative resection is greatly reduced, and responsiveness to conventional oncological treatment options is poor. Although chemotherapy has improved prognosis in many malignancies, its impact on pancreatic cancer is limited. The same is true for intraoperative or external radiotherapy, antihormonal treatment, and immunotherapy. Due to the lack of effective adjuvant treatment protocols, median survival time following diagnosis of nonresectable tumors is only about 4–6 months. For cancers without distant metastases, resectability rates have increased steadily during the past several decades, due in part to improved diagnostic techniques and lower postoperative mortality and morbidity at centers experienced in pancreatic surgery and having a high case load (>40 procedures/year]. However, long-term survival after resection continues to be low. Recent studies indicate that the 5-year survival rate following resection for pancreatic cancer is only around 10%, with a range between 0.4 and 33% [2]. Despite this, the fact remains that pancreatic resection represents the only chance for cure, and often also the best chance for palliation. It has been possible in recent years to substantially reduce mortality and morbidity following pancreatic resection by improving surgical skill and perioperative care. Many specialized centers have reported mortality rates after Whipple resection around or even below 5%. However, the postoperative complication rate after pancreatic resection is still between 30 and 40%.

Morbidity results from surgical and nonsurgical postoperative complications, which can be subdivided into early and late events in the postoperative course. The so-called nonsurgical complications include mainly cardiopulmonary disturbances, renal failure, and metabolic disorders, such as pancreatic exocrine and endocrine insufficiency. These postoperative complications are common

W. Siquini (Ed.), *Surgical Treatment of Pancreatic Diseases.*
©Springer-Verlag Italia 2009

sequelae of major operations and have had an impact on mortality and morbidity since surgery in pancreatic cancer patients has improved and thus reduced the number of surgical complications. The most feared surgical complications are leakage of the pancreaticointestinal anastomosis and hemorrhage. Nevertheless, the other leading causes of postoperative morbidity, such as pancreatic fistula, intra-abdominal abscess, and delayed gastric emptying, are major factors in reducing quality of life and extending hospitalization time and therefore increase health costs [3].

Calvien and associates in cooperation with the Baltimore group have proposed that surgical complications following pancreatic surgery be classified as follows:

Grade I: Any deviation from the normal postoperative course without pharmacologic treatment or surgical, endoscopic, or radiological intervention. Allowed therapeutic regimens are: drugs as antiemetics, antipyretics, analgesics, diuretics, electrolytes, and physiotherapy. This grade also includes wound infections opened at bedside.

Grade II: Any deviation requiring pharmacologic treatment with drugs other than those allowed for grade I complications. Blood transfusion and total parenteral nutrition are also included.

Grade III: Any deviation requiring surgical, endoscopic, or radiologic intervention; IIIa (intervention not under general anesthesia); IIIb (intervention under general anesthesia). *Grade IV:* Life-threatening complication (including central nervous system complications) requiring intensive care management; IVa (single-organ dysfunction including dialysis); IVb (multiorgan dysfunction).

Grade V: Death of the patient.

Suffix "d": If a patient is suffering from a complication at the time of discharge, the suffix "d" (for disability) is added to the respective grade of complication (including resection of the pancreatic remnant). This suffix indicates the need for follow-up to fully eliminate the complication [4].

This chapter reviews the major surgical postoperative complications, discusses their prevention and treatment, and finally evaluates whether the chosen surgical technique influences the frequency and severity of complications following pancreatic resection.

Intraoperative Accidents

Various events may occur performing pancreatic surgery. Some are related to general surgical risk (e.g., previous surgery, adhesions), while others are associated with the pancreatic surgery itself. One major point of concern during pancreatic surgery is the dissection of the pancreatic neck from its vascular axis (portal vein) due to inflammatory or neoplastic adhesions. Moreover, it is important to remember that venous compression of the portal vein by the pancreatic tumor can generate portal hypertension that increases the risk of intraoperative bleeding and endangers the resection itself [5].

Vascular accidents can be classified as arterial or venous. In 10–15% of patients the hepatic artery arises from the superior mesenteric artery (SMA) and is in direct contact with the retroportal lamina. This malformation can be recognized during hepatic ligament dissection when preparing the posterolateral side of the common bile duct. If the surgeon resects this artery to achieve an R0 (curative) resection, he or she has to reconstruct the vessel by making a direct anastomosis with the gastroduodenal artery stump or by patching it with the great saphenous vein. An even rarer event is the presence of a common hepatic artery arising from the SMA, which during dissection may be mistaken for the gastroduodenal artery. To prevent this we apply a bulldog clamp before ligating the gastroduodenal artery to verify the presence of flow in the hepatic artery. In the case of celiac axis stenosis the only blood supply to the liver is backflow from the gastroduodenal artery and its resection can generate hepatic ischemia. In such a case it might also be useful to clamp the vessels with a bulldog before ligation. In the case of celiac trunk stenosis the trunk should be carefully dissected to identify the arcuate ligament, which in the majority of the cases causes the stenosis [5].

More common are venous accidents. As already described, neoplastic or inflammatory infiltration of the portal vein or superior mesenteric vein is frequent, and the difficulty involved in dissecting the posterior face of the pancreas from these structures is proportional to the extent of infiltration. In some cases bleeding from the portal/mesenteric vein can be significant and pose a serious risk for the patient. In our experience small defects can be treated with a hemostatic matrix (such as FloSeal) applied directly to the lesion. Major defects can be sutured with monofilament 5-6/0. The anterior approach with direct resection of the pancreas can be used for anterior wall venous invasion or adhesion until the front wall of the vein is reached. Suspension stitches placed on the resection margins make it possible to control any bleeding from marginal pancreatic vessels and facilitate dissection of the pancreas from the anterior portal vein wall. In the case of infiltration of the lateral/posterior wall of the portal vein a vein resection can be considered to obtain an R0 resection. The portal vein can be partially resected using a vascular clamp or completely resected. In this case vessel continuity is restored with a direct end-to-end anastomosis or with a prosthesis (e.g., Teflon, polytetrafluoroethylene) [6]. In some cases, the portal vein stumps can be physiologically elongated by closing the splenic vein; this is possible without a splenectomy, but may require direct anastomosis [6].

Postoperative Complications

Postoperative complications can be classified as early or late events.

Pancreatic Fistulas and Leakage of the Pancreaticointestinal Anastomosis

For a discussion of these complications please see Chapter 30.

Intra-abdominal Abscess

Intra-abdominal abscesses are mostly the consequence of pancreatic fistulas and/or leakage of the pancreaticointestinal or biliary anastomosis and are seen in 10% of patients after pancreaticoduodenectomy. They are often associated with increased morbidity due to the development of sepsis. In an abdominal CT image care should be taken to not confuse intra-abdominal fluid collection, which is a common condition in the early postoperative course after pancreaticoduodenectomy, and the serious finding of an abscess. The former is generally insignificant and will resolve spontaneously. Rarely, abscesses can also occur due to insufficiency of the hepaticojejunostomy, gastrojejunostomy, or jejunojejunostomy [7]. These abscesses are localized mainly in the right subhepatic region or under the left diaphragm. The treatment of choice is drainage via a percutaneous catheter that is introduced under ultrasonographic or CT guidance. In addition, appropriate intravenous antibiotics should be administered. Most patients can be successfully treated by these means if the underlying cause (fistula leakage) is also controlled [7]. If there is no improvement in the patient's clinical condition, surgical reintervention should be launched with extensive lavage and placement of drains. If there is any sign of anastomosis leakage as the underlying problem, a "completion pancreatectomy" or sufficient drainage of the leakage is the therapy of choice [7].

Postpancreatectomy Hemorrhage

After leakage of the pancreaticointestinal anastomosis, the second most feared complication after pancreaticoduodenectomy is postpancreatectomy hemorrhage (PPH) [8]. The literature reports hemorrhage in 5–16% of postpancreatectomy patients [9]. In cases of pancreaticointestinal anastomosis leakage, the occurrence of postoperative hemorrhage is associated with a mortality rate between 15 and 58% [9]. Blanc and associates defined hemorrhage as postoperative bleeding from the surgical site with a drop in hemoglobin concentration of ≥ 3 g/dl in 24 h, evidence of bleeding ≥ 200 ml through either the surgical drain or the nasogastric tube, a blood transfusion requirement of ≥ 2 units of packed red blood cells during resuscitation, or evidence of peripheral circulatory impairment. Sentinel bleeding was defined as any kind of minor hemorrhage that required no intervention and often preceded major hemorrhage [10].

PPH can be subdivided into two groups of different origin: intra-abdominal bleeding (mostly from the retroperitoneal operation field) and gastrointestinal bleeding (intraluminal). Furthermore, early postoperative bleeding within the first 24 h is distinguished from late bleeding, which occurs in the 2nd or 3rd postoperative week. Bleeding occurring within the first 24 h postoperatively is mostly caused by insufficient intraoperative hemostasis, as can happen after any major abdominal operation. By monitoring the output of the drains, hemoglobin levels, and the patient's vital signs, postoperative bleeding can be recognized early [11]. If the first sign is bloody output of the nasogastric tube and/or melena, a careful gastroscopy is the first diagnostic procedure to be performed. Suture line bleeding is often easily recognized in this way. If endoscopic intervention fails and stabilization is not achieved by administering blood and fresh frozen plasma, reoperation is the therapy of choice. "Stress" ulcers are always feared but rarely seen following pancreaticoduodenectomy.

A major cause of early postoperative bleeding is diffuse hemorrhage from the retroperitoneal operation field. Blanc and associates found the most frequent source of bleeding in the retroportal pancreatic lamina [10]. A recent study found no difference between jaundiced and nonjaundiced patients in the incidence of diffuse operative field bleeding [11]. Therefore, coagulation disturbances, which are frequently seen in jaundiced patients, seem not to be the reason for early diffuse bleeding. The higher incidence of gastrointestinal bleeding in jaundiced patients is the subject of contradictory findings. Some groups have shown that high serum bilirubin levels correlate with a higher frequency of bleeding complications following pancreatic surgery. Other studies did not find such a correlation. A multicenter trial concerning this topic (DROP trial) is currently under way [12].

Patients should be closely monitored for hemorrhage in the later postoperative course. Anastomotic suture bleeding or marginal ulcers can be the reasons for late postoperative bleeding. However, gastrointestinal hemorrhage often masks erosive bleeding from retroperitoneal vessels ("sentinel bleeding"), which is caused by leakage of the pancreatic anastomosis. If gastroscopy does not demonstrate a clear source of gastrointestinal (intraluminal) bleeding, the integrity of the pancreatic anastomosis must be carefully evaluated. If there is any suspicion of leakage of the anastomosis, or if there is already a known fistula, reoperation is imperative. Tien et al. [13] reported outcomes in 402 patients undergoing pancreaticoduodenectomy. Using univariate logistic regression analysis they concluded that signs of clinical infection and bile in the drainage fluid were associated with the development of massive hemorrhage. Moreover, Choi et al. [14] noted delayed hemorrhage more frequently in patients with abdominal complications including pancreatic fistula, biliary fistula, and intra-abdominal abscess. The direct cause is thought to be erosion of the vasculature in the area adjacent to the surgical anastomosis required after pancreaticoduodenectomy. This results in formation of pseudoaneurysms or arterial bleeding. Indeed, pseudoaneurysms account for 30 to 43% of delayed hemorrhages in the three most recent reports. The hemorrhage site is the gastroduodenal artery, the hepatic artery, or the splenic artery [9].

Angiography is presumed to be the most sensitive and most specific diagnostic test for pseudoaneurysm and late postoperative bleeding. However, de Castro and associates [9] found that angiography was successful in diagnosing the source of hemorrhage in only eight of the 17 patients in whom it was employed. In that study, CT was more accurate in detecting cases of pseudoaneurysm, identifying it as the source of bleeding in nine of 11 patients. One reason why angiography may not be accurate is that a clot in the pseudoaneurysm can obscure visualization even while the patient is actively bleeding.

Management of delayed intra-abdominal hemorrhage can include operative intervention or, as more recently reported, treatment with imaging-guided techniques including transarterial embolization or the insertion of covered stents to occlude the orifice of the bleeding vessel. Which treatment is employed depends on the hemodynamic stability of the patient, the imaging findings, and the potential cause of the bleeding. In the case of delayed intra-abdominal hemorrhage, exploration is warranted in the unstable patient. The results of transcatheter treatment are encouraging but not always successful. The report by Blanc et al. [10] combined with other recent reports provides fair (level II) evidence to support the following treatment recommendations for patients developing postoperative intra-abdominal hemorrhage after pancreaticoduodenectomy:

1. Patients with hemorrhage in the first 3 postoperative days should undergo urgent re-exploration to achieve hemostasis.
2. Patients with delayed hemorrhage who cannot be stabilized with resuscitation require urgent surgery for hemostasis.
3. Patients with delayed intra-abdominal hemorrhage following pancreaticoduodenectomy, who are either stable or resuscitated to a stable state, should undergo CT angiography to potentially identify a pseudoaneurysm.
4. Stabilized patients with delayed hemorrhage secondary to pancreaticoduodenectomy and pseudoaneurysm detected by CT angiography should undergo arteriography and imaging-based treatment with either transarterial embolization or covered stents. Treatment failure should be followed by prompt exploration unless the bleeding subsides with conservative management [9].

In conclusion, the best way to prevent postoperative hemorrhage is through good surgical practice and careful hemostasis. Skillful management of the pancreatic stump is of special importance in order to prevent pancreatic anastomosis leakage and the consequent danger of erosive bleeding.

The consensus definition of postpancreatectomy hemorrhage developed by the International Study Group of Pancreatic Surgery (ISGPS), which was founded in the spring of 2006, is as follows:

Time of onset: Early hemorrhage (≤24 h after completion of the index operation), late hemorrhage (>24 h after completion of the index operation).

Location: Intraluminal (intraenteric, e.g., anastomosis suture line at stomach or duodenum, or pancreatic surface at anastomosis, stress ulcer, pseudoaneurysm), extraluminal (extraenteric, bleeding into the abdominal cavity, e.g., from arterial or venous vessels, diffuse bleeding from resection area, anastomosis suture lines, pseudoaneurysm).

Severity of hemorrhage:
- *Mild:* Small- or medium-volume blood loss (from drains, nasogastric tube, or on ultrasonography; drop in hemoglobin concentration by <3 g/dl) – mild clinical impairment of the patient, no therapeutic intervention, or at most the need for noninvasive treatment with volume resuscitation or blood transfusions (2–3 units packed cells within 24 h of termination of the operation or 1–3 units if later than 24 h after the operation) – no need for reoperation or interventional angiographic embolization; endoscopic treatment of anastomotic bleeding may occur provided the other conditions apply.
- *Severe:* Large-volume blood loss (hemoglobin level drops by ≥3 g/dl) – clinically significant impairment (e.g., tachycardia, hypotension, oliguria, hypovolemic shock), need for blood transfusion (>3 units packed cells) – need for invasive treatment (interventional angiographic embolization, or relaparotomy).

To summarize the various factors influencing PPH and establish a clinical grading system, three PPH grades (grades A, B, and C) are defined according to the time of onset, location, and severity of the hemorrhage taking into consideration the cumulative overall risk and clinical severity of the hemorrhage. *Grade A PPH* results in only a temporary and marginal variation of the standard postoperative course of the patient after pancreatectomy. In general, PPH Grade A has no major clinical impact, and its occurrence should not be associated with a major delay in the patient's hospital discharge. *Grade B PPH* requires adjustment of a given clinical pathway, including further diagnostics and intervention; this PPH grade will call for therapeutic intervention such as transfusion, re-admission to an intermediate or intensive care unit, and potential invasive therapeutic interventions, such as relaparotomy or embolization. Most likely, the occurrence of grade B PPH will prolong the patient's hospital stay. *Grade C PPH* will entail severe impairment of the patient and should always be considered potentially life-threatening. Immediate diagnostic and therapeutic steps are mandatory. The hospital stay of this group of patients is always prolonged and sometimes involves a longer stay in the intensive care unit [8].

Delayed Gastric Emptying

Delayed gastric emptying is the leading cause of postoperative morbidity after pancreaticoduodenectomy [15]. Although it is not associated with higher mortality, its occurrence results in longer hospitalization, reduced quality of life, and increasing health costs. It occurs in about one-third of patients following pancreaticoduodenectomy (a range of 25–70% is described in the literature) [16]. The wide range of incidence of delayed gastric emptying in several studies is probably based on various definitions of this complication. We define delayed gastric emptying as persistent secretion via the gastric tube of more than 500 ml/day over more than 5 days after surgery, or recurrent vomiting in combination with swelling of the gastrojejunostomy/duodenojejunostomy and dilatation of the stomach in the contrast medium passage [16].

The incidence of delayed gastric emptying does not seem to increase with preservation of the pylorus, as initially thought. The most important risk factors for delayed gastric emptying are the presence of intra-abdominal complications and the radicality of the resection (lymph node dissection) [17, 18]. Horstmann et al. [19] demonstrated that the incidence of delayed gastric emptying increases from 1% in patients without complications to 28% in patients with moderate complications (wound infection, pulmonitis) and 43% in patients with fistula or leak of the anastomosis; these results were confirmed by others [20–22]. Cameron et al. [23] demonstrated that after extended retroperitoneal lymphadenectomy, delayed gastric emptying is significantly increased (16% vs. 4%, $p = 0.03$). This observation supports the general idea that delayed gastric emptying is caused by gastric atony resulting from disruption of the gastroduodenal neural network. Another hypothesis postulates that the circulating levels of motilin, a hormone that stimulates gastric motility and is mainly produced in the duodenum and the proximal jejunum, are significantly reduced by resection of the duodenum [24]. Based on this hypothesis, a prospective, randomized, placebo-controlled study that administered the motilin agonist erythromycin found a tendency (not significant) toward reduced postoperative delayed gastric emptying (19% vs. 30% in the verum group) [25]. Other treatment options are prokinetic agents, such as metoclopramide and/or cisapride. However, none of them has been tested in randomized controlled trials, and therefore their efficacy in treating delayed gastric emptying is not proven.

It should be noted that erythromycin is not allowed to be administered in combination with cisapride in the treatment of delayed gastric emptying. Furthermore, decompression of the stomach via the nasogastric tube and nutritional support via the parenteral or enteral route should be performed. In most cases, delayed gastric emptying resolves with these measures within 2–4 weeks. It is most important not to lose patience and to reassure the patient that it is only a matter of time until the stomach adapts to the new situation.

A consensus classification was developed by the International Study Group of Pancreatic Surgery (ISGPS). It identifies mild, moderate, and severe forms of delayed gastric emptying after pancreatic resection in grades A, B, and C on the basis of their clinical impact:

- *Grade A* delayed gastric emptying (DGE) should be considered if a nasogastric tube is required between postoperative days (POD) 4 and 7, or if reinsertion of a nasogastric tube was necessary owing to nausea and vomiting after removal by PODent is unable to tolerate a solid diet on POD 7, but resumes a solid diet before POD 14.
- *Grade B* DGE is present if the nasogastric tube is required from POD cannot tolerate unlimited oral intake by POD 14, but is able to resume a solid oral diet before POD 21.
- *Grade C* DGE is present when nasogastric intubation cannot be discontinued or has to be reinstated after POD 14, or if the patient is unable to maintain unlimited oral intake by POD 21.

In grade A DGE, vomiting is uncommon, whereas in grades B and C, there is usually vomiting, perhaps indicating that a trial should be considered of pro-kinetic drugs (such as metoclopramide or erythromycin), as used in idiopathic or diabetic gastroparesis. In grade A DGE, nutritional support (enteral or parenter-al) may or may not be required in the first 14 postoperative days. By contrast, nutritional support is required in grade B DGE in the first 3 weeks postopera-tively, whereas in grade C DGE prolonged nutritional support is required for more than 3 weeks postoperatively. In grade C DGE, the commencement of adjuvant therapy is delayed [26].

Exocrine and Endocrine Insufficiency after Pancreatic Surgery

The pancreas has a central function in digestion and control of glucose home-ostasis. In the interdigestive phase pancreatic secretion is closely coordinated with the migrating motor complex (MMC), and bursts of enzyme and bicarbon-ate secretion occur in association with MMC phase III every 80–120 min. The physiological role of interdigestive pancreatic secretion (complemented by bile secretion) is believed to be that of a housekeeper that allows the small bowel to be cleaned of bacterial overgrowth and other detrimental collections within the luminal site. Obviously, both the digestive and interdigestive functions of the exocrine pancreas as well as pancreatic hormone production are strongly affect-ed by major pancreatic surgery. It is unpredictable whether postoperative changes are purely procedure-related or a sequela of the preexisting disease. In most cases they are likely to be a combination of both. In patients with chronic pancreatitis the fate of exocrine and endocrine pancreatic function is usually progressive impairment. By the time surgery is required, many patients have developed mechanisms of compensation that vary from dietary habits, a shift in the site of maximal nutrient digestion from the duodenum to the more distal small intestine, to partial compensation of enzyme production from extrapancre-atic enzyme sources (such as gastric lipase) [27]. In pancreatic cancer the tumor growth in the pancreatic head gradually obstructs the main pancreatic and com-mon bile ducts. Usually there is little time for functional adaptation in this con-dition and patients deteriorate rapidly [27].

Exocrine Pancreatic Function

The main clinical effect of impaired exocrine pancreatic function is the presence of steatorrhea (fat excretion in stool in excess of 6 g/day). By association, there can also be a deficit of vitamins A, D, E, and K. Only limited data are available on the effect of pancreatic resection on exocrine function. These data come mostly from a series of patients suffering from chronic pancreatitis. Further deterioration of exocrine pancreatic function is a frequent but not obligatory consequence of pancreatic resection. The degree of pancreatic function impair-ment is related to the extent of pancreatic parenchyma resection and the functional state of the residual pancreas. An important additional factor that influences not only exocrine function but also the digestive process in its complexity is gastrectomy. Even partial gastrectomy causes impaired release of gastrin, pancreatic polypeptide, and cholecystokinin and also brings on postcibal asynchrony. This contributes to further deterioration in the digestive process, with maldigestion as the clinical result.

The influence of different types of surgery on the course of exocrine pancreatic function has been studied in only a few comparative investigations. In patients who underwent pylorus-preserving pancreaticoduodenectomy, various types of pancreaticoenterostomy (either pancreaticogastrostomy or pancreaticojejunostomy) were compared. A significant deterioration of pancreatic exocrine function occurred in patients who underwent pancreaticogastrostomy. Early deactivation of pancreatic enzymes by gastric acid is the suggested cause of this phenomenon. This problem can be overcome by administering a proton pump inhibitor (PPI). We would argue that the main determinant of the postoperative course of pancreatic function in chronic pancreatitis is, in addition to the extent of resection, either the inflammatory activity or the fibrotic tissue replacement within the remaining portion of the pancreas. For practical reasons pancreatic enzyme supplementation starts with 40–120,000 IU of lipase in minimicrospheres. If enzyme administration is not sufficient to compensate the exocrine insufficiency, additional diagnostic procedures and additional treatment directed at other forms of malabsorption are mandatory. In clinical routine the administration of pancreatic enzymes is recommended in all cases following resectional pancreas surgery. In pylorus- and duodenum-preserving procedures additional PPIs are mandatory to prevent early inactivation of orally given pancreatic enzymes by gastric acid. The most important reason for the inadequacy of acid neutralization is impaired bicarbonate production, but increased acid secretion has also been reported [21, 27, 28].

Endocrine Pancreatic Function

The incidence of postoperative diabetes mellitus after Whipple's resection ranges from 20 to 50%. The most significant challenge in these patients is posed by recurrent attacks of hypoglycemia. Postoperative insulin sensitivity increases because of the simultaneous decrease in glucagon secretion. Hypoglycemia due to glucagon deficiency causes a substantial number of deaths and brain damage. In particular in patients with alcoholic chronic pancreatitis and insulin-dependent diabetes mellitus it is hypoglycemic complications that put the main limitations on life expectancy. Comparing pylorus- and duodenum-preserving pancreatic head resection (DPPHR), the pylorus-preserving procedure shows a more pronounced impairment of endocrine function than does the duodenum-preserving procedure. Possible explanations are a smaller amount of resected pancreatic parenchyma and maintenance of the enteroinsulin axis by preserving the duodenum [28].

Peptic Ulcer

Peptic ulcers occur in around 5% of patients after pancreatic surgery. Limited resection of the gastric oxyntic compartment together with a decrease in pancreatic bicarbonate secretion and consequent inadequate acid buffering is the most plausible explanation. Mixing of bicarbonate secreted into the ascending loop with the chyme is impaired, which favors ulcer formation. A higher prevalence of peptic ulcer after Whipple's procedure is reported than after left pancreatic resection. Ongoing PPI therapy, which is also required to prevent acidic inactivation of orally given pancreatic enzyme preparations, is the treatment of choice. In patients with *Helicobacter pylori* infection of the gastric mucosa, *H. pylori* eradication therapy should be carried out first [29].

Ascending Cholangitis

After extensive pancreatic head resections an anastomosis is made between the extrahepatic bile duct and a small intestinal loop. This condition favors recurrent acute or chronic cholangitis in a subset of patients. In patients with an anastomotic stricture, transhepatic intervention or surgical reintervention becomes mandatory. In patients with bacterial overgrowth of the excluded loop connected to the biliary system, intermittent antibiotic therapy is often very helpful and may completely control the relapsing episodes of cholangitis. We have good experience of adding prokinetics in the form of interval therapy [30].

Wound Infection

Patients who have undergone preoperative biliary stenting are at major risk of wound infection after surgery [31].

Classical vs. Pylorus-Preserving Whipple or Standard vs. Radical Resection in Pancreatic Cancer: Influence on Postoperative Complications

Two resection procedures are mainly used today in pancreatic cancer surgery, the classical Whipple resection and the pylorus-preserving Whipple resection. The classical Whipple resection was introduced by Kausch in 1909 and reintroduced by Whipple in 1935. It was for a long time the standard surgical therapy for malignant processes in the pancreatic head region [31]. With the intention of reducing postoperative morbidity without compromising adequate radicality, various modifications of the original Whipple procedure have been proposed. The most important was the introduction of the pylorus-preserving Whipple resection by Traverso and Longmire, which was first performed by Watson in 1945 [32]. By preserving the stomach, the pylorus, and the first part of the duodenum, the pylorus-preserving Whipple resection protects against gastric dumping, marginal ulceration, and bile-reflux gastritis [21]. Whether this operation is sufficiently radical to treat pancreatic cancer is still debated. However, several retrospective studies were not able to show any difference in postoperative survival between the classical and the pylorus-preserving Whipple in pancreatic cancer patients [21]. With regard to postoperative mortality and morbidity, the pylorus-preserving Whipple resection shows similar or even better results. In addition, quality of life appears to be better following the pylorus-preserving Whipple resection than after the classical Whipple resection. As the pylorus-preserving Whipple resection includes a significant reduction in operating time, intraoperative blood loss, and the consequent need for blood substitution, it should become the procedure of choice in treating pancreatic head cancer if oncological radicality is not compromised [16]. Regarding the surgical technique, the antecolic gastro/duodenojejunal anastomosis seems to be associated with a low incidence of complications [16, 33].

In 1973, Fortner performed a so-called "regional pancreatectomy" by resecting the entire pancreas with en-bloc removal of the surrounding soft tissue and the regional lymph nodes. The idea of extended radicality was mainly supported and further developed by several Japanese groups in the past decade. By providing an extended retroperitoneal lymphadenectomy they reported improvement of the 5-year survival rate to up to 40% in retrospective and non-randomized studies [17, 34]. Two recently published prospective randomized trials in Europe and the United States reported no significant survival benefit for extended resection procedures. There seems to be a distinct trend toward longer survival, but longer follow-up is needed for a definitive conclusion. In this context it remains to be discussed whether more radical and extended operations are the cause of higher perioperative mortality and morbidity. Does the additional retroperitoneal lymphadenectomy cause more postoperative complications? There are reports of disabling watery diarrhea as a new common postoperative complication after extended resection for pancreatic cancer. The two randomized trials demonstrated no difference in mortality and morbidity between standard and extended resection [17, 23]. The presently available data provide evidence that a pancreaticoduodenectomy with extended retroperitoneal lymphadenectomy can be performed safely in specialized centers, without additional risk for postoperative complications [17]. Whether radical resection provides a survival benefit for patients in comparison to standard resection must be investigated in future randomized studies. With regard to vascular resection it is clear that venous resection must be performed only with the intent to complete an R0 resection [35].

References

1. Jemal A, Siegel R, Ward E (2007) Cancer statistics, 2007. CA Cancer J Clin 57:43–66
2. Birkmeyer JD, Sun Y, Wong SL, Stukel TA (2007) Hospital volume and late survival after cancer surgery. Ann Surg. 245:777–783
3. Ujiki MB, Talamonti MS (2007) Guidelines for the surgical management of pancreatic adenocarcinoma. Semin Oncol 34:311–320
4. DeOliveira ML, Winter JM, Schafer M et al (2006) Assessment of complications after pancreatic surgery: a novel grading system applied to 633 patients undergoing pancreaticoduodenectomy. Ann Surg 244:931–937
5. Kurosaki I, Hatakeyama K, Nihei KE, Oyamatsu M (2004) Celiac axis stenosis in pancreaticoduodenectomy. J Hepatobiliary Pancreat Surg 11:119–124
6. Sakorafas GH, Friess H, Balsiger BM et al (2001) Problems of reconstruction during pancreatoduodenectomy. Dig Surg 18:363–369
7. Berberat PO, Friess H, Kleeff J et al (1999) Prevention and treatment of complications in pancreatic cancer surgery. Dig Surg 16:327–336
8. Wente M, Veit J, Bassi C et al (2007) Postpancreatectomy hemorrhage (PPH) – an International Study Group of Pancreatic Surgery (ISGPS) definition. Surgery 142:20–25
9. de Castro SM, Busch OR, Gouma DJ (2004) Management of bleeding and leakage after pancreatic surgery. Best Pract Res Clin Gastroenterol 18:847–864
10. Blanc T, Cortes A, Goere D et al (2007) Hemorrhage after pancreaticoduodenectomy: when is surgery still indicated? Am J Surg 194:3–9
11. Yekebas EF, Wolfram L, Cataldegirmen G et al (2007) Postpancreatectomy hemorrhage: diagnosis and treatment: an analysis in 1669 consecutive pancreatic resections. Ann Surg 246:269–280
12. van der Gaag NA, de Castro SM, Rauws EA et al (2007) Preoperative biliary drainage for periampullary tumors causing obstructive jaundice DRainage vs. (direct) OPeration (DROP trial). BMC Surg 7:3
13. Tien YW, Lee PH, Yang CY et al (2005) Risk factors of massive bleeding related to pancreatic leak after pancreaticoduodenectomy. J Am Coll Surg 201:554–559
14. Choi SH, Moon HJ, Heo JS et al (2004) Delayed hemorrhage after pancreaticoduodenectomy. J Am Coll Surg 199:186–189
15. Paraskevas KI, Avgerinos C, Manes C et al (2006) Delayed gastric emptying is associated with pylorus-preserving but not classical Whipple pancreaticoduodenectomy: a review of the literature and critical reappraisal of the implicated pathomechanism. World J Gastroenterol 12:5951–5958
16. Muller MW, Friess H, Beger HG et al (1997) Gastric emptying following pylorus-preserving Whipple and duodenum-preserving pancreatic head resection in patients with chronic pancreatitis. Am J Surg 173:257–263
17. Pedrazzoli S, DiCarlo V, Dionigi R et al (1998) Standard versus extended lymphadenectomy associated with pancreato-duodenectomy in the surgical treatment of adenocarcinoma of the head of the pancreas: a multicenter, prospective, randomized study. Lymphadenectomy Study Group. Ann Surg 228:508–517
18. Seiler CA, Wagner M, Bachmann T et al (2005) Randomized clinical trial of pylorus-preserving duodenopancreatectomy versus classical Whipple resection – long term results. Br J Surg 92:547–556
19. Horstmann O, Markus PM, Ghadimi MB, Becker H (2004) Pylorus preservation has no impact on delayed gastric emptying after pancreatic head resection. Pancreas 28:69–74
20. Jimenez RE, Fernandez-del Castillo C, Rattner DW et al (2000) Outcome of pancreaticoduodenectomy with pylorus preservation or with antrectomy in the treatment of chronic pancreatitis. Ann Surg 231:293–300

21. Beger HG, Buchler M (1990) Duodenum-preserving resection of the head of the pancreas in chronic pancreatitis with inflammatory mass in the head. World J Surg 14:83–87
22. Schmidt U, Simunec D, Piso P et al (2005) Quality of life and functional long-term outcome after partial pancreatoduodenectomy: pancreatogastrostomy versus pancreatojejunostomy. Ann Surg Oncol 12:467–472
23. Yeo CJ, Cameron JL, Sohn TA et al (1999) Pancreaticoduodenectomy with or without extended retroperitoneal lymphadenectomy for periampullary adenocarcinoma: comparison of morbidity and mortality and short-term outcome. Ann Surg 229:613–622
24. Strommer L, Raty S, Hennig R et al (2005) Delayed gastric emptying and intestinal hormones following pancreatoduodenectomy. Pancreatology 5:537–544
25. Yeo CJ, Barry MK, Sauter PK et al (1993) Erythromycin accelerates gastric emptying after pancreaticoduodenectomy. A prospective randomized, placebo-controlled trial. Ann Surg 218:229–237
26. Wente MN, Bassi C, Dervenis C et al (2007) Delayed gastric emptying (DGE) after pancreatic surgery: a suggested definition by the International Study Group of Pancreatic Surgery (ISGPS). Surgery 142:761–768
27. Kahl S, Malfertheiner P (2004) Exocrine and endocrine pancreatic insufficiency after pancreatic surgery. Best Pract Res Clin Gastroenterol 18:947–955
28. Gouma DJ, van Geenen RC, van Gulik TM et al (2000) Rates of complications and death after pancreaticoduodenectomy: risk factors and the impact of hospital volume. Ann Surg 232:786–795
29. Grace PA, Pitt HA, Longmire WP (1990) Pylorus preserving pancreatoduodenectomy: an overview. Br J Surg 77:968–974
30. Gutknecht DR (2001) Cholangitis and pneumobilia after a Whipple procedure. Am J Emerg Med 19:87–88
31. Whipple AO, Pearson WB, Mullins CR (1935) Treatment of carcinoma of the ampulla of Vater. Ann Surg 102:763–769
32. Traverso LW, Longmire WP Jr (1978) Preservation of the pylorus in pancreaticoduodenectomy. Surg Gynecol Obstet 146:959–962
33. Lemaire E, O'Toole D, Sauvanet A et al (2000) Functional and morphological changes in the pancreatic remnant following pancreaticoduodenectomy with pancreaticogastric anastomosis. Br J Surg 87:434–438
34. Fortner JG (1973) Regional resection and pancreatic carcinoma. Surgery 73:799–800
35. Mann O, Strate T, Schneider C et al (2006) Surgery for advanced and metastatic pancreatic cancer – current state and perspectives. Anticancer Res 26(1B):681–686

Chapter 33

Pancreas Transplantation

Andrea Risaliti, Nicola Cautero, Fabrizio di Francesco, Stefano De Luca

Introduction

Pancreas transplantation, developed to provide a self-regulated endogenous source of responsive insulin to the usual feedback systems, is the only therapy able to establish euglycemic status and standardization of glycosylated hemoglobin in diabetic patients [1, 2]. Despite exogenous insulin support, metabolic control is usually incomplete in diabetic patients, and in the long run diabetes causes many complications, such as retinopathy, sensitive and motorial neuropathy, vascular disease and, in 20–30% of cases, nephropathy.

The main predictive event, from the renal standpoint, and an early indicator of increased risk of cardiovascular morbidity and mortality, is microalbuminuria (>30 mg/dl). Without a specific therapy, within 10–15 years 80% of persons with type 1 diabetes with microalbuminuria will develop clear nephropathy with related arterial hypertension. About 30% of diabetic patients with end-stage renal failure who underwent kidney transplantation show a low incidence of coronary heart disease, whereas the increase of cardiovascular morbidity in patients on dialysis translates into a yearly increase in mortality risk of about 10%.

Although appropriate insulin and antihypertensive therapy can reduce both the albuminuria and the average of progression of the renal pathology, currently, although very invasive, pancreas transplantation, with or without concomitant kidney transplantation (in cases of chronic renal failure), is the only available option to obtain long-term independence from insulin [3, 4].

Indications

Currently, combined kidney and pancreas transplantation – whether the pancreas is transplanted at the same time as the kidney or immediately after – is considered the best available option for patients with type 1 diabetes mellitus and chronic renal failure. The reasons for this are:
- Standardization of the excellent results obtained from pancreatic transplantation

W. Siquini (Ed.), *Surgical Treatment of Pancreatic Diseases.*
©Springer-Verlag Italia 2009

- A functioning pancreas makes the patient euglycemic and insulin-free, preventing or stabilizing complications due to diabetes mellitus
- If the patient already has a transplanted kidney, and is already on immunosuppressant therapy, additional pancreas transplantation does not increase the oncologic, infectious, and immunologic risks of surgery. Furthermore, thanks to the effective protection given by the pancreas to the new kidney and to the other target organs, a significant improvement in the long-term outcome is possible

There are many options available for transplant surgery. The pancreas transplantation can be performed simultaneously with the cadaveric kidney transplantation (simultaneous pancreas–kidney or SPK), or simultaneously with a living donor kidney transplantation (SPLK); it can be sequential, after a previously performed kidney transplant (pancreas after kidney, PAK); or it can be transplanted as an isolated organ (pancreas transplantation alone, PTA).

An interesting option which particularly addresses the specific case of diabetic patients is simultaneous transplantation of the pancreatic body/tail segment and the kidney, both coming from a single living donor. SPK and PTA transplants are traditionally the most common options to treat uremic patients suffering from type 1 diabetes mellitus and in some selected type 2 cases. Since the kidney has a sentinel function in relation to pancreatic rejection (90% of rejections in SPK also involve the kidney, while only 10% are related to just the pancreas) [5], SPK is the most used of these techniques because it consists of a single operation and offers immunologic benefit to the recipient.

Indications for SPK Transplantation

SPK is considered the gold standard for those patients who suffer from type 1 diabetes mellitus and clear nephropathy, i.e., patients who are about to start dialysis treatment or who are already undergoing dialysis, patients with a creatinine clearance of <30 ml/min and/or severe nephritic syndrome, and patients in dialysis following functional exhaustion of a previous kidney transplant. Timing is the basic element for a good outcome of a SPK transplant, and current available data indicate a consistent benefit if the transplantation is performed before dialysis is started. The goal of this choice is to obtain the maximum benefit from the transplant, achieve survival for the patient and the graft, a better cost-benefit ratio, and more rapid postoperative rehabilitation with lower post-transplant morbidity.

Apart from SPK transplantation, another therapeutic option, preferable for many when a living kidney donor is available, is sequential transplantation of the pancreas (from a cadaveric donor) following renal transplantation. The benefits of this option include a reduced waiting time with better outcomes for the transplanted kidney function in both the short and the long run. The only disadvantage is the need for the correct timing in order to coordinate kidney procurement from the living donor with pancreas procurement from the cadaveric donor in the shortest possible time.

Indications for PAK Transplantation

Diabetic patients with an existing functioning renal transplant and stable immunosuppressive therapy may be candidates for pancreas transplantation using the PAK method without any further immunologic risk. Poorer functional outcomes compared with those registered after a SPK transplant are related to the fact that, in combined transplants, the parameters by which renal functionality is monitored cannot be used as a tool to foresee and treat pancreatic rejection at the very beginning, because the organs come from different donors.

Indications for PTA

Indications for PTA can be found in diabetic patients who do not present rapidly evolving nephropathy and in those who have a critical failure of glucose metabolism, marked by hypoglycemic episodes which are uncontrollable by insulin therapy and which critically compromise patients' relationships and social life. It is estimated that PTA reduces the diabetic patient's risk of cardiovascular accidents, particularly when there is not optimal glycemic compensation. Evident benefits have been demonstrated on neuropathy, retinopathy, saturation of LDL, and LDL blood concentration.

A new indication for PTA concerns the presence of an initial nephropathy that can be stopped by eliminating the diabetes. Data from the literature show high mortality in diabetic patients waiting for a renal transplant with a 15–29 ml/min glomerular filtration rate. It has been calculated that this mortality can be reduced to 45 % if the transplant is performed before the patient starts dialysis.

Another piece of gradually emerging knowledge relates to the effective benefit deriving from the transplant for patients suffering from type 2 diabetes mellitus. In functional terms, these insulin-treated patients are totally comparable to type 1 diabetics and have a cardiovascular risk multiplied by long-term diabetes and nephropathy. Therefore, the transplant may be appropriate as a therapy for the type of patient who is already critically compromised by pathologic complications, but most of all as a therapeutic option which must be taken into consideration by the physician during the natural development of the diabetic disease, before the onset of irreversible organ compromise.

Recipient Selection

Most healthcare facilities offer SPK mainly to type 1 diabetics and only in 5% of cases to those with type 2 diabetes, although the results obtained in each group are completely superimposable. For recipient selection, the presence and criticality of diabetic complications, cardiovascular status, and probable nephropathy (creatinine clearance <30 ml/min and/or severe nephritic syndrome) are the main elements to be considered in the case of patients needing to be selected for a combined transplant before dialysis (preemptive renal transplant), Currently, being older than 45 and having a reduced coronary functional reserve are the major determining factors of poorer survival after SPK; for this reason, in order to achieve an accurate assessment of cardiovascular risk it is very often necessary to resort to myocardial scintigraphy and probably related coronary arteriography. In regard to PTA, creatinine clearance higher than 70 ml/min is necessary to ensure that the nephrotoxic effects of the immunosuppressant drugs do not create latent renal failure.

Just as for all other types of transplant, preoperative assessment is multidisciplinary and is carried out by a team of anesthesiologists, cardiologists, surgeons, diabetes specialists, and nephrologists. Once the feasibility of transplantation has been assessed, the goal of screening is to rule out the presence of infections and hidden neoplasms together with further risk factors such as obesity, drug addiction, untreated psychiatric illness, and lack of compliance with medical treatment.

The Ideal Pancreas Donor

The high incidence of complications associated with pancreas transplantation in the past has required such a strict selection of potential pancreas donors that the total number of registered donors reported in the literature is 80% of those needed for liver, 35% for heart, and only 24% for pancreas. Although general contraindications are the same as for other organs, there are some leading characteristics that a pancreas donor has to have in order to be considered suitable, including: age between 10 and 40 years, no obesity, and stable hemodynamic and euglycemic status. Survival rates after 1 year for patients who received a SPK transplant between 1999 and 2001 were 89% when the donor was younger than 16, 84% when the donor was between 16 and 45 years old, and 73% when the donor was aged over 45. A donor body mass index of over 30 and pancreatic parenchymal fatty infiltration correlate with an increased risk of graft loss, whereas temporary hyperglycemia and hypertransaminasemia do not influence the outcome during the stay in the intensive care unit. Pancreas assessment of donors with abdominal trauma, carried out by a procurement expert, must rule out the presence of traumatic or degenerative lesions, which do not allow the pancreas to be used, whereas parenchymal edema does not necessarily exclude it.

Due to the chronic lack of available organs, some strategies have been put into practice in order to expand the available donor pool. Among these, in some selected cases, living donor pancreas procurement allows a good donor/recipient immunologic match and an effective reduction of the waiting time. In such cases, usually a pancreas caudal-body segment is used together with the living donor's kidney, or the living donor's pancreas segment is used in a patient who has already gone through a cadaveric kidney transplantation. In relation to the first option, data collected by Gruessner show absence of mortality, a noticeable incidence of complications in the donors (glucose intolerance, splenectomies, abdominal abscesses and pseudocysts), and survival rates of 98% for pancreas and 100% for kidney after 1 year.

Pancreas Procurement Techniques

Although there are many procurement techniques, the basic principle to observe is to avoid any kind of gland manipulation and, bearing in mind that the procurement is nearly always a multiple-organ one, the best technique is to remove abdominal organs complete and then separate them on the surgical table. This makes it possible to minimize the procurement time (avoiding the limitations related to the donor's unstable hemodynamic status) and visceral manipulation and cold ischemia, reducing as far as possible the "struggle" for vascular segments between the different surgical teams.

Conventional Procurement Technique

Isolated pancreas procurement is performed after liver procurement and before kidney procurement. After performing visceral hypothermic perfusion via the aorta, cold dissection starts by carrying out a duodenal kocherization and by mobilizing the pancreatic head. The choledochus and gastroduodenal artery are ligated and the portal vein dissected within the splenomesenteric confluence. The upper mesenteric and splenic arteries, isolated up to the aorta, are left adhering to the pancreas in order to be used during the surgery. The pancreas is detached from the peritoneal lax tissue starting from the tail and the spleen is used as a traction point. Mesenteric root dissection, performed in the lower margin of the pancreas and followed by an extensive duodenal mobilization, completes graft procurement using both the spleen and the duodenum (Fig. 33.1).

When the transplantation starts, preparation of the pancreatic graft at the surgical table consists in performing a splenectomy, perfecting vascular hemostatic ligation, shortening the duodenal cap adequately, and extending the arterial peduncle (splenomesenteric) by implantation of an iliac Y graft procured directly from the donor (Fig. 33.2). This reconstruction is not necessary if the pancreas procurement maintained the arterial, splenic, and mesenteric ostium united in an aortic Carrel's patch. Usually the portal trunk is not extended by means of venous implantation in order to minimize the risk of postoperative thrombosis.

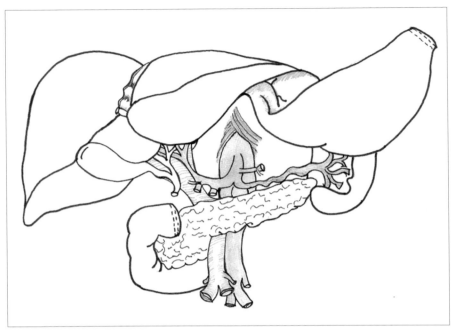

Fig. 33.1 On the *left* the visceral bloc (pancreas, duodenum, and spleen) during organ procurement is depicted. The composite graft is removed by section of the splenic artery and superior mesenteric vessels at their origin (gastroduodenal artery, biliary duct, and duodenum have already been sectioned)

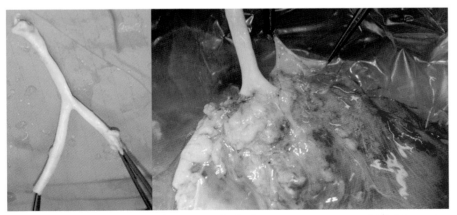

Fig. 33.2 The superior mesenteric artery and splenic artery are anastomosed (*right*) to a single inflow by interposition of an iliac artery Y graft from the same cadaveric donor (*left*)

Multiple-Organ Procurement Technique

This technique allows procurement of the visceral bloc formed by liver, pancreas, and kidneys all at once. The preliminary stages consist in visceral exploration and splanchnic refrigeration via the aorta.

The next steps consist in a wide coloepiploic detachment, opening of the lesser omentum and dissection of the pylorus and duodenum, through which it is possible to reflect the stomach cranially. Total dissection of the mesocolon, behind the viscera, allows it to be reflected caudally, creating a space for removal of the visceral bloc, which starts with iuxtavescical section of the ureters.

The operation continues with dissection of the two hemidiaphragms of the posterior chest wall, reaching the prevertebral plane so as to be able to move the multiple-organ bloc both sides, in a median direction, as far as the vertebral column. Through the dissection of the mesenteric roof, the small intestine is displaced caudally (this maneuver is not performed if there is simultaneous intestinal procurement, postponing creation of the upper mesenteric pedicle to the surgical table) and the visceral bloc formed by liver, pancreas, and kidneys is retrieved all together in one piece by detaching it from the prevertebral band. The procedure is completed with procurement of arteries and iliac veins.

At the surgical table, organ partition is carried out from the back (Fig. 33.3) by opening the aortic wall and separating the celiac tripod, the upper mesenteric

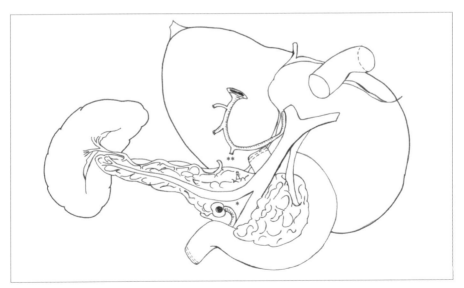

Fig. 33.3 Posterior view of a composite graft (liver and pancreas) after removal of the kidneys. The origins of the superior mesenteric artery (*) and splenic artery (**) are exposed and ready for back-table surgery

artery, and the ostium of the renal arteries. After renal vein dissection at the caval confluence, the kidneys can be separated from the hepatopancreatic bloc. Separation of the pancreas from the liver starts with detachment of the ostia of the upper mesenteric artery and the celiac tripod, isolating the common hepatic artery up to the origin of the splenic artery. Dissection of the gastroduodenal artery and portal trunk allows the final separation between pancreas and liver. As described above, pancreas surgery is carried out at the table to procure the isolated pancreas.

Pancreas Transplantation Techniques

The transplantation consists in the implantation of the entire gland and duodenal "C" used to derive exocrine secretion. The main variables relating to drainage of exocrine secretion (cystic versus enteral) and venous drainage (systemic versus portal) are addressed differently by different healthcare centers according to team experience, graft quality, and the vascular anatomy of the recipient. The most usual surgical access is via a median laparotomy from the pubis to above the navelwith intraperitoneal implantation performed into the right ilio-cavity or, as recently described, behind the right colon. Pancreatic segmental transplantation, by ductal injection of neoprene, remains a practicable option for selected patients with cysticor enteral diversion. In most cases, arterial anastomosis is performed on the recipient's iliac axis (less frequently on the aorta) with an end-to-end anastomosis with the iliac Y graft or with Carrel's aortic patch (when present).

Venous Drainage

Although the majority of pancreas transplantations have been, or are, performed by anastomosis between graft portal vein and recipient iliocaval axis (Figs. 33.4 and 33.5) – and therefore within the patient's systemic circulation – "portal" reconstruction by anastomosis on the recipient's portal axis tributary vein is considered the most physiologically appropriate. This way, the insulin discarded into the portal circulation will avoid hyperinsulinemia and will normalize C-peptide levels as well as lipoprotein composition. Furthermore, such a reconstruction allows the donor's antigens to be released into the portal system with a consequent decrease of alloreactivity towards the graft and therefore a related decrease in the overall rejection rate.

Exocrine Secretion Drainage

Cystic and enteral derivations are the most used techniques (Figs. 33.4 and 33.5). In the early experience with pancreatic transplantation, when exocrine

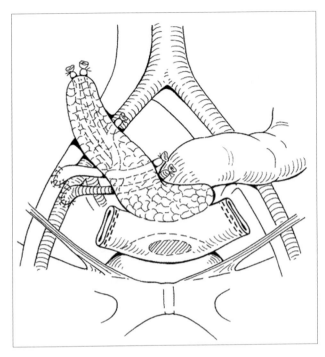

Fig. 33.4 Schematic representation of a pancreas transplantation alone (PTA) with enteric-cystic diversion. The vascular anastomoses are located on the right iliac vessel of the recipient

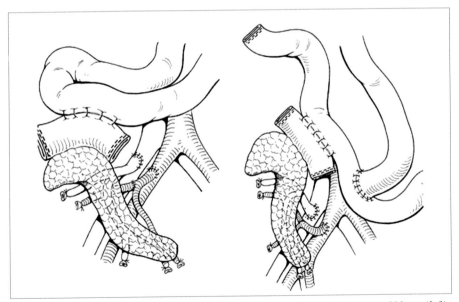

Fig. 33.5 PTA with enteric diversion with direct anastomosis or with Roux-en-Y loop (*left*). On the *right* a surgical view of vascular anastomosis performed on the recipient's vena cava and common right iliac artery

drainage was obtained through an anastomosis between the graft duodenum and the recipient's intestine, the major complication was the high incidence of infections caused by anastomotic dehiscence, often due to faulty technique. Sclerosis of the exocrine component of a pancreatic caudal–body segment, by means of intraductal injection of neoprene, represented a subsequent but temporary improvement of transplantation technique. The technique of cystic exocrine diversion was first described in 1987, and from 1995 it was used in more than 90% of the transplants in the USA. This happened because cystoduodenal anastomosis was technically easier, and safer from the point of view of infection, being made up between nonfunctional (graft duodenum) and sterile viscera (bladder). Furthermore, the possibility of maintaining cystic detention by catheterization allowed tension-free anastomotic cicatrization. From a functional standpoint, cystic diversion allowed the monitoring of graft function monitoring on the basis of urinary amylase concentration and early identification of rejection manifestations. The main disadvantages of cystic drainage reflect the method's nonphysiological function: all patients develop severe metabolic acidosis, hyponatremia, and volume depletion. In about 24–40% of cases urologic complications appear, and 0.4–1% of recipients develop reflux pancreatitis at such a level that enteral drainage conversion is required.

The cystic option feels the effect of vessel position and of cystic wall trophism and, in general, a large distance between duodenal patch and bladder calls for the making up of an enteric diversion. This represents the most physiologic reconstructive option, which has come back into favor for all three transplant categories (77% for SPK, 54% for PAK, and 54% for PTA). This technique, although liable to the effects of an initial learning curve and characterized by a certain incidence of fistula, abscesses, and peritonitis, allows greater flexibility in the vascular anastomosis even though it does not allow monitoring of pancreatic secretions for early recognition of an acute rejection. Enteric diversion can be performed through a direct anastomosis between graft duodenum and recipient ileal loop or through a Roux-en-Y anastomosis (Fig. 33.5).

Immunosuppression in Pancreas Transplantation

In addition to improvement in surgical techniques and to better selection of patients, the success of pancreas transplantation has also been due to the perfecting of immunosuppressive therapy, which has allowed the incidence of acute rejection to drop from 70–80% of cases in the early 1990s to the current 10%.

In most healthcare centers, post-transplantation immunosuppressive therapy consists of a combination of several types of drugs. In addition to basic steroid therapy, nearly all groups carry out an induction treatment using antilymphatic serums (about 70% of SPK, 80% of PAK, and 85% of PTA). The antibodies used, polyclonal (Thymoglobulin) and monoclonal (ATGAM or OKT3), can provoke lymphatic depletion. Antibodies such as daclizumab or basiliximab do not provoke this as they are better tolerated and carry reduced risks of iatrogenic morbidity. The rest of the combination involves calcineurin inhibitors (cyclosporine and tacrolimus), antimetabolites (mycophenolate mofetil), and mTOR inhibitors (sirolimus, everolimus). The decrease in the incidence of rejection, especially in patients with an enteric drainage, has immediately translated into a noticeable improvement in survival at 2 years, which is now 86% compared to 80% in absence of antibody induction. Steroid therapy is gradually reduced until it is either suspended within 3–6 months from transplant or is maintained long-term at a low rate. The most frequent immunosuppressive plan is therefore a quadruple type with induction (steroids + basiliximab) combined with a calcineurin inhibitor and mycophenolate mofetil. PTA seems to be the most liable to rejection (8% vs. 7% for PAK and 2% for SPK) [4–8].

Rejection

Immunologic alloreactivity in the recipient generally starts in the exocrine parenchymal component and, at a different time, in the B-cell population, so that a rejection diagnosis based only on hyperglycemia is late and often denotes irreversible damage of the gland. For this reason the first biochemical parameters to be monitored are acinar. From a clinical perspective, pancreatic edema can cause the pain and swelling in the transplant site. This symptom is accompanied by hyperamylasemia and hyperlipidemia and, in the case of cystic diversion, also hypoamylasuria. The differential diagnosis includes vascular complications and reflux pancreatitis. The diagnostic gold standard is a percutaneous, transcystoscopy or minilaparotomic graft biopsy. In case of post-SPK transplant rejection, the transplanted kidney becomes the best indicator as creatinemia increases and urinary flow decreases. Pharmacological treatment consists of bolus administration of steroid or the initiation of antilymphatic immunotherapy, which, if the diagnosis comes early enough, is successful in more than 90% of cases [6].

Surgical Complications

Pancreas transplantation is exposed to a high risk of complications owing to the fragility of the parenchyma, its susceptibility to ischemia–reperfusion damage, and the complex table surgery. The most dangerous complications are vascular thrombosis, graft pancreatitis, anastomotic fistulas, urologic complications, and intra-abdominal infections.

Vascular thrombosis appears within 24–48 hours from transplantation and frequently involves venous reflux of a still not entirely understood etiology. Some of the causes are technical error in the anastomosis, pancreatitis by reperfusion, and blood flow abnormalities caused by back-table splenectomy. Hemorrhagic pancreatitis, infarct, and he accompanying parenchymal necrosis lead to graft death and to the risk of thrombosis propagation on recipient's iliac axis. Clinical symptoms are local pain, hematuria, hyperamylasemia, and decreasing amylasuria, hyperglycemia, and low limb edema. Diagnosis is by ultrasonography and, if necessary, can be confirmed by CT scan or traditional angiography. In the case of partial thrombosis, surgical recanalization of the vessel or anticoagulative therapy can be attempted, but for total thrombosis an urgent explant is necessary. According to the literature, although in the long run thrombotic complications have been reduced from 12% to an average of 5–6% up to 0.8% for SPK transplant, they are statistically more frequent in SPK transplants with enteric diversion and in PAK with vesical drainages compared to PTA where they occur with the same frequency in the two types of exocrine diversion. Decreasing the risk of thrombosis relies on a meticulous surgical technique for the anastomosis wrapping and on adequate anticoagulant prophylaxis.

Graft pancreatitis can rarely cause new-pancreas loss. A certain level of pancreatitis may be found in most patients after transplantation and can be documented by a modest and temporary increase of serum amylase concentrations for 48–72 h in the absence of evident graft alterations on ultrasound. Infrequent, and difficult to diagnose early, is pancreatitis due to stenosis of loop–duodenum anastomosis in the case of enteric diversion, or pancreatitis due to cystic reflux, where the suspect element is distension of the Wirsung duct.

After cystic diversion, anastomotic fistulas usually appear within 2–3 months of the transplantation and begin with pain, temperature, and hyperamylasemia. Urine leakage at the level of the anastomosis can be diagnosed by cystography or CT scan, and its treatment consists in reviewing the anastomosis or enteric conversion or, in the most critical cases, in removal of the graft. In cases of enteric diversion, the appearance of anastomotic fistulas (within 1–6 months) can bring further complications because of intestinal bacterial load with the appearance of typical intra-abdominal abscesses. Radiologic diagnosis combined with percutaneous drainage, followed by bacterial catheterization, are the first treatment steps, which may be followed by surgical review of the anastomosis combined with drainage of the abscesses. An incomplete abdominal toilette exposes the immune-compromised patient to sepsis and multiple organ failure or to the appearance of vascular anastomotic aneurysms with a high risk of hemorrhage. In such cases, the sacrifice of the transplanted pancreas is mandatory in order to protect recipient's survival.

The most frequent urologic complications after cystic diversion include recurrent urinary infections; acute hematuria due to hemorrhage from anastomotic rima; late hematuria due to cystoduodenal ulcerative lesions or anastomotic granuloma. Ureteral fistulas and stenoses may necessitate conversion to enteric exocrine diversion.

Intra-abdominal infections may be the result of anastomotic fistulas or mycotic infection of peripancreatic fluid collections, which are frequently observable after transplantation. Chronic immunosuppression supports these kinds of complications, the incidence of which may reach 20%. Diagnosis is clinical-instrumental and treatment is by surgical or percutaneous drainage [5, 6].

Pancreas Transplantation Results

According to data of the International Pancreas Transplantation registry, at the end of 2004, more than 23,000 transplants had been performed, 17,000 of them in the USA. Stratifying the types of transplant it is possible to observe how, between 1988 and 2003, graft survival at 1 year has improved from 75 to 85% for SPK, from 55 to 78% for PAK, and from 45 to 77% for PTA, with patient survival at 1 year for all categories higher than 95%. This was possible because of a reduction in technical failure rates (from 12 to 6% for SPK, from 13 to 8% for PAK, and from 24 to 7% for PTA, with a higher incidence in cases of enteric diversion and in a statistically significant way only for SPK) and in immunologic rejection rates (from 7 to 2% for SPK, from 28 to 7% for PAK, and from 38 to 8% in the cases of PTA, with about a 15% incidence in cases of enteric diversion compared to cystic diversion 5%). In most cases enteric diversion was used (81% for SPK, 67% for PAK, and 56% for PTA), and among these portal venous drainage was used in 20% of SPK, 23% of PAK, and 35% of PTA. No matter what kind of exocrine diversion is used, it does not result in significant differences in graft survival at 1 year (with an average of 85% vs. 87% for SPK, 77% vs. 80% for PAK, and 72% vs. 79% for PTA), nor does it make any difference to the functionality of the transplanted kidney. The cystoenteric conversion rate was 9% at 1 year and 17% at 3 years. In addition to antibody induction and basic steroid treatment, the maintenance immunosuppressive plan has been based on mycophenolate mofetil and tacrolimus for all categories, with an average graft functionality at 1 year of 80% or greater. In non-USA countries the majority of transplants are of the SPK type, with patient, kidney, and pancreas survival at 1 year of 94, 92, and 87% respectively. Although isolated transplant is not much used now, it shows a yearly survival rate equal to 85% for PAK and 76% for PTA.

Intestinal Transplantation for Pancreatic Cancer

Ductal adenocarcinoma of the pancreas represents one of the most aggressive tumors, as demonstrated by the 3- and 5-year survival rates. It is well established that the most common obstacle to achieving clean surgical margins during pancreatoduodenectomy is tumor involvement of the superior mesenteric artery and vein. Based on this concept, any improvement in the resection rate can potentially lead to an increase in the survival rate. Many reports in the literature describe ex vivo resection of tumor in heart, liver, and kidney surgery. In these techniques, the organ is removed from the surgical field with its vascular pedicle, perfused on the back table with cold preservation solution, and then subjected to parenchymal dissection of the tumor in a safe bloodless condition. To date very few published reports are available in terms of intestinal autotransplantation for various lesions of the pancreas involving the mesenteric root [9–11]. In all cases the decision to undertake this surgical option derived from major invasion of the mesenteric root by the tumor, from the absence of liver and peritoneal metastasis, the excellent clinical status and young age of the patients at the time of diagnosis, and, finally, from the patient's willingness and motivation to undergo a high-risk, critical, but potentially curative procedure, although with a very low success rate.

As described elsewhere [10], ex situ perfusion and dissection can help provide an adequate tumor-free margin in the mesenteric pedicle and in the retroperitoneal pancreatic bed, which are frequently invaded by neoplastic tissue even in the case of small neoplasms. The analysis of the cases performed so far shows that no perioperative mortality occurred, ensuring that in highly selected patients and in centers with intestinal transplantation experience, this surgical option can be performed with acceptable rates of mortality and morbidity. Because of the rarity of intestinal autotransplantation, is very difficult to settle the border between palliation and cure, and further studies are required to assess the real benefit of this approach.

References

1. Sutherland DE (1989) Coming of age for pancreas transplantation. West J Med 150:314–318
2. Coosemans W, Pirenne J (2003) Pancreatic transplantation. Acta Chir Belg 103:73–80
2. Steinman TI, Becker BN, Frost AE et al (2001) Clinical Practice Committee, American Society of Transplantation. Guidelines for the referral and management of patients eligible for solid organ transplantation. Transplantation 71:1189–1204
4. Di Carlo A, Odorico JS, Sollinger HW (2004) Pancreas transplantation: an overview. Transplantation Review 1:54
5. Boggi U, Mosca F (2001) I trapianti di pancreas. ETS edizioni, Pisa
6. Stuart FP, Abecassis MM, Kaufman DB (2000) Il trapianto d'organo. Excerpta Medica, Milan
7. Gruessner AC, Sutherland DE (2005) Pancreas transplant outcomes for United States (US) and non-US cases as reported to the United Network for Organ Sharing (UNOS) and the International Pancreas Transplant Registry (IPTR) as of June 2004. Clin Transplant 19:433–455
8. Vessal G, Wiland AM, Philosophe B et al (2007) Early steroid withdrawal in solitary pancreas transplantation results in equivalent graft and patient survival compared with maintenance steroid therapy. Clin Transplant 21:491–497
9. Lai DT, Chu KM, Thompson JF et al (1996) Islet cell carcinoma treated by induction regional chemotherapy and radical total pancreatectomy with liver revascularisation and small bowel autotransplantation. Surgery 119:112–114
10. Tzakis AG, Tryphonopoulos P, De Faria W et al (2003) Partial abdominal evisceration, ex vivo resection, and intestinal autotransplantation for the treatment of pathologic lesions of the root of the mesentery. J Am Coll Surg 197:770–776
11. Quintini C, Di Benedetto F, Diago T et al (2007) Intestinal autotransplantation for adenocarcinoma of pancreas involving the mesenteric root. Pancreas 34:266–268

Chapter 34

Endoscopic Palliation of Pancreatic Cancer: Biliary and Duodenal Stenting

Giuseppe Feliciangeli, Giampiero Macarri, Silvia Taffetani,
Antonio Benedetti

Ductal pancreatic adenocarcinoma is the second most common malignant neoplasm of the gastrointestinal tract and the fifth most common cause of neoplasia-related death in USA [1, 2]. Although progress in diagnosis and in medical and surgical treatment has been made, the median survival is less than 6 months and the survival rate at 5 years is 3–5%. At diagnosis most patients already have locally advanced disease with vascular invasion and/or metastatic lesions, which rule out a curative surgical approach. In the minority of patients in whom radical surgery is possible, survival at 5 years is still 15–20%. For these reasons, palliation is the cornerstone of treatment for most patients with pancreatic adenocarcinoma.

There are many palliative options: chemotherapy, surgery, interventional radiology, and endoscopy. The last is the most widespread. Endoscopic palliative treatment is at the moment fundamental to the management of the most frequent complications that occur in patients with pancreatic neoplasia:
- Obstructive jaundice
- Gastric outlet obstruction
- Intractable abdominal pain from neoplastic invasion of nerves and from obstruction of the pancreatic duct

In recent years, endoscopic positioning of biliary, enteral, and pancreatic stents has proved highly effective in alleviating these symptoms. At present, thanks to recent technological progress, endoscopy represents the first-line approach in the management of inoperable pancreatic neoplasms [3, 4].

Palliation of Obstructive Jaundice

Between 70 and 80% of patients with pancreatic adenocarcinoma develop a biliary obstruction, resulting in jaundice, itching, cholangitis, hepatic failure, and coagulopathy. Biliary drainage may be achieved through endoscopy, surgery, or a percutaneous approach. In patients with advanced disease, the first line remains endoscopy alone.

The first step in correct biliary drainage is to perform a complete cholan-

W. Siquini (Ed.), *Surgical Treatment of Pancreatic Diseases.*
©Springer-Verlag Italia 2009

giogram to locate the stricture. Especially in the case of hilar strictures, before performing endoscopic retrograde cholangiopancreatography (ERCP) it is useful to carry out magnetic resonance cholangiopancreatography (MRCP), which will give a first indication of the location of the stricture(s).

Once the stricture has been characterized from an imaging point of view, it is useful to characterize it anatomopathologically. This can be done during ERCP (brushing, intraductal biopsy) or, alternatively, by endoscopic ultrasonography (EUS) combined with cytohistological sampling (fine-needle aspiration, FNA).

Positioning of a Biliary Stent

In much carefully selected cases, before positioning a biliary stent it may be useful to perform a pneumatic dilatation. Many techniques for stent positioning exist; the most widespread consists of the positioning of a catheter with radiopaque markers on an introducer wire. The plastic stent is pushed on this catheter with a push catheter, that is a catheter that is coaxial with the introducer wire. Once the stent is in the desired position, the catheters are removed. Other systems exist, such as the Oasis system (Cook Medical Inc, Bloomington, USA), where the stent is premounted.

Generally, sphincterotomy is not necessary, but it can be done to simplify stent replacement or the positioning of another stent in parallel.

One question that remains unanswered is the question about whether to drain all the hepatic segments or just a single one.

Stent Types

Plastic Stents

Plastic biliary stents were introduced in 1979 [5] and are very widely used because they are easy to position and are low cost. There are fundamentally two types of plastic stent: straight and curved with little wings at the ends to avoid dislocation.

The major problem of stents is occlusion [6]. Stent occlusion starts with the deposition of sludge and a biofilm on the internal surface of the stent. This biofilm is composed of bacterial microcolonies in a matrix of extracellular material. Many methods to prolong stent patency have been studied (administration of mucolytics, bile acids, antibiotics) without noteworthy results. Special materials have been used to make stent surfaces that are as smooth as possible, or that have been soaked with substances with bactericidal activity. The shape has been modified, such as in the Teflon Tannenbaum stents, which are without side holes; this is because these holes could cause microturbulence that can make it easier for material to be deposited and thus for occlusion to occur. A new type of stent makes provision for the absence of a central lumen. However, the easiest way was to make a stent with a larger diameter. Comparison between 5- to 7-Fr stents and 10-Fr stents does indeed shows longer-lasting patency of the larger stents. The difference is not significant in the comparison between 10-Fr and 11.5-Fr stents, and therefore the diameter used is 10 Fr [5].

Plastic stents still have a tendency to occlude, making it necessary periodically to exchange them. There are three strategies: (1) to replace the stent every 3–4 months; (2) to test the cholestasis indices and replace the stent when the alkaline phosphatase value starts to rise; (3) to replace the stent when the occlusion became clinically evident [5]. The first and the second may lead to an unnecessary rise in the number of endoscopies; the third can lead to the risk of severe cholangitis. At present, there are no studies showing that any one of the above strategies is better than the others, so the most useful approach is to individualize the strategy based on the patient characteristics.

Biliary Self-Expandable Metallic Stents

To overcome the problem of the short length of plastic stents, towards the end of the 1980s self-expandable metallic stents (SEMS) were introduced [5, 6]. Many types of SEMS stents exist (Table 34.1). All have an initial diameter of 7–8 Fr in their collapsed configuration. Wallstents are the most widespread.

Stents are introduced using a 0.035-inch introducer wire and are positioned in the stricture under fluoroscopic guidance helped by radiopaque markers [7]. The Wallstent, once completely expanded, can reach 30 Fr diameter [5]. The stent embeds itself in the biliary duct wall, thus inducing a superficial necrosis that, through the inflammatory reaction, imprisons the stent, limiting its migration.

In spite of their larger diameter, these stents too tend to become occluded, for many reasons: (1) tumor ingrowth within the stent meshes; (2) tumor overgrowth at the ends of the stent; (3) biliary epithelial hyperplasia; (4) sludge formation [5, 6]. The consequence of all this is that the stent remains patent in only 50% of the patients. Recanalization can be achieved by inserting a new metallic or plastic stent inside the first. Another technique is to debulk the obstructing tissue [5, 8].

To obviate to the above problems, coated metallic stents have been introduced. These stents, however, tend to dislocate more easily and can be obstructed by bacteria sticking to the stent coat. Moreover, the doubt remains that the coated stent could block the cystic duct.

Recently, a comparison has been made between the endoscopic approach with positioning of a SEMS and surgical palliation. The results suggest the endoscopic approach for patients with a life expectancy of less than 6 months [9].

A transabdominal radiologic approach is always a second choice to an endoscopic approach.

The use of endoscopic stent placement before surgery remains controversial [5, 6, 8].

Table 34.1 Some of the self-expanding metallic stents commercially available at present for the treatment of biliary strictures

Stent	Brand/manufacturer	Dimensions of open stent (mm)	
		Length	Diameter
Sx Ella biliary	Ella Stent; Ella CS, Hradec Králové, Czech Republic	26, 34, 50, 74 22, 32, 52, 72	8 10
Wallstent biliary stent	Boston Scientific-Microvasive, Natick, MA, USA	40, 60, 80, 100	8, 10
Wallstent biliary stent with Permalume	Boston Scientific-Microvasive, Natick, MA, USA	40, 60, 80,	8, 10
Biliary stent	Endo-Flex GmbH, Voerde, Germany	60, 80	10
Zilver stent	Wilson-Cook, Winston-Salem, NC, USA	40, 60, 80,	6, 8, 10
SHIM-Hanarostent biliary	MI Tech Co., Ltd., Seoul, South Korea	60, 80, 100	10
Hanarostent biliary	MI Tech Co., Ltd., Seoul, South Korea	60, 80, 100	10
Biliary stent	Taewoong-Medical Co., Ltd., Seoul, South Korea	Covered or uncovered, 50, 60, 70, 80, 90, 100	10

Comparison of Plastic Stent and SEMS

Self-expanding metallic stents have a longer functioning half-life than plastic stents. However, plastic stents are less expensive. A cost-effectiveness analysis shows that SEMS are preferable if the life expectancy is more than 3–4 months [5, 6]. Unfortunately, the stent type has no influence on the patient's survival. To identify patients at risk of early SEMS occlusion can help avoid the placement of unnecessary SEMS and thus save money. A recent study has shown that SEMS patency does not depend on neoplasm type, stricture morphology, stent length, patient age, or bilirubin value. One factor that correlates with the patency duration is the degree of stent expansion. Plastic and metallic stent patency rates remain similar for the first 3 months, than diverge in favor of SEMS [5, 6]. A second useful factor for making the choice is the presence of hepatic metastases, which suggest the use of a plastic stent [5].

Palliation of Gastric-Outlet Obstruction

Gastric-outlet obstruction (GOO) is a mechanical or functional obstruction that obstructs passage of the gastric content into the small bowel. Symptoms include early satiety, postprandial abdominal pain, nausea, vomiting, and weight loss [8, 10, 11].

GOO is a late complication of pancreatic neoplasm. About 10–15% of pancreatic neoplasms cause a GOO. Until a few years ago, surgery (bypass) was the only option for restoring continuity between the stomach and the bowel [8, 10]. Although surgical bypass is still the gold standard (now performed laparoscopically), the positioning of a duodenal SEMS is a valid alternative, especially in patients with an advanced neoplasm.

First outcomes date back to the early 1990s [8]. The SEMS target for GOO is to restore the functional continuity between the stomach and the bowel, thus allowing oral nutrition and the resolution of all problems related to the obstruction [8, 12].

An enteral SEMS can be positioned either by the endoscopist or by the interventional radiologist. Endoscopic positioning has the advantage of obtaining easier access to the duodenum with the possibility of passing the stent through the operative channel of the endoscope. Enteral SEMS are composed of a variety of metallic alloys and are available in various shapes and length [5, 13]. There are also covered and uncovered stents to avoid neoplastic ingrowth (Table 34.2) [13].

Positioning Technique

The first step in positioning a duodenal SEMS is to define the shape and length of the stricture by a radiologic study. Sometimes, especially in the case of a tight, complete strictures, endoscopy allows a more precise diagnosis [5].

The patient is positioned in left decubitus to avoid aspiration of gastric contents. Sometimes the patient is intubated in deep sedation. Once the stricture is reached with the endoscope (some use a gastroscope, others a duodenoscope because it gives an operative channel with a larger diameter), an attempt is made to pass it with the endoscope, although it is preferable to avoid forcing the stricture or dilating it because of the risk of perforation. If the endoscope passes easily through the stricture, a guide wire with a soft end is positioned. If it is impossible to pass the stricture with the endoscope, a biliary catheter is passed with a hydrophilic guide wire previously mounted beyond the stricture. Contrast is injected downstream of the stricture to confirm the patency of the intestinal lumen downstream and to evaluate the length and the morphology of the stricture. Then the hydrophilic guide wire is replaced by a more rigid one [5].

A SEMS is selected that is 4 cm longer than the stricture [8]. The stent is passed on the guide wire through the endoscopic operative channel and is released starting from the distal margin under fluoroscopic and endoscopic control, trying to maintain the nearer margin in the desired position. With non-

Table 34.2 Some of the enteral self-expanding metallic stents, at the present commercially available for the treatment of enteral strictures

Stent	Brand/manufacturer	Dimensions of open stent (mm)	
		Length	Diameter
Ella Stent	Ella CS, Hradec Králové, Czech Republic	82–90–113–135	20–22–25
Wallstent duodenal stent	Boston Scientific-Microvasive, Natick, MA, USA	60, 90	20, 22
WallFlex duodenal stent	Boston Scientific-Microvasive, Natick, MA, USA	60, 90, 120	Ends: 27 Midportion 22
Duodenal stent covered, uncovered, partially covered	Endo-Flex GmbH, Voerde, Germany	80	18–20
Hanarostent duodenal/ partially covered	MI Tech Co., Ltd., Seoul, South Korea	90, 110	Ends: 18 Midportion 24
TTS Niti-S pyloric stent	Taewoong-Medical Co., Ltd., Seoul, South Korea	Covered, uncovered: 60, 80, 100	Ends: 18 Midportion 24
Hanarostent duodenal/ uncovered	MI Tech Co., Ltd., Seoul, South Korea	80, 110, 140	Ends: 18 Midportion 24

through-the-scope (TTS) stents the endoscope needs to be withdrawn and the positioning is done exclusively under fluoroscopic guidance [8]. After the stent is released it must be checked by fluoroscopy. If one end is not completely expanded, this may mean that the stent does not cover the entire length of the stricture. At this point it is useful to position a second stent to completely pass beyond the stricture.

During stent expansion, macro and micro changes occur in the surrounding tissue. Due to necrosis secondary to the pressure, stent meshes migrate into the mucosa and submucosa where there is a fibrotic reaction that merges the stent with the fibrotic tissue and the newly deposited collagen [8].

In some patients there may be a coexisting biliary obstruction. In this case three situations are possible depending on whether the duodenal stricture is proximal or distal to or at the level of the papilla (Fig. 34.1). Generally the biliary stricture shows itself before the GOO. Sometimes, however, a biliary obstruction can occur as a complication of the duodenal SEMS positioning for the GOO [8, 9, 11].

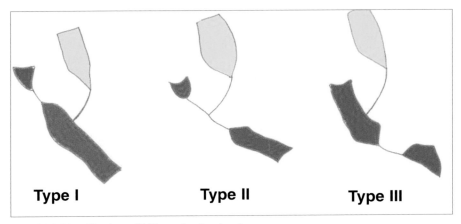

Fig. 34.1 Classification of biliary–duodenal strictures

If the biliary stricture is synchronous with the duodenal one, it is recommended to position the biliary SEMS before the duodenal one. If the biliary stricture occurs after positioning of the duodenal stent, usually the biliary drainage is done through the percutaneous route even if endoscopic positioning is possible. In this case the duodenoscope is introduced through the SEMS as far as the papillary region and an attempt is made to reach the biliary tree through the metallic meshes of the SEMS. A gap is made in the meshes either with a bile duct balloon or by ripping with a foreign-body forceps or by burning with the argon plasma coagulator. Then a biliary SEMS is positioned that leads to the duodenal SEMS (Fig. 34.2).

The technical success rate in duodenal SEMS positioning for GOO varies between 90 and 100% with a clinical success rate of 80–90% [12–14].

Two retrospectives studies have compared SEMS placement with surgery. Treatment with a SEMS is cheaper and involves a shorter hospital stay. Moreover, more than a half of the surgical patients developed delayed gastric emptying, while patients with a duodenal SEMS can fed a semisolid diet the day after stent positioning. No differences in survival have been recorded [7].

In this case there is a element of timing in the choice of surgery or endoscopy. For patients with a life expectancy shorter than 6 months, SEMS placement is preferable.

Failure of a duodenal SEMS placement for a GOO often is the consequence of a stricture that is not reachable endoscopically or that cannot be passed with the guide wire.

If an improvement of the GOO is not seen after placement of an enteral SEMS, this may be explained by the presence of lower intestinal strictures, by the presence of intestinal carcinosis, or by neuronal infiltration (by the primitive neoplasm) of the celiac plexus.

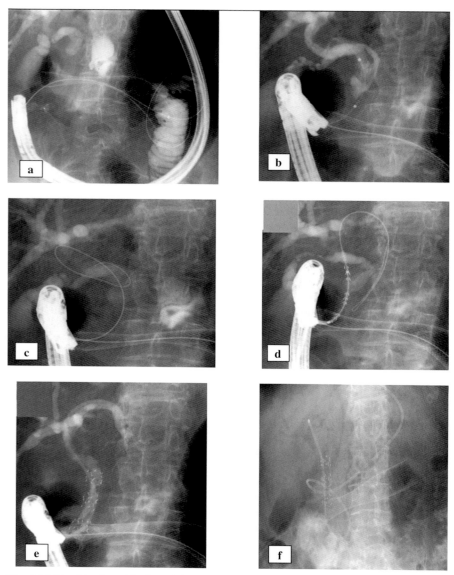

Fig. 34.2 Combined positioning of duodenal and biliary SEMS. After the duodenal stent is positioned (**a**), access to the biliary tract is obtained (**b,c**). Then the biliary SEMS is positioned, still closed (**d**), and finally it is opened (**e,f**). (Courtesy of Prof. M. Mutignani, Digestive Endoscopy Unit, University Hospital A. Gemelli, Catholic University, Rome, Italy)

Contraindications to duodenal SEMS placement are suspicion of an intestinal ischemia, perforation, peritonitis and pneumoperitoneum, and impossibility of passing a guide wire through the stricture. Early complications (within a few days of placement) includes aspiration, bleeding, and perforation. Late complications include bleeding, fistula formation, migration, and obstruction due to tumor ingrowth, reactive hyperplasia, tumor overgrowth, and/or a food bolus. Late perforation is rare [7, 15].

Symptomatic SEMS occlusion requires the positioning of a new stent within the occluded one. Another possibility is to attempt disobstruction with argon plasma [7, 12].

Pancreatic Stenting

Pain related to pancreatic duct obstruction is recorded in 15% of patients with advanced pancreatic neoplasms. Usually, the pain is postprandial and is associated with a rise in pancreatic enzymes. Sometimes, the pain is so severe it can be difficult to control even with opiates. Neoplastic compression of the duct of Wirsung leads to ductal obstruction with an upstream dilatation and associated ductal hypertension that causes pain. Positioning a stent across the stricture reduces the hypertension and thus mitigates the pain. Approximately 50–60% of patients cut down on opiate use after pancreatic stent positioning. Complications related to the stent placement are rare. The timing of the placement remains to be defined [5, 6].

Progress in the Palliation Using Stents

Recent progress in the endoscopic palliation with stents is represented by the introduction of SEMS coated with a membrane incorporating paclitaxel, an antitumor drug. Progress has also been made with plastic stents. Recently, a study from Hamburg has shown an improvement of the stents made using the nanotechnology for the inner covering [16].

References

1. Sanders M, Papachristou GI, McGrath KM, Slivka A (2007) Endoscopic palliation of pancreatic cancer. Gastroenterol Clin N Am 36:455–476
2. Michaud DS (2002) The epidemiology of pancreatic, gallbladder, and other biliary tract cancers. Gastrointest Endosc 56:S195–S200
3. Hawes RH (2002) Diagnostic and therapeutic uses of ERCP in pancreatic and biliary tract malignancies. Gastrointest Endosc 56:S201–S205
4. Baron TH, Mallery JS, Hirota WK et al (2003) The role of endoscopy in the evaluation and treatment of patients with pancreaticobiliary malignancy. Gastrointest Endosc 58:643–649
5. Shah JN, Muthusamy R (2005) Endoscopic palliation of pancreaticobiliary Malignancies.

Gastrointest Endoscopy Clin N Am 15: 513–531

6. Raijman I (2003) Biliary and pancreatic stents. Gastrointest Endosc Clin N Am 13:563–592
7. Holt AP, Patel M, Ahmed MM (2004) Palliation of patients with malignant gastroduodenal obstruction with self-expanding metallic stents: the treatment of choice? Gastrointest Endosc 60:1010–1017
8. Simmons DT, Baron TH (2005) Technology Insight: enteral stenting and ney technology. Nat Clin Pract Gastroenterol Hepatol 2:365–374
9. Mutignani M, Tringali M, Shah SG et al (2007) Combined endoscopic stent insertion in malignant biliary and duodenal obstruction. Endoscopy 39:440–447
10. Van Hooft J, Mutignani M, Repici A et al (2007) First data on the palliative treatment of patients with malignant gastric outlet obstruction using the WallFlex enteral stent: a retrospective multicenter study. Endoscopy 39:434–439
11. Dormann A, Meisner S, Verin N et al (2004) Self-expanding metal stents for gastroduodenal malignancies: systematic review of their clinical effectiveness. Endoscopy 36:543–550
12. Graber I, Dumas R, Filoche B et al (2007) The efficacy and safety of duodenal stenting: a prospective multicenter study. Endoscopy 39:784–787
13. Tierney W, Chuttani R, Croffie J et al (2006) Technology Status Evaluation Report: Enteral stents. Gastrointest Endosc 63:920–926
14. Baron TH, Harewood GC (2003) Enteral self-expandable stents. Gastrointest Endosc 58:421–433
15. Del Piano M, Ballarè M, Montino F et al (2005) Endoscopy or surgery for malignant GI outlet obstruction? Gastrointest Endosc 61:421–426
16. Seitz U, Block A, Schaefer AC et al (2007) Biliary stent clogging solved by nanotechnology? In vitro study of inorganic-organic sol-gel coatings for teflon stents. Gastroenterology 133:65–71

Chapter 35

Unresectable Pancreatic Neoplasms: Endoscopic and Surgical Palliation

Antonio Crucitti, Luigi Ciccoritti

Introduction

Pancreatic adenocarcinoma is the fifth most common cause of deaths from cancer in Europe, with a mortality rate close to 95%. At about 65,000 deaths per year, it represents 5.5% of the total number of deaths from cancer [1].

Anorexia, weight loss, abdominal pain, and nausea are the early symptoms in pancreatic carcinoma but they are extremely nonspecific, so that diagnosis is almost always delayed. The majority (70%) of all these neoplasms grow in the head of the pancreas and lead to obstructive jaundice, due to involvement of the intrapancreatic hepatic duct, which is the main specific sign of clinical presentation. Unfortunately, upon diagnosis, radical resection can be performed only in a small percentage of cases (15–20%), since about 40% of the patients already have locally advanced cancer with vascular invasion and 40–45% present with distant metastasis [2]. Still, even palliative treatment has strategic relevance in the majority of these patients, as it helps to solve the jaundice syndrome and the duodenal occlusion, and to achieve pain control, ultimately improving the quality of life.

Surgical Palliation

Surgery has for decades been the only choice for palliation of unresectable pancreatic tumors, and has been based on bilioenteric and gastroenteric bypass. Morbidity and mortality rates initially reported after surgical bypass [3, 4] were 10–20% and 33%, respectively. Today, authors report significantly lower percentages [5–7], with for example the Johns Hopkins Medical Institutions reporting 3.1% morbidity and 22% mortality [8].

Surgical strategies for obstructive jaundice treatment consist of anastomoses between the gallbladder, the main hepatic duct, and the duodenum or a jejunal loop. Due to the high morbidity rates reported, procedures based on bilioduodenal anastomosis were abandoned many years ago; hepaticojejunostomy (Fig. 35.1) is currently the treatment of choice in biliary duct occlusion, even preferred to cholecystoenterostomy, mostly because of its good long-term results.

W. Siquini (Ed.), *Surgical Treatment of Pancreatic Diseases.*
©Springer-Verlag Italia 2009

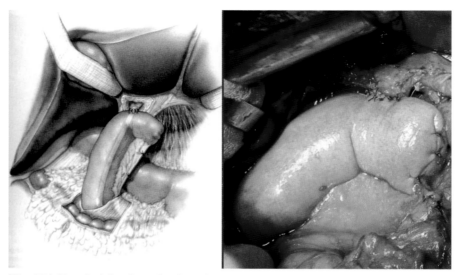

Fig. 35.1 Hepaticojejunal termino-lateral anastomosis

The main advantage of this type of bypass is the significantly lowered risk (four times) of any subsequent additional surgery for recurrent jaundice. The more distant this surgical bypass is from the gallbladder duct, the less likely it is to be involved early in the progression of the disease [4, 9–12]. Tarnasky et al., in a retrospective study, reported on an early 90% gallbladder duct occlusion after the ERCP procedure because of recurrent neoplastic jaundice [13].

Hepaticojejunostomy is commonly hand-sewn in an end-to-side fashion on the antimesenteric jejunal loop, lifted up via the transmesocolic loop, and then fashioned in an omega or a Roux-en-Y loop. Although the omega loop is much less time-consuming than the Roux-en-Y loop, the latter results in less anastomotic tension and exclusion from the gastrointestinal tract, with a significantly lower risk of leakage and cholangitis.

Specific complications after surgical palliation can be immediate or late. Among the former are delayed gastric emptying (7–9%), biliary leakage (5%), and the presence of an intra-abdominal abscess (4%); among the latter recurrent jaundice (4–13%) and cholangitis are the most frequent (2%) [4, 6, 8].

As to duodenal occlusion, about 30–50% of patients with pancreatic adenocarcinoma complain of nausea and vomiting at the time of diagnosis, and in one-third of them a stenosis will certainly develop sooner or later.

In fact it is well known overall that gastrojejunostomy, although it prolongs surgical time, does not have any effect on morbidity or mortality or on postoperative hospital stay [14]. Many retrospective studies on patients who did not undergo prophylactic gastric bypass show that 10–25% of them developed obstruction and required new surgery to restore bowel transit. Moreover, almost 20% of them die with clinical evidence of bowel obstruction.

After all these observations, many authors suggest performing a double bypass, both gastric and hepaticojejunal (Fig. 35.2) early on, even in patients with less than 6 months' life expectancy [14–16].

In the past, the gastrojejunal anastomosis was performed in the antecolic position, trying to avoid close contiguity with the tumor bed. Currently, however, the transmesocolic option is widely used because of the reported lower risk of delayed gastric emptying [10]. The gastrojejunal bypass is generally sewn on the posterior wall of the major curvature of the stomach, preserving the vagal nervous fibers and without performing the Roux-en-Y jejunal loop.

There have been reports in the literature of the possibility of performing a palliative pancreaticoduodenectomy, with increasing improvement in early or late results. In a retrospective study, Lillemoe et al. [17] found that, in selected cases of locally advanced pancreatic neoplasms, pancreatic resection, even with microscopically or macroscopically infiltrated margins (R1 or R2), leads to a higher survival rate than biliogastric bypass alone. However, this option, proposed by a single referring institution, needs to be further proved before being adopted in general clinical practice.

The laparoscopic approach to surgical palliation, although attractive, remains controversial. A clear distinction must be made between those minimally invasive surgical procedures that relate to jaundice and those carried out for duodenal obstruction. While gastric bypass performed via the laparoscopic approach [18] has been widely reported with good early and long-term outcome, no such encouraging results have been reported for laparoscopic biliary bypass.

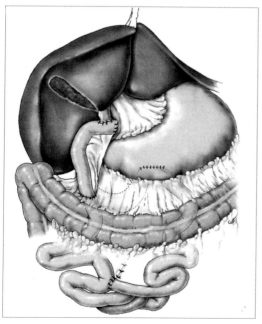

Fig. 35.2 Double by-pass: hepaticojejunal T-L anastomosis and gastrojejunal T-L anastomosis

Sometimes after a laparoscopic approach, to overcome some technical difficulties, it becomes necessary to chose options that have currently been abandoned, even in open surgery. For example, the choice of a mechanical cholecystojejunostomy, the most often adopted solution in laparoscopic palliation – also much easier than hepaticojejunostomy [19] – led to the same negative results as in open surgery and has now been abandoned.

Pain control is another major step in improving the quality of life of all these patients. Although only 30–40% of them complain of a moderate to severe pain at the time of diagnosis, more than 80% of them will develop more severe pain later on.

Alcoholization of the celiac plexus at laparotomy, with a 50% alcohol solution, is efficacious both in preventing and in controlling the neoplastic pain [20].

Endoscopic Palliation

Alternative options to surgical palliation might be required in high-risk patients (aged, weak, American Society of Anesthesiologists class 3 or 4) and, because of the assessed high likelihood of morbidity and mortality, in individuals with locally advanced disease or with metastatic disease and short life expectancy.

At the beginning of the 1970s, transhepatic percutaneous cholangiography was very helpful with the application of external stents or biliary endoprostheses, increasing the percentage of patients who were eligible for palliative treatment. However, in 1976 Nagai and Cotton et al. [21–23] introduced the first nasobiliary stents placed by the endoscopic approach and reported good external drainage, thus stimulating a rapid spread in the use of this method. Since then, due also to the improvement in the materials used, exponential technological progress has been achieved in the endoscopic approach to these patients and has completely replaced percutaneous stenting [24], becoming as it is now the most widely used method for nonsurgical palliation in these patients.

Biliary drainage is obtained through retrograde placement into the neoplastic stenosis of an endoprosthesis, under X-ray guidance and under the guidance of hydrophilic wires, which are preferred today to Teflon ones (Fig. 35.3).

In any case a preliminary study of the entire biliary tree is mandatory for the most efficacious treatment. After ultrasound confirmation of a dilatation in the biliary system, ERCP allows better definition of the segmental branch distribution. In more advanced cases, if the neoplastic stenosis also involves the hepatic hilum, magnetic resonance cholangiopancreatography (MRCP) can be more useful. In addition, MRI, without the direct injection of contrast through the neoplastic stenosis, significantly reduces the risk of cholangitis.

Biliary endoscopic sphincterotomy, although not mandatory, is performed in the majority of cases, mostly when more than two endoprostheses have to be positioned; however, in patients with coagulation disorders this procedure is strongly contraindicated.

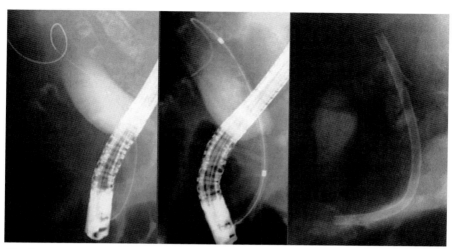

Fig. 35.3 ERCP. From left to right: guide wire through the neoplastic stenosis; stent placement; contrast-enhanced mean flow after the procedure

In some instances balloon dilatation of the neoplastic stenosis has to be performed before endoscopic stenting [25]. In addition, brushing or direct biopsy for histotyping are easy to perform during this procedure.

Endoscopic palliation is successful for resolution of jaundice in about 90% of cases; the main problem is not the stenting procedure in itself but rather the high and early rate of occlusion (about 3–5 months) and the recurrent jaundice and cholangitis [26]. The stent occlusion starts with an internal film made of biliary pigments and bacterial colonies, which progressively reduce the draining function of the stent, so that in 30–60% of cases it has to be replaced [27]. Differences in plastic materials, presence of turbulence, and hole distribution have to be considered in order to explain the short life of these endoprostheses [26]. Meanwhile – while we wait for new stent profiles and new materials – the first strategy to try to make the stents last longer has been to enlarge their size.

In fact, after the first low-cost 7-Fr stents, which also were much easier to apply, the 10-Fr polyethylene or Teflon stents were preferred, when possible, thus obtaining a longer efficacy (20–32 and 10–12 weeks, respectively). No statistically significant differences were demonstrated with larger stents (11.5 Fr) [28–30]. An approach that is still the subject of controversy in the literature is the option of a scheduled stent removal every 3 months, even if no occlusion or cholangitis has occurred. Using this protocol, on one hand we could protect the patient from severe infections, on the other hand it is much more cost effective. Self-expanding metal stents (Fig. 35.4) were introduced into clinical practice in 1989, also with the purpose of reducing the risk of occlusion; these prostheses, from an initial size of 7–8 Fr, can reach a maximum diameter of 30 Fr and demonstrate a lower occlusion rate (21–51% after 48 weeks) than plastic stents [31, 32]. However, even with a longer useful life, metal stents are more expen-

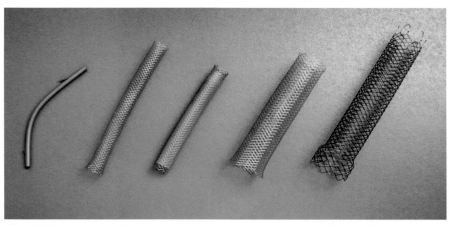

Fig. 35.4 Examples of biliary and enteric endoprostheses (last two from left)

sive and are more difficult to place endoscopically. In addition, this kind of prosthesis causes an inflammatory reaction of the biliary endothelium until the prosthesis becomes part of the main hepatic duct. When this happens, it is true that the stent will never migrate, but if it malfunctions, it will be impossible to remove and the only solution will be to "stent" the metal stent again with a new, smaller device [26]. For all these reasons, some authors suggest the use of self-expanding metal stents only in patients with life expectancy of 3 or more months [33, 34].

For duodenal occlusion, too, the application of self-expanding metal stents is increasingly used as a valid alternative to surgery, mostly in high-risk patients (Fig. 35.5). Enteric stents can reach 2–3 cm in diameter, are very flexible and show an efficacy rate of 90–100%, at least so far [26]. The first enthusiastic reports were tempered by the report of relevant complications such as mucosal ulceration, duodenal perforation, migration, and, last but not least, ingrowth of cancer and occlusion. In patients with longer life expectancy a surgical palliative bypass has been the only solution that gives a better quality of life [16].

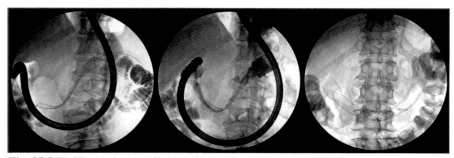

Fig. 35.5 ERCP: duodenal wall stent placement

Since 1995, the endoscopic approach to cancer-related pain has been adopted. The procedure, guided by endosonography, is neurolysis of the celiac plexus by means of transgastric delivery of an alcoholic solution [35]. However, no comparative studies have been published to confirm that the endoscopic approach is better than the surgical, percutaneous, or radiological (CT-guided) approaches.

Discussion

The availability of many therapeutic options for palliative treatment of unresectable pancreatic neoplasms can make it difficult to choose the appropriate one (Fig. 35.6).

It is widely accepted in the literature that symptom relief is achieved equally with all the different methods [12, 26], and that none of the therapeutic options has any effect on overall survival, which today is about 8–10 months in patients without metastases who have received palliative treatment and 4–5 months in those with metastases or who have not received treatment [4, 6, 8, 36]. Other parameters need to be considered in regard to the choice of palliation, such as: prevalence of immediate- or late-onset complications, duration of recovery, procedure-related costs and reproducibility on a wide scale, and, last but not least, the quality of life of the patients.

Morbidity rate and early complications (2.7 and 15%) and also median hospital stay (about 7–8 days) are certainly less for the endoscopic approach than

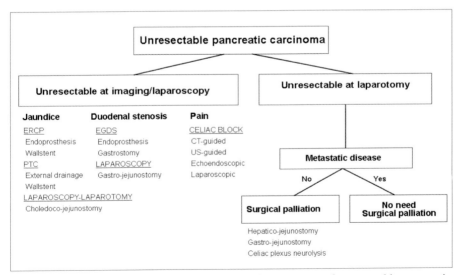

Fig. 35.6 Flow chart for decision making in palliative treatment of unresectable pancreatic cancer (modified from [12])

for the surgical one (4.4 and 30%, with a 15-day median hospital stay). However, the late-onset complication rate is higher for endoscopic treatment (25% vs. 10% for surgical treatment) and patients often need to be readmitted to hospital [4–8, 12, 27–31, 37, 38].

On the other hand, surgical palliation offers some advantages in comparison with other methods: treatment of jaundice, resolution of duodenal occlusion, and pain control can be obtained at the same time [12], and late-onset complications are less frequent, arising in most cases shortly before death.

In conclusion, the meta-analytic studies suggest that the endoscopic approach should be preferred for patients with a life expectancy of less than 3 months, i.e., the majority, while the surgical palliation should be reserved for longer-surviving patients [39].

Conclusions

The evolution of noninvasive methods of palliation on the one hand and the short median survival of patients with unresectable pancreatic cancer on the other have contributed to a reduction in surgical approaches. Recent developments in oncology and radiation therapy have contributes to prolong the survival even of patients with locally advanced and metastatic disease. In addition, there are the recent benefits achieved in patients treated with gemcitabine or capecitabine protocols, with or without conformational radiation therapy: a small advantage in terms of survival, but a big one in terms of the quality of the patient's remaining life, as reported in the literature [2, 40].

Although we need more and larger trials to confirm these preliminary results, there is no doubt that a moderate improvement in the median survival in these patients has to be matched by an increased number of surgical palliations. A multidisciplinary approach for the treatment of cancer is the only solution in almost all these patients, and if we think this should be true for patients with operable pancreatic cancer, it must also be so for the patient whose pancreatic cancer is locally advanced, unresectable, or metastatic. Unfortunately, the progress of technology and the experience of the referring hospitals do not represent a real opportunity for any patient.

In conclusion, choosing the most appropriate therapeutic strategy in pancreatic cancer palliation means considering what the most effective options might be, knowing the skills of the available personnel and the experience of the center in which they work.

References

1. Ferlay J, Autier P, Boniol M et al (2007) Estimates of the cancer incidence and mortality in Europe in 2006. Ann Oncol 18:581
2. Richard K, Muhammad WS (2007) Is there an optimal neoadjuvant therapy for locally advanced pancreatic cancer? JOP 8:279

3. Sarr MG, Cameron JL (1984) Surgical palliation of unresectable carcinoma of the pancreas. World J Surg 8:906
4. Singh SM, Longmire WP Jr, Reber HA et al (1990): Surgical palliation for pancreatic cancer. The UCLA experience. Ann Surg 212:132
5. Potts JR 3d, Broughan TA, Hermann RE (1990) Palliative operations for pancreatic carcinoma. Am J Surg 159:72
6. deRooij PD, Rogatko A, Brennan MF (1991) Evaluation of palliative surgical procedures in unresectable pancreatic cancer. Br J Surg 78:1053
7. Lillemoe KD, Sauter PK, Pitt HA et al (1993) Current status of surgical palliation of periampullary carcinoma. Surg Gynecol Obstet 176:1
8. Sohn TA, Lillemoe KD, Cameron JL et al (1999) Surgical palliation of unresectable periampullary adenocarcinoma in the 1990s. J Am Coll Surg 188:658
9. Sarfeh IJ, Rypins EB, Jakowatz JG et al (1988) A prospective, randomized clinical investigation of cholecystoenterostomy and choledochoenterostomy. Am J Surg 155:411
10. Watanapa P, Williamson RC (1992) Surgical palliation for pancreatic cancer: developments during the past two decades. Br J Surg 79:8
11. Urbach DR, Bell CM, Swanstrom LL et al (2003) Cohort study of surgical bypass to the gallbladder or bile duct for the palliation of jaundice due to pancreatic cancer. Ann Surg 237:86
12. House MG, Choti MA (2005) Palliative therapy for pancreatic/biliary cancer. Surg Clin North Am 85:359
13. Tarnasky PR, England RE, Lail LM et al (1995) Cystic duct patency in malignant obstructive jaundice. An ERCP-based study relevant to the role of laparoscopic cholecystojejunostomy. Ann Surg 221:265
14. Sarr MG, Cameron JL (1982) Surgical management of unresectable carcinoma of the pancreas. Surgery 91:123
15. Lillemoe KD, Cameron JL, Hardacre JM et al (1999) Is prophylactic gastrojejunostomy indicated for unresectable periampullary cancer? A prospective randomized trial. Ann Surg 230:322
16. Espinel J, Vivas S, Munoz F et al (2001) Palliative treatment of malignant obstruction of gastric outlet using an endoscopically placed enteral Wallstent. Dig Dis Sci 46:2322
17. Lillemoe KD, Cameron JL, Yeo CJ et al (1996) Pancreaticoduodenectomy: does it have a role in the palliation of pancreatic cancer? Ann Surg 6:718
18. Choi YB (2002) Laparoscopic gastrojejunostomy for palliation of gastric outlet obstruction in unresectable gastric cancer. Surg Endosc 16:1620
19. Ravindra SD, Siriwardena AK (2004) Laparoscopic biliary bypass and current management algorithms for palliation of malignant obstructive jaundice. Ann Surg Oncol 11:815
20. Lillemoe KD, Cameron JL, Kaufman HS et al (1993) Chemical splanchnicectomy in patients with unresectable pancreatic cancer. A prospective randomized trial. Ann Surg 217:447
21. Nagai N, Toli F, Oi I et al (1976) Continuous endoscopic pancreatocholedochal catheterization. Gastrointest Endosc 23:78
22. Cotton PB, Chapman M, Whiteside CG et al (1976) Duodenoscopic papillotomy and gallstone removal. Br J Surg 63:709
23. Cotton PB, Chapman M, Whiteside CG et al (1976) Proceedings: Duodenoscopic papillotomy and gallstone removal. Gut 17:395
24. Speer AG, Cotton PB, Russell RCG et al (1987) Randomized trial of endoscopic versus percutaneous stent insertion in malignant obstructive jaundice. Lancet 2:57
25. Costamagna G, Pandolfi M (2004) Endoscopic stenting for biliary and pancreatic malignancies. J Clin Gastroenterol 38:59
26. Sanders M, Papachristou GI, McGrath KM et al (2007) Endoscopic palliation of pancreatic cancer. Gastroenterol Clin N Am 36:455
27. Smith AC, Dowsett JF, Russell RCG et al (1994) Randomized trial of endoscopic stenting versus surgical bypass in malignant low bile duct obstruction. Lancet 344:1655

28. Speer AG, Cotton PB, MacRae KD (1988) Endoscopic management of malignant biliary obstruction. Stents of 10 French gauge are preferable to stents of 8 French gauge. Gastrointest Endosc 34: 412
29. Pedersen FM (1993) Endoscopic management of malignant biliary obstruction. Is stent size of 10 French gauge better than 7 French gauge? Scand J Gastroenterol 28:185
30. Pereira-Lima J, Jakobs R, Maier M et al (1996) Endoscopic biliary stenting for the palliation of pancreatic cancer: results, survival predictive factors and comparison of 10 Fr with 11.5 Fr gauge stents. Am J Gastroenterol 91:2179
31. Prat F, Chapat O, Ducot B et al (1998) A randomized trial of endoscopic drainage methods for inoperable malignant strictures of the common bile duct. Gastrointestinal Endosc 47:1–7
32. Dumonceau JM, Cremer M, Auroux J et al (2000) A comparison of Ultraflex Diamond stents and Wallstents for palliation of distal malignant biliary strictures. Am J Gastroenterology 95:670–676
33. David PHP, Groen AK, Rauws EA et al (1992) Randomized trial of self-expanding metal stents versus polyethylene stents for distal malignant biliary obstruction. Lancet 340:1488
34. Kaassis M, Boyer J, Dumas R et al (2003) Plastic or metal stents for malignant stricture of the common bile duct? Results of a randomized prospective study. Gastrointest Endosc 57:178
35. Wiersema MJ, Wiersema LM (1996) Endosonography-guided celiac plexus neurolysis. Gastrointest Endosc 44:656
36. Baron TH (2006) Palliation of malignant obstructive jaundice. Gastroenterol Clin N Am 35:101
37. Andersen JR, Sorensen SM, Kruse A et al (1989) Randomised trial of endoscopic endoprosthesis versus operative bypass in malignant obstructive jaundice. Gut 30:1132
38. Shepherd HA, Royle G, Ross APR et al (1988) Endoscopic biliary endoprosthesis in the palliation of malignant obstruction of the distal common bile duct: A randomized trial. Br J Surg 75:1166
39. Taylor MC, McLeod RS, Langer B (2000) Biliary stenting versus bypass surgery for the palliation of malignant distal bile duct obstruction: A meta-analysis. Liver Transpl 6:302
40. Alberts SR, Gores GJ, Kim GP et al (2007) Treatment options for hepatobiliary and pancreatic cancer. Mayo Clin Proc 82:628

Chapter 36

Interventional Radiology for Pancreatic Disease

Leonardo Costarelli, Enrico Paci, Ettore Antico

Interventional radiology is a discipline whereby diagnostic and/or therapeutic procedures are carried out either endovascularly or percutaneously, using the guidance of imaging systems (including conventional X-rays, ultrasonography, CT, and MRI). If employed on appropriate indication, it reduces the need for conventional surgery with consequently reduced morbidity [1].

Diagnostic Role

Percutaneous Fine-Needle Aspiration/Biopsy

Percutaneous fine-needle biopsy is a first-line procedure for a variety of clinical conditions and, in particular, in diagnostic procedures for pancreatic pathology. The technique, using a fine 20- to 22-gauge needle (fine-needle aspiration biopsy, FNAB) plays a well-established role in the differential diagnosis between cystic tumors and pseudocystic tumors (90% of fluid-filled lesions found in the pancreas) and in differentiating between sterile and infected fluid collections (fine-needle aspiration, FNA). When a fluid-filled lesion in the pancreatic area is studied, a firm diagnosis of pseudocyst is the end of a clinical and instrumental process. Taking a sample of the fluid is a necessary step, especially if the decision has been made to treat the patient in a noninvasive ("wait and see" approach) or minimally invasive way (percutaneous or endoscopic).

Ultrasound-guided needle aspiration with a Chiba needle (20–22 gauge) must avoid any potentially contaminating route (transgastric or transduodenal); the ultrasound-endoscopic path, if routinely employed in clinical practice, is effective in drastically reducing the risk of contamination (seeding) [2]. The fluid is then tested for the following: viscosity, microbiological culture, cytology, amylase, lipase, and tumor markers (CEA).

The quantity of intracystic CEA gives good diagnostic accuracy in differentiating between mucinous cystoadenoma (values >5 ng/ml) and serous cystoadenoma (values <5 ng/ml); using a cut-off of 400 ng/ml the technique reaches a sensitivity of 50% and a specificity of 100% in the differential diagnosis between pseudocysts and cystic tumors.

W. Siquini (Ed.), *Surgical Treatment of Pancreatic Diseases.*
©Springer-Verlag Italia 2009

Core biopsy using an 18- to 20-gauge coaxial needle is carried out for confirmation and typing of tumor lesions and possibly for better diagnostic framing of focal aspects in cases of chronic pancreatitis [3]. Currently percutaneous biopsy has the following indications:

- Differentiation of nodular lesions/masses of uncertain interpretation with imaging techniques (i.e., differential diagnosis between inflammatory nodules and tumors)
- Firm diagnosis of locally advanced cancers (therefore inoperable) and/or metastatic lymph nodes (which would avoid explorative laparotomy and surgical biopsies)
- Diagnosis of tumor recurrences and/or of metastatic lymph nodes shown during postoperative radiology check-ups

For guidance, any imaging system which provides the optimum detection of the lesion and resolution of the surrounding structures, can be used. Ultrasonography has numerous advantages such as real-time and 3D imaging; it also offers the possibility of choosing different angles; it is cheap, quick and easy to use. It is precise and allows a very accurate choice of needle path. Its main limitation is the effect of the presence of intestinal gases on the image.

CT as a guide is time-consuming; furthermore, the needle is introduced without direct visual control and its position is checked via a series of scans. Such an approach is justified only in cases where ultrasound imaging cannot be used because of intestinal meteorism, or where the lesions under investigation are tiny (i.e., pancreatic tail, or lesions located close to large blood vessels).

Contraindications are lack of secure access because of anatomical structures such as intestine or blood vessels, coagulation problems, and poor collaboration from the patient with the risk of needle malpositioning and consequent damage to adjacent organs.

The risk of complications ranges from 3 to 6.7% depending on the needle gauge. The most frequent complication is postbiopsy pancreatitis, which is caused by passing through healthy pancreatic tissue. Less frequent complications are hemorrhage, acute pancreatic duct leak, and neoplastic spreading along the route of the needle. The potential spreading of neoplastic cells along the needle route and/or intraperitoneal spreading have been described in the literature; however, they have often been related to multiple needle passes through the lesion [2]. If biopsy is unavoidable, it is best practice for the biopsy pathway to follow the same line as the subsequent surgical incision.

Accuracy will depend on a number of factors: experience, collaboration between radiologist and pathologist, patient size, the size and location of the lesion, needle gauge, and number of samples; range is from 50 to 94% (the latter with the use of CT-guided biopsy in the presence of a pathologist). Biopsy under CT scan guidance using a coaxial needle would be the gold standard procedure in terms of accuracy and diagnostic reliability and because of its impact on future patient management (Fig. 36.1). Close co-operation with the pathologist for immediate examination of the tissue samples means that decisions about further aspiration in the same or surrounding areas can be made on the spot,

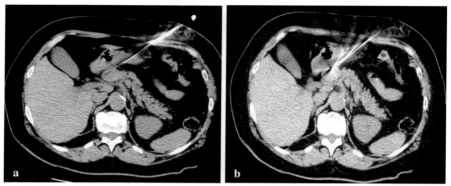

Fig. 36.1 CT-guided biopsy of expansive lesion of the pancreatic head (**a, b**)

thereby avoiding biopsy of purulent or necrotic material, fibrous tissues, or inflammatory cells. The majority of false negative reports in neoplastic pathology are caused by sampling errors due to difficulty in identifying the core of the lesion because of the presence of necrotic tissue or peritumoral desmoplastic changes, or because of acute localized pancreatitis caused by the obstruction of pancreatic ducts adjacent to the lesion.

Diagnostic Angiography

Digital subtraction angiography is currently used as an emergency procedure for detection of postpancreatitis acute bleeding due to pseudoaneurysms of the splenic or gastroduodenal artery. As an elective procedure, it can be necessary for more precise evaluation of vascular lesions, in conjunction with noninvasive angiographic studies to be carried out, such as multislice CT angiography or MR angiography.

The "traditional" role of conventional angiography in the diagnosis of endocrine tumors of the pancreas has now been virtually abandoned and is limited to cases in which a detailed study of the local vasculature is indicated with a view to a possible percutaneous embolization procedure (neuroendocrine tumors).

Another complex technique, which however now is virtually relegated to history, can be used when all other methods have proved inconclusive. This is the "selective arterial stimulation test," which consists of catheterization of the right hepatic vein accessed through the femoral vasculature and concomitant selective catheterization of the pancreatic arteries; secretion-stimulating substances are injected selectively into the various pancreatic arterial branches and samples are then withdrawn from the veins every 1–2 min following the initial injection into the arteries; the difference in variation of neuroendocrine peptides in the various arterial branches can indicate the location of the tumor with good approximation [4].

Therapeutic Role

Percutaneous Drainage

It is essential to distinguish needle aspiration from permanent catheterization of fluid collections of pancreatic origin. Direct needle aspiration of the pseudocyst is beneficial both from the diagnostic point of view, enabling one to determine the nature of the fluid (differential diagnoses between cystic or ductal tumors with acute presentation, or in the search for superinfections), and, from the therapeutic point of view, enabling evacuation of the fluid; a procedure which can then be repeated several times. Direct needle aspiration has however lost its therapeutic value over time, given its poor results. [5]. "Percutaneous drainage" means the positioning of a catheter directly inside the fluid-filled space, which can then be left in situ for variable periods of time. The first record of this procedure, used to treat two infected pseudocysts of the pancreas, dates back to 1979 [6].

Catheterization can be carried out using an ultrasound-fluoroscopic probe or under CT guidance. The first step involves diagnostic puncture, sterile aspiration, and direct evaluation of the physical characteristics of the liquid evacuated (appearance, color, clarity, viscosity, odor) and its subsequent laboratory analysis (enzymes, markers, cytology, cultures); any obvious presence of blood leads to immediate discontinuation of the procedure and arrangement of other tests to evaluate the presence of pseudoaneurysms of the local arteries. Needle aspiration must be extraintestinal to avoid contamination of the fluid and to avoid false positivity of the microbiology culture. In cases where the nature of the material obtained through aspiration, is not immediately obvious, it is permissible to wait a few days, delaying the drainage procedure until results of the tests on the aspirated fluid become available.

There are three different methods of percutaneous drainage:

– *External drainage* or percutaneous extraintestinal catheterization via ultrasound or CT-guided skin needle insertion, when a peritoneal or extraperitoneal route is followed, avoiding passing through the stomach.
– *External–internal drainage* or percutaneous transvisceral (through the stomach) catheterization: A catheter is inserted into the cavity and through the stomach, with the intention of actively creating a fistula between the stomach and the pseudocyst which will continue to evacuate the cyst's contents even after removal of the catheter. This procedure is conducted under ultrasound or CT guidance and, sometimes, with endoscopic control.
– *Internal drainage* or percutaneous cystogastrostomy is the positioning of an internal prosthesis which links the stomach and cavity; it can be a second step in the external–internal procedure described above.

Cystogastrostomy is a difficult procedure and has a 10% chance of failure, even in very expert hands.

External or external–internal drainage offer some benefits: displacement of the prosthesis is uncommon, and it is easily replaceable if it becomes obstructed; also, imaging with contrast and monitoring of the quantity and type of material drained (allowing early diagnosis in the case of hemorrhage) are easily performed.

For external drainage the same accesses are used as for needle aspiration. For multiple, unconnected lesions, multiple catheters of different diameters ranging from 10 to 16 Fr are used. The catheter is left in situ for 6–7 weeks, with daily evaluation of the flow rate and amylase level. The flow rate usually slowly decreases; this trend is favored by parenteral feeding and the administration of somatostatin analogues. A flow rate which does not show any tendency to reduce is a good indication for further investigations including transcatheter contrast studies or endoscopic retrograde cholangiopancreatography, in order to check for the presence of stenoses of the pancreatic duct due either to inflammation, lithiasis, or tumors. When the flow of the fluid evacuation reaches zero (or at least drops to less than 10 ml daily), or if there has been no fluid accumulation in the cavity 48–72 h after its clamping, the catheter can be removed.

Not all pancreatic cysts or fluid collections have to be subjected by definition to percutaneous evacuation: a correct timing factor is involved, and some lesions respond best to a certain type of drainage procedure, whilst others do not respond at all (the 1992 Atlanta Consensus Conference was the first to issue some guidelines for the percutaneous evacuation of pancreatic cysts or fluid collections) [7].

Acute Pancreatic Inflammation

The severity of acute pancreatitis can be evaluated by adopting clinical (Ranson criteria and APACHE II score) or radiological criteria (Balthazar score). The Balthazar system [8], used to evaluate the severity and prognosis of acute pancreatitis, is based on parameters linked to CT imaging and, in particular, to the number and distribution of fluid collections, combined with an estimated degree of pancreatic necrosis (0–33%, 33–50%, >50%).

Complications of pancreatitis can be systemic (shock, acute renal failure, adult respiratory distress syndrome) or localized (fluid collections, pseudocysts, necrosis and abscess). Mortality in the presence of infected necrosis is between 30–35% compared with 10–15% for sterile necrosis. Mortality in the case of abscess is less than for infected necrosis (10–25%).

CT scanning is the imaging technique of choice both for diagnosis and often also for treatment.

The objectives of CT imaging are:
– Differential diagnosis with mesenteric infarction or intestinal perforation
– Severity scoring (evaluation of the degree and extension of the inflammation outside the pancreas, associated with the presence of parenchymal necrosis)
– Detection of complications (necrosis, pseudocysts, abscesses, ascites)

The purpose of medical treatment is to reduce morbidity and mortality by limiting systemic and local complications (necrosis and infection), treating the inflammation, and re-addressing risk factors (cholelithiasis, etc.).

Guidelines for the surgical management of pancreatitis have been issued by the International Association of Pancreatology [9]. This issued 11 recommendations, amongst which those of interest to us are "grade B" recommendations:
- FNA is indicated for differentiating between sterile necrosis and infected necrosis in the presence of sepsis
- Infected pancreatic necrosis in patients with symptoms and signs of sepsis is an indication for surgical treatment and/or percutaneous drainage
- The patient with sterile necrosis (negative after FNA) should receive only conservative treatment
- Early surgery (within 14 days) is not recommended in necrotizing pancreatitis.

The terminology used to describe surgically treatable complications was defined by the International Symposium in Atlanta in 1992 [7].

Acute Fluid Collections

Acute fluid collections present early on in 30–50% of cases of acute pancreatitis, within or around the pancreas; they do not have well-defined walls, and in half of the cases can spontaneously regress. They are associated with a high level of amylase content (if the level is low they are pseudopseudocysts. Yeo and Sarr [10] introduced the concept of pseudopseudocyst, as an early fluid collection due to reaction to underlying acute pancreatitis which tends to spread within the omental sac: pseudopseudocysts are characterized by a low amylase level and a tendency to resolve spontaneously).

Treatment of the fluid collection is usually unnecessary: should the FNA procedure show any infection, percutaneous drainage would be indicated. If the fluid collection persists for over 4–6 weeks and a peripheral wall becomes apparent, a pseudocyst or abscess (if infected) is developing and as such requires treatment [11].

Pseudocysts

A pseudocyst is a collection of pancreatic secretions and fibrin surrounded by a fibrotic wall or by granulation tissue, without an epithelial layer. It can originate from (acute or chronic) inflammation or from trauma, because of two possible different mechanisms:
- In acute pancreatitis the mechanism is self-digestion of parenchyma and ducts with both inter- and periglandular extravasation of secretion (another mechanism would be the liquefaction of areas of parenchyma necrosis).
- In chronic pancreatitis the most likely mechanism is secondary ductal hypertension due to ductal stenosis, which is caused by an accumulation of intraglandular secretion and subsequent rupture of the ducts.

Histologically, the two forms are identical, and chronic pancreatitis seems to be nothing more than the result of multiple episodes of acute pancreatitis.

The pseudocyst contains amylase at high concentration, a sign of the presence of links with the ducts. If infected, it is considered an abscess. Those smaller than 5 cm can heal spontaneously and should just be monitored (CT or ultrasound).

Treatment options include percutaneous needle aspiration and drainage, internal drainage (surgical or endoscopic), and surgical resection. The efficacy of these methods has yet to be assessed and compared in controlled trials. The percutaneous option represents the first choice, although it is associated with high chances of recurrence. The surgical option (cystogastrostomy or cystoduodenostomy) is very effective, with little chance of recurrence. The endoscopic option can be chosen when the pseudocyst closely adheres to the posterior aspect of the stomach.

Since in the majority of cases the cyst is not infected, initial treatment is usually simple needle aspiration, which can also be curative even if the initial cause is a ruptured duct. Should the cyst recur, which is usually caused by linkage with a duct, a catheter should be placed and left in place until the secretions stop.

Indications for percutaneous drainage are: diameter greater than 5 cm, infection, temperature, pain, increase in volume, biliary or gastrointestinal obstruction, and duration over 2 months [12] (Fig. 36.2a).

Drainage should be placed following the simplest and most direct route; sometimes more complex approaches are needed, such as the transgastric or transhepatic routes [13]. The catheter can be removed when secretion reduces to less than 10 ml/24 h for 2 consecutive days. Before removal, a transcatheter X-ray study with contrast and a CT scan should be performed; if neither fluid collections nor links with ducts or intestine are identified, the procedure is curative in 90% of cases, with results similar to those of surgical treatment (Fig. 36.2b).

Infection due to the positioning of drainage within a sterile pseudocyst is described in 5% of cases, although a subclinical colonization is usually more common. For the small subgroup of patients with fistulas of the pancreatic ducts who do not respond to prolonged drainage, surgical resection of the pancreatic tail or endoscopic stenting remains an option.

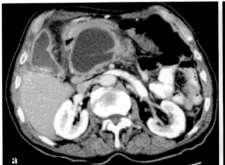 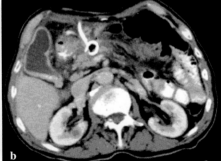

Fig. 36.2 a CT scan with intravenous contrast enhancement of pseudocysts from acute pancreatitis. **b** Complete resolution after percutaneous treatment with pig-tail type catheter

Surgery is indicated in cases of drainage failure, when complications occur, or because of the cholecystolithiasis which causes pancreatitis, or in cases where possible percutaneous access routes are identified as too risky [14].

Pancreatic Necrosis

Pancreatic necrosis appears either as diffuse or localized areas of nonviable pancreatic tissue, often associated with areas of peripancreatic steatonecrosis. CT imaging shows absence of contrast enhancement; the degree of necrosis represents a good indicator of the severity of the pancreatitis according to the Balthazar scale (Fig. 36.3a).

Crucial to the outcome of therapy is the distinction between sterile and infected necrosis. The presence of gas bubbles in areas of necrosis seen under CT scan is highly specific for infection, which can be confirmed by FNA and subsequent microbiology culture studies.

In sterile necrosis the majority of studies favor conservative medical treatment (intravenous fluids, hyperalimentation, antibiotics, pain relief, nutritional support). The few retrospective studies which have compared medical conservative treatment with debridement of sterile necrotic tissue have not shown any benefit from the surgical approach, even if, in theory, the removal of uninfected pancreatic necrosis might prevent both the systemic effects of necrosis and the mortality associated with superimposed infections [15].

The role of percutaneous drainage in the treatment of sterile necrosis is also controversial; the principal argument against it being the possibility of introducing infection into the fluid collection, although in the majority of cases bacterial colonization remains at a subclinical level (Fig. 36.3b).

Colliquative necrosis can be treated by percutaneous drainage, which can also represent a definitive cure; drainage reduces postsurgical morbidity, or can allow postponement of the operation to a more favorable time.

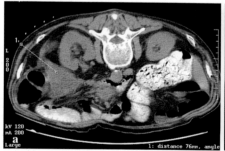 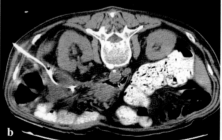

Fig. 36.3 Sterile pancreatic necrosis. **a** Preliminary CT scan with positioning of cutaneous target points and calculation of both the depth of the lesion and the angle of insertion of the needle. **b** Positioning of a pig-tail type percutaneous catheter

Traditionally, infected necrosis is a direct indication for surgical treatment – debridement and/or surgical necrosectomy [16], which can be carried out either with closed evacuation or by using the packing technique (which requires multiple subsequent abdominal explorations).

Currently the tendency towards less invasive therapies associated with more aggressive interventional radiology techniques has led to a broader range of new indications [17]:

- Diagnostic aspiration, often of multiple sites, can ascertain or rule out infection
- Successful outcome can be achieved by drainage of liquefactive necrosis, whether sterile or infected, when located in easily accessible sites which can be easily evacuated
- Drainage can postpone surgery; furthermore, it does not close the door on surgery altogether and can in fact optimize its timing.

Pancreatic Abscess

A pancreatic abscess is a collection of pus delimited by connective reactions, resulting from acute pancreatitis or trauma, usually 4 weeks after clinical presentation with or without minimal necrotic component content. The term includes infected pseudocysts, recently infected fluid collections, and postsurgery collections. The degree of necrosis must be minimal, since infected necrosis has double the mortality rate of an abscess. More or less infected pancreatic fluid collections, which complicate pancreatic surgery, should be defined as "postoperative pancreatic abscesses."

Controversy surrounds the timing of treatment, the type of operation (percutaneous or surgical), and the method of treatment [18]. The percutaneous approach is beginning to play a crucial role thanks to the use of multiple catheters (to drain all cavities) of large caliber (from 12 to 30 Fr; Fig. 36.4).

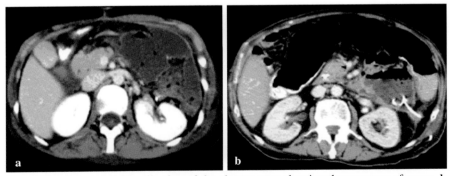

Fig. 36.4 a Infected fluid collection of the abscess type showing the presence of gases. **b** Reduction of the abscess after percutaneous drainage

Surgery is reserved for when these less invasive treatments fail. Percutaneous drainage, indicated as a first line of therapy, represents a diagnostic/therapeutic step in the context of a complex pluridisciplinary approach.

Chronic Pancreatic Inflammation

In 50% of cases treatment is essentially medical: alcohol is banned, and pancreatic extract supplements and analgesics are administered.

Surgical treatment is based on Wirsung-jejunum by-pass (when the duct of Wirsung is dilated) or resectioning (when the Wirsung duct is not dilated). The main indications for surgery are frequent attacks of pain, nonresponse to pain-control therapies, and complications (cholecystitis, gallbladder duct or duodenum obstructions, etc.).

Over the past few years more gentle treatments have been suggested, the most important being percutaneous or endoscopic evacuation of the pseudocysts. External-internal or internal drainage grants good results in cases of chronic disease, especially where there is partial obstruction of the pancreatic duct.

Other Procedures not Directly Correlated to Pancreatic Pathology

Drainage of Pleural Fluid

Positioning of a catheter in the thorax, a role usually performed by the thoracic surgeon, involves the interventional radiologist in cases where removal of fluid collections might require ultrasound or CT guidance (Fig. 36.5).

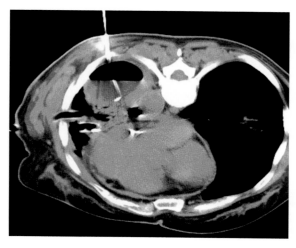

Fig. 36.5 CT-guided positioning of percutaneous drain to evacuate a fluid collection in the pleural space (empyema)

Positioning of Nasoduodenal Catheter under Fluoroscopic Control for Enteral Feeding

Positioning of a jejunal catheter, combined with the use of antibiotics, reduces bacterial spread and therefore limits the risk of superinfection within the necrotic areas.

Treatment of Vascular Complications

One of the worst vascular complications of pancreatic pathology is pseudoaneurysm of the splenic or gastroduodenal artery due to necrosis of the vascular walls through contact with proteolytic enzymes; contact with the septic or infected focus is inevitable.

The risk of hemorrhage (which occurs in 1–3% of cases of acute pancreatitis) makes angiography and subsequent embolization necessary; the latter is considered the treatment of choice given its success rate of 78–100% [19] (Fig. 36.6).

The infected necrosis often causes recurrence of bleeding; it is possible to treat postsurgery bleeding with the same technique.

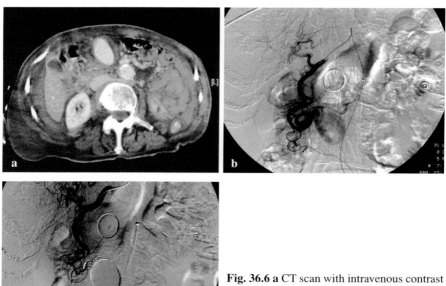

Fig. 36.6 a CT scan with intravenous contrast enhancement of pseudoaneurysm of the gastroduodenal artery. **b** Digital angiographic scan of the lesion. **c** Postembolization check reveals complete stemming of the hematic flow from the pseudoaneurysm pouch

Treatment of Obstructive Icterus

Jaundice complicates 80–90% of tumors of the pancreatic head (Fig. 36.7a). Surgical biliary–digestive anastomosis carries a significant risk of morbidity (20–60%) and mortality (2.5–30%). Treatment is often palliative. Percutaneous and/or endoscopic palliative treatment is associated with very much less morbidity (15–35%) and practically zero mortality. These latter techniques have to be considered the treatment of choice, although surgery may be considered as a valid alternative [20].

External Biliary Drainage

External biliary drainage (EBD) represents the preliminary step before surgery or before an external–internal biliary drainage (EIBD) or internal biliary drainage (IBD); it also represents the only palliative treatment in cases of inoperable neoplastic stenosis. Absolute contraindications are noncorrectable coagulation impairment or multiple intrahepatic obstructions. Used over prolonged periods EBD can cause electrolyte depletion and malabsorption, since the entire liver system is bypassed. The most common complications are malpositioning (15–25%) and cholangitis (3–15%). Hemobilia has a low incidence (2–5%).

External-Internal Biliary Drainage

EIBD can be carried out as first choice or in a subsequent step, following EBD in cases where it has not been possible to overcome a blocked stenosis. Its goal is definitive biliary decompression. The distal end of the catheter is positioned in the duodenum. Due to the positioning of the holes of the catheter over the lesion, the bile flow follows a physiological direction, cleansing the entire biliary circuit (Fig. 36.7c).

Bleeding complications are slightly more frequent than after EBD (5–7%).

Internal Biliary Drainage

IBD uses an 8- to 10-Fr plastic endoprosthesis, which is positioned at the level of the stenosis deemed to be inoperable. It takes place after EBD, when decompression has already been achieved and having secured the intrahepatic route. IBD makes it possible to bypass problems related to the management of the cutaneous end of the EIBD, but does not provide direct access to the system should any correction of complications be required, such as displacement (3–4%) and blockage (5%). Occlusion is caused by the deposition of a protein biofilm on the wall of the prosthesis, where bacteria adhere and easily proliferate; they then are responsible for calcium salt deposits or calcium bilirubinate, which through precipitation end up blocking the prosthesis.

Stent

Today, the use of a percutaneous plastic endoprosthesis is almost unheard of, given the possibility of using metal prostheses of larger diameter, generally 7–10 mm rather than the 8- to 10-Fr of the plastic prosthesis (around 3 mm) (Fig. 36.7d).

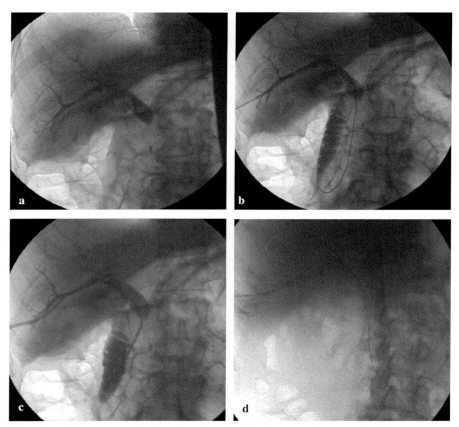

Fig. 36.7 a Percutaneous cholangiography showing "mouse tail" stenosis of the common bile duct due to cancer of the pancreatic head. **b** Overcoming the stenosis using a transpapillary guidewire. **c** Positioning an external–internal percutaneous transpapillary catheter with its distal end in the duodenum. **d** Subsequent positioning of a self-expanding metal stent

Compared to plastic prostheses, stents cause less trauma, even though other systems use a smaller gauge (6–10 Fr); furthermore, their wider caliber reduces the chances of blockage, almost tripling the time they stay open. The disadvantages are the higher costs compared to the plastic prosthesis (5:1), the impossibility of their surgical removal, and the possible infiltration by part of the tumor growth. The obstruction of metal stents is mainly due to the growth of neoplastic tissue over the metallic mesh.

Postsurgical Complications

Pancreatic surgery involves various procedures depending on the type and severity of the pathology (neoplastic or infectious).

An early postsurgical complication is arterial bleeding in the area that has undergone to the procedure. Interventional management of this complication requires very accurate diagnosis in terms of origin of the bleeding, which can be determined via an angiogram or CT angiography; these complications can then be treated via embolization with metal nonmagnetic microspirals or with the implantation of a stent-graft.

Follow-up is essential to identify subsequent peripancreatic fluid collections; if the collections display features of low internal pressure (i.e., a nonspherical shape and no dislocation of nearby organs) they will tend to resolve spontaneously [21]. Failure to self-heal and/or eventual abscess formation requires treatment via the positioning of a percutaneous drain.

A level of amylase in the fluid collection three times higher than the serum amylase concentration raises the suspicion of pancreatic fistula, which can be treated at the beginning by positioning a percutaneous drain of the pig-tail type [22].

If, after the 3rd postoperative day, more than 10 ml/day secretion continues to drain from the peripancreatic catheter, with amylase concentration three times that of the serum amylase, a diagnosis of pancreatic fistula can be made. This condition should be managed with substitution of the surgical drainage with a percutaneous one of lower gauge, less invasive but of higher drainage capacity. Another possibility would be to attempt closure of the fistula with surgical glue (N-butyl-cyanoacrylate) [23].

Biliary fistulas or bile collections (biloma) can also be treated by inserting a drain or prosthesis into the bile duct system [24].

References

1. Adam A (1998) The definition of interventional radiology. Eur Radiol 8:1014–1015
2. Linder JD, Geenen JE, Catalano MF (2006) Cyst fluid analysis obtained by EUS-guided FNA in the evaluation of discrete cystic neoplasms of the pancreas: a prospective single-center experience. Gastrointest Endosc 64:697–702
3. Gupta S, Ahrar K, Morello FA Jr et al (2002) Masses in or around the pancreatic head: CT-guided coaxial fine-needle aspiration biopsy with a posterior transcaval approach. Radiology 222:63–69

4. Kalra MK, Maher MM, Mueller PR et al (2003) State of the art imaging of pancreatic neoplasms. Br J Radiol 76:857–865
5. Van Sonnenberg E et al (2001) Percutaneous abscess drainage: update. World J Surg 25:362–369
6. Gerzof SG, Robbins AH, Birke TT et al (1979) Percutaneous catheter drainage of abdominal abscesses guided by ultrasound and CT. AJR Am J Roentgenol 133:1–8
7. Bradley EL (1993) A clinically based classification system for acute pancreatitis. Summary of the International Symposium on Acute Pancreatitis Atlanta, 11–13 September 1992. Arch Surg 128:586–590
8. Balthazar EJ (2002) Acute pancreatitis: assessment of severity with clinical and CT evaluation. Radiology 223:603–613
9. Uhl W, Warshaw A, Imri C et al (2002) IAP guidelines for the surgical management of acute pancreatitis. Pancreatology 2:565–573
10. Yeo CJ, Sarr MG (1994) Cystic and pseudocystic diseases of the pancreas. Curr Probl Surg 31:165–252
11. Neff R (2001) Pancreatic pseudocysts and fluid collections: percutaneous approaches. Surg Clin North Am 81:399–403
12. Kumbasar AB, Acunas B (2001) Interventional radiology in inflammatory pancreatic disease. Eur J Radiol 38:133–136
13. Brugge WR (2004) Approaches to the drainage of pancreatic pseudocysts. Curr Opin Gastroenterol 20:488–492
14. Nealon WH, Walser E (2005) Surgical management of complications associated with percutaneous and/or endoscopic management of pseudocyst of the pancreas. Ann Surg 241:948–957
15. Bradley EL, Howard TJ, van Sonnenberg E et al (2008) Intervention in necrotizing pancreatitis: an evidence-based review of surgical and percutaneous alternatives. J Gastrointest Surg 12:634–639
16. Buchler MW, Gloor B, Mueller CA et al (2000) Acute necrotizing pancreatitis: treatment strategy according to the status of infection. Ann Surg 232:619–626
17. Lee JK, Kwak KK, Park JK et al (2007) The efficacy of nonsurgical treatment of infected pancreatic necrosis. Pancreas 34:399–404
18. Rodriguez JR, Razo AO, Targarona J et al (2008) Debridement and closed packing for sterile or infected necrotizing pancreatitis: insights into indications and outcomes in 167 patients. Ann Surg 247:294–299
19. Yamakado K, Nakatsuka A, Tanaka N et al (2000) Transcatheter arterial embolization of ruptured pseudoaneurisms with coils and n-butyl cyanoacrylate. J Vasc Interv Radiol 11:66–72
20. Shankar S, VanSonnenberg E, Silverman SG et al (2004) Imaging and percutaneous management of acute complicated pancreatitis. Cardiovasc Intervent Radiol 27:567–580
21. Baker TA, Aaron JM, Borge M et al (2008) Role of interventional radiology in the management of complications after pancreaticoduodenectomy. Am J Surg 195:386–390
22. Yamazaki S, Kuramoto K, Itoh Y (2003) A minimally invasive approach for postoperative pancreatic fistula. Cardiovasc Intervent Radiol 26:580–582
23. Findeiss LK, Brandabur J, Traverso LW et al (2003) Percutaneous embolization of the pancreatic duct with cyanoacrylate tissue adhesive in disconnected duct syndrome. J Vasc Interv Radiol 14:107–111
24. Singh AK, Gervais DA, Alhilali LM et al (2006) Imaging-guided catheter drainage of abdominal collections with fistulous pancreaticobiliary communication. AJR Am J Roentgenol 187:1591–1596

Chapter 37

Chemotherapy and Radiotherapy in Pancreatic Cancer

Mario Scartozzi, Chiara Pierantoni, Alessandra Pagliacci, Stefano Cascinu

Introduction

Pancreatic cancer continues to be a highly lethal disease, with approximately 37,000 estimated new cases in the USA in 2007 in both sexes, representing the fourth leading cause of cancer death [1]. Surgery remains the only treatment with a curative potential for local disease, but only 15–20% of patients have resectable disease at the time of diagnosis [2], and the median survival of radically resected patients is approximately 20 months, with a 2-year survival rate ranging from 20 to 40%. Adjuvant chemotherapy or radiotherapy has been assessed in several trials in an attempt to improve patients' prognosis.

At the time of diagnosis 80% of patients are ineligible for surgical resection due to local spread or metastatic disease. Thus, most patients receive palliative treatment with the aim of improving their quality of life. Patients with advanced disease treated with the best supportive care have a median survival of approximately 3–4 months. Gemcitabine became the standard of care for patients with advanced disease after showing superiority over fluorouracil about 10 years ago [3].

The need for further improvement in the treatment represents a major challenge at all stages of pancreatic cancer. In this chapter we will discuss the advances in the adjuvant treatment of pancreatic cancer and the results of innovative approaches in the treatment of advanced pancreatic cancer. The differences in terms of treatment strategy between locally advanced and metastatic cancer will also be addressed and reviewed.

Adjuvant and Neoadjuvant Treatment for Pancreatic Cancer

Chemoradiotherapy

Postoperative adjuvant therapy has been evaluated in the attempt to improve outcome for patients with pancreatic cancer who are undergoing radical surgery. In this patient population, micrometastasis and local recurrence are the main cause

W. Siquini (Ed.), *Surgical Treatment of Pancreatic Diseases.*
©Springer-Verlag Italia 2009

of failure of surgical treatment. From 1980 on, a few randomized studies of adjuvant treatment have been conducted, usually with controversial results mainly related to suboptimal treatment regimens (chemo- and radiotherapy), small patient numbers, and heterogeneous sites of primary disease.

In 1985 the Gastrointestinal Tumor Study Group reported that the median survival of patients undergoing radical resection could be improved by postoperative chemoradiation [4]. In this trial 49 patients were randomly assigned to observation or radiotherapy combined with 5-fluorouracil (5-FU) bolus after resection. 5-FU 500 mg/m^2 daily for 3 days was given concurrently with radiotherapy (standard split course 4000 cGy). The 5-FU regimen was continued weekly for 2 years. A significant survival advantage was observed in treated patients (median survival 21 months vs. 10.9 months; $p = 0.03$). Adjuvant chemoradiotherapy was adopted in North America as the standard treatment after curative resection of pancreatic cancer based on the results of this small study. This survival advantage was not confirmed in a large-powered randomized trial by the European Organization for Research and Treatment of Cancer (EORTC), designed to test the efficacy of a combination of 5-FU with split-course radiotherapy compared with no postoperative treatment after radical surgery of pancreatic carcinoma and carcinoma of the periampullary region [5]. One of the main criticisms of this trial was that it allowed enrollment of non-pancreatic cancer patients; in fact, when patients with cancer of the pancreatic head were analyzed as a subgroup, a significant benefit from adjuvant chemoradiation was observed [6] (Table 37.1).

In 2003 a phase II study on adjuvant chemoimmunoradiation with external-beam irradiation (4500–5400 cGy) and three-drug chemotherapy (continuous infusion of 5-FU, weekly intravenous bolus of cisplatin, and subcutaneously administered interferon-α) suggested that overall survival may be improved for patients with adenocarcinoma of the pancreatic head using an adjuvant-interferon-based protocol. At 31.9 months' follow-up, 67% of the patients were alive [7]. On the basis of this trial a phase III study is ongoing with the aim of comparing chemoimmunotherapy with cisplatin, interferon-α-2b, and 5-FU combined with external radiotherapy with chemotherapy (5-FU plus folinic acid) for six cycles [8].

In a nonrandomized but comparative single-institution trial Yeo et al. reported a survival benefit in patients receiving adjuvant chemoradiotherapy after radical surgery, with a median survival of 19.5 months vs. 13.5 months ($p = 0.003$) [9].

The RTOG9704 trial is a randomized study assessing the role of gemcitabine in combination with postoperative adjuvant 5-FU chemoradiotherapy in patients with radically resected pancreatic cancer. Chemotherapy with either gemcitabine or fluorouracil was given for 3 weeks before and 12 weeks after chemo-radiation. Gemcitabine significantly improved overall survival (median survival 20.6 months vs. 169 months) in a subgroup of 381 patients with pancreatic head tumors [10], but unfortunately this study was not able to elucidate the role of radiation therapy.

Table 37.1 Comparative studies of adjuvant chemoradiotherapy in resected pancreatic cancer

Study	No. of patients	Survival (months)		p
		RCT/5-FU	Observation	
GITSG (1985) [4]	49	21	10.9	0.005
EORTC (1999) [5]	114	17.1	12.6	0.099
ESPAC-1 (2004) [14]	289	15.9	17.9	

RCT, Chemoradiotherapy; *5-FU*, fluorouracil; *GITSG*, Gastrointestinal Tumor Study Group; *EORTC*, European Organization for Research and Treatment of Cancer; *ESPAC*, European Study Group for Pancreatic Cancer

Chemotherapy

The role of chemotherapy alone in the adjuvant setting has been a subject of controversy during the last 20 years. In most randomized trials, fluorouracil-based regimens have been compared with observation after pancreatic surgery.

Norwegian investigators evaluated the combination of chemotherapy with fluorouracil, doxorubicin, and mitomycin C after surgery with surgery alone in a small, randomized trial involving 61 patients. Chemotherapy resulted in a significant advantage in median survival (23 vs. 11 months; $p = 0.02$) but was not able to improve 5-year survival [11].

In a later controlled trial 158 patients were randomized to receive fluorouracil plus mitomycin or not, with a significant advantage showing for 5-year survival only in patients with gallbladder carcinoma, not for those with pancreatic cancer [12].

The results of a large randomized controlled trial of adjuvant chemotherapy (CONKO-001) were recently published. Three hundred sixty-eight patients with R0 or R1 pancreatic resection were randomized to undergo adjuvant chemotherapy with gemcitabine for six cycles or observation. Gemcitabine significantly improved disease-free survival (13.4 vs. 6.9 months; $p < 0.001$), with the beneficial effect evident for both R0 and R1 resection. However, no differences in overall survival were observed (22.1 vs. 20.2 months; not significant) [13] (Table 37.2).

The ESPAC-1 trial used a two-by-two factorial design in which 289 patients were randomized to receive chemoradiotherapy (20 Gy over 2 weeks plus fluorouracil); chemotherapy with fluorouracil alone (six cycles of the Mayo Clinic schedule); chemoradiotherapy followed by chemotherapy (both defined previously); or no treatment (observation). Based on the study design, two separate comparisons were performed. The first was between chemotherapy (chemoradiotherapy followed by chemotherapy or chemotherapy alone) versus no chemotherapy (observation or chemoradiotherapy without subsequent chemotherapy). The second comparison was between those patients who

Table 37.2 Randomized studies of adjuvant chemotherapy in resected pancreatic cancer

Study	No. of patients	Treatment	Median survival (months)	5-Year survival (%)
Bakkevold et al. (1993) [11]	61	AMF	23	4
		Observation	11	8
Takada et al. (2002) [12]	158	FU/MitC	–	11.5
		Observation	–	18
Oettle et al. (2007) [13]	368	Gem	22.1	22.5
		Observation	20.2	11.5

AMF, Doxorubicin–mitomycin C–fluorouracil; *FU*, fluorouracil; *MitC*, mitomycin C; *Gem*, gemcitabine

received chemotherapy or chemoradiotherapy alone and those who did not (observation or chemotherapy alone). After 47 months' median follow-up, a highly significant difference in median survival in favor of chemotherapy was reported (20.1 vs. 15.5 months; $p = 0.009$). The 2-year and 5-year survival times for chemotherapy versus no chemotherapy were estimated at 40% and 21%, and 30 and 8%, respectively. On the other hand, adjuvant chemoradiotherapy did not show any substantial benefit, and the patients who received this treatment had a higher chance of deleterious effects than those who did not receive chemoradiotherapy (median survival 15.9 vs. 17.9 months; $p = 0.05$). The 2-year and 5-year survivals for chemoradiotherapy versus no chemoradiotherapy were respectively 29 and 10% vs. 41 and 20% [14].

These results seem to be confirmed by a meta-analysis including several studies demonstrating that adjuvant chemotherapy may result in a survival advantage, whereas chemoradiotherapy seems not to be effective except in patients with positive resection margins (R1 resection) [15].

In conclusion, there is strong evidence for the role of adjuvant chemotherapy. Gemcitabine or fluorouracil for 6 months may be used. Adjuvant chemoradiotherapy may be a choice after pancreatic surgery with R1 resection.

A critical point remains the difficulties of pancreatic cancer patients in receiving adjuvant chemotherapy, mainly due to surgical sequelae. Furthermore, the need for tumor down-staging in locally advanced pancreatic cancer, possibly resulting in an increase in radical resection, suggests a crucial role for neoadjuvant therapy.

Neoadjuvant therapy in patients with potentially resectable tumors has been evaluated in a few small studies. Spitz et al. compared preoperative versus postoperative radiochemotherapy using fluorouracil. No differences in survival or toxicity were observed; moreover, 25% of patients did not receive postoperative treatment because of surgical complications [16]. In a phase II trial 86 patients were treated preoperatively with gemcitabine plus radiotherapy; 71 patients underwent surgery and 74% of them had a resectable tumor. Median survival in patients who underwent radical resection was 36 months, whereas 7 months was the median survival in nonresected cases [17]. Overall, neoadjuvant therapy for potentially resectable pancreatic cancer remains experimental as evidence of its role from large randomized trials is lacking.

Advanced Disease

Although new strategies have been explored in the past few years to improve the outcome of patients with advanced pancreatic cancer, their prognosis remains poor, with a median survival ranging from 6–10 months in locally advanced to 3–6 months in metastatic disease [18]. As is clear from the statistics just cited, advanced pancreatic cancer is made up of two different clinical conditions: locally advanced disease and metastatic disease. They are different in terms of prognosis and require different treatment approaches.

Chemoradiotherapy in Locally Advanced Disease

Locally advanced unresectable pancreatic cancer is defined as a tumor that encases a vascular structure, such as the superior mesenteric artery, celiac axis, or superior mesenteric vein or the portal confluence, in the absence of distant metastases. Tumors associated with bulky peripancreatic lymphadenopathy are also to be considered locally advanced. Since surgical resection of the primary tumor remains the only potentially curative treatment for pancreatic carcinoma, preoperative approaches have been investigated with the aim of downstaging localized disease in order to allow radical surgical resection and thus, hopefully, prolong survival.

Along these lines, several trials have reported an intriguing percentage of patients who undergo resection of the primary tumor after chemoradiation, with rates ranging between 12 and 22%, and a small but significantly longer survival following chemoradiotherapy (10 months) as compared with chemo- or radiotherapy alone (6–9 months). In the 1960s, the Mayo Clinic had already documented the efficacy of combined chemoradiotherapy in a small randomized study. This trial indicated an improvement in median survival from 6.3 months in patients treated with radiotherapy to 10.4 months in patients treated with radiotherapy in those treated with chemoradiotherapy [19]. These results were confirmed in two further randomized studies carried out in the 1980s by the Gastrointestinal Tumor Study Group (GITSG). The first study randomized 194 patients with locally advanced pancreatic cancer to receive high-dose radiotherapy (HDRT) alone (6000 cGy) or HDRT plus chemotherapy (5-FU) or low-dose radiotherapy (4000 cGy) plus chemotherapy (5-FU). Both 5-FU-containing regimens (6000 or 4000 cGy + 5-FU) produced a highly significant survival improvement when compared with radiation alone (6000 cGy), with median survivals of 40.3, 42.2, and 22.9 weeks respectively ($p < 0.01$). However, differences in survival between the two 5-FU-containing regimens were not significant [20]. A further GITSG trial, comparing a multidrug chemotherapy regimen including streptozocin, mitomycin, and 5-FU (SMF) with radiation combined with 5-FU followed by SMF, showed improved median survival for the combined-modality therapy (42 weeks) compared with chemotherapy alone (32 weeks). One-year survival rates were 41 and 19% respectively for the two regimens (p <0.02) [21]. The GITSG studies suggested that combined-modality therapy may be superior to either optimal radiotherapy or chemotherapy alone.

The Eastern Cooperative Oncology Group (ECOG) randomized 91 patients with locally unresectable pancreatic cancer to receive chemotherapy alone with 5-FU or radiotherapy plus 5-FU followed by a maintenance treatment with 5-FU and showed no differences between the two treatment arms in terms of time to progression and survival. Furthermore, the combined-modality arm proved to be more toxic, as 27% of patients treated with 5-FU and 51% of those treated with combination therapy experienced hematological toxicity [22].

Recently, Chauffert et al. have reported the results of a phase III trial that compared chemoradiation (60 Gy in 6 weeks concomitant with 5-FU and cisplatin at 1–5 weeks) followed by gemcitabine, as maintenance treatment, with gemcitabine alone to assess whether chemoradiotherapy improves survival in patients with locally advanced pancreatic cancer. An intermediate analysis showed that survival was better in patients receiving chemotherapy alone (14.3 versus 8.4 months, respectively, p <0.014), and the study was stopped after 119 patients had been included [23]. The reasons for these results are currently under discussion. However, the failure of chemoradiotherapy as first approach may be considered a consequence of the approximately 30% of locally advanced pancreatic cancer patients who progress early because they had occult metastatic disease at diagnosis. This group of patients does not receive any clinical benefit from locoregional treatment. The toxicity experienced by patients in the combined treatment resulted in lower administered doses of systemic chemotherapy with gemcitabine and may be another reason for the premature stop to the study. Randomized phase III studies with chemoradiotherapy for locally advanced pancreatic cancer are summarized in Table 37.3.

Gemcitabine, a potent radiosensitizer, has been investigated in locally advanced pancreatic cancer in association with radiotherapy mainly in phase I–II clinical trials [24–26]. Gemcitabine 440–600 mg/m^2 per week given as a once-weekly infusion concurrent with conventional radiotherapy of 50.4–55.8 Gy in 1.8-Gy/day fractions was reported to be reasonably well tolerated.

Crane et al., in a retrospective study comparing the toxicity and efficacy of gemcitabine-based chemoradiation versus 5-FU-based chemoradiation in patients with unresectable pancreatic cancer, showed no significant differences between two regimens in terms of local and distant progression rates and 1-year overall survival. However, patients receiving gemcitabine developed a significantly higher rate of severe toxicity than those receiving 5-FU [27].

A small randomized trial of 34 patients has shown that gemcitabine-based concurrent chemoradiotherapy significantly improves survival, time to progres-

Table 37.3 Randomized phase III studies of radiochemotherapy of locally advanced unresectable pancreatic cancer

Study	No. of patients	Treatment	Median survival (months)	p
Moertel et al. (1969) Mayo Clinic [19]	69	35–40 Gy 35–40 Gy + 5-FU	6.3 10.4	Significant
Moertel et al. (1981) GITSG [20]	194	40 Gy split + 5-FU 60 Gy split + 5-FU 60 Gy split	9.6 9.2	Significant 5.2
Klassen et al. (1985) ECOG [22]	91	40 Gy + 5-FU 40 Gy	8.8 8.2	Not t significan
Douglass et al. (1988) GITSG [21]	43	54 Gy + 5-FU Sq SMF SMF	10.5 8.0	Significant
Chauffert et al. (2006) [23]	119	60 Gy + 5-FU/CDDP Sq Gem Gem	8.4 14.3	Significant

CDDP, Cisplatin; *5-FU*, 5-fluorouracil; *Gem*, gemcitabine; *Sq*, sequential; *SMF*, streptozocin–mitomycin–5-fluorouracil; *GITSG*, Gastrointestinal Tumor Study Group; *ECOG*, Eastern Cooperative Oncology Group

sion, response rate, and quality of survival (in terms of symptom control) compared with 5-FU-based chemoradiotherapy in patients with locally advanced pancreatic cancer. The median survival and median time to progression were respectively 14.5 and 7.1 months for the gemcitabine combination versus 6.7 and 2.7 months for 5-FU combination (p <0.027 and p <0.019) [28]. These results obviously need further confirmation in larger clinical trials.

A small study confirmed that chemoradiotherapy (radiotherapy with concurrent infusion of 5-FU) may improve survival and quality of life as compared to no treatment, providing a palliative benefit for patients with unresectable pancreatic cancer [29].

Taken together these studies seem to suggest that the combination of chemoradiotherapy and radioterapy improves survival and quality of life over supportive care alone, with radiotherapy being less effective than chemoradiation. However, the role of chemotherapy alone in comparison with chemoradiotherapy is still not well defined. In addition, we should also take into account that some patients with locally advanced disease may show rapid tumor progression and develop metastatic disease within few weeks, whatever type of treatment they receive. In addition, an intensive approach may be difficult to tolerate, mainly because of the proximity of radiosensitive structures to the pancreatic bed and the poor performance status of patients with advanced pancreatic cancer. This treatment should thus be reserved for selected patients who might benefit from it (i.e., those with good performance status and no evidence of metastatic disease).

The French Groupe Coopérateur Multidisciplinaire en Oncologie (GER-COR) has proposed a different strategy for locally advanced pancreatic cancer. They suggest starting the treatment with chemotherapy for at least 3 months. In patients whose disease has not progressed and who have a good performance status, chemoradiotherapy should then be performed. This suggestion rises from a retrospective analysis of 181 patients with locally advanced pancreatic cancer enrolled in prospective phase II and III GERCOR studies. This analysis compared the survival of patients receiving chemoradiotherapy after initial disease control with chemotherapy alone. Among the 128 patients who had no disease progression after 3 months of chemotherapy, 72 (56%) received chemoradiotherapy and 56 (44%) continued chemotherapy. Patients who received the combined treatment had significantly better survival than those who continued with chemotherapy alone; the median overall survival times were 15 and 11.7 months respectively ($p = 0.0009$) [30]. Although we need to await results from phase III randomized trials, these findings seem to suggest a more advantageous treatment strategy in locally advanced pancreatic cancer patients. In fact this approach is potentially effective for a well-selected subgroup of patients without early metastatic spread who can potentially benefit from chemoradiotherapy, and would prevent giving useless and toxic treatment (radiotherapy) to patients who will rapidly progress.

Chemotherapy in Advanced Disease

Chemotherapy is never curative for metastatic disease, and its potentially palliative benefit must be carefully weighed against its toxic effects.

Chemotherapy vs. Best Supportive Care

The role of chemotherapy as palliative treatment in advanced pancreatic cancer has been demonstrated in several clinical trials in recent years. In 1996, Glimelius et al. reported the results of a small randomized phase III trial that compared chemotherapy (5-FU/leucovorin combined with etoposide or the same regimen without etoposide in elderly patients and those with poor performance status) in addition to best supportive care (BSC) to BSC alone in patients with advanced pancreatic and biliary cancer [31]. Chemotherapy significantly improved both quality of life (EORTC-QLQ-C30) ($p < 0.01$) and survival compared with BSC. Median survival was 6 months in the chemotherapy plus BSC group and 2.5 months in the BSC alone group ($p < 0.01$).

Improvements in quality of life and survival with palliative chemotherapy compared to BSC was also reported by Palmer et al. comparing a FAM [5-FU, doxorubicin (formerly adriamycin), mitomycin C] regimen with BSC. The results from this trial showed a median survival of 8.3 months for the FAM regimen and 3.8 months for the BSC arm [32].

Finally, a recent published meta-analysis of chemotherapy for locally and metastatic pancreatic cancer confirmed that overall survival is significantly better in patients who receive chemotherapy compared with those who receive BSC alone, with the risk of death reduced by 36% in patients who received chemotherapy [33].

Fluoropyrimidines

5-FU has been studied using a variety of doses and schedules, but the response rate rarely exceeded 20% and no consistent effect on survival has been demonstrated [34]. Combination chemotherapy of 5-FU with mitomycin C, doxorubicin, and streptozotocin (FAM and SMF regimens) showed promising activity with 30–50% response rate in phase II studies, but these findings were not confirmed in subsequent phase III trials. Protracted 5-FU infusion combined with cisplatin was shown to be superior to 5-FU in terms of progression-free survival, but not for overall survival [35]. Capecitabine is an oral fluoropyrimidine that has demonstrated a single-agent activity in advanced pancreatic cancer, with a clinical benefit response (24%) and overall response rate (9.5%) similar to those observed for single-agent gemcitabine and a tolerable safety profile [36].

Gemcitabine

Gemcitabine is a nucleoside analogue with activity across a broad range of solid tumors [37]. Its activity in advanced pancreatic carcinoma was assessed in early phase II trials. These studies reported an improvement in disease-related symptoms among patients with responding or stable disease. This improvement, which appeared greater than expected from the objective tumor response rate, consisted of decreased pain severity with a consequent reduction of opioid analgesics use and improved performance status. The "clinical benefit response" was then introduced as an end point for the evaluation of gemcitabine efficacy [38, 39].

In a randomized phase III trial, Burris et al. showed that gemcitabine as single agent was superior to 5-FU bolus monotherapy in terms of improved clinical benefit and survival. One hundred twenty-six patients with advanced pancreatic cancer were randomized to receive gemcitabine (1000 mg/m^2 given once weekly for 7 consecutive weeks, followed by 1 week rest and then weekly for 3 consecutive weeks every 4 weeks) or 5-FU (600 mg/m^2 bolus given once weekly). Clinical benefit was experienced by 23.8% of gemcitabine-treated patients, with a median duration of response of 18 weeks, compared with 4.8% of 5-FU-treated patients with a median duration of 13 weeks ($p < 0.0022$). Gemcitabine also showed a modest but significant survival advantage over 5-FU (1-year survival:

18% in the gemcitabine arm versus 2% in the 5-FU arm; median survival: 5.65 versus 4.41 months respectively, p <0.0025) [3].

As a result, gemcitabine has become the standard first-line treatment for advanced pancreatic cancer. However it should also be noted that the clinical superiority of gemcitabine over more active 5-FU schedules such as 5-FU infusion or 5-FU/folinic acid in this setting has never been demonstrated. A multicenter randomized phase III trial comparing protracted venous infusion (PVI) of fluorouracil with PVI fluorouracil plus mitomycin in 208 patients with advanced pancreatic cancer showed similar results to gemcitabine in terms of median survival (5.1 versus 6.5 months respectively). Although this comparison cannot be considered correct, these results confirm the potential role of 5-FU as an acceptable alternative to gemcitabine in the treatment of pancreatic cancer [40].

Clinical studies suggested that the infusion rate of gemcitabine may be important for its efficacy. Gemcitabine is a prodrug which must be phosphorylated to its active metabolites gemcitabine diphosphate and triphosphate to induce cellular apoptosis. However, there is evidence that standard gemcitabine infusion over 30 min could saturate the rate of intracellular accumulation of triphosphate. Alternatively, administration of gemcitabine at a fixed dose rate (FDR) at 10 mg/m^2 per minute could maximize intracellular concentrations of the active phosphorylated forms and enhance its cytotoxicity.

In a phase II randomized trial, Tempero et al. have shown that FDR infusion of gemcitabine results in improved efficacy, compared to a standard infusion (30 min) at a higher dose. In fact, although time to progression and response rate were comparable in both arms of this study, a modest overall improvement in survival along with higher rates of hematological toxicity were found in the FDR infusion arm [41]. However, a randomized phase III study comparing the FDR and the standard 30-min gemcitabine infusion failed to demonstrate superiority of the FDR regimen in terms of overall survival [42].

Combination Chemotherapy

Several phase III trials tested the combination of gemcitabine with other chemotherapeutic agents such as cisplatin, oxaliplatin, 5-FU, capecitabine, and irinotecan, mostly in doublets, with the aim of improving the outcome of patients with advanced pancreatic cancer. The results of these studies have failed to demonstrate convincingly the superiority of doublets over single-agent gemcitabine in terms of increased survival. However, it should also be noted that most randomized clinical trials were not adequately powered to detect small survival differences.

Berlin et al. showed a favorable impact of gemcitabine combined with 5-FU bolus versus gemcitabine alone on response rate and time to progression, but failed to demonstrate improved overall survival [43]. Similar results were reported from other studies that evaluated the efficacy of gemcitabine combinations including cisplatin [44, 45], oxaliplatin [46], capecitabine [47], irinotecan [48], exatecan [49, 50], and pemetrexed [51].

In a phase III study Reni et al. compared gemcitabine monotherapy to a multidrug combination including cisplatin, epirubicin, 5-FU, and gemcitabine (PEFG) and showed higher response rate (38.5% vs. 8.5%, p <0.0008), better progression-free survival (5.4 vs. 3.3 months, p <0.0033) and better 2-year overall survival (11.5% vs. 2.1 %, p <0.033) in the PEFG arm. However, more patients had grade 3–4 neutropenia and thrombocytopenia in the PEFG group than in the gemcitabine group (p <0.0001) [52]. Table 37.4 presents a summary of phase III trials comparing gemcitabine alone to gemcitabine in combination with other cytotoxic compounds.

Table 37.4 Phase III trials comparing gemcitabine alone to combination with other compounds

Study	Treatment	No. of patients	PFS/TTP		OS	
			Time	p	Time/ percentage	p
Berlin et al. [43]	Gem	327	2.2 mo.	0.022	5.4 mo.	NS
	Gem + 5-FU		3.4 mo.		6.7 mo.	
Cunningham et al. [53]	Gem	533	3.9 mo.	NS	6.0 mo.	0.026
	Gem + cape		4.3 mo.		7.4 mo.	
Herrmann et al. [47]	Gem	319	3.9 mo.	NS	7.2 mo.	NS
	Gem + cape		4.3 mo.		8.4 mo.	
Heinemann et al. [44]	Gem	198	2.5 mo.	0.16	6.0 mo.	NS
	Gem + cis		4.6 mo.		7.6 mo.	
Colucci et al. [45]	Gem	107	1.9 mo.	0.048	4.7 mo.	NS
	Gem + cis		4.7 mo.		7 mo.	
Louvet et al. [46]	Gem	313	3.7 mo.	0.04	7.1 mo.	NS
	Gem + ox		5.8 mo.		9.0 mo.	
Rocha Lima et al. [48]	Gem	360	3.0 mo.	NS	6.6 mo.	NS
	Gem + CPT-11		3.4 mo.		6.3 mo.	
Stathopoulos et al. [50]	Gem	145	2.9 mo.	NS	6.5 mo.	NS
	Gem + CPT-11		2.8 mo.		6.4 mo.	
Richards et al. [51]	Gem	565	3.9 mo.	NS	6.3 mo.	NS
	Gem + pem		3.3 mo.		6.2 mo.	
Abou-Alfa et al. [49]	Gem	349	3.8 mo.	NS	6.2 mo.	NS
	Gem + ex		3.7 mo.		6.7 mo.	
Reni et al. [52]	Gem	97	3.3 mo.	<0.0033	2.1%	<0.033
	PEFG		5.4 mo.		11.5% (2-year OS)	

Gem, Gemcitabine; *cape*, capecitabine; *PEFG*, cisplatin–epirubicin–fluorouracil–gemcitabine; *PFR*, progression-free survival; *TTP*, time to progression; *OS*, overall survival; *NS*, not significant; *mo.*, months; *cis*, cisplatin; *ox*, oxaliplatin; *pem*, pemetrexed; *ex*, exatecan

In part contrast to this, a large phase III study involving 533 patients and comparing the combination of gemcitabine and capecitabine with gemcitabine monotherapy has shown significantly improved median (7.4 vs. 6 months) and 1-year survival (26 vs. 19%) in of the combination arm (p <0.026) but with a good toxicity profile [53]. However, more recently Hermann et al., evaluating the same combination, have reported significantly improved survival only in the subgroup of patients with good performance status (Karnofsky performance status score 90–100) [47].

The ECOG 6201 study compared standard gemcitabine (1000 mg/m^2 over 30 min weekly for 7 out of 8 weeks and for 3 out of 4) to a fixed-dose-regimen gemcitabine (1500 mg/m^2 over 150 min weekly for 3 out of 4 weeks) and gemcitabine (1000 mg/m^2 over 100 min on day 1) combined with oxaliplatin (100 mg/m^2 on day 2) every 14 days. This trial, which enrolled 833 patients, was not able to show a significant improvement in overall survival. Both the fixed-dose-regimen and the gemcitabine plus oxaliplatin arms showed a median survival 1 month longer than the gemcitabine alone arm, but this difference was not statistically significant (1-year survival respectively 17% vs. 21% vs. 21%) [42].

Milella et al., in a large pooled analysis of 5561 patients, demonstrated that the addition of a platinum compound to gemcitabine improved overall response rate and progression-free survival in advanced pancreatic cancer, justifying the use of a platinum-based chemotherapy with gemcitabine in these patients, but failed to show an overall survival advantage [54]. However, a meta-analysis of 3687 patients with advanced pancreatic cancer suggested a small survival benefit for the gemcitabine combination with platinum analogues in comparison with gemcitabine alone in younger patients with a good performance status. By contrast, combination chemotherapy in patients with poor performance status appeared to be ineffective or even harmful. This latter group of patients should be then considered optimal candidates for monotherapy [55].

A recently published meta-analysis involving 9970 patients with locally advanced or metastatic pancreatic cancer confirmed a significant survival benefit for chemotherapy over best supportive care and for gemcitabine-based combination over single-agent gemcitabine. A subgroup analysis supports the use of gemcitabine in combination with a platinum agent or capecitabine [33]. Taken together these observations seem to suggest that a combination chemotherapy with a platinum analogue or capecitabine may be of some benefit in specific subgroups of patients (only young patients with good performance status), while elderly patients or those with poor performance status may be optimal candidates for gemcitabine monotherapy.

Second-Line Chemotherapy

Approximately half of patients in whom first-line treatment fails present good performance status and could be candidates for further treatment. Two recent retrospective studies suggested that selected patients may benefit in terms of disease-related symptom control and time to progression from a salvage chemotherapy after first-line chemotherapy has failed. According to these data, younger patients with good performance status and progressive disease at least 6 months after up-front treatment could be candidates for a second-line therapy [56, 57]. Furthermore, patients who responded to first-line gemcitabine chemotherapy seemed more likely to obtain a stable or partial remission after a second-line treatment [58]. However, only limited information on second-line treatment of patients with pancreatic cancer is available, and there is no consensus on salvage therapy regimens for patients with failing first-line therapy.

Recently, small phase II trials showed that patients whose disease had progressed after gemcitabine chemotherapy could benefit from a second-line treatment including 5-FU and oxaliplatin. The combination of oxaliplatin, 5-FU, and leucovorin was well tolerated with manageable toxicity, offering encouraging activity in pretreated gemcitabine patients; a subjective improvement of cancer-related symptoms was also noticed [59, 60].

Second-line treatment in gemcitabine-refractory disease may include as alternatives the combination of capecitabine with oxaliplatin [61] or capecitabine monotherapy. Both regimens have been shown to be active in this setting [62].

In a phase II study, the combination of gemcitabine and oxaliplatin proved to be a well-tolerated and active regimen in patients with advanced pancreatic cancer after progression following standard gemcitabine treatment [63].

The CONKO 003 phase III trial is currently evaluating treatment with 5FU/leucovorin versus 5-FU/leucovorin plus oxaliplatin in patients with advanced pancreatic cancer refractory to gemcitabine [64].

Several studies (mostly phase I and II trials) have been conducted to test the efficacy and toxicity profiles of other salvage therapy regimens such as monotherapy with irinotecan, pemetrexed, or raltitrexed, doublets (e.g., capecitabine and docetaxel; pemetrexed and irinotecan; raltitrexed and irinotecan), and multidrug combination (e.g., G-FLIC regimen: gemcitabine, 5-FU, leucovorin, irinotecan, and cisplatin), but results so far are too early to define their role in this particular setting.

Targeted Therapy in Advanced Pancreatic Cancer

Therapeutic options for advanced pancreatic cancer are limited. The need for an improved patient outcome along with the availability of new biologically targeted agents has generated a large number of clinical trials investigating new treatment options.

Matrix Metalloproteinase Inhibitors

Marimastat, a metalloproteinase inhibitor, was compared in three different doses with gemcitabine in a phase III trial. Four hundred fourteen patients were randomized but no difference in overall survival was observed between the two treatment arms [65]. In a successive randomized trial gemcitabine plus marimastat was compared with gemcitabine plus placebo; 239 patients were randomized in this study but there were no apparent differences in overall and progression-free survival and overall response rate between the two arms [66].

Farnesyl Transferase Inhibitors

Van Cutsem et al. compared a combination of gemcitabine plus tipifarnib (farnesyl transferase inhibitor) with gemcitabine plus placebo. Six hundred eighty-eight patients were randomized with no advantage in overall survival shown for the tipifarnib-based treatment [67].

Antiangiogenic Drugs

Interest in tumor angiogenesis and angiogenic factors has led to an increased number of clinical trials investigating antiangiogenic drugs. In the CALGB80303 study, the addition of bevacizumab to gemcitabine did not seem to improve survival in patients with advanced pancreatic cancer patients when compared to gemcitabine plus placebo [68]. Even sorafenib, an inhibitor of PDGF (platelet-derived growth factor) and VEGF (vascular endothelial growth factor) receptor kinase, was not able to show an improved outcome when added to gemcitabine [69].

Epidermal Growth Factor Receptor Inhibitors

A small but significant survival advantage was demonstrated for erlotinib. The addition of this EGFR (epidermal growth factor receptor) tyrosine kinase inhibitor to gemcitabine improved median survival, progression-free survival, and 1-year survival (median survival: 6.24 months vs. 5.91 months, $p = 0.038$; progression-free survival: 3.75 months vs. 3.55 months, $p = 0.004$; 1-year survival: 23% vs. 17%, $p = 0.03$) in patients with advanced pancreatic tumors [70]. The results of a phase II trial with gefitinib plus gemcitabine were presented at the 2007 American Society of Clinical Oncology meeting, with findings comparable to those seen with erlotinib plus gemcitabine with respect to median and 1-year survival [71]. Among anti-EGFR treatment strategies, the use of cetuximab, a monoclonal antibody directed against the extracellular domain of the EGFR, showed encouraging results in preliminary trials.

Unfortunately, the SWOG S0205 study, which compared gemcitabine plus cetuximab (anti-EGFR antibody) to gemcitabine alone in patients with locally advanced or metastatic pancreatic cancer, failed to demonstrate a clinically significant advantage of the addition of cetuximab to gemcitabine for overall survival, progression-free survival, and response. The results, in fact, showed a median survival of 6 months in the gemcitabine arm and 6.5 months in the gemcitabine plus cetuximab arm ($p = 0.14$); the progression-free survival was 3 and 3.5 months, respectively ($p = 0.058$), and the confirmed response probabilities were 7% in each arm [72] (Table 37.5). Other authors explored the combination of cetuximab, gemcitabine, and a platinum analogue with contrasting results. Cetuximab did not seem to interact positively with gemcitabine and cisplatin in a GISCAD phase II trial [73], whereas the addition of cetuximab to gemcitabine and oxaliplatin exhibited a high response rate of 38%, with a 54% 6-month survival [74]. Indeed, these results were quite comparable with those achieved in the phase II study of gemcitabine and oxaliplatin by GERCOR [75], calling into question the impact of patient selection in phase II trials.

Numerous trials with new and "old" target agents are ongoing to improve pancreatic cancer patients' outcome. In these trials and in past trials the selection of patients for molecular markers may be a crucial key for better and further insights into the biology of this highly deadly disease.

Table 37.5 Studies with biological agents in advanced pancreatic cancer

Study	Treatment	Median survival (months)	1-Year survival (%)	p
Bramhall et al. (2001) [65]	Marimastat Gemcitabine	169 d. 160 d.	30 25	NS
Van Cutsem et al. (2004) [67]	G + tipifarnib G + placebo	193 d. 182 d.	27 24	NS
Kindler et al. (2007) [68]	G + bevacizumab G + placebo	5.7 mo. 6 mo.		NS
Wallace et al. (2007) [69]	G + sorafenib	4 mo.	23 (6-month survival)	NS
Moore et al. (2007) [70]	G + erlotinib Gemcitabine	6.24 mo. 5.91 mo.	23 17	S
Philip et al. (2007) [72]	G + cetuximab Gemcitabine	6.5 mo. 6 mo.		S

G, Gemcitabine; *NS*, not significant; *S*, significant; *mo.*, months; *d.*, days

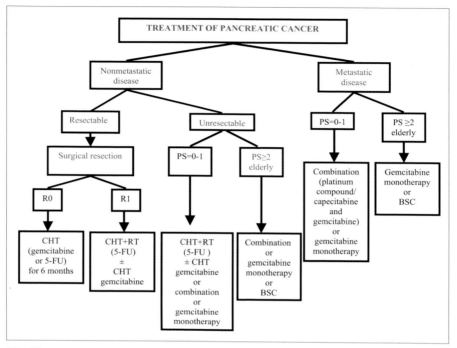

Fig. 37.1 Algorithm of pancreatic cancer treatment. *BSC*, Best supportive care; *PS*, performance status; *CHT*, chemotherapy; *RT*, radiotherapy

References

1. Jemal A, Siegel R, Ward E et al (2007) Cancer statistics 2007. CA Cancer J Clin 57:43–66
2. Li D, Xie K, Wolff R, Abruzzese JL (2004) Pancreatic cancer. Lancet 363:1049–1057
3. Burris III HA, Moore MJ, Andersen J et al (1997) Improvements in survival and clinical benefit with gemcitabine as first-line therapy for patients with advanced pancreas cancer: a randomized trial. J Clin Oncol 15:2403–2413
4. Kalser MH, Ellemberg SS (1985) Pancreatic cancer: adjuvant combined radiation and chemotherapy following curative resection. Arch Surg 120:899–903
5. Klinkenbjil J, Jekel J, Sahmoud T et al (1999) Adjuvant radiotherapy and 5-fluorouracil after curative resection of cancer of the pancreas and periampullary region: phase III trial of the EORTC Gastrointestinal Tract Cancer Cooperative Group. Ann Surg 230: 776–784
6. Garofalo MC, Regine WF, Tan MT (2006) On statistical reanalysis, the EORTC trial is a positive trial for adjuvant chemoradiation in pancreatic cancer. Ann Surg 244:332–333
7. Picozzi VJ, Kozarak RA, Traverso LW (2003) Interferon-based adjuvant chemoradiation therapy after pancreaticoduodenectomy for pancreatic adenocarcinoma. Am J Surg 185:476–480
8. Knaebel HP, Marten A, Schmitz-Winnenthal H et al (2005) Phase III trial of postoperative cisplatin, interferon alpha-2b and 5-FU alone for patients with resected pancreatic adenocarcinoma. CapRI: study protocol [ISRCTN6286675P]. BMC Cancer 5:37
9. Yeo CJ, Abrams RA, Grochow LB et al (1997) Pancreaticoduodenectomy for pancreatic adenocarcinoma: postoperative adjuvant chemoradiation improves survival. A prospective, single-institution experience. Ann Surg 225:621–636

10. Regine WF, Winter KW, Abrams R et al (2006) RTOG9704 a phase III study of adjuvant pre and postchemoradiation (CRT) 5-FU vs. gemcitabine (G) for resected pancreatic adenocarcinoma. J Clin Oncol 24(Suppl 18s):4007

11. Bakkevold KE, Arnesjø B, Dahl O et al (1993) Adjuvant combination chemotherapy (AMF) following radical resection of carcinoma of the pancreas and papilla of Vater results of a controlled, prospective, randomized multicentre study. Eur J Cancer 29A:698–703

12. Takada T, Amano H, Yasuda H et al (2002). Is postoperative adjuvant chemotherapy useful for gallbladder carcinoma? A phase III multicenter prospective randomized trial in patients with resected pancreaticobiliary carcinoma. Cancer 95:1685–1695

13. Oettle H, Post S, Neuhaus P et al (2007) Adjuvant chemotherapy with gemcitabine vs. observation in patients undergoing curative-intent resection of pancreatic cancer. JAMA 3:267–277

14. Neoptolemos JP, Stocken DD, Friess H et al (2004). A randomized trial of chemotherapy and chemotherapy after resection of pancreatic cancer. N Engl J Med 350:1200–1210

15. Stocken DD, Büchler MW, Dervenis C et al (2005) Meta-analysis of randomized adjuvant therapy trials for pancreatic cancer. Br J Cancer 92:1372–1381

16. Spitz FR, Abruzzese JL, Lee JE et al (1997) Preoperative and postoperative chemoradiation strategies in patients treated with pancreaticoduodenectomy for adenocarcinoma of the pancreas. J Clin Oncol 15:928–937

17. Varadhachary GR, Evans DE, Crane C et al (2002) Initial results of preoperative gemcitabine based chemoradiation for resectable pancreatic adenocarcinoma. Proc Am Soc Clin Oncol 21:Abs 516. Available at www.asco.org

18. Evans DB, Abruzzese JL, Willett CG (2001) Cancer of the pancreas. In: Devita VT Jr, Hellman S, Rosenberg SA (eds) Cancer. Principles and practice of oncology, 6th edn. Philadelphia: Lippincott Williams and Wilkins, pp 1126–1161

19. Moertel CG, Childs DS Jr, et al (1969) Combined 5-fluorouracil and supervoltage radiation therapy of locally unresectable gastrointestinal cancer. Lancet 2:865–867

20. Moertel CG, Frytak S, Hahn RG et al (1981) Therapy of locally unresectable pancreatic carcinoma. A randomized comparison of high dose (6000 rads) radiation alone, moderate dose radiation (4000 rads + 5-fluorouracil), and high dose radiation + 5-fluorouracil: The Gastrointestinal Tumor Study Group. Cancer 48: 1705–1710

21. Douglass HO (1988) Treatment of locally unresectable carcinoma of the pancreas: comparison of combined-modality therapy (chemotherapy plus radiotherapy) to chemotherapy alone; Gastrointestinal Tumor Study Group. J Natl Cancer Inst 80:751–755

22. Klassen J, John M, MacIntyre Met al (1985) Treatment of locally unresectable cancer of the stomach and pancreas: a randomized comparison of 5-fluorouracil alone with radiation plus concurrent and maintenance 5-fluououracil. An Eastern Cooperative Oncology Group Study. J Clin Oncol 3:373–378

23. Chauffert B, Mornex F, Bonnetain F et al (2006) Phase III trial comparing initial chemoradiotherapy (intermittent cisplatin and infusional 5-FU) followed by gemcitabine vs. gemcitabine alone in patients with locally advanced non metastatic pancreatic cancer: A FFCD-SFRO study. J Clin Oncol 24(Suppl 18):A4008

24. McGinn CJ, Zalupski MM, Shureiqi I et al (2001) Phase I trial of radiation dose escalation with concurrent weekly full-dose gemcitabine in patients with advanced pancreatic cancer. J Clin Oncol 19:4202–4208

25. Blackstok AW, Bernard SA, Richards F et al (1999) Phase I trial of twice-weekly gemcitabine and concurrent radiation in patients with advanced pancreatic cancer. J Clin Oncol 17:2208–2212

26. Epelbaum R, Rosenblat E, Nasrallah S et al (2002) Phase II study of gemcitabine (GEM) combined with radiation therapy (RT) in localized, unresectable pancreatic cancer. J Surg Oncol 81:138–143

27. Crane CH, Abbruzzese JL, Evans DB et al (2002) Is the therapeutic index better with gemcitabine based chemoradiation than with 5-fluorouracil based chemoradiation in locally advanced pancreatic cancer? Int J Radiat Oncol Biol Phys 52:1293–1302

28. Li CP, Chao Y, Chi KH et al (2003) Concurrent chemoradiotherapy treatment of locally advanced pancreatic cancer: gemcitabine versus 5-fluorouracil, a randomized controlled study. In J Radiat Oncol Biol Phys 57:98–104

29. Shinchi H, Takao S, Noma H et al (2002) Length and quality of survival after external-beam radiotherapy with concurrent continuous 5-fluorouracil infusion for locally unresectable pancreatic cancer. Int J Radiat Oncol Biol Phys 53:146–150

30. Huguet F, Andrè T, Hamel P et al (2007) Impact of chemoradiotherapy after disease control with chemotherapy in locally advanced pancreatic adenocarcinoma in GERCOR Phase II and III studies. J Clin Oncol 25:326–331

31. Glimelius B, Hoffman K, Sjoden PO et al (1996) Chemotherapy improves survival and quality of life in advanced pancreatic and biliary cancer. Ann Oncol 7:593–600

32. Palmer KR, Cereda S, Passoni P et al (1994) Chemotherapy prolongs survival in inoperable pancreatic carcinoma. Br J Surg 81:882–885

33. Sultana A, Smith CT, Cunnigham Det al (2007) Meta-analyses of chemotherapy for locally advanced and metastatic pancreatic cancer. J Clin Oncol 25:2607–2615

34. Hansen R, Quebbman E, Ritch Pet al (1988) Continuous 5-fluorouracil infusion in carcinoma of the pancreas. Am J Med Sci 295:91–93

35. Ducreux M, Rouguer P, Pignon JP et al (2002) A randomized trial comparing 5-FU with 5-FU plus cisplatin in advanced pancreatic carcinoma. Ann Oncol 13:1185–1191

36. Cartwright TH, Cohn A, Varkey JA et al (2001) Phase II study of oral capecitabine in patients with advanced or metastatic pancreatic cancer. J Clin Oncol 20:160–164

37. Abbruzzese JL (1996) Phase I studies with the novel nucleoside analogue gemcitabine. Semin Oncol 23:25–31

38. Casper E, Green M, Kelsen D (1994) Phase II trial of gemcitabine (2,2-difluorodeoxycytidine) in patients with adenocarcinoma of the pancreas. Invest New Drugs 12:29–34

39. Carmichael J, Fink U, Russel RCG et al (1996) Phase II study of gemcitabine in patients with advanced pancreatic cancer. Br J Cancer 73:101–105

40. Maisey N, Chau I, Cunningham D et al (2002) Multicenter randomized phase III trial comparing protracted venous infusion (PVI) fluorouracil (5-FU) with PVI 5-FU plus mitomycin in inoperable pancreatic cancer. J Clin Oncol 20:3130–3136

41. Tempero M, Plunkett W, Ruiz Van Haperen V et al (2003) Randomized phase I comparison of dose-intense gemcitabine. Thirty-minute infusion and fixed dose rate infusion in patients with pancreatic adenocarcinoma. J Clin Oncol 21:3402–3408

42. Poplin E, Levy D, Berlin J et al (2006) Phase III trial of gemcitabine (30 min infusion) versus gemcitabine fixed-dose rate infusion (FDR) versus gemcitabine + oxaliplatin (GEMOX) in patients with advanced pancreatic cancer (E6201). J Clin Oncol 24(Suppl 18):LBA4004

43. Berlin JD, Catalano P, Thomas JP et al (2002) Phase III study of gemcitabine in combination with fluorouracil versus gemcitabine alone in patients with advanced pancreatic carcinoma: Eastern Cooperative Oncology Group trial E2297. J Clin Oncol 20:3270–3275

44. Heinemann V, Qietzsch D, Gieseler F et al (2006) Randomized phase III trial of gemcitabine plus cisplatin compared with gemcitabine alone in advanced pancreatic carcinoma. J Clin Oncol 24:3946–3952

45. Colucci G, Giuliani F, Gebbia V et al (2002). Gemcitabine alone or with cisplatin for the treatment of patients with locally advanced and/or metastatic pancreatic carcinoma. A prospective randomized phase III of the Gruppo Oncologico dell'Italia Meridionale. Cancer 94:902–910

46. Louvet C, Labianca R, Hammel P et al (2005) Gemcitabine in combination with oxaliplatin compared with gemcitabine alone in locally advanced or metastatic pancreatic cancer: results of a GERCOR and GISCAD phase III trial. J Clin Oncol 23:3509–3516

47. Herrmann R, Bodoky G, Rushstaller T et al (2007) Gemcitabine (G) plus capecitabine versus G alone in locally advanced or metastatic pancreatic cancer: a randomized, multicenter, phase III trial of the Swiss Group for Clinical Cancer Research (SAKK) and the Central European Cooperative Oncology Group (CECOG). J Clin Oncol 25:2212–2217

48. Rocha Lima CM, Green MR, Rotche R et al (2004) Irinotecan plus gemcitabine results in

no advange compared with gemcitabine monotherapy in patients with locally advanced or metastatic pancreatic cancer despite increased tumor response rate. J Clin Oncol 22:3776–3783

49. Abou-Alfa GK, Letourneau R, Harker G et al (2006) Randomized phase III study of exatecan and gemcitabine compared with gemcitabine alone in untreated advanced pancreatic cancer. J Clin Oncol 24:4441–4447

50. Stathopoulos GB, Syrigos K, Aravantinos G et al (2006) A multicenter phase II trial comparing irinotecan–gemcitabine (IG) with gemcitabine (G) monotherapy as first-line treatment in patients with locally advanced or metastatic pancreatic cancer. Br J Cancer 95:587–592

51. Richards D, Oettle H, Ramanathan RK et al (2005) A phase III trial of pemetrexed plus gemcitabine versus gemcitabine in patients with unresectable or metastatic pancreatic cancer. Ann Oncol 16:1639–1645

52. Reni M, Cordio S, Milandri C et al (2005) Gemcitabine versus cisplatin, epirubicin, fluorouracil and gemcitabine in advanced pancreatic cancer: a randomized controlled multicentre phase III trial. Lancet Oncol 6:369–376

53. Cunningham D, Chau I, Stocken D et al (2005) Phase III randomized comparison of gemcitabine (GEM) versus gemcitabine plus capecitabine (GEM-CAP) in patients with advanced pancreatic cancer. Eur J Cancer 3:4 (PS11)

54. Milella M, Bria E, Carlini P et al (2006) Does a second drug added to gemcitabine (G) improve outcome over G in advanced pancreatic cancer APC? A pooled analysis of 5561 patients enrolled in 16 phase II trials. Ann Oncol 17(Suppl 9): abstract 10740, ESMO 2006

55. Heinemann V, Hinke A, Bock S et al (2006) Meta-analysis of randomized trials. Evaluation of benefit of chemotherapy from combination chemotherapy applied in advanced pancreatic cancer. Ann Oncol 17(Suppl 9): abstract 10730

56. Reni M, Manbrini A, Pasetto L (2006) Salvage therapy in advanced pancreatic adenocarcinoma. Ann Oncol 17(Suppl 9) Abs P1132

57. Herrmann T, Jaeger D, Stremmel SW et al (2007) Second-line chemotherapy in advanced pancreatic cancer: A retrospective, single center analysis. ASCO 2007, abstract 15187. Available at www.ASCO.org, accessed 28 June 2008

58. Mancuso A, Sacchetta S, Saletti P et al (2007) Clinical and molecular determinants of survival in pancreatic cancer patients treated with second line chemotherapy: results of an Italian/Swiss multicenter survey. J Clin Oncol 25: abstract 4622

59. Gebbia V, Maiello E, Giuliano F et al (2007) Second line chemotherapy in advanced pancreatic carcinoma: a multicenter survey of the Gruppo Oncologico Italia Meridionale on the activity and safety of the FOLFOX4 regimen in clinical practice. Ann Oncol 18:124–127

60. Tsavaris N, Kosas C, Sopelitis H et al (2005) Second line treatment with oxaliplatin, leucovorin and 5-fluorouracil in gemcitabine pre-treated advanced pancreatic cancer: A phase II study. Invest New Drugs 23:369–375

61. Xiong HQ, Wolff RA, Hess KR et al (2006) A phase II trial of oxaliplatin plus capecitabine (xelox) as second line therapy for patients with advanced pancreatic cancer. J Clin Oncol 24(20): abstract 4119

62. Boeck SH, Wilkowski R, Bruns CJ et al (2007) Oral capecitabine in pre-treated gemcitabine patients with advanced pancreatic cancer: a single center study. J Clin Oncol 24(18): abstract 15085

63. Demols A, Peeters M, Polus M et al (2006). Gemcitabine and oxaliplatin (GEMOX) in gemcitabine refractory advanced pancreatic adenocarcinoma: a phase II study. Br J Cancer 94:481–485

64. Riess H, Pelzer U, Stieler J et al (2007) A randomized second line trial in patients with gemcitabine refractory advanced pancreatic cancer-CONKO 003. J Clin Oncol 24(18) abstr. 4119

65. Bramhall SR, Rosemurgy A, Brown PD et al (2001) Marimastat as first line therapy for patients with unresectable pancreatic cancer: a randomized trial. J Clin Oncol 19:3447–3455

66. Bramhall SR, Schulz J, Nemunaitis J et al (2002) A double-blind placebo-controlled, ran-

domized study comparing gemcitabine and marimastat with gemcitabine and placebo as first line therapy in patients with advanced pancreatic cancer. Br J Cancer 87:161–167

67. Van Cutsem E, Van de Velt H, Karasek P et al (2004) Phase III trial of gemcitabine plus tipifarnib compared with gemcitabine plus placebo in advanced pancreatic cancer. J Clin Oncol 22:1430–1438

68. Kindler HL, Niedzwiecki D, Hollis D et al (2007) A double blind, placebo-controlled, randomized phase III trial of gemcitabine (G) plus bevacizumab (B versus gemcitabine plus placebo (P) in patients (pts) with advanced pancreatic cancer (PC): a preliminary analysis of Cancer and Leukemia Group B (CALGB)80303. Gastrointestinal Cancers Symposium abstract 108. Available at www.ASCO.org, accessed 28 June 2008

69. Wallace JA, Locker G, Nattam S et al (2007) Sorafenib (S) plus gemcitabine (G) for advanced pancreatic cancer (PC): a phase II trial of the University of Chicago Phase II Consortium. Gastrointestinal Cancers Symposium abstact 137. Available at www.ASCO.org, accessed 28 June 2008

70. Moore MJ, Goldestein D, Hamm J et al (2007) Erlotinib plus gemcitabine compared with gemcitabine alone in patients with advanced pancreatic cancer: a phase III trial of the National Cancer Institute of Canada Clinical Trials Group. J Clin Oncol 25:1960–1966

71. Fountzilas G, Murray S, Xiros N et al (2007) Hellenic Cooperative Oncology Group (HeCOG). Gemcitabine (G) combined with gefitinib in patients with inoperable or metastatic pancreatic cancer. A phase II trial. ASCO abstract 15016. Available at www.ASCO.org, accessed 28 June 2008

72. Philip PA, Benedetti J, Fenoglio-Preiser C et al (2007) Phase III study of gemcitabine (G) plus cetuximab versus gemcitabine alone in patients (pts) with locally advanced or metastatic pancreatic adenocarcinoma (P): SWOGs0205 study. ASCO abstr. LBA4509. Available at www.ASCO.org, accessed 28 June 2008

73. Cascinu S, Berardi R, Siena S et al (2007) The impact of cetuximab on the gemcitabine/cisplatin combination in first line treatment of EGFR-positive advanced pancreatic cancer (APC): a randomized phase II of GISCAD. ASCO abstract 4544. Available at www.ASCO.org, accessed 28 June 2008

74. Kullmann F, Hollerbach S, Dollinger M et al (2007) etuximab plus gemcitabine/oxaliplatin (GEMOXCET) in 1st line metastatic pancreatic cancer. First results from a multicenter phase II study. Gastrointestinal Cancers Symposium abstract 137

75. Louvet C, Andrè T, Liedo G et al (2002) Gemcitabine combined with oxaliplatin in advanced pancreatic adenocarcinoma: final results of a GERCOR multicenter phase II study. J Clin Oncol 20:1512–1518

Chapter 38

Pain Relief in Unresectable Pancreatic Cancer and After Pancreatic Surgery

Erica Adrario, Paola Verdenelli, Lorenzo Copparoni, Paolo Pelaia

Introduction

Cancer pain is an important problem from the health and social points of view. Thirty percent of patients affected by cancer have pain at diagnosis, and this percentage increases to 85% in the advanced stages of the disease. Yet, cancer pain can be efficiently controlled in most patients with an integrated program of pharmacological treatments for analgesia and anticancer therapies (radiotherapy, chemotherapy, and hormone therapy) [1].

In particular in the terminal stages of the disease, the pain takes on *global* features, characterized by the simultaneous presence of physical, psychological, and social components. The pain is not an isolated symptom; nausea, vomiting, asthenia, and deterioration of the cognitive faculties contribute to worsen the global suffering of the ill person. For this reason, therapy for cancer pain must take into account the close bond between the organic source of the pain and the psychological one [2], with a wider approach to the evaluation and treatment of the whole setting of the person's suffering.

The simultaneous presence of several pain syndromes in the same patient is very frequent:
- 1 patient in 5 presents just one type and/or cause of pain
- 4 patients in 5 complain 2 or more types and/or causes of pain
- 1 patient in 3 presents 4 or more types and /or causes of pain

Innervation of the Pancreas

Pancreas is innervated by *efferent pathways* from the sympathetic and parasympathetic system and by *afferent sensory pathways*.

The sympathetic nerves of the pancreas originate in preganglionic fibers located in the thoracic and upper lumbar segments of the spinal cord (T5–T9, sometimes even T10–T11). The myelinated axons of these cells traverse the ventral roots to form the white communicating rami of the thoracic and lumbar

W. Siquini (Ed.), *Surgical Treatment of Pancreatic Diseases.*
©Springer-Verlag Italia 2009

nerves, which reach the paravertebral sympathetic chain, travel through the splanchnic nerves, and reach the celiac and mesenteric ganglia, which give off postganglionic fibers that eventually reach the vascular pathways nearest to the pancreas.

The parasympathetic innervation travels within the vagus nerve (cranial nerve X), and through the hepatic, gastric, and celiac branches of the vagus; it reaches intrapancreatic ganglia that are dispersed in the exocrine tissue.

Pancreas sensory afferents are amyelinic nociceptive fibers (C fibers) that transmit noxious visceral information to the central nervous system by synapsing on second-order neurons of the dorsal horn of the spinal cord. They leave the pancreas along capsular and interstitial sympathetic fibers to the celiac plexus without interruption; they continue within the splanchnic nerves to the dorsal root ganglia, mainly at the level of the lower thoracic segments of the spinal cord located between T5 and T12: second-order neurons to the central nervous system within the anterolateral spinothalamic tract.

Pain Relief in Patients with Unresectable Pancreatic Cancer

All pancreatic nervous fibers, both afferent and efferent pathways, cross the celiac plexus, so its excision causes complete denervation of the gland. Pancreatic pain is essentially a deep, undefined, unlocatable visceral pain; its pathogenesis is due to mechanical compression or neoplastic invasion of the nervous plexuses and/or to the presence of metastases involving nearby organs, and/or to inflammation during enzymatic autodigestion.

When inflammatory or neoplastic processes progress beyond the parenchyma of the gland and beyond the capsule, involving the parietal peritoneum and posterior muscle plane, parietal somatic sensory fibers are stimulated, and this evokes the metameric, well-locatable and defined, persistent and recurrent somatic pain that is completely unaffected by splanchnic fiber neurolysis.

Particularly in unresectable pancreatic cancer, pain can be due to tumor compression on nervous structures or on adjacent organs, with infiltration of cave organs and skeletal apparatus.

Deep psychological distress is often observed in patients with pancreatic cancer. Depression is due to the awareness that they have a disease with very low survival rate; anxiety and nervousness can be evident with the worsening of symptoms, and pain can be barely controllable. Furthermore, the psychological status of pancreatic cancer patient can be influenced by related symptoms such as anorexia, vomiting, asthenia, and constipation due to opioid treatment. Clever pain management can help the patient to adopt adjustment strategies in order to face the disease. Pain management includes the following steps:
1. Evaluation
2. Explanation
3. Treatment
4. Re-evaluation

Evaluation

Evaluation of the intensity of the pain is very important. Multidimensional questionnaires employing visual analogue scales (VAS), numeric scales (NRS), or verbal scales (VRS) can be used (0: no pain – 10: worst pain imaginable) even in the less articulate patient. A score of 5 defines a pain that interferes with the quality of life; scores 1–4 are for mild pain, scores 5–6 are for moderate pain, while scores 7–10 are for severe pain (Fig. 38.1).

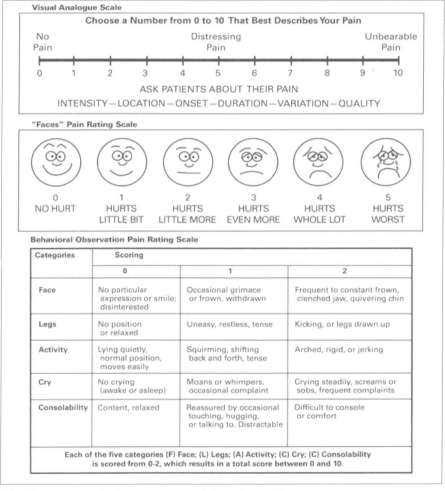

Fig. 38.1 Methods of pain measurement. (adapted rom [3])

Explanation

Explanations to the patient aim to:
- Decrease anxiety
- Involve the patient/relatives/other carers
- Improve the patient's mental state

"Suffering doesn't destroy man, a nonsense suffering destroys him [4].

Treatment

The step-by-step objectives of treatment are: increase of sleep painless periods, and decrease of pain in the standing position or during common daily activities. Pharmacological treatment is the basis: it can control pain in at least 90% of patients, with only a few percent of patients needing more invasive treatment (spinal neurolytic and neuroablative treatment). Despite this, pain is underestimated and inadequately treated.

Rational therapy is based on correct initial diagnosis of the origin, type, and intensity of the pain, so that the best analgesic agent can be identified for each specific clinical situation. The WHO guidelines for cancer pain relief [5] uses three pain levels as a way to choose the best analgesic agent (Fig 38.2). Anti-

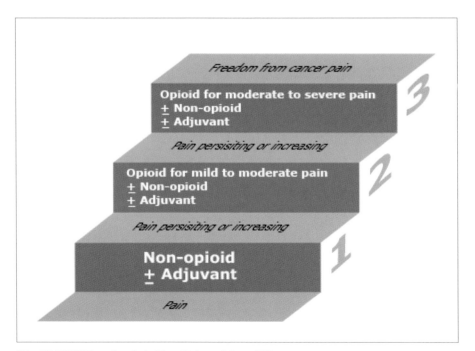

Fig. 38.2 WHO analgesic ladder. (Adapted from [3])

inflammatory agents, weak opioids, and morphine [6] are used sequentially at personalized dosages according to the patient's needs and permit neoplastic pain control in most cases. These guidelines have the advantage of indicating the best analgesic agent for each specific clinical situation and the additional advantage of indicating the pain level at which to changing treatment modalities without any interference with quality of life. First-step patients present with mild to moderate pain and can be treated by nonopiate analgesic agents including salicylates, nonsteroidal anti-inflammatory drugs (NSAIDs), and paracetamol. If moderate pain persists despite the first-step therapy, second-step drugs can be used: weak opioids (codeine, tramadol). The third step, in cases of severe pain, includes the use of strong opiates (morphine, methadone, fentanyl).

Efficient analgesic therapy should be *simple to administer:* oral administration is the most physiological and the least invasive for long-term treatment. Efficient analgesic therapy should be *able to prevent the onset of pain*, it *should be rapidly modified* in the case of failure or side effects, and it should be *personalized to the patient's needs*.

Drugs in Use

NSAIDs. NSAIDs (Table 38.1) are a various group with analgesic, antipyretic, and antiphlogistic action due to their inhibition of prostaglandin synthesis. They are very useful in cancer pain, above all in the control of pain due to mechani-

Table 38.1 Nonsteroidal anti-inflammatory drugs. (From: [6])

Active principle	Half-life (h)	Average oral dosages	Daily maximum dose
Acetylsalicylic acid	3–12	500 mg every 4–6 h	6 g
Paracetamol	1–4	500 mg every 4–6 h	4 g 2.6 g in long-term therapy
Ibuprofen	2,5	400 mg every 6–8 h 600 mg every 8–12 h	1800 mg
Naproxen	12–15	225–550 mg every 12 h	1100 mg
Ketoprofen	2–3	50–75 mg every 8 h 150 mg every 12 h	300 mg
Flurbiprofen	5–6	50–100 mg every 8–12 h 200 mg every 24 h	300 mg
Indomethacin	2–3	50 mg every 6–12 h	200 mg
Diclofenac	2	50 mg every 8 h 75 mg every 12 h 100 mg every 24 h	200 mg
Piroxicam	45	20 mg every 24 h	40 mg
Nimesulid	12	100–200 mg every 12 h	400 mg

cal compression of muscles, tendons, periosteum, bony tissue, and subcutaneous tissue. The limitation of these drugs is the "roof effect": once the limit dosage is reached, no further dose increase can improve the analgesic effect, so second-step drugs have to be used. The main side effects of NSAIDs are gastritis, coagulation defect, functional renal failure, and granulocytopenia. In order to minimize gastric side effects, it is recommended that NSAIDs be taken after meals and accompanied by antacids and gastroprotective agents.

Adjuvant Drugs. Adjuvant drugs are a heterogeneous group of drugs (Table 38.2) with various structures and actions and they are used for cancer pain as coanalgesic drugs. They can have a direct or indirect analgesic effect, increasing the efficacy or decreasing the side effects of the other analgesic drugs. This category includes anticonvulsants, antidepressants, corticosteroids, local anesthetics, myorelaxants, etc.

Opioids. The biological effects of opium-derived drugs (Table 38.3) depend on their interaction with one or more subtypes of specific receptors called μ, δ, and κ by reducing transmission of nociceptive impulses at a supraspinal, spinal, or peripheral level. On the basis of the receptors interaction, pure agonist, partial agonist, or agonist–antagonist drugs can be distinguished. Weak opioids for medium-intensity pain are *codeine* and *tramadol*, which unlike pure agonists have low intrinsic activity, a low "roof effect," and low efficacy (duration 28–45 days) despite having minor side effects.

In the case of severe cancer pain, the first-choice drug is morphine [7], the standard opioid of the third-step drugs and available in a wide variety of forms fororal administration. It seems to have no clinically significant "roof effect" for analgesia. If the patient cannot manage oral morphine administration, the subcutaneous route can be used, otherwise even intravenous administration can be used. The success of opioid therapy depends partly on control of the side effect such as constipation, nausea, sedation, sleepiness, respiratory depression, itching, cognitive disturbances, and urinary retention (Table 38.4). Several side effects disappear after prolonged use due to the onset of tolerance. A small percentage of patients experience intolerable side effects with oral morphine [8]; alleviation can be attempted in such cases by reducing the dosage, or changing the mode of administration, or using another third-step drug such as methadone, fentanyl, hydromorphone, or oxycodone [9].

Although several studies have demonstrated the absolute validity of the WHO guidelines for cancer pain relief, the SIAARTI group has proposed a fourth step to include pain management intervention for neurolysis, neuroablation, and neuromodulation (Table 38.5) [10].

Spinal Analgesic Treatment

Spinal administration (epidural or subarachnoid) is indicated for those patients who suffer intolerable side effects due to systemic administration of opioids or in case other drugs such as local anesthetics or agonists are used for adequate analgesia.

Table 38.2 Adjuvant drugs. (From [6])

Drug	Indications	Dosage	Notes
Anticonvulsants			
Carbamazepine	Neuropathic pain, especially lancinating flash pain	100 mg an evening, increasing every week if necessary, up to 400 mg every 12 h	Response after some days; anticonvulsant doses; myelotoxicity risk; monitoring blood concentration of carbamazepine
Gabapentin	Continuous burning pain associated with dysesthesia	300 mg an evening, increasing 300 mg/day every 3 days up to 400 mg every 8 h (dosage increasing up to 3600 mg/day)	High dosages for good response
Antidepressants			
Amitriptyline Newest antidepressants (bicyclic and SSRIs) are also effective in neuropathic pain	Neuropathic pain, especially if continuous and associated with dysesthesia	10 mg (1 drop = 2 mg) an evening, increasing up to 10 mg every 3 days, if necessary, up to 75 mg/day. Response after 4–7 days.	May be combined with anticonvulsants
Corticosteroids			
Dexamethasone	Peritumoral edema pain – Compression of nerves, plexuses, or spinal cord – Organ infiltration with compression of vascular, capsular, and/or ductal structures Cephalalgia caused by endocranial hypertension	16–24 mg/day p.o., i.m., or i.v. for at least 5–7 days; decrease dosage by 2 mg/day to achieve the minimum dosage that will control symptoms.	Anti-inflammatory and antiemetic, increases mood and appetite Morning administration is recommended – less interference with ACTH-cortisol system – or 2 administrations a day within 18 h to avoid insomnia Various interactions and side effects: (hyperglycemia, fluid retention, gastric pathology, oral candidiasis) Psychotic reaction and insomnia

continue ↑

continue **Table 38.2**

Table 38.2 Adjuvant drugs. (From [6])

Drug	Indications	Dosage	Notes
Local anesthetics			
Flecainide (second-line vs. anticonvulsants and antidepressants)	Neuropathic pain	100 mg every 12 h	Mexiletine in patients with ventricular impairment or myocardial ischemia: 150 mg/day increasing up to 200 mg every 8 h
Neuroleptics (antipsychotics)			Analgesic effect even for indirect factors
Levomepromazine	These drugs have possible efficacy for: tenesmus, ghost sensation following rectal amputation, or cystectomy	12.5 mg every 8 h, increasing gradually, up to 100 mg every 8 h.	such as increased sleep, decreased anxiety, and decreased nausea
Haloperidol		2 mg every 8 h, increasing gradually up to 6–8 mg every 8 h	

SSRI, Selective serotonin reuptake inhibitor; *p.o.,* per os/orally; *i.m.,* intramuscularly; *i.v.,* intravenously

Table 38.3 Classification of opium derived drugs based on their interaction with receptors (From [6])

Pure agonist	Partial agonist	Agonist-antagonist
Morphine	Dextropropoxyphene	Pentazocin
Metadone	Codeine	
Hydromorphone	Bupremorphine	
Fentanyl	Tramadol	
Oxycodone		
Meperidin		

Antalgic Neurolytic Therapy

Antalgic neuroablative therapy [11] aims to interrupt nociceptive impulse transmission by irreversibly destroying central or peripheral nervous pathways using mechanical, physical, or chemical agents. Neurolytic block of the celiac plexus [12] and splanchnic nerves can be indicated in visceral pain of the upper abdominal quadrants, particularly in patients with pancreatic cancer or chronic pancreatitis. The efficacy of antalgic neuroablative therapy varies from 10–24% if used alone to 70–80% if combined with other treatments. It should be performed in the early phases of pain that is still strictly visceral; if tumor reaches extravisceral structures, extravisceral nociceptive somatic impulses will be present that will be poorly controlled by neuroablative therapy alone. Various techniques have been described: the transaortic approach of Ischia [13, 14] and anterior approach of Gadde and Miller [15] permit neurolytic block of the celiac plexus, while the posterior approaches of Moore or Boas [16, 17] permit neurolytic block of the splanchnic nerves.

Possible complications of this procedure are orthostatic hypotension, diarrhea due to sympathetic denervation, pneumothorax, transient hematuria, diaphragmatic paralysis, and in rare cases flaccid paraplegia due to ischemic myelopathy caused by injury to the anterior spinal artery (artery of Adamkiewicz).

Re-evaluation

Re-evaluation is very important in order to correlate symptoms to patient response to therapy (dosage titration and changing characteristics of pain). If necessary, the whole therapeutic plan can be reviewed.

Table 38.4 Side effects of opioid drugs and their possible treatments. (From [6])

Side effect	Prevention	Precaution	Treatment
Nausea and emesis	Hydration	Rotation of the route of administration and/or of the opioid	Antiemesis: metoclopramide, haloperidol, prochlorpromazine, chlorpromazine, 5-HT$_3$ antagonists
Constipation	Hydration	Rotation of the route of administration and/or of the opioid (trial of transdermal fentanyl or of methadone)	High-fiber diet, senna or lactulose, macrogol, oral naloxone (under experimentation)
Sedation	Hydration, reduce opioid dosage, stop or reduce hypnotic drugs, benzodiazepines, NSAIDs and other drugs that act on the CNS	Rotation of the route of administration and/or of the opioid	Adjuvant drugs: methylphenidate (not available in Italy), caffeine Do not use naloxone
Cognitive dysfunction	Hydration, reduce opioid dosage, stop or reduce hypnotic drugs, benzodiazepines, NSAIDs, ranitidine, and other drugs that act on the CNS	Rotation of the opioid drug	Adjuvant drugs: haloperidol, methotrimeprazine, chlorpromazine, midazolam s.c. or c.i.
Myoclonia	Hydration	Rotation of the opioid drug	Adjuvant drugs: baclofen, diazepam, clonazepam, spinal bupivacaine, midazolam, sodium valproate, dantrolene sodium

continue ↑

continue **Table 38.4**

Itching	Hydration	Rotation of the route of administration or/and opioid drug	Adjuvant antihistamine drugs Experimental: naloxone/naltrexone, intranasal butorphanol, propofol, 5-HT$_3$ antagonists
Respiratory depression	Reduce or stop administration of opioid drugs Reduce or stop all drugs that act on the CNS	Assisted ventilation: If RR <8/min If cyanosis is present If patients is in coma	Dilute naloxone 400 µg in 10 ml PS, administer 0.5 ml (20 µg) i.v. every 2 min to achieve satisfactory breathing; if necessary administer other boluses because of the short half-life of naloxone

RR, Respiratory rate; *CNS*, central nervous system; *PS*, physiological solution; *s.c.*, subcutaneous; *c.i.*, continuous infusion; *i.v.*, intravenously

Table 38.5 Changes proposed by SIAARTI

Do not interpret WHO ladder in a mechanistic way
The first and second steps are completed into one step
The third step is supported by a fourth step to include pain management interventions for neurolysis/neuroablation and neuromodulation

Pain Therapy After Pancreatic Surgery

Postoperative pain [18] is a subjective, complex, and multifactorial phenomenon: it depends on the histological type of cancer lesion, site of cancer lesion and type of surgery. Pain intensity is high after major surgery such as pancreatic surgery: tissue injury causes the release of powerful inflammatory and pain mediators which cause hormonal stress response that leads to catabolic phenomena, impairment of immunologic function, immunodepression, impairment of platelet function with hypercoagulability, and activating sympathetic hypertonia with centralization of blood flow, increase in oxygen consumption, increase in heart rate, and fluid retention. Pain may cause superficial breathing and depression of cough, followed by retention of pulmonary secretions causing hypoxia and infection. If pain treatment is delayed, central and peripheral sensitization may occur, making subsequent pain control and suppression difficult [19]. It has been observed that adequate postoperative pain control improves patient outcome, reducing mortality and postoperative complications, improving early mobilization, and reducing hospitalization.

Many drugs are used for postoperative pain control, divided into four main classes: NSAIDs, opioids, local anesthetics, and adjuvant drugs. The choice of specific drug and technique (administration route) depends on the seriousness of the disease and on the patient's clinical status. Nowadays acute postoperative pain is thought to be best controlled by *multimodal therapy* with a combination of various drugs acting synergetically: in this way the best pain control and reduction of side effects can be obtained.

Analgesic drugs are preferably administered intravenously in continuous mode in order to maintain a constant level of analgesia. This can be done by an elastomeric pump, a kind of balloon filled with the drug that is slowly released at a preselected speed. Patient-controlled analgesia (PCA) is a sophisticated and innovative technique which permits self-administration of analgesia and experimentation with its effect during the onset of pain. The patient is able to evaluate pain intensity and adjust the level of analgesia to as much as he needs. This technique involves informing the patient about how the administering instrument functions.

Postoperative pain after pancreatic surgery can be well controlled by local anesthesia technique in the form of continuous peridural block. Several studies have demonstrated the advantages of peridural anesthesia [20]: it decreases the neuroendocrine effects of surgical stress, decreases cardiovascular response, improving heart oxygenation (even in cardiac patients), and reduces blood loss and thromboembolism during major surgery. Furthermore, the integration of local and general anesthesia in the blended anesthesia technique has been shown to be the best method for postoperative protection and functional recovery. Epidural analgesia is obtained by the use of local anesthetics and low doses of opioids (morphine, fentanyl, sufentanyl, buprenorphine) in continuous infusion with infusional pumps, PCA systems, or elastomeric systems.

The only actual contraindication to locoregional peridural anesthesia is the presence of coagulation defect because of the risk of spinal hematoma. Unlike in other European or American countries, intra-hospital acute pain "quality control" does not exist in Italy. The introduction of a method for controlling the efficacy of postoperative pain treatment is needed. An "acute pain service" could be created; it could be a valid organizational model with a simple and safe protocol for analgesia with precise objectives in order to guarantee adequate information for patients by recording the side effects of the various therapies and discussing cost-benefit ratios interactively.

References

1. Venuti FS, Filoni G, Interlandi F, Taglieri D (2001) Trattamento farmacologico del dolore da cancro. Nuove strategie terapeutiche e Qualità di Vita in Oncologia: dalla clinica alla bioetica. Messina. 9–10 March 2001
2. Carney CP, Jones L, Woolson RF et al (2003) Relationship between depression and pancreatic cancer in the general population. Psychosom Med 65:884–888
3. Wick JY (2007) Pain in special populations: the cognitively impaired. Pharmacy Times
4. Frankl V (1987) La sofferenza di una vita senza senso. Psicoterapia per l'uomo di oggi. LDC, Turin
5. World Health Organization (1986) Cancer pain relief with a guide to opioid availability. World Health Organization, Geneva
6. Servizio Sanitario Regione Emilia-Romagna (2005) Indications for evaluation and treatment of cancer pain – guideline. Regional Health Service Emilia Romagna, Italy
7. Hanks GW, Conno F, Cherny N et al; Expert Working Group of the Research Network of the European Association for Palliative Care (2001) Morphine and alternative opioids in cancer pain: the EAPC recommendations. Br J Cancer 84:587–593
8. Hanks GW (1991) Opioid-responsive and opioid-non-responsive pain cancer. Br Med Bull 47:718–731
9. Hanks GW, De Conno F, Cherny N et al (2003) Morphine and alternative opioids in cancer pain. J Clin Oncol 21(9 Suppl):87–91
10. Ambrosio F, Paoletti F, Savoia G et al; SIAARTI (2003) Recommendations on the assessment and treatment of chronic cancer pain. Minerva Anestesiol 69:697–716; 717–729
11. Sabersky L, Ligham D (1997) Neuroablative techniques for cancer pain management. Techn Reg Anaesth Pain Manag 1:53–58
12. Mercadante S (1993) Celiac plexus block versus analgesics in pancreatic cancer pain. Pain 52:186–192
13. Ischia S, Luzzani A (1983) A new approach to the neurolytic block of the celiac plexus:the transaortic technique. Pain 16:333–341
14. Ischia S, Ischia A (1992) Three posterior percutaneous celiac plexus block techniques. A

prospective, randomized study in 61 patients with pancreatic cancer pain. Anestesiology 76:534–540

15. Gadde PK, Miller DL (1984) CT guidance for celiac plexus neurolysis: posterior and anterior approaches. Reg Anest 9:49
16. Moore DC, Bush W, Burnett LL (1978) Celiac plexus block: a roentgenographic, anatomic study of technique and spread of solution in patients and corpses. Anesth Analg 60:369–379
17. Boas RA (1978) Sympathetic blocks in clinical practice. Int Anesthesiol Clin 16:149–157
18. Ready LB, Edwards WT (1999) Management of acute pain: a practical guide, task force on acute pain, international associate for the study of pain. JASP Press, Seattle
19. Dahl JB (1993) The value of pre-emptive analgesia in the treatment of post-operative pain. Br J Anaesth 70:434–439
20. Liu S, Carpenter R, Neal JM et al (1995) Epidural anaesthesia and analgesia. Their role in postoperative outcome. Anesthesiology 82:1474–1506

Subject Index

Printed in Italy in September 2008

WITHDRAWN